Slimming
AND
Tasty

Slimming AND Tasty

100 Delicious, Low-Calorie Recipes and Healthy Fakeaways

LATOYAH EGERTON

CREATOR OF THE SUGAR PINK FOOD BLOG

greenfinch

CONTENTS

a little bit about me

For as long as I can remember, people have told me how unusual my name is. 'I've never met another Latoyah before!', they would say. When I was younger, I hated that people made such a big deal about it. Substitute teachers would struggle to pronounce it, prompting laughter from the rest of the class.

Fast-forward to 2014 and a conversation with friends turned to domain names on the internet, and how most people's names would already have been purchased by now. We went through everyone's names and the only domain name that was still available to purchase was mine: www.latoyah.co.uk. I purchased it immediately, and it lay there for a while with nothing on it. I didn't really have any plans for it at the time, and if you had told me then that in 2022 I would be writing my own cookbook based on the recipes I shared on that website, I would never have believed you!

I have always loved cooking and grew up obsessing over TV chefs, religiously watching them create delicious meals. The early 2000s saw an influx of TV chefs, with Nigella Lawson and Jamie Oliver particularly captivating me.

When I left home at 18, I found cooking to be such a therapeutic form of relaxation. I loved creating new meals and dishes and had to be extremely resourceful with ingredients as money was tight at the time. I created some amazing recipes, but my style of cooking was very experimental and a little bit 'chuck it in and see'. This meant it was pretty hard to recreate the same dish twice.

So, after a while of owning www.latoyah.co.uk, I decided that I wanted to use the space to develop and save my recipes – mainly for myself, so that I could remember how to recreate the good ones, and as a way to share recipes with friends. At the time, Sugar Pink was my username for everything, and so Sugar Pink Food was born. (Sugar Pink is a pale pink hue that I have always been obsessed with. After all, pink isn't a colour, it's a way of life!)

At first the recipes I posted weren't aimed at anyone in particular. But I had always

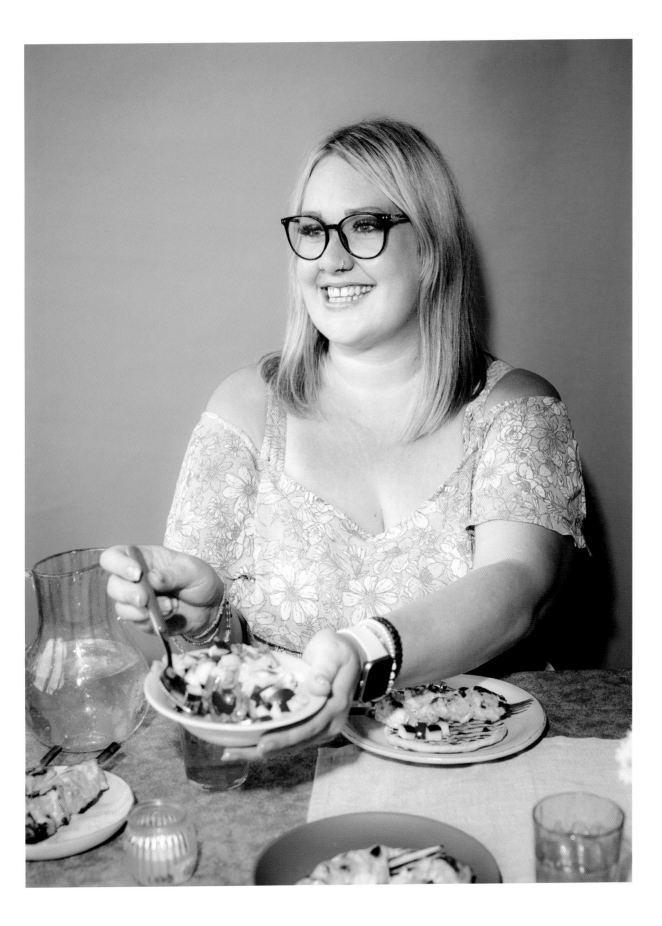

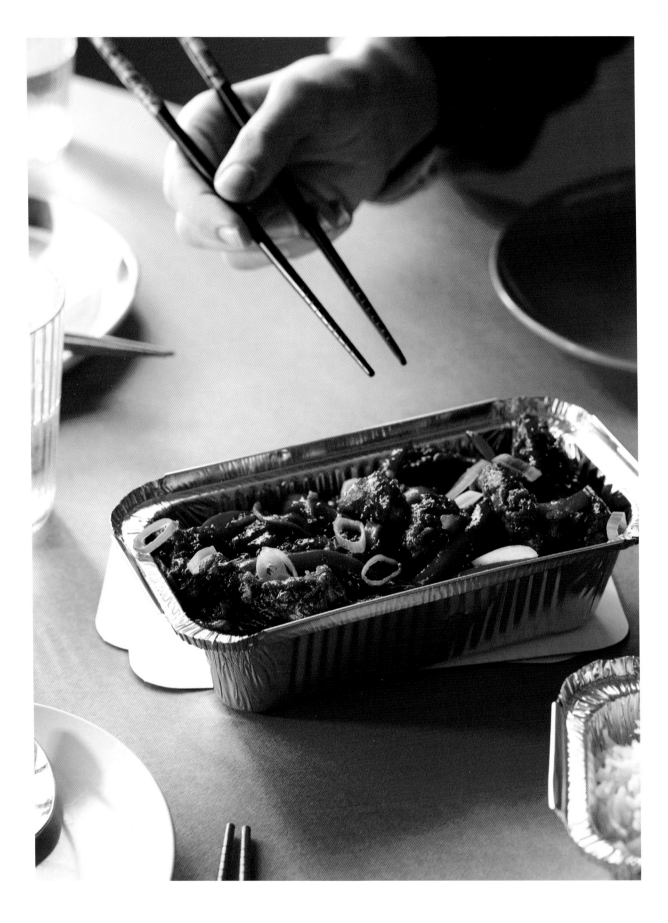

struggled with my weight and found it really hard to stick to a diet. I had tried diet clubs and plans, but it just wasn't for me. I hated how most diet food lacked any real flavour, and that I had to make separate meals for partners and friends as they didn't want to eat 'diet dishes'.

I started posting recipes that were low in fat and calories and without added sugar, but that – most importantly – were packed with flavour, easy to make and could feed everyone in the family, because you would never be able to tell that they are 'healthy'. It was when I started sharing these recipes that I really started to build a following on my humble recipe blog. After I ditched the diet clubs and focused on healthy home cooking, I shed five stone (31kg).

When I started posting 'fakeaway' recipes, I gained even more momentum. People loved them. I tried to recreate every different cuisine that I could think of. After the pandemic hit in 2020 and many restaurants were shut for a brief period, my fakeaway recipes were picked up

by the national press as people could recreate their favourite takeaway dishes in the comfort of their own homes.

My recipes are aimed at people who like to cook flavourful food with minimum effort, because eating delicious meals shouldn't have to be hard work. I am all for an easy life, so utilize things like tray baking, prepping lunches and breakfasts ahead of time, and making food that is super easy to prepare, even for the most unconfident of cooks.

I am so excited to be able to share these recipes that I have worked so hard on, especially as so many of them are brand new and have not been shared on my website. I hope that you enjoy making them all as much as I have enjoyed creating them.

how to make your slimming journey a tasty one

What makes a recipe 'slimming'? It's not just about eating less, and it shouldn't be about cutting out the things you love.

When I have followed slimming clubs before I have found them very restrictive, with certain foods off-limits. I think that life is too short to deny yourself the food you like, so my motto is that everything should be allowed in moderation.

I follow these principles when developing recipes:

Look for lean meat
One easy, healthy choice you can make is to use lean meats when cooking, such as skinless chicken breast, lean beef or lean turkey mince that is 5 per cent fat or less. For any meats that are naturally fattier, you can trim any excess fat off.

For some fatty cuts of meat like bacon, you can search out an alternative like bacon medallions instead of trimming off the excess, as this also saves on waste.

Swap in low-fat cheese and dairy
A simple swap you can make is to change your cheese to a low-fat alternative and use low-fat cream cheese as a replacement for cream. Low-fat cream cheese helps to make deliciously creamy sauces without as much fat as using butter and cream.

Use as little sugar as possible
I try to use as little sugar as possible in my cooking. Of course, some foods naturally contain sugars, such as fruit, but I try to avoid adding additional sugar to my recipes. A simple swap from sugar to sweetener is easy when making things like BBQ sauce.

Swap oil for low-fat cooking spray
Another great way to save on calories is to replace butter or oil in your frying pan with low-calorie cooking spray.

Fill up on vegetables
Vegetables are low-calorie and high in fibre and nutrients, so they're great for filling you up. All of my main meals are low enough in calories that you can serve them with a big portion of vegetables or salad. This helps to keep you fuller for longer and helps keep nutrition balanced.

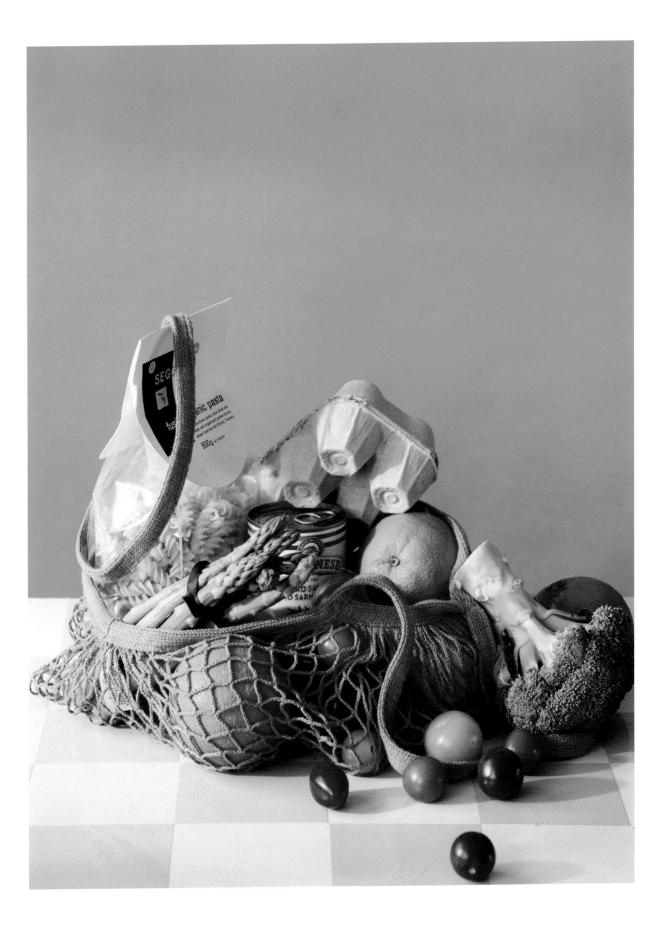

Eat smaller portions

I find it is better to have smaller portion sizes of a core dish, which you can then bulk out with extra vegetables. For years I ate absolutely huge plates of food, thinking that I was being good because it was slightly lower in fat. The bigger the portion, the more calories you take in.

Stick to under 600 calories per meal

The majority of the recipes in this book are in fact under 500 calories, but I always aim to create meals that are 600 calories or less.

Drink two litres of water every day

One of the most important things – which I cannot stress enough – is how drinking water helps you lose weight. When your body starts burning fat, you need to flush the fat out, and the easiest way to do so is by drinking enough water. At first it will seem hard to do, but the more you make sure you're drinking enough, the better you will feel.

Prep ahead – and make use of leftovers

My recipes are split into portion sizes, which means you can either serve multiple people from each meal or portion it up to save the leftovers for another day. One thing that I have always taken pride in is that my meals are so tasty, that you wouldn't realize that they are 'slimming'. This means that the whole family can enjoy them without you needing to make separate meals. This saves you from having to prepare another meal and from calculating calories again.

Some of the breakfast and lunch recipes are designed specifically for prepping ahead. If you have any of those takeaway plastic boxes kicking around, they are absolutely perfect for storing food that you have prepped ahead, as well as any leftovers. If not, you can pick them up very cheaply, and there are endless amounts of food storage containers available online.

Slimming and tasty is the title of this book and the main principle of all my recipes. If you're not enjoying what you eat, you're missing out on one of life's simple pleasures!

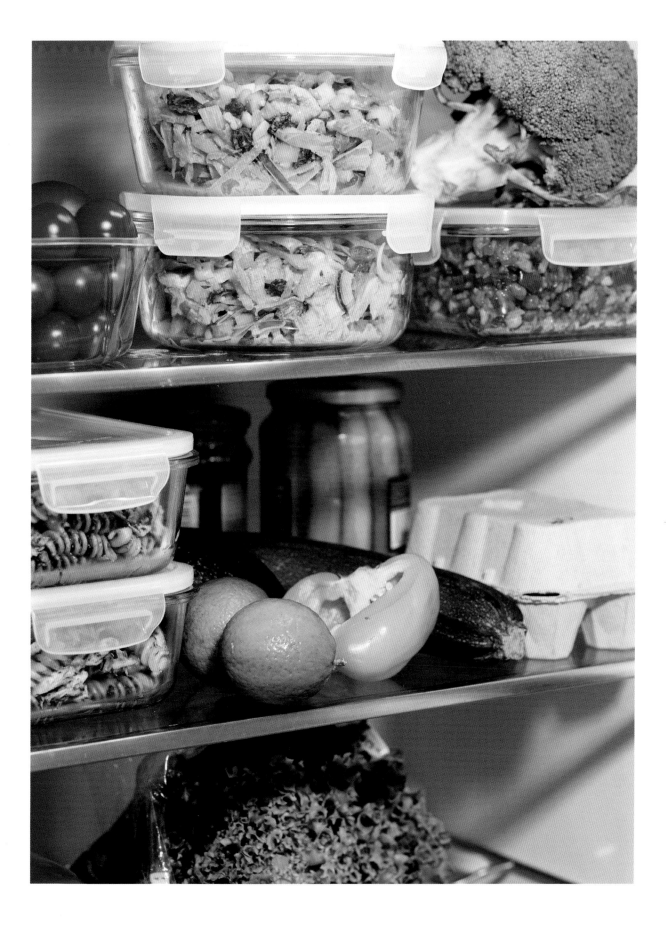

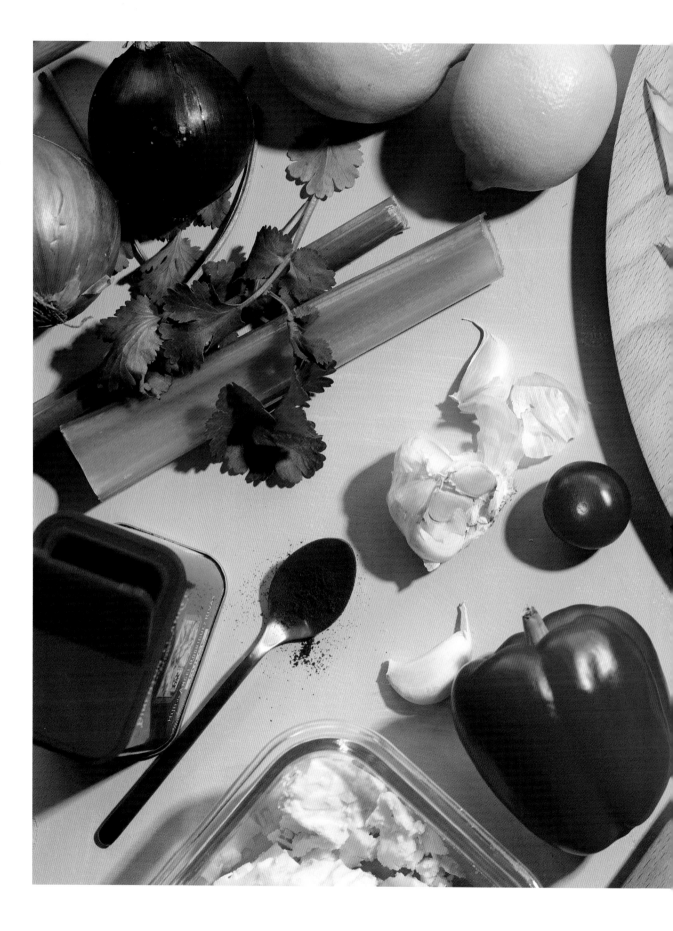

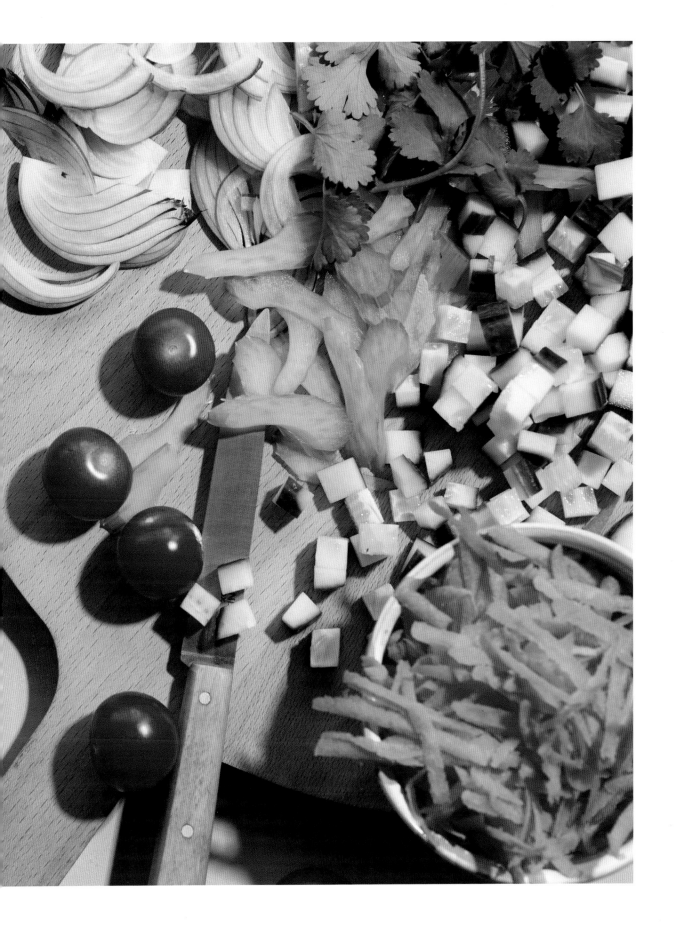

before you get started

While I have calculated **calories** to the best of my ability, there is always room for variables based on the particular brands that you may use or small variations in weight. I always recommend double-checking the calories if you deviate from the recipe or are following a strict calorie plan.

Ovens and hobs vary, even if cooking at the same temperature. Make sure to preheat your oven before cooking and always check food is fully cooked before eating, especially for fish, seafood and meat. The best way to check if chicken is cooked is to make sure it is no longer pink in the middle. If using a meat thermometer, chicken should register 75–80°C (167–176°F) in the thickest part.

Chicken breast weights and sizes can vary, but I work on the general rule of one breast per person. When chicken is used, make sure it is always skinless as this makes it as lean as possible.

All **eggs** used are medium-sized, and I find that you cannot beat the quality of a free-range egg.

There are loads of **low-calorie cooking sprays** on the market, and you can use any based on your preference. The majority are zero calories per spray. You can also get olive oil sprays, which allow you to use real oil, but much less of it. Double-check the calories on these and adjust when required.

I find that the easiest way to follow a recipe is to **prep all of the ingredients beforehand** – so get everything peeled and chopped, out of the fridge and within arm's reach, set out ready to go.

Most of my recipes can be stored in the refrigerator if you have **leftovers**, and each recipe has a specific note about this. When refrigerating food, leave it to cool to room temperature first, and if reheating, make sure it is piping hot in the middle before serving.

Eating food is all about the flavour, and I couldn't be without my **herbs and spices**. I use a lot of dried herbs and spices as I always have them in my cupboard, and they last forever. Dried basil, smoked paprika, chilli flakes, sea salt and black pepper are probably the most useful to always have to hand. Passata (sieved tomatoes) and chopped tomatoes are an absolute staple and go on my shopping list every time. There are so many tasty meals you can create using a base of passata or chopped tomatoes!

For **traybakes**, I love using an enamel oven tray that isn't too deep. The deeper the tray, the longer the ingredients inside it will take to cook. The key to traybakes is not overcrowding the tray so that everything cooks evenly, so the larger the tray, the better.

A **slow cooker** has to be one of my favourite appliances to use in the kitchen. Not only can you add ingredients into it in the morning and let your dinner cook away during the day, but it cooks meat slowly so that it is extra succulent and melts in the mouth. They don't cost a lot to buy, but once you have one you will use it over and over again. If you don't have one yet, though, don't worry – I have provided instructions for cooking on the hob or in the oven, too.

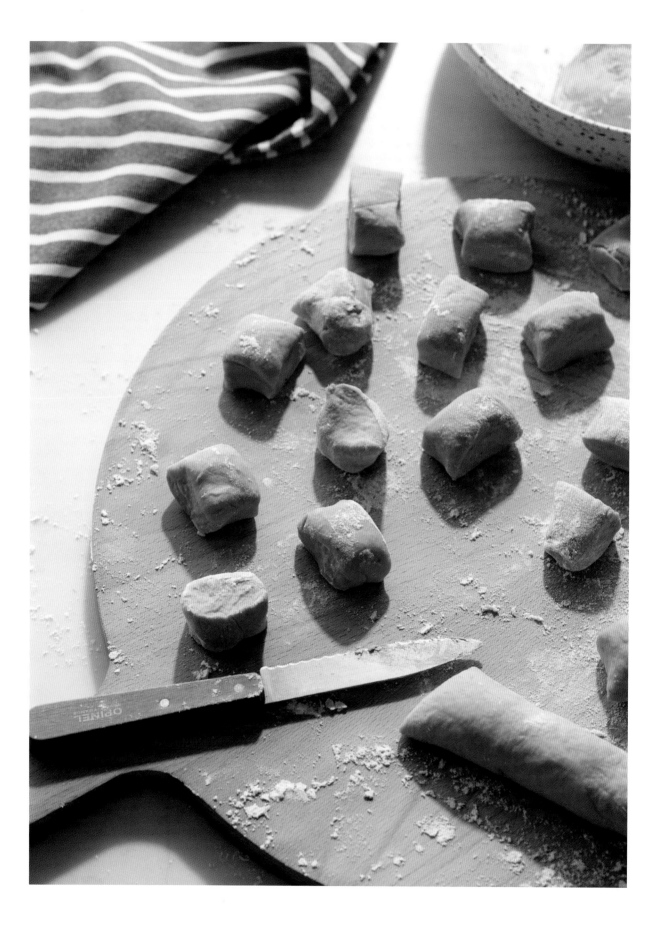

how to use this book

This book has plenty of delicious breakfast, lunch and dinner recipes as well as over 20 fakeaway treats. I have split the chapters so that navigating the book to find the recipe that best suits your needs is as easy as possible. You can choose from speedy weekday breakfasts (see page 20) that can be made ahead of time or thrown together quickly, or lazy weekend brunches (see page 34) to make from scratch and enjoy slowly. Then there's soups and salads (see page 56) and prep-ahead lunchboxes (see page 76) that are perfect to make ahead of time so that lunch is ready when you are, or if you have a little more time, leisurely lunches (see page 98), which are delicious midday meals that you can cook up when at home. For dinner you can turn to hearty dinners (see page 118) for delicious recipes that the whole family will love, or go for a simple and tasty traybake (see page 156) for an easy weeknight option that saves on washing up. Finally, you can recreate some of your favourite takeaway dishes in the comfort of your own home by whipping up a fakeaway (see page 182) that has all the flavour of the original but fewer calories.

Meal plans

I have created two meals plans using the recipes in the book, one for a working week (see page 228) that allows you to prep ahead, and one for all the family (see page 230), where a little more preparation is required.

The meal plans are based on eating 1500 calories per day, but with plenty of space for snacks. If you are not trying to stick to 1500 calories, you can easily adjust to larger portion sizes.

Icons

The following icons are used in the book:

- Vegetarian
- Vegan
- Gluten-free
- Dairy-free

Where a recipe can be easily adapted to become vegetarian, I have included notes and suggested swaps. You may need to adjust the calorie count based on what ingredients you use.

SPEEDY

WEEKDAY BREAKFASTS

Breakfast is the most important meal of the day, so we're told. For years I substituted a healthy balanced breakfast for a massive coffee instead. I never used to be hungry in the mornings, and could easily make it until lunchtime before desiring any food. I convinced myself that I was 'saving calories' by not eating in the mornings.

The truth is that eating a good breakfast in the morning kick-starts your metabolism for the day. If you don't eat, your metabolism doesn't get started until you eat at lunchtime. Your metabolism is responsible for using up the energy you obtain from eating food, so the better your metabolism is working, the easier it is to lose weight and keep it off long term. Have you ever noticed that when you eat breakfast that you're always much more hungry by lunchtime than when you don't? This is because your metabolism has kicked in.

If you have to leave the house really early in the mornings or don't feel hungry when you first get up, breakfast is the last thing that you want to think about preparing. These speedy weekday breakfast recipes are perfect for either prepping ahead the night before or cooking up and portioning out for the week ahead. This means you can take breakfast with you to work and eat it as soon as you're ready.

These recipes are tasty, easy to prepare, and will help you survive the working week with a balanced breakfast every day.

tiramisu overnight oats

The literal translation of *tiramisu* from Italian into English is 'pick-me-up', and we all need a bit of a pick-me-up in the mornings! This tiramisu-inspired recipe can be prepared the night before and left in the refrigerator so that your 'pick-me-up' is ready when you are. It's your breakfast and morning cup of coffee, all rolled into one!

MAKES 1 PORTION

40g (1½oz/⅓ cup) porridge oats

120ml (4fl oz/½ cup) strong black coffee

3 tablespoons fat-free vanilla Greek yoghurt

A small squirt of 'light' squirty cream

½ teaspoon cocoa powder

Prep time 5 minutes, plus chilling time | **Calorie count** 309 calories per portion

Put the oats into a small bowl, pour over the coffee and mix well. Add half a tablespoon of the fat-free yoghurt and mix until combined.

I like to use a mason jar to prep the overnight oats in, but any glass will do. Make layers in the jar by adding some of the oat mixture, then some fat-free yoghurt and then more oats until you get to the top of the jar/glass.

Add a small squirt of low-fat squirty cream on the top, then sprinkle with the cocoa powder to finish.

Chill in the refrigerator overnight, or for at least 3 hours.

Note Works best if you leave overnight, but if you can't wait that long to tuck in, a few hours will do.

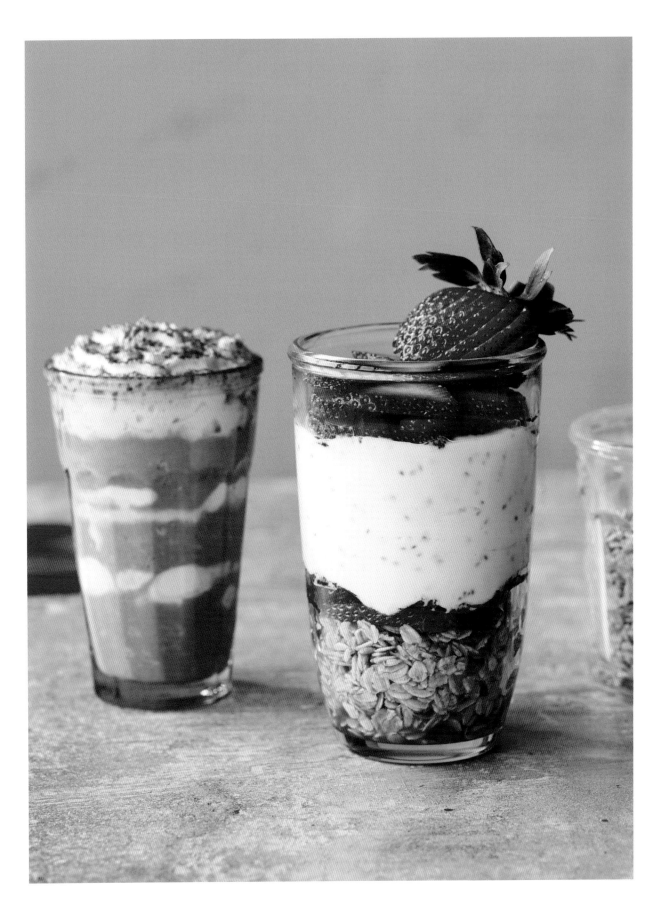

strawberry cheesecake overnight oats

Overnight oats are just so simple to prepare, and it is great to know that your breakfast is sitting in the refrigerator waiting for you when you wake up! Strawberry cheesecake is an elite cheesecake flavour, so works as a great inspiration for this recipe.

MAKES 1 PORTION

40g (1½oz/⅓ cup) porridge
   oats
1 tablespoon maple syrup
4 strawberries, sliced
3 tablespoons fat-free
   vanilla Greek yoghurt
1 tablespoon low-fat cream
   cheese
1 tablespoon chia seeds

Prep time 5 minutes, plus chilling time | **Calorie count** 380 calories per portion

Put the porridge oats into the base of a sealable container or mason jar. Add the maple syrup to the oats, then press them down to form a base like a cheesecake.

I like to double layer the strawberries, so add a layer of strawberry slices on top of the base.

Mix together the yoghurt, cream cheese and chia seeds, then pour this over the top, using a spatula to smooth the surface. Add a layer of strawberry slices to finish.

Seal the container and refrigerate overnight, or for at least 3 hours.

overnight banoffee-bix

When I first posted this video recipe it went viral all over my socials, with thousands of people commenting. Overnight Weetabix is a great twist on overnight oats, and you can use the wheat biscuits as a base to make it a little more like a banoffee pie. It's like having a treat for breakfast!

MAKES 1 PORTION

1 wheat biscuit (such as
   Weetabix)
120ml (4fl oz/½ cup) skimmed
   milk
1 tablespoon biscuit spread
   (such as Biscoff)
1 banana, sliced
200g (7oz/scant 1 cup)
   fat-free vanilla protein
   yoghurt

Prep time 10 minutes | **Cook time** 2 minutes, plus chilling time | **Calorie count** 420 calories per portion

Start by crushing up the wheat biscuit until it becomes crumbs, then add it to a resealable container. Add the milk and mix well, pressing down on the mixture with the back of a fork to create the base of the banoffee pie in the container.

Melt the biscuit spread in the microwave on high and drizzle most of it over the base, saving a little for the top

Add half of the banana slices on top of the biscuit base, then top with the yoghurt, smoothing out the surface with a spatula.

Top with the rest of the banana slices and drizzle with the reserved melted biscuit spread.

Seal the container and refrigerate overnight, or for at least 3 hours.

Note This recipe calls for low-fat protein yoghurt as it is made with cream cheese, but this can be substituted with quark instead.

microwave mini cinnamon rolls

I absolutely adore cinnamon buns and cinnamon rolls, but I certainly don't adore the calories that come with them! This recipe is for a super speedy, microwavable mug cake that is ready in just 60 seconds. There are only five main ingredients as well, making them really cheap to make, too.

MAKES 4 ROLLS

120g (4¼oz/½ cup) fat-free Greek yoghurt

100g (3½oz/⅔ cup) self-raising (self-rising) flour, plus extra for dusting

1 teaspoon baking powder

6 tablespoons biscuit spread (I use Biscoff)

2 teaspoons ground cinnamon

Low-calorie cooking spray

Prep time 5 minutes | **Cook time** 60 seconds
Calorie count 383 calories per cinnamon roll

In a mixing bowl, mix the yoghurt, flour and baking powder together until combined. Keep mixing to bring it all together until it forms a dough. If it looks a little sticky, you may need to add a little more flour – don't forget to adjust the calories accordingly though.

Divide the dough into 4 balls. Flour your work surface, then roll out the dough into 4 thin strips, about the thickness of a one-pound coin.

In a small jug or cup, melt the biscuit spread in the microwave for 30 seconds.

Spread a tablespoon of the biscuit spread over each strip of dough, then sprinkle some ground cinnamon over each strip. Roll the strips up with the spread and cinnamon on the inside.

Spray a microwaveable cup or dish with some low-calorie spray to stop it from sticking, then place the rolls into the mug.

If you don't want to eat the rolls right away, wrap them up and refrigerate it at this stage.

Microwave for 60 seconds on high, then pour the remaining biscuit spread over the top.

Note If you don't want to eat the rolls right away, you can store them uncooked in the refrigerator for up to 2 days.

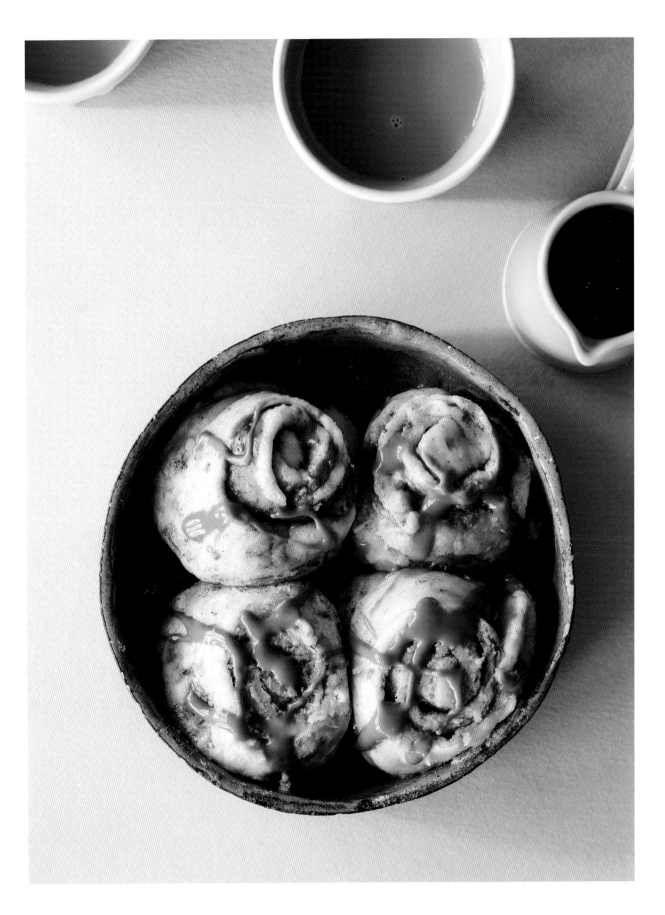

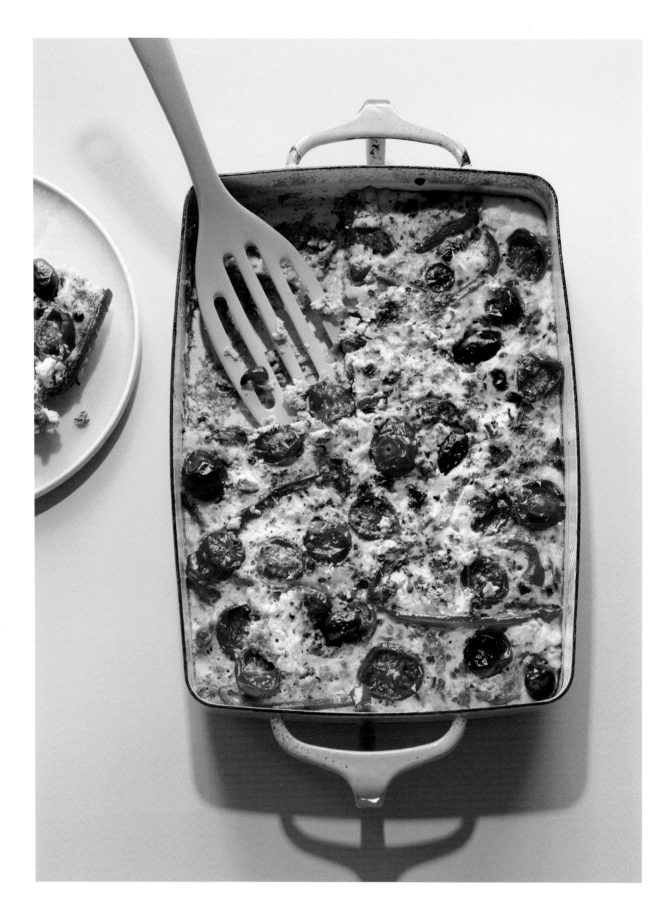

sunny breakfast casserole

I call this a 'sunny' breakfast casserole because I love having this when the sun is shining. With Greek-inspired flavours, it truly is a touch of sunshine on your plate. Perfect for prepping ahead and serving each morning during a working week, by either reheating or eating it cold.

MAKES 4 PORTIONS

500g (1lb 2oz) extra lean minced (ground) turkey
1 red (bell) pepper, sliced into strips
1 red onion, finely diced
300g (10½oz) cherry tomatoes, halved
2 tablespoons pitted black olives, halved
6 eggs
100ml (3½fl oz/⅖ cup) skimmed milk
120g (4¼oz) reduced-fat feta cheese, crumbled
2 teaspoons dried oregano
Low-calorie cooking spray
Sea salt and freshly ground black pepper

Notes Cool completely before placing slices into a resealable container. Can be kept for 3-4 days in the refrigerator. If reheating make sure it's cooked all the way through when serving.

Prep time 10 minutes | **Cook time** 45 minutes
Calorie count 445 calories per portion

Preheat the oven to 220°C/200°C fan/425°F/Gas mark 7.

Heat a frying pan over a medium heat and spray with low-calorie cooking spray. Add the turkey mince and fry for 2–3 minutes until the turkey has browned.

Spray an ovenproof dish with low-calorie cooking spray and transfer the browned turkey mince to the dish. Spread the pepper, onion, tomatoes and olives on top.

Whisk the eggs with the milk in a bowl or jug and add the feta, oregano and a pinch of salt and pepper and whisk again.

Pour the milk mixture over the mince and vegetables and stir so that everything is spread evenly throughout the dish.

Bake for 35 minutes, or until the egg has set. This can be served immediately, or leave it to cool completely before cutting into slices and storing in a sealable container.

MAKE IT VEGGIE
Instead of turkey mince, use a meat-free alternative or soy mince.

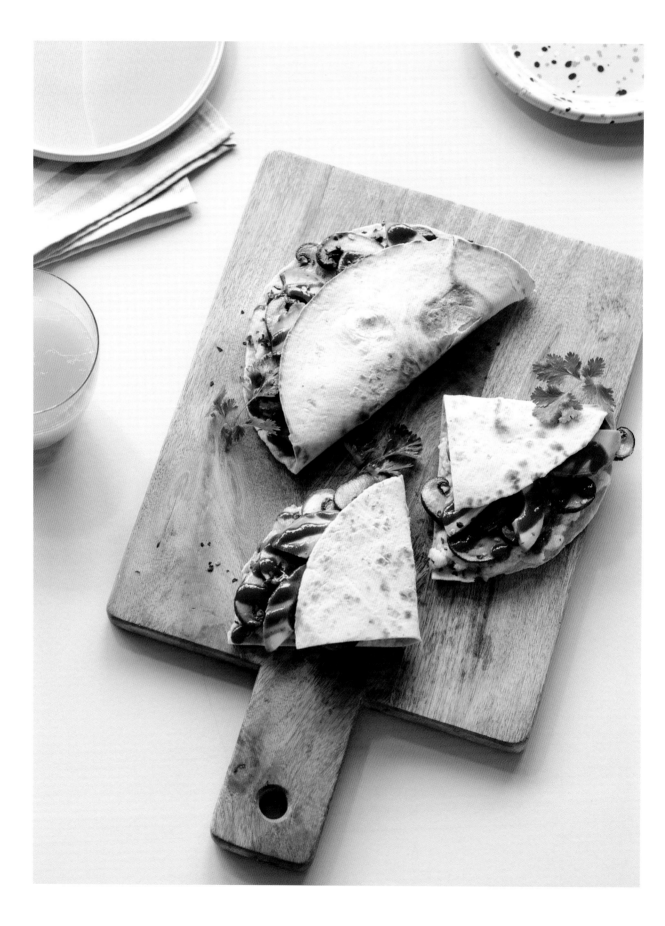

breakfast quesadillas

A quesadilla is a Mexican dish consisting of a fried tortilla wrap that is folded in half with a filling. This recipe is a great twist on some traditional breakfast ingredients, with a cheeky kick! I love an avocado and egg combination, and this recipe is one of my favourite ways to enjoy it.

**MAKES 2 QUESADILLAS
(2 PORTIONS)**

100g (3½oz) mushrooms, sliced

2 eggs

½ teaspoon dried chilli flakes

80g (3oz) low-fat Cheddar cheese

2 tortilla wraps

1 avocado, stoned (pitted) and sliced

Drizzle of sriracha chilli sauce

Low-calorie cooking spray

Coriander (cilantro), to serve

Sea salt and freshly ground black pepper

Prep time 5 minutes | **Cook time** 10 minutes
Calorie count 480 calories per quesadilla

Place a frying pan over a medium heat and spray with low-calorie cooking spray. Add the mushrooms and fry for 4 minutes, then remove them from the pan and set aside.

To prepare the scrambled eggs, crack both eggs into a mixing bowl and whisk. Season with salt and pepper and the chilli flakes, then grate the Cheddar into the bowl.

Heat the frying pan you used for the mushrooms and spray with some more low-calorie cooking spray. Add the whisked eggs and use a spatula to fold the eggs, moving the spatula from the outside of the pan into the centre of the pan.

Repeat the folding for about 3 minutes, until the eggs are fluffy and cooked. Remove from the heat and set aside.

Spray a clean frying pan with low-calorie cooking spray and add the tortilla wrap. Cook over a medium heat on one side for 2 minutes, then flip the tortilla over.

Add the mushrooms, avocado, a drizzle of sriracha and the scrambled eggs to one half of the tortilla, then fold over to close the filling inside. (If you are preparing ahead of time, remove it from the heat and wrap it up at this stage.)

Cook for 2 minutes, then flip over and cook the other side. Repeat with the second tortilla, then serve sprinkled with a few coriander leaves.

Note Quesadilla can be prepped ahead of time and toasted in the morning when ready to eat.

make-ahead english breakfast muffins

The beauty of these muffins is that you can prep them ahead of time, freeze them, then just take them out the night before to defrost. Just pop them in the microwave for 45 seconds when you're ready to eat them. Of course, you can also eat these straight away too!

MAKES 5 BREAKFAST MUFFINS

5 eggs

5 English muffins

5 cheese slices (you can use the American cheese slices or slices of low-fat Cheddar)

Low-calorie cooking spray

For the sausage patties

500g (1lb 2oz) low-fat minced (ground) pork (5% fat or less)

½ teaspoon dried sage

1 teaspoon Italian mixed herbs

¾ teaspoon garlic powder

¾ teaspoon onion powder

½ teaspoon sea salt

½ teaspoon black pepper

Prep time 15 minutes | **Cook time** 20 minutes
Calorie count 464 calories per muffin

Preheat the oven to 220°C/200°C fan/425°F/Gas mark 7. Spray 5 ovenproof ramekin dishes with low-calorie cooking spray.

Prepare the sausage patties by mixing the minced pork, sage, Italian herbs, garlic powder, onion powder, salt and pepper together in a large bowl. Mix well, then use your hands to mould them into 5 round patties. If you wanted to double up, make them into 10 smaller patties and have 2 in each muffin.

Whisk the eggs together in a bowl or jug and divide them evenly between the 5 ramekins. Bake for 10 minutes until the egg is cooked. Alternatively, the eggs can be microwaved on high for 1 minute 30 seconds.

Spray a large frying pan with low-calorie cooking spray and set over a medium heat. Add the patties and cook for about 6 minutes on each side, checking that there is no pink left in the middle of each patty.

Assemble the muffins by adding the patties, then a cheese slice, then the egg. Wrap in foil immediately, then allow to cool before freezing. You can also eat one right away if you would like!

Leave to defrost fully overnight before reheating. When you're ready to eat them, unwrap, then pop them in the microwave on high for 45 seconds.

MAKE IT VEGGIE
Instead of pork mince, use a meat-free alternative or soy mince. Alternatively, fill your muffins with spinach, egg and cheese.

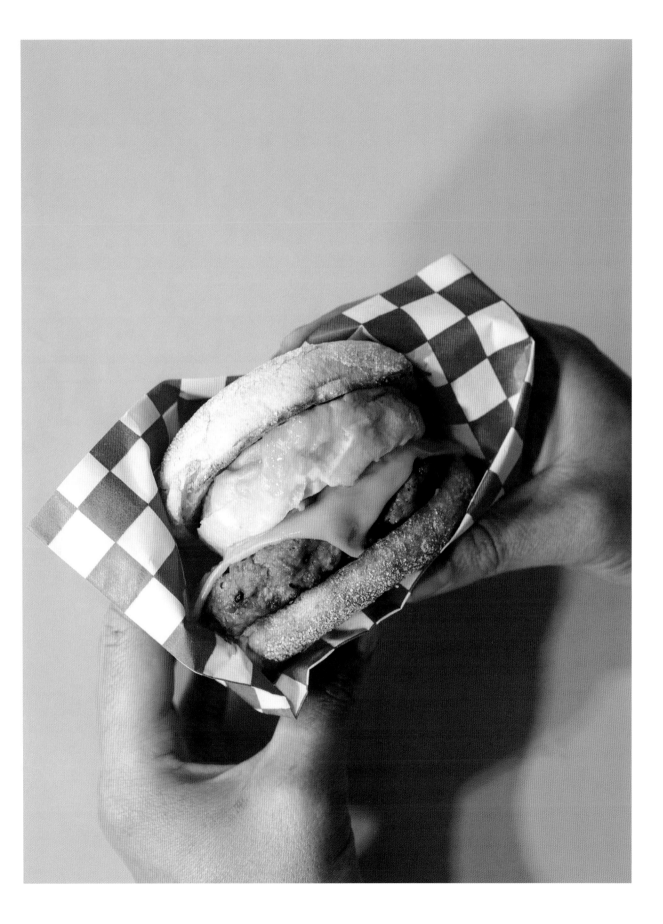

LAZY

WEEKEND BRUNCHES

Sometimes you just have to let yourself sleep in, clear the diary of activities for the day, and enjoy a lazy weekend brunch and a day of relaxation. We all lead such busy lives, and one thing I have learned recently is the importance of a bit of self-care.

What is a lazy brunch recipe? It is a delicious morning meal that you can prepare when you have the time to cook something properly in the kitchen. When it's not quite early enough to be classed as breakfast and not quite late enough to be considered lunch, lazy brunch recipes are the perfect solution.

I absolutely love throwing a brunch together at the weekend, and these recipes are some of my favourites. They require a little bit of prepping and cooking but they are still calorie-conscious while packing loads of flavour.

For years my house would be the place where everyone would gather at the weekend for some delicious food in the mornings, and these recipes are all tried and tested on my friends over the years.

I find all of these recipes extremely comforting and love planning which one I am going to prepare at the weekend. It gives me a little something to look forward to during the week!

I hope that your household finds a new favourite to enjoy every week, too!

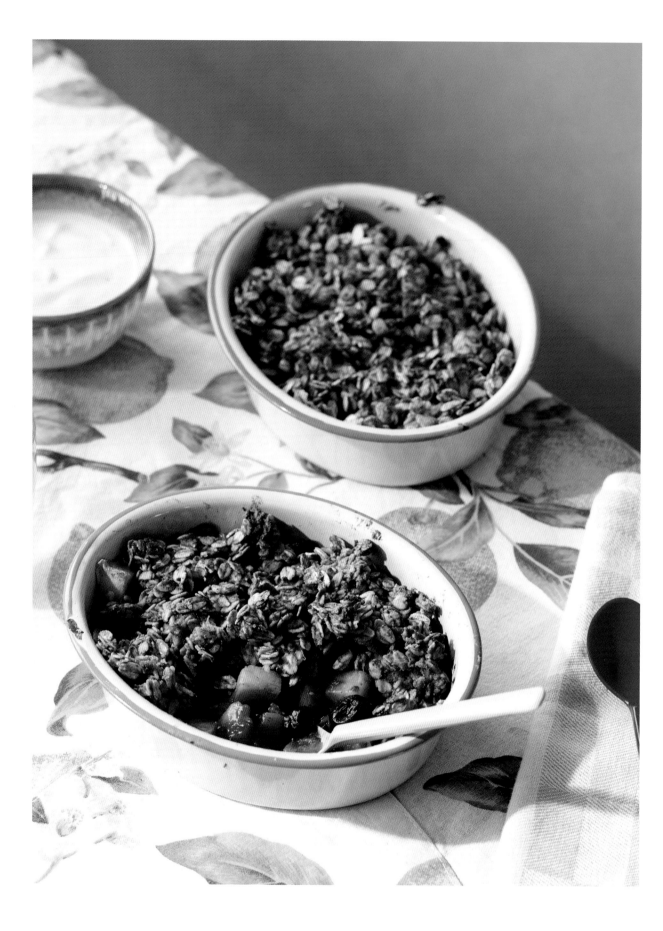

blueberry and apple breakfast crumble

You can't beat an apple crumble! Well, actually you can – an apple crumble that you can eat for breakfast, guilt-free! This recipe switches butter for almond butter and doesn't use any added sugar. A mashed banana helps to make the crumble topping absolutely perfect.

MAKES 2 PORTIONS

80g (3oz/⅔ cup) porridge
   oats
½ teaspoon ground cinnamon
1 ripe banana, mashed
1 tablespoon almond butter
   (or any other nut butter)
1 tablespoon maple syrup
Fat-free vanilla yoghurt,
   to serve

For the filling

250g (9oz/2 cups)
   blueberries
2 apples, peeled, cored and
   diced
½ teaspoon ground cinnamon
1 teaspoon plain
   (all-purpose) flour

Prep time 10 minutes | **Cook time** 40 minutes
Calorie count 481 calories per portion

Preheat the oven to 200°C/180°C fan/400°F/Gas mark 6.

For the oat crumble topping, mix the oats and cinnamon together in a mixing bowl. Add the banana to the oat mixture along with the almond butter and the maple syrup and mix everything together.

To make the filling, mix the blueberries, apples, cinnamon and flour together in an ovenproof dish.

Top with the oat crumble topping and spread it out evenly over the fruit.

Bake for 40 minutes until the oats are golden and the filling is bubbling. Make sure you cook the dish for long enough as while the oats may look ready, the filling needs the full cooking time.

Serve with some fat-free vanilla yoghurt.

Notes This recipe makes 2 portions, which you can either prepare in separate dishes and cook each one when ready to eat, or in one large dish. Store it in the refrigerator in a sealed container for up to 3 days. You could also prep this ahead of time and cook it in the morning.

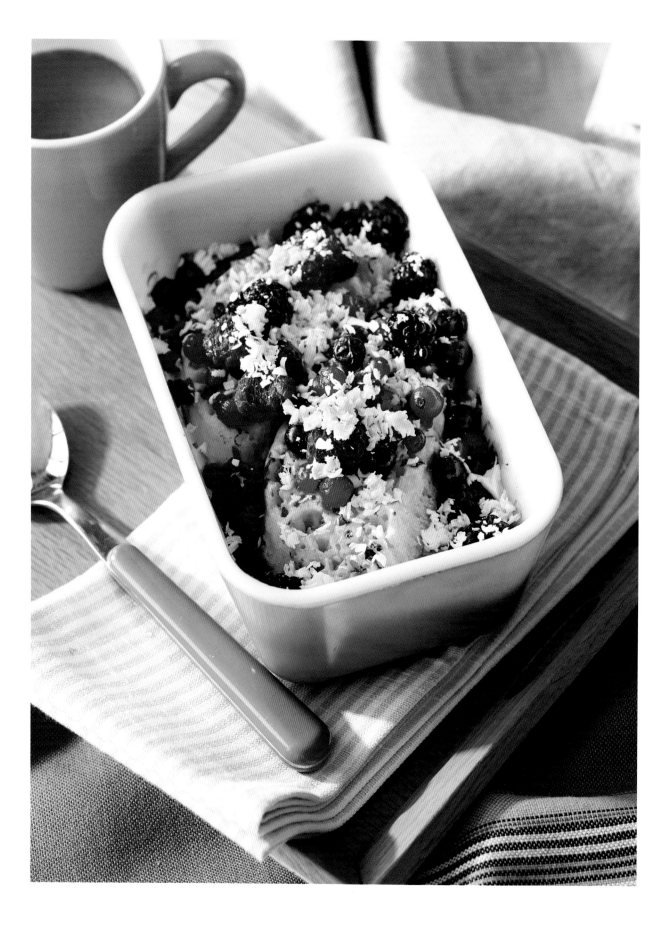

white chocolate summer fruits baked crumpets

Take your brunch to the next level with this tasty baked crumpets recipe. Boring buttered crumpets are a thing of the past with this delicious idea. You can vary the fruit toppings and flavours as you perfect this dish. This flavour combination is my personal favourite, though.

MAKES 1 PORTION

1 egg
50ml (3½ tablespoons)
    semi-skimmed milk
1 teaspoon granulated
    sweetener
2 crumpets
A handful of frozen
    mixed berries (such
    as strawberries,
    raspberries, blueberries)
25g (¾oz) white chocolate
Low-calorie cooking spray

Prep time 5 minutes | **Cook time** 20 minutes
Calorie count 400 calories per portion

Preheat the oven to 200°C/180°C fan/400°F/Gas mark 6.

Spray a 450g (1lb) loaf tin or ovenproof dish with low-calorie cooking spray.

In a mixing bowl whisk together the egg, milk and sweetener.

Cut the crumpets into halves, then dip each section into the egg mixture.

Arrange the crumpet halves in the greased tin/dish, then pour the leftover egg mixture over the top of the crumpets. Scatter the mixed berries evenly over the top of the crumpets.

Bake for 15–20 minutes until the crumpets are golden and the egg mixture has set.

Grate the white chocolate over the top of the dish when ready to serve.

Note Dip the crumpets into the eggy mixture and make sure it is all well coated for best results.

balsamic roasted tomatoes on toast with whipped chilli cream cheese

The fluffy, light, slightly spicy whipped chilli cream cheese takes this breakfast up to 'epic' levels! The sweetness of the roasted tomatoes with balsamic is perfectly paired with the kick of the chilli cheese. This is one of my go-to weekend breakfasts.

MAKES 2 PORTIONS

330g (11½oz) plum tomatoes (or cherry tomatoes), halved

1 teaspoon honey

3 tablespoons balsamic vinegar

½ teaspoon dried basil

1 garlic clove, peeled but left whole

Sea salt and freshly ground black pepper

2 slices of wholemeal bread, toasted, to serve

For the whipped cream cheese

100g (3½oz) full-fat cream cheese (see note)

1 tablespoon sparkling water

1 teaspoon dried chilli flakes (adjust depending on how spicy you like it)

Prep time 10 minutes | **Cook time** 35 minutes
Calorie count 472 calories per portion

Preheat the oven to 200°C/180°C fan/400°F/Gas mark 6.

For the roasted tomatoes, put the tomato halves into an ovenproof dish. Drizzle them with the honey and balsamic vinegar, season with salt and pepper and then sprinkle over the basil and add the garlic. Give everything a mix with a spoon so the tomatoes are coated in the honey and seasoning.

Bake for 35 minutes, stirring the tomatoes halfway through.

When ready to serve, add all of the whipped cheese ingredients to a mixing bowl. Use a hand mixer to whip up the cream cheese. It does start off looking a little watery, but keep mixing for at least 5 minutes and it should thicken up and start to have a thicker 'whipped' texture. You should be able to run a spoon through the middle and have the mixture stay where it is on either side of the bowl.

Remove the tomatoes from the oven, then crush the garlic clove with the back of a fork and mix in with the tomatoes.

Layer the toast with half of the whipped cream cheese on each slice and top with the roasted tomatoes, drizzling any leftover juice from the tomatoes over the top.

Note I have tried this recipe with low-fat cream cheese, but the whipping just doesn't seem to work. I recommend using full-fat cheese and taking the calorie hit, or if you prefer to use low-fat cream cheese, spread it on the toast rather than whipping it up. Whipping it makes it go further, so you actually use less than you would if you were spreading it.

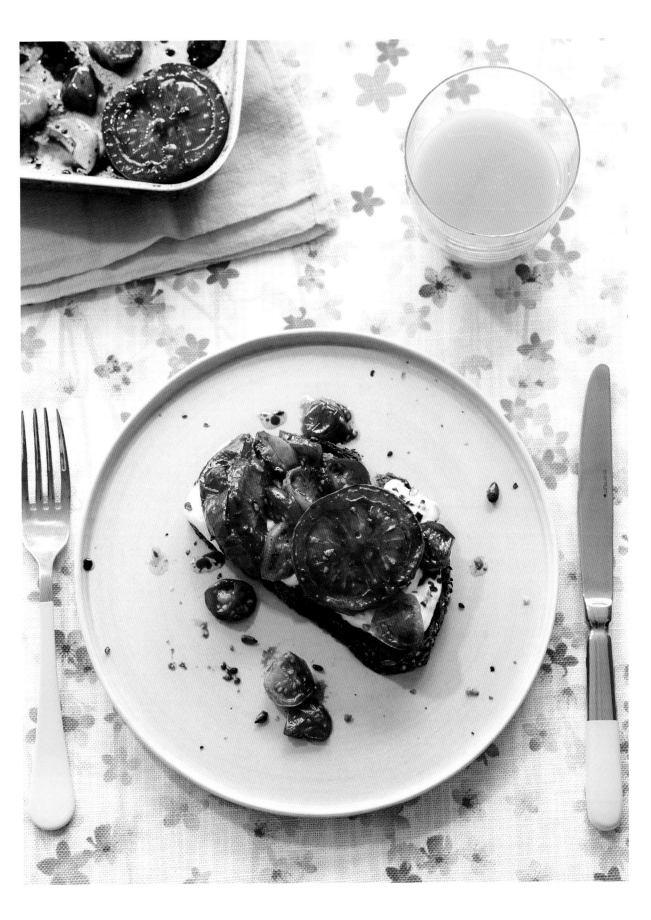

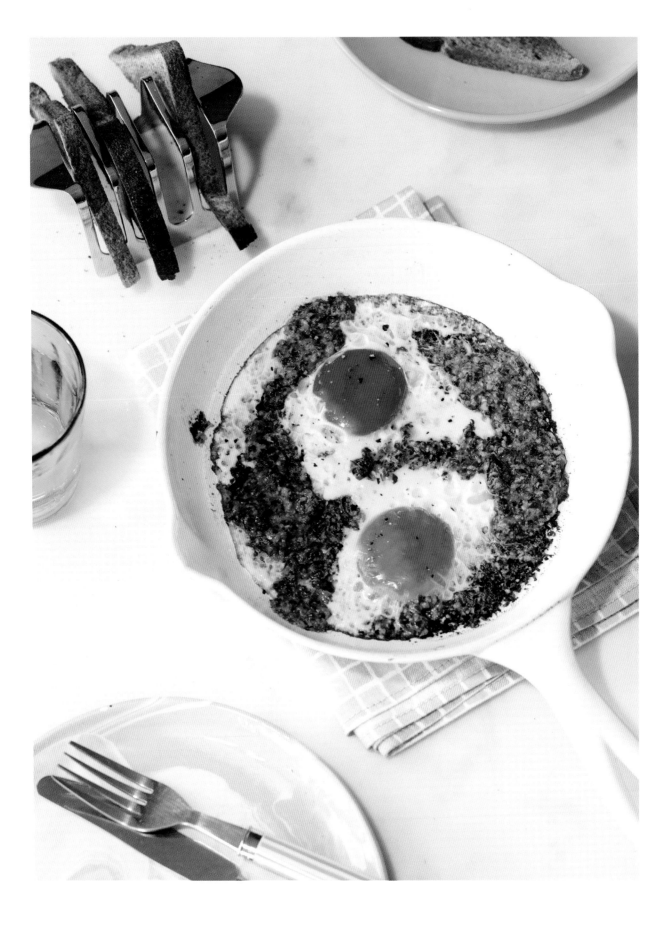

perfect pesto eggs

I love pesto, but it contains a lot of oil if you buy it ready-made in a jar. With this tasty recipe, you can save some fat and calories, while still enjoying the pesto flavours. This is my version of the viral pesto eggs craze, and I think you will love it as much as I do.

MAKES 2 PORTIONS
30g (1oz) basil leaves
½ tablespoon olive oil
2 tablespoons pine nuts
1 garlic clove
1 tablespoon grated Parmesan
Low-calorie cooking spray
Sea salt and freshly ground
    black pepper

To serve
2 eggs
2 slices of wholemeal bread,
    toasted

Prep time 5 minutes | **Cook time** 10 minutes
Calorie count 424 calories per portion

First make the pesto. Put the basil, oil, pine nuts, garlic clove, Parmesan and a pinch of salt and pepper in a food processor or blender. Blitz the ingredients until smooth, adding a teaspoon of water at a time to make a smoother consistency. You shouldn't need any more than 3 teaspoons, but add as required to get a pesto-like texture.

Heat a frying pan over a medium heat and spray with low-calorie cooking spray. Add 3 tablespoons of the pesto to the pan and spread it out in the pan with a spoon.

Crack the eggs on top of the pesto and cook for 3 minutes until the white has set.

Scoop some of the excess pesto on top of the eggs, then cover the pan with a lid and leave to cook for a further minute. If you don't want runny eggs, cook for an additional 2 minutes.

Scoop the eggs onto the toast along with the excess pesto in the pan and serve.

Note Any leftover pesto can be used as a dip for vegetables, or stored in the refrigerator in a sealable container.

BBQ bean and cheese bake

I love dipping toast into this smoky, cheesy bean bake. There is something about the smoky barbecue flavours and cheese that are perfect together. This breakfast tastes like you are consuming more calories than you actually are – which is always a winner!

MAKES 2 PORTIONS

1 onion, finely diced

1 red (bell) pepper, cut into cubes

1 x 415g (14oz) tin of baked beans

½ teaspoon mustard powder

1 teaspoon smoked paprika

1 teaspoon Worcestershire sauce

1 teaspoon balsamic vinegar

60g (2oz) low-fat mozzarella cheese, pulled into small chunks

4 slices of wholemeal bread, toasted

Low-calorie cooking spray

Prep time 5 minutes | **Cook time** 15 minutes
Calorie count 400 calories per portion (including bread)

Preheat the oven to 200°C/180°C fan /400°F/Gas mark 6.

Spray a frying pan with low-calorie cooking spray and add the onion and pepper. Cook for 2–3 minutes over a medium heat until the onion has softened.

Transfer the onion and pepper to an ovenproof dish along with the baked beans, mustard powder, smoked paprika, Worcestershire sauce and balsamic vinegar. Stir and then top with the mozzarella.

Bake for 15 minutes until the beans are bubbling and the cheese has melted.

Serve with wholemeal toast and get dipping!

Note Ensure the Worcestershire sauce you use is vegetarian friendly.

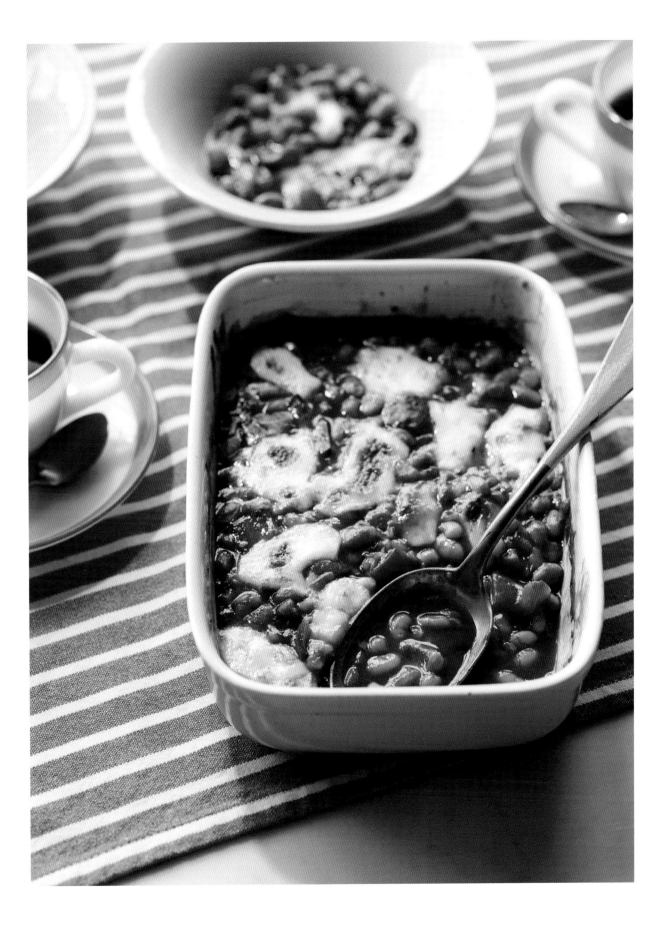

sweet potato eggs in a hole with sour cream and chives

There is something about the sour cream and chive flavour with the sweet potato that means I simply cannot get enough of this dish. The great thing about this recipe is that once you have perfected the sweet potato eggs in hole, you can let your imagination run wild with different toppings.

MAKES 2 PORTIONS

1 medium sweet potato, peeled and grated
½ red onion, grated
1 teaspoon garlic powder
1 teaspoon smoked paprika
2 tablespoons plain (all-purpose) flour
3 eggs
1 tablespoon olive oil
Sea salt and freshly ground black pepper

For the topping

3 tablespoons reduced-fat sour cream
1 tablespoon chopped fresh chives

Note I find that these come out best when using proper olive oil in the pan. You can substitute for low-calorie cooking spray, but it is more likely to stick.

Prep time 15 minutes | **Cook time** 11 minutes
Calorie count 450 calories per portion

Put the grated sweet potato and onion into a clean tea towel and wrap it around to squeeze out all the extra moisture over a bowl or the sink. The more moisture you remove the crispier it will be.

Put the sweet potato and red onion into a mixing bowl, then add the garlic powder, smoked paprika, flour and some salt and pepper. Mix well. Add one of the eggs and stir. This should bring all the mixture together.

Use your hands to make 2 balls with the sweet potato mixture, then press down to make a flat patty. Use a small cutter to make a hole for the egg, or use a knife to cut out a circle.

Heat a large frying pan over a medium heat with a tablespoon of olive oil.

Add both the sweet potato patties and fry for 3 minutes, then flip over to cook the other side for a further 3 minutes. I also fried the 'holes' that you cut out so that there is no waste, and added them on the side when serving.

Crack the eggs into the holes, then season the yolk with salt and pepper. Cover with a lid and cook for 5 minutes (adjust cooking time depending on how you like to have your eggs).

To make the topping, mix the sour cream with the fresh chives while the eggs are cooking.

Serve the sweet potato eggs in hole with a big dollop of sour cream.

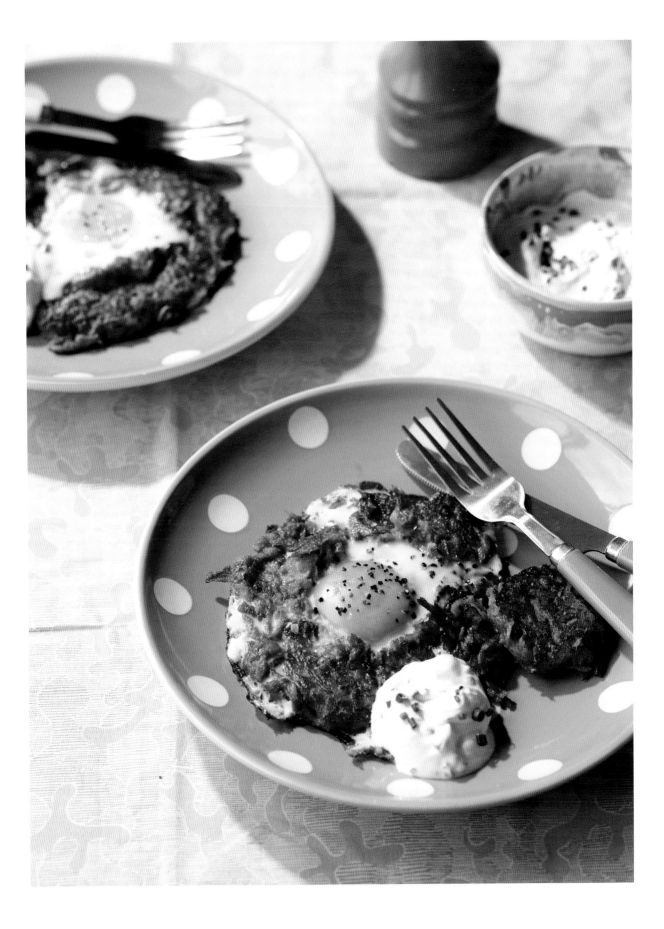

wholegrain mustard roasted potatoes with spinach and feta

I love making this dish on a lazy Sunday morning. It is absolutely delicious served on its own, or served with some fluffy scrambled egg. It is also the perfect side dish, fit for any breakfast plate! The potatoes are crispy and crunchy, perfectly balanced with the warm feta and spinach. The trick to the crunch of these potatoes is all in the seasoning and adding the oil to the potatoes rather than to the tray. This also helps to reduce the total amount of oil in the dish, too.

MAKES 2 PORTIONS

2 medium potatoes, peeled
   and sliced into 1cm (½in)
   cubes
1 tablespoon of extra virgin
   olive oil
1 teaspoon wholegrain
   mustard
1 teaspoon dried parsley
1 teaspoon smoked paprika
60g (2oz) reduced-fat feta
   cheese, crumbled up
90g (3¼oz) spinach
Sea salt and freshly ground
   black pepper

Notes The calorie count is for the potatoes, spinach and feta only. Don't forget to adjust the calories if serving with scrambled eggs. This dish is best served right away while the feta is still warm.

Prep time 10 minutes | **Cook time** 35 minutes
Calorie count 330 calories per portion

Preheat the oven to 200°C/180°C fan /400°F/Gas mark 6.

Put the cubed potatoes into a saucepan and bring to the boil. Once boiling, turn the heat down to low and leave to simmer for 5 minutes.

Drain the potatoes, then return them to the pan. Give the pan a shake so that the potatoes get fluffy on the outside – this helps them capture the added flavourings and also helps to get them crispy.

Add the olive oil, wholegrain mustard, parsley, smoked paprika and a pinch of salt and pepper to the potatoes. Use a large spoon to mix well and make sure all the potatoes are covered in the flavours and oil.

Lay the potatoes out evenly in a shallow roasting tin and bake for 20 minutes, or until they start to get golden.

After the potatoes have been in the oven for 20 minutes, remove the tray from the oven and add the crumbled feta. Return to the oven for a further 5 minutes, then remove and scatter the spinach over the top. Give everything a good stir, then return to the oven for a final 5 minutes – just long enough for the spinach to wilt.

Remove from the oven and stir well again to disperse all the ingredients evenly before serving.

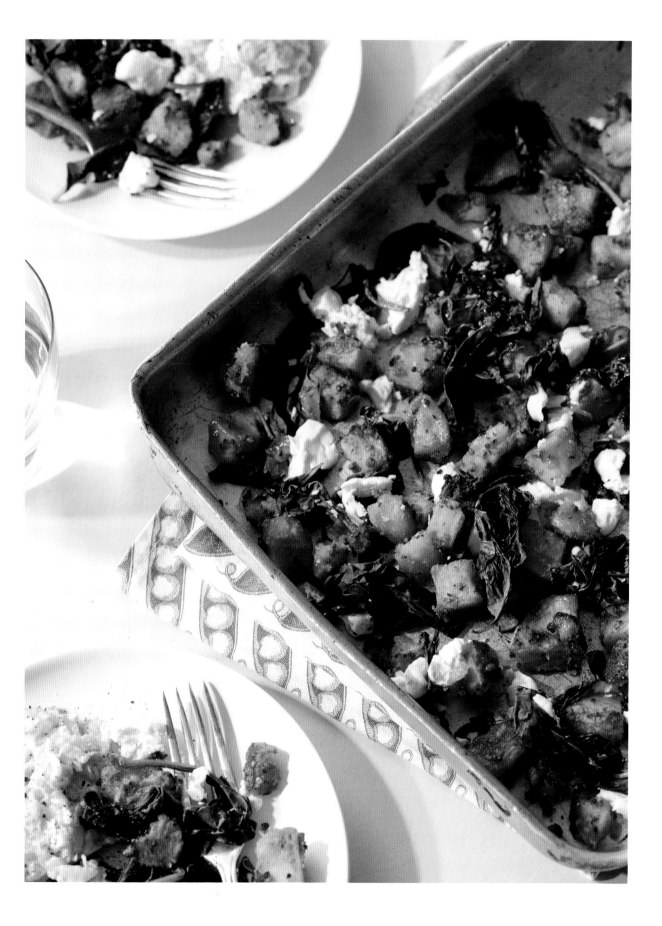

cheesy bacon hash brown waffles

I have a waffle iron machine and I swear I've only used it to make actual waffles once! Hash brown waffles are even better in my opinion. Instead of waffle batter, I use grated potatoes to make the easiest hash browns ever. The bacon and melted cheese are hidden in the middle of the hash brown waffle, which is a real treat when you cut into it.

**MAKES 2 WAFFLES
(1 WAFFLE PER PORTION)**

2 large potatoes, peeled and
    grated
½ onion, grated
1 egg, beaten
1 teaspoon smoked paprika
½ teaspoon garlic powder
4 cooked bacon medallions,
    fat removed and chopped
80g (3oz) extra light
    Cheddar cheese, grated
Low-calorie cooking spray
Sea salt and freshly ground
    black pepper

Prep time 5 minutes | **Cook time** 8 minutes
Calorie count 450 calories per waffle

Preheat the waffle iron.

Place the grated potatoes and onion in a clean tea towel. Squeeze out all the excess moisture in the potatoes by wrapping the towel around and squeezing it over a bowl or into your sink. The more moisture you can get out, the crispier the hash browns will be.

Transfer the grated potatoes to a mixing bowl and add the beaten egg, smoked paprika, garlic powder and some salt and pepper. Mix well and then split into 4 equal portions.

Spray the waffle iron with low-calorie cooking spray and add one of the portions of hash brown mix and spread out to cover the waffle iron.

Scatter half of the chopped bacon medallions over the top, along with half of the cheese. Add one of the other hash brown potato portions on top to cover the cheese and bacon. Close the lid of the waffle iron and cook for 8 minutes, or until the potato is golden and crispy. Repeat this process to make the other waffle.

Note This recipe uses a waffle machine, however, if you don't have one you can use a silicone waffle mould, or a round cake tin, and bake in an oven preheated to 200°C/180°C fan/400°F/Gas mark 6 for 25 minutes until the hash browns are golden and crispy.

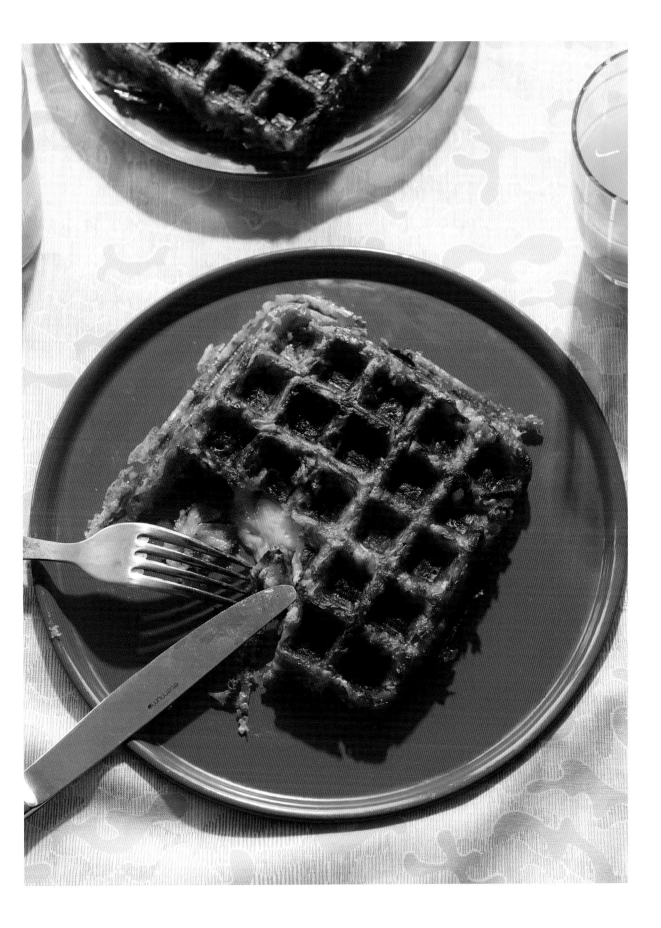

smoky bacon shakshuka

Shakshuka is a dish in which eggs are poached or baked in a smoky tomato-based sauce. It is often topped with feta cheese and made with chorizo, but I have created this recipe with bacon instead. This saves on some fat and calories, and I think it tastes just as good. This breakfast can be prepared in one large frying pan with a lid, saving you some washing up, too.

MAKES 4 PORTIONS

1 large red onion, sliced

1 large red (bell) pepper, sliced

1 large yellow (bell) pepper, sliced

3 garlic cloves, peeled and diced

200g (7oz) cherry tomatoes, chopped

6 smoked bacon medallions, all fat removed and cut into strips

1 x 400g (14oz) tin of chopped tomatoes

500g (1lb 2oz) passata (sieved tomatoes)

1 beef stock cube

2 tablespoons tomato purée (paste)

1 teaspoon ground cumin

2 teaspoons smoked paprika

½ teaspoon cayenne pepper

1 teaspoon dried coriander

1 teaspoon dried parsley

4 eggs

120g (4¼oz) feta cheese

Low-calorie cooking spray

Sea salt and freshly ground black pepper

Roughly chopped flat-leaf parsley, to serve

Prep time 10 minutes | **Cook time** 30 minutes
Calorie count 345 calories per portion

Spray a large frying pan (skillet) with a lid with low-calorie cooking spray and set over a medium heat. Add the onion and peppers and cook for around 8 minutes until softened.

Add the garlic, cherry tomatoes and bacon strips and cook for a further 3 minutes.

Add the chopped tomatoes, passata, crumbled beef stock cube, tomato purée and some salt and pepper and stir well.

Add the cumin, smoked paprika, cayenne pepper, coriander and parsley. Stir well, cover and simmer over a low heat for 15 minutes to reduce.

Once the sauce has reduced, create a well in the sauce for however many eggs you are using. Crack the egg into the well and sprinkle the feta over the top. Cover and heat over a low heat for 7 minutes, or until the eggs are cooked as you like them. Sprinkle with the parsley before serving.

Notes The recipe makes 4 portions, but if you aren't eating it all at once, just add the number of eggs you need for that time, and reheat the mixture when ready to eat the next portion and add a poached egg when serving. You could also prepare this in a slow cooker. Just adjust the cooking time to 4 hours on high or 8 hours on low, and add the eggs for the last 20 minutes of cooking.

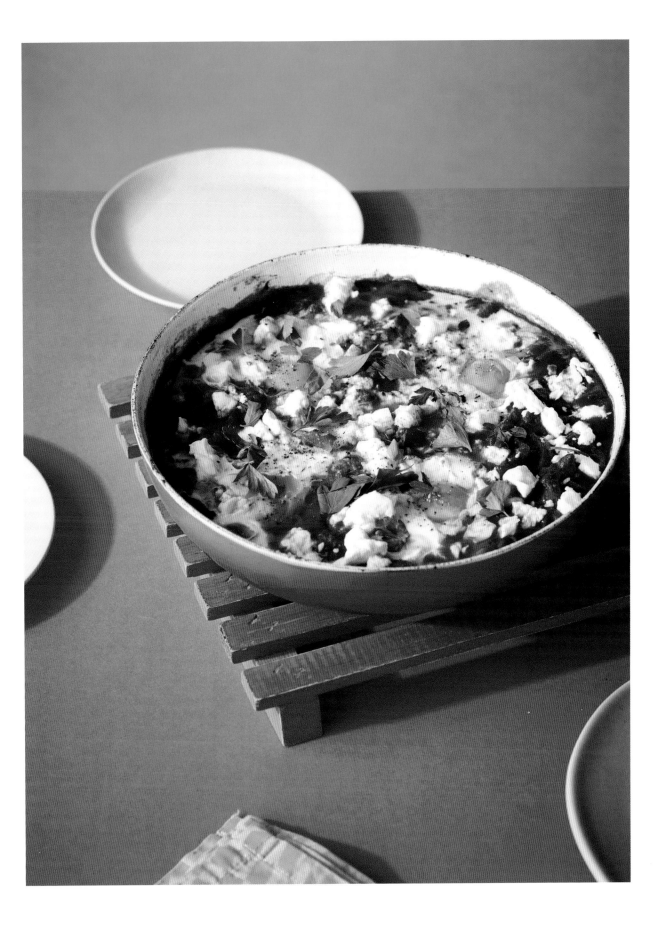

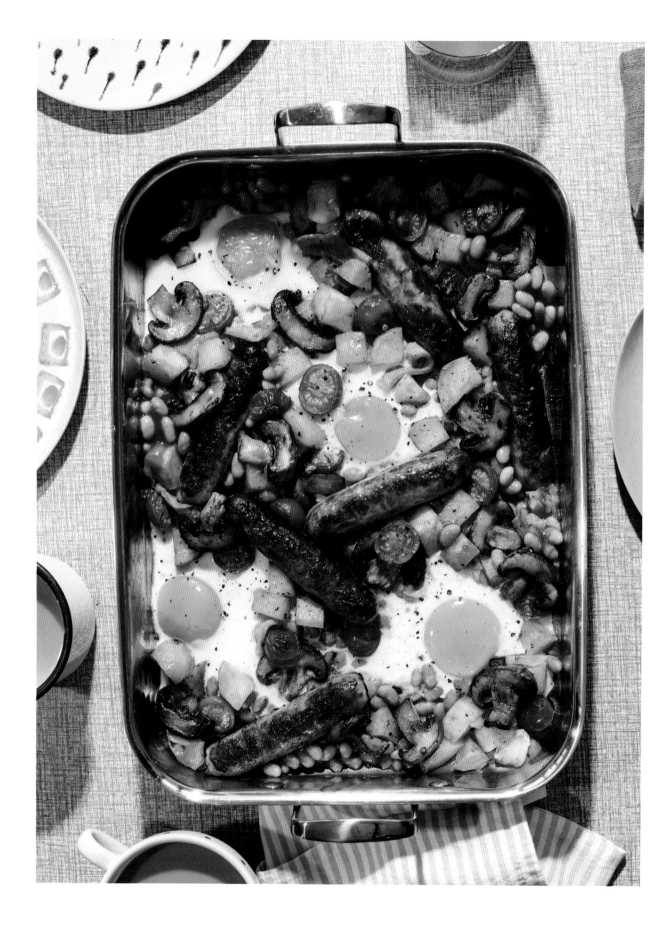

bumper breakfast traybake

I have always preferred to make 'oven-ups' instead of fry-ups – it's easier and means less washing up! I like to have my bacon crispy and my sausages well done. This recipe lets you have all the best bits from a traditional fry-up, all cooked together in one tray and without all the oil from frying. This is the easiest 'fry-up' that you can make!

MAKES 4 PORTIONS

2 large potatoes, peeled and cut into 1cm (½in) cubes

2 teaspoons olive oil

6 low-fat lean sausages, halved in the middle

4 bacon medallions, fat removed and cut into thin strips

1 garlic clove, finely chopped

12 cherry tomatoes, halved

200g (7oz) mushrooms, sliced

½ x 400g (14oz) tin of baked beans

1 teaspoon dried sage

4 eggs

Sea salt and freshly ground black pepper

Note There are lots of low-fat sausages available on the market; lean chicken sausages are also tasty and low in fat. Don't forget to double-check the calories depending on the sausage you use and adjust accordingly.

Prep time 10 minutes | **Cook time** 35 minutes
Calorie count 545 calories per portion

Preheat the oven to 200°C/180°C fan/400°F/Gas mark 6.

Put the cubed potatoes in a mixing bowl and add the olive oil. Season with salt and pepper, then stir well to ensure that the potato cubes are evenly coated in the oil and seasoning.

Add the potatoes to a baking tray along with the sausages and bake for 20 minutes.

In a mixing bowl, mix together the bacon, garlic, tomatoes, mushrooms, beans and sage. After the potatoes and sausages have cooked for 20 minutes, remove from the oven and give the potatoes a good stir.

Add the ingredients in the bowl to the tray, spreading everything out evenly. Return to the oven for 10 minutes.

Remove the tray from the oven, make 4 spaces for the eggs and crack them in. Return the tray to the oven and cook for another 3–4 minutes, depending on how runny you like your eggs.

MAKE IT VEGGIE
You can easily swap the sausages for vegetarian sausages, and either omit the bacon or use a meat-free alternative.

SOUPS

AND
SALADS

Soups and salads have gained a rather bad reputation over the years, but I am hoping to change that.

We are all so used to easy tinned soups, but soup can be so much more than your standard sugar-packed tomato soup in a tin. And salads have the potential for so much more flavour than a soggy bit of lettuce and salad cream. There are so many flavour combinations you can create, without the need for lashings of heavy dressing.

What's more, if you're trying to eat healthily, tinned soups often have a lot of extra sugar and fats in them. It's the same with pre-made salads - a lot of the dressings can be full of oil or fat, which means your healthy salad may not be as healthy as you think.

My salads are light, fresh and filling and pack loads of flavour. The soups are comforting, delicious warmers that are perfect to keep in the refrigerator for lunches throughout the week. They can be enjoyed as part of a 'take-to-work lunch' or made fresh to be enjoyed at home. They are anything other than plain and ordinary!

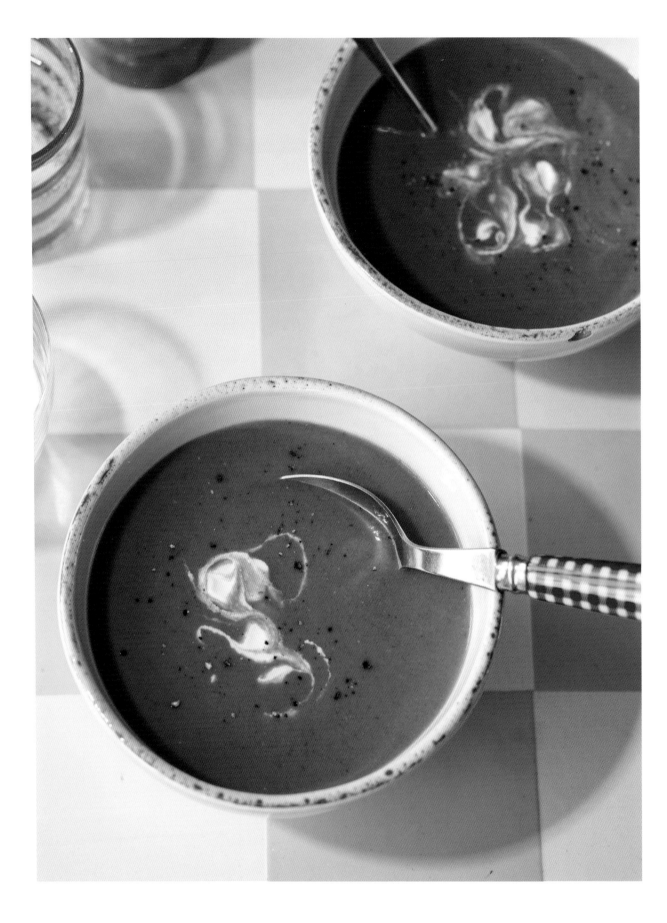

slow cooker creamy spicy tomato and vodka soup

Is there anything better than being able to throw all of the ingredients into a slow cooker and let it do its thing? You could leave the slow cooker to cook this overnight and then leave it on warm until you're ready to eat at lunch. Don't be put off by the vodka in this recipe – it helps to bring the dish together, balance the flavours and make the dish extra creamy and zesty. It won't make you tipsy!

MAKES 4 PORTIONS

300g (10½oz) cherry
  tomatoes, halved
300g (10½oz) plum tomatoes,
  halved
1 red chilli, finely diced
1 red onion, finely diced
500g (18fl oz/1lb 2oz)
  passata (sieved tomatoes)
25ml (1fl oz) vodka
1 vegetable stock cube
Sea salt and freshly ground
  black pepper
2 tablespoons low-fat cream
  cheese, to serve

Prep time 5 minutes | **Cook time** 4 hours/8 hours depending on whether you put it on low or high. | **Calorie count** 175 calories per portion

Put all of the ingredients for the soup into the slow cooker with 100ml (3½fl oz/⅓ cup) water and cook on high for 4 hours, or on low for 8 hours.

When ready to serve, add the cream cheese and stir through the soup until it has completely melted. Transfer the mixture to a food processor or blender and blitz to a tasty, smooth soup.

Notes If you don't own a slow cooker, I really recommend you get one! But if you're making this recipe without, chuck everything into an ovenproof dish and cook in an oven preheated to 180°C/160°C fan/350°F/Gas mark 4 for 45 minutes instead. Store extra portions in a sealed container in the refrigerator for up to 7 days.

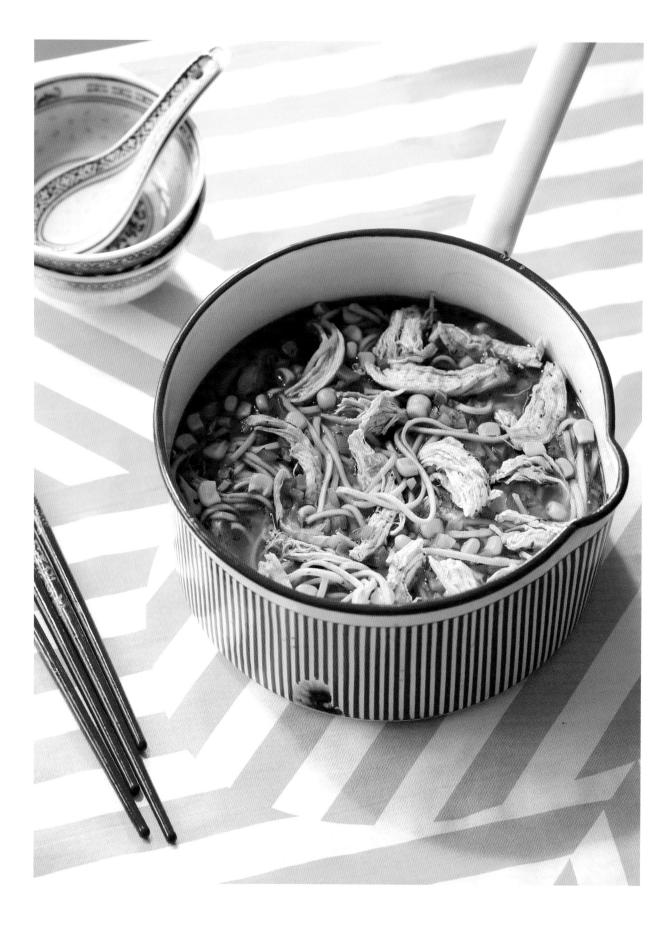

chicken noodle soup

This is a really hearty, rustic, delicious soup. It is like having a hug in a bowl when you slurp on it! It's what I call proper comfort food, which you can also freeze so that you're never without it. You could also experiment and add as many different vegetables as you like.

MAKES 4 PORTIONS

1 carrot, finely diced
1 onion, finely diced
1 celery stick, finely diced
1 garlic clove, finely diced
½ teaspoon smoked paprika
½ teaspoon dried thyme
850ml (29fl oz/3½ cups)
   chicken stock
1 x 198g (7oz) tin of
   sweetcorn
2 skinless and boneless
   chicken breasts
100g (3½oz) dried egg
   noodles
Low-calorie cooking spray
Sea salt and freshly ground
   black pepper

Prep time 5 minutes | **Cook time** 30 minutes
Calorie count 200 calories per portion

Spray a large saucepan with low-calorie cooking spray and add the carrot, onion, celery and garlic. Cook for 6 minutes over a medium heat until the vegetables soften.

Add the smoked paprika and thyme and cook for 2 minutes. Add the chicken stock and sweetcorn and reduce the heat to a low simmer. Add a pinch of sea salt and pepper and the chicken breasts and make sure they are fully submerged in the stock. Cover and leave to simmer for 20 minutes.

Remove the chicken breasts from the soup and check that they are fully cooked. Use 2 forks to pull the chicken breasts apart and shred them up.

Add the noodles to the soup along with the shredded chicken and cook for another 10 minutes until the noodles are fully cooked.

Note Leave to cool fully before putting in a sealed container and storing in the refrigerator for up to 5 days.

roasted leek, potato and horseradish soup

Leek and potato is one of my favourite soup flavours, but the horseradish in this recipe really adds something special. It isn't too powerful and adds an extra creaminess and depth of flavour to the soup.

MAKES 5 PORTIONS

500g (1lb 2oz) potatoes, peeled and roughly chopped into chunks
2 large leeks, sliced
1 onion, finely diced
1 garlic clove, finely diced
500ml (18fl oz/2 cups) vegetable stock
1 tablespoon low-fat crème fraîche
1 tablespoon horseradish sauce
Low-calorie cooking spray
Sea salt and freshly ground black pepper

Prep time 10 minutes | **Cook time** 45 minutes
Calorie count 150 calories per portion

Preheat the oven to 200°C/180°C fan/400°F/Gas mark 6. Spray a roasting dish with low-calorie cooking spray.

Put the potatoes, leeks and onion into the prepared roasting dish and sprinkle the garlic on top.

Season with salt and pepper, give everything a spray with low-calorie cooking spray, then bake for 40–45 minutes until the potatoes are cooked.

Once cooked, transfer the roasted potatoes and leeks in batches to a food processor or blender and blitz. Once all the potato and leeks have been blended, transfer it to a saucepan.

Add the stock, crème fraîche and horseradish and stir to combine and create a smooth soup. You may need to add more stock if you like your soup to be thinner.

Serve straight away or leave to cool completely and store in a sealed container.

Notes Store in a sealable container in the refrigerator for up to 5 days. Can also be frozen. Reheat to serve by heating in the microwave or on a saucepan over a medium heat.

tuna crunch pasta salad

This is my go-to, quick, easy, prep-ahead lunch. I make a huge batch up on a Sunday so that it is always to hand during the week. I try to add as many salad items as I can to make it extra filling. The mix of half yoghurt and half mayo helps to make it extra creamy and light.

MAKES 5 PORTIONS

250g (9oz) dried pasta shape of your choice (I usually use penne)

½ red onion, finely diced

1 x 198g (7oz) tin of sweetcorn

1 cucumber, finely diced

150g (5oz) cherry tomatoes, halved

100g (3½oz) spinach

2 x 145g tins of tuna in spring water, drained

2 tablespoons fat-free Greek yoghurt

2 tablespoons low-fat mayonnaise

½ teaspoon mustard powder

100g (3½oz) reduced-fat feta cheese, cut into cubes

Sea salt and freshly ground black pepper

Prep time 10 minutes | **Cook time** 10 minutes
Calorie count 360 calories per portion

Cook the pasta in a saucepan of salted boiling water according to the packet instructions, while you prepare the rest of the salad.

Put the red onion, sweetcorn, cucumber and tomatoes into a large bowl with the spinach.

In a separate bowl, put the drained tuna, Greek yoghurt, mayonnaise, mustard powder and some salt and pepper and mix well.

Once the pasta has cooked, drain it and run it under the cold tap until it is completely cooled. Shake off the excess water, then add the pasta to the bowl with the spinach, sweetcorn and tomatoes.

Add the tuna mixture to the rest of the salad and mix everything together well.

Note This can be portioned up and kept in the refrigerator in a sealable container for up to 5 days.

sugar pink super salad

You'd be forgiven for thinking that salads can be boring and unappetizing, but this salad is anything but! The sweetness of the fruit mixed in with the crunchy, fresh lettuce combined with the saltiness of the feta cheese means you will want to make this over and over again. It also contains one of my favourite things, a little splash of pink!

MAKES 4 PORTIONS

For the salad
½ head of iceberg lettuce, shredded
1 red onion, finely diced
½ cucumber, finely diced
50g (1¾oz) cherry tomatoes, halved
100g (3½oz) spinach, shredded
200g (7oz) rocket (arugula)
3 slices of pickled beetroot, cut into small cubes
50g (1¾oz) strawberries, sliced
120g (4¼oz) reduced-fat feta cheese
80g (3oz) pomegranate seeds

For the dressing
3 tablespoons balsamic vinegar
1 teaspoon dried oregano
Sea salt and freshly ground black pepper

Notes Store in a sealable container in the refrigerator for up to 5 days with the dressing separate. If portioning up for lunches, keep the dressing separate and pour over when ready to eat.

Prep time 10 minutes | **Calorie count** 175 calories per portion

Put the shredded lettuce, red onion, cucumber and tomatoes into a bowl with the spinach, rocket, beetroot, strawberries and feta cheese, then top with the pomegranate seeds. Give everything a good mix.

Mix the dressing ingredients together in a small bowl and drizzle it all over the salad and give it a good mix before serving.

MAKE IT VEGAN
Remove the feta cheese or replace it with a vegan alternative.

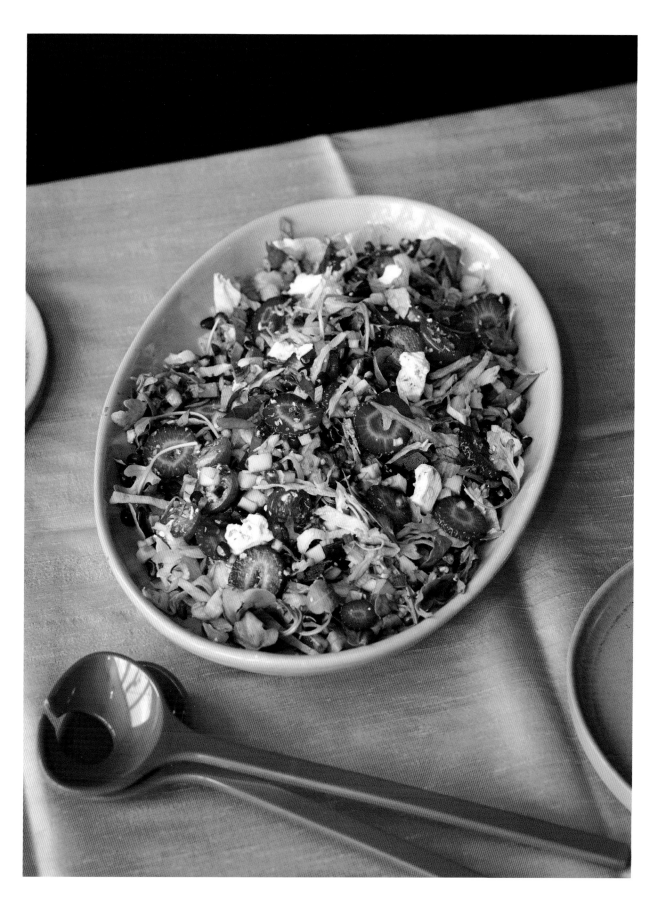

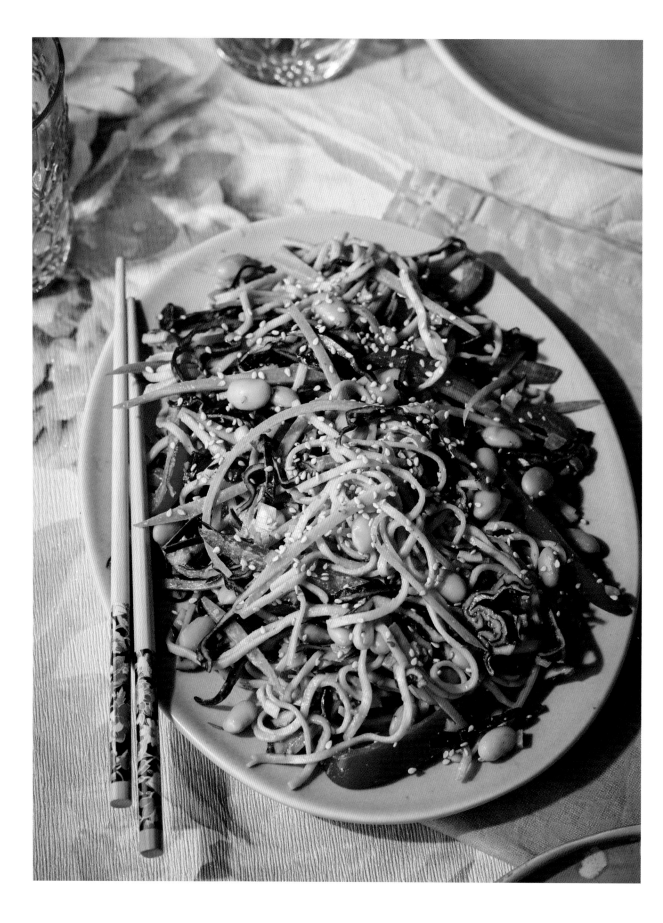

cold noodle salad

There is something so refreshing about a cold noodle salad. They're super easy to put together and are something a little different to have for a 'take-to-work' lunch.

Prep time 10 minutes | **Cook time** 5 minutes
Calorie count 280 calories per portion

Cook the noodles in a saucepan of boiling water according to the packet instructions. Once cooked, drain and set aside to cool.

For the dressing, whisk all the ingredients together in a small bowl or jar, then put it into a mixing bowl with the noodles, carrot, cabbage, pepper, edamame beans and spring onions. Pour over the dressing and give everything a good mix.

Serve immediately or portion up into sealed containers and refrigerate for up to 5 days.

MAKES 4 PORTIONS

50g (1¾oz) dried egg noodles (about 1 nest)

1 carrot, peeled and grated

½ red cabbage, sliced into thin strips

1 red (bell) pepper, sliced into thin strips

100g (3½oz) podded edamame beans

3 spring onions (scallions), chopped

1 tablespoon sesame seeds

For the dressing

1 tablespoon peanut butter

1 tablespoon soy sauce

1 tablespoon rice wine vinegar

Juice from 1 lime

1 teaspoon sriracha

½ teaspoon honey

½ teaspoon of 'lazy ginger' (ginger that's in a jar, ready prepared)

Sea salt and freshly ground black pepper

Notes Store in a sealed container for up to 5 days in the regrigerator. This salad also works well with some cooked shredded chicken.

MAKE IT VEGAN
Swap the honey for maple syrup.

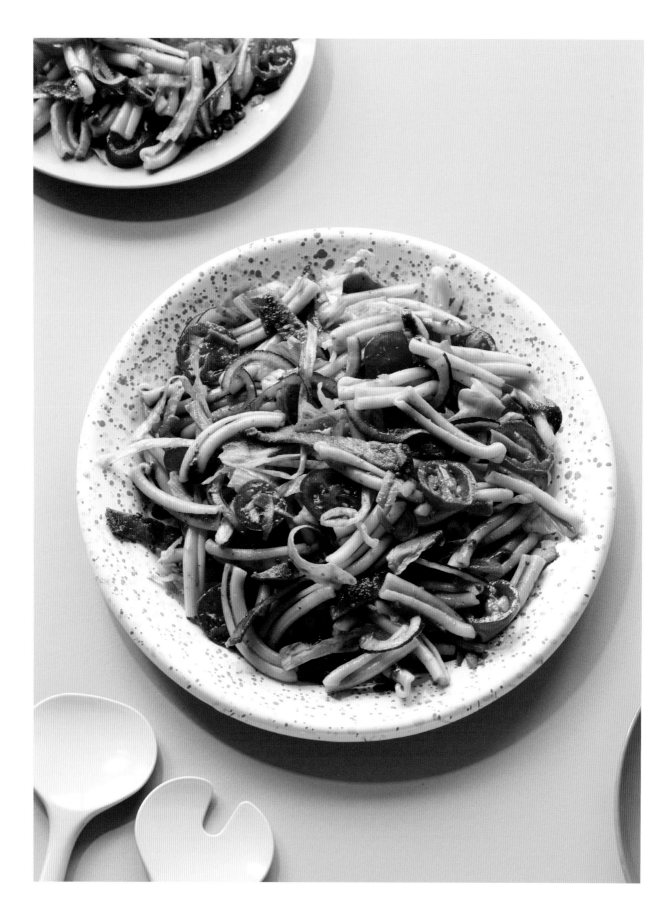

bumper BLT pasta salad

This is a twist on a very old recipe of mine, but new and improved. This salad is perfect to make ahead as a 'take-to-work' lunch and is a showstopper to present at any kind of summer barbecue. It is light, filling and has all the flavours of the classic sandwich that we all know and love, but without the bread.

MAKES 4 PORTIONS

5 bacon medallions, all fat
   removed
250g (9oz) dried pasta
   shapes of your choice
120g (4¼oz) cherry tomatoes,
   sliced
½ head of iceberg lettuce,
   sliced into strips
½ red onion, sliced into
   thin strips
1 carrot, grated
Low-calorie cooking spray

For the dressing

1 tablespoon olive oil
1 tablespoon wholegrain
   mustard
2 tablespoons balsamic
   vinegar
½ small garlic clove
Sea salt and freshly ground
   black pepper

Prep time 10 minutes | **Cook time** 5 minutes
Calorie count 407 calories per portion

Spray a frying pan (skillet) with low-calorie cooking spray. Add the bacon medallions and fry over a medium heat until cooked, turning regularly. Remove the bacon from the pan and then cut it into thin strips.

Cook the pasta in a saucepan of salted boiling water according to the packet instructions, then drain, set aside and leave to cool.

Make the dressing by whisking together the olive oil, mustard, balsamic vinegar, garlic and some salt and pepper in a small bowl or jar until combined.

If serving straight away, add all of the remaining ingredients to a mixing bowl with the drained pasta and bacon strips, drizzle with the dressing, mix well and serve.

Notes If you want to take this to work throughout the week, keep the dressing in a separate container and pour over the salad when ready to serve.

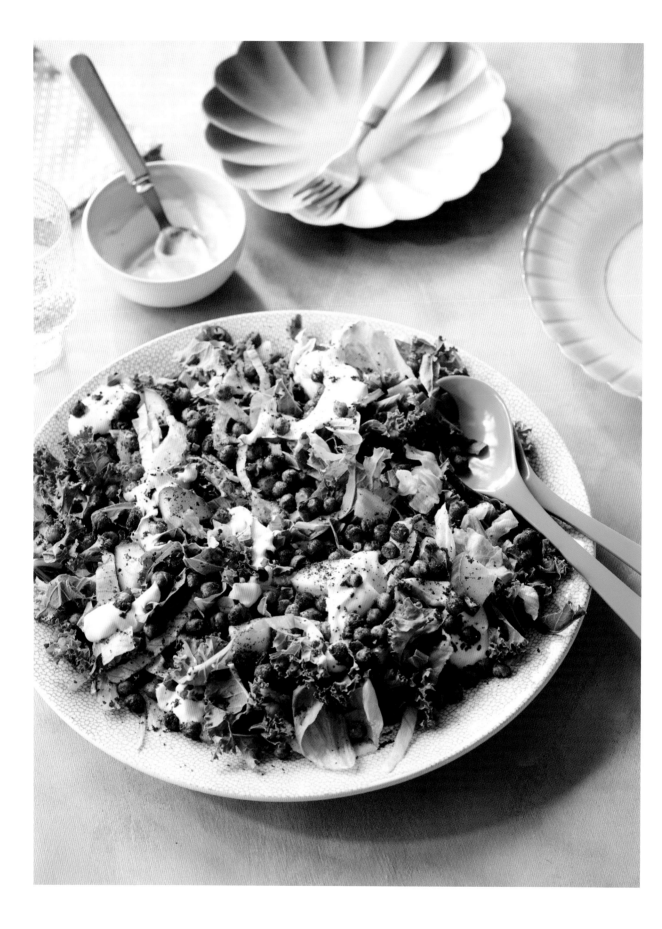

crunchy chickpea salad

When I think of what to do with chickpeas my first thought is usually to make hummus to serve with bread or vegetables, but actually, chickpeas can be the star of the show. If seasoned and cooked correctly, they come out so crunchy and delicious, and this salad certainly shows them off.

MAKES 2 PORTIONS

1 x 400g (14oz) tin of
   chickpeas, drained
2 teaspoons smoked paprika
1 teaspoon ground cumin
2 teaspoons ground coriander
½ teaspoons cayenne pepper
Low-calorie cooking spray
Sea salt and freshly ground
   black pepper

For the dressing

3 tablespoons fat-free Greek
   yoghurt
1 garlic clove, finely diced

For the salad

100g (3½oz/2½–3 cups) kale,
   roughly chopped
½ head of iceberg lettuce,
   roughly chopped
½ cucumber, chopped into
   cubes

Prep time 10 minutes | **Cook time** 35 minutes
Calorie count 450 calories per portion

Preheat the oven to 200°C/180°C fan/400°F/Gas mark 6.

Put the chickpeas into a bowl and spritz them with low-calorie cooking spray. Sprinkle over the smoked paprika, cumin, coriander, cayenne pepper and some salt and pepper. Give the chickpeas a good mix around so that they are all evenly coated with the flavours.

Spread the chickpeas out on a baking tray (sheet) and bake for 35 minutes, giving them a shake halfway through cooking.

Mix the ingredients together for the dressing and add a pinch of salt and pepper.

Put the kale, lettuce and cucumber in a serving dish and drizzle with some of the dressing. Add the chickpeas and drizzle with some more of the dressing to finish.

rainbow buddha bowls

Buddha bowls are vegetarian bowls filled with a balanced and healthy portion of rice and veggies. I love the process of loading my bowl up with all my favourite veggies, and find it so satisfying and filling to eat. I love seeing a bit of colour on my plate, too, so the more variety you can pack into this dish, the better. It's up to you how pretty you make this dish when preparing it, you can either chuck it all in or present it nicely so it is fit for the 'gram!

MAKES 2 PORTIONS

80g (3oz/⅓ cup) brown rice
100g (3½oz) podded edamame
    beans
1 yellow (bell) pepper,
    sliced
1 cucumber, sliced
½ x 400g (14oz) tin of
    chickpeas, drained
½ a red onion, finely diced
1 carrot, grated
100g (3½oz) spinach, roughly
    chopped
50g (1¾oz/½ cup) stoned
    (pitted) black olives,
    roughly chopped
Juice of 1 lime
Sea salt and freshly ground
    black pepper

Prep time 10 minutes | **Cook time** none
Calorie count 504 calories per portion

Bring a large saucepan of water to the boil and cook the rice according to the packet instructions, then drain.

To assemble the buddha bowls, divide the cooked rice between two bowls, then arrange the edamame beans, pepper, cucumber, chickpeas, red onion, carrot, spinach and olives in sections over the top.

Drizzle with lime juice and add a sprinkling of salt and pepper before serving.

Notes You can add as many different vegetables on top as you like. If you like, you can also include some feta cheese or a vegan alternative, but you will need to recalculate the calorie count accordingly.

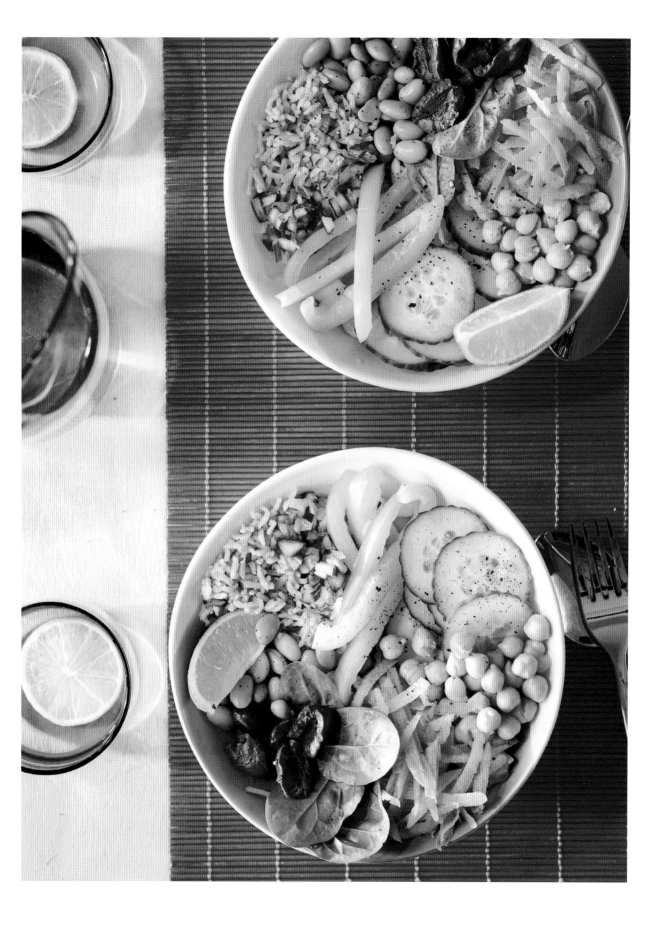

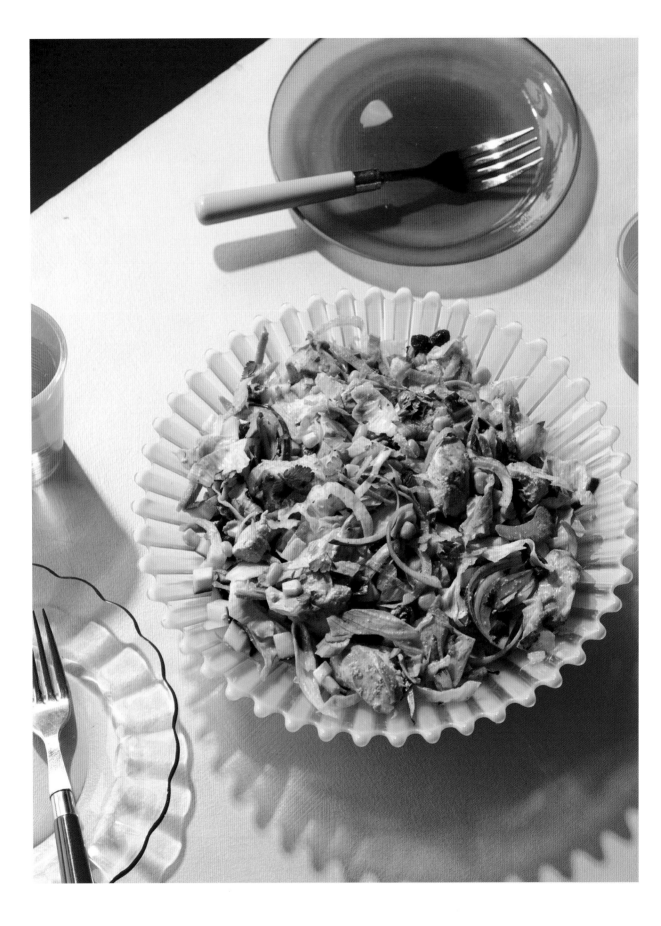

curried chicken salad

This salad is my take on Coronation chicken, and can easily be prepared on the weekend and stored in the refrigerator for 'take-to-work' lunches. It's light, super filling and the perfect mix of sweet and spicy.

MAKES 4 PORTIONS

2 large skinless and
    boneless chicken breasts,
    diced
2 carrots, grated
40g (1½oz/⅓ cup) raisins
1 celery stick, sliced
1 red onion, sliced
1 cucumber, cubed
1 x 198g (7oz) tin of
    sweetcorn
Small handful of freshly
    chopped coriander
    (cilantro)
1 large iceberg lettuce,
    sliced into strips

For the dressing

120g (4¼oz/½ cup) fat-free
    Greek yoghurt
2 tablespoons low-fat
    mayonnaise
Juice of 1 small lemon
2 teaspoons curry powder
½ teaspoon honey
1 teaspoon smoked paprika

Notes Store in a
sealable container in
the refrigerator for up
to 5 days.

Prep time 15 minutes, plus 30 minutes marinating
Cook time 35 minutes | **Calorie count** 250 calories
per portion

Preheat the oven to 220°C/200°C fan/425°F/Gas mark 7.

For the dressing, mix all of the ingredients together in a bowl.

Place the chicken in a bowl and add 2 tablespoons of the dressing. Mix together so that the chicken is coated and then leave it to marinate for 30 minutes.

Put the marinated diced chicken into an ovenproof dish and bake for 25 minutes until the chicken is cooked all the way through.

Put the carrots, raisins, celery, red onion, cucumber, sweetcorn and coriander into a mixing bowl and mix with the remaining dressing.

Once the chicken is cooked, leave it to cool for a few minutes, then add it to the rest of the salad, mixing everything together so that it is fully combined.

MAKE IT VEGGIE
You can easily adapt this to be vegetarian by replacing the chicken with tofu or a meat-free alternative.

PREP AHEAD

LUNCH BOXES

Do you struggle with ideas for lunches that you can either eat on the go or take with you to work? Finding your soggy sandwich more unappetizing than ever? Stuck on the same old salads?

I find that lunch can be the hardest meal of the day to keep on track if you're following a healthy eating plan. If you don't plan or prep ahead it can be so easy to grab something on the go that isn't particularly healthy, especially if you're out at work all day. Popping to the kitchen to cook up a tasty lunch for yourself may be out of the question, but making the same old sandwiches over and over again can be so boring - enough to stop you from prepping your lunch ahead of time at all.

These prep-ahead lunches are perfect to take to work, and can either be made in a big batch at the weekend to last the week or made the night before and kept in the refrigerator. These recipes will have you looking forward to your lunch break once again.

Making a big batch of some of the recipes in this chapter at the weekend before you start your working week can be the secret to keeping you on track throughout the day. And above all else, lunch doesn't have to be the most boring meal of the day anymore!

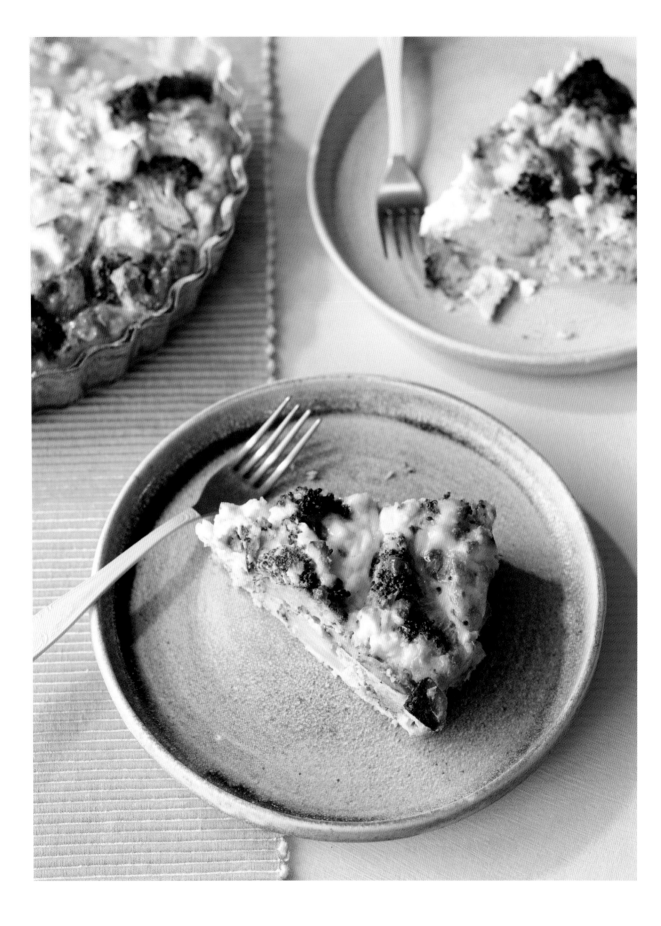

bacon, broccoli and feta crustless quiche

Quiche is such a classic lunch, but I find they can be quite heavy with the pastry. Without the crust, you can easily save some calories. I think that this quiche is just as delicious without any pastry, though, and can be enjoyed on its own or with a salad. Perfect for prep-ahead ready portioned lunches, too!

MAKES 4 PORTIONS

6 bacon medallions, all
    fat removed and cut into
    strips
2 garlic cloves, finely
    diced
1 teaspoon mixed Italian
    herbs
1 small head of broccoli,
    cut into small florets
75g (2¾oz) 'lighter'
    mascarpone cheese
8 eggs
100g (3½oz) feta cheese
Low-calorie cooking spray
Sea salt and freshly ground
    black pepper

Note Store in a sealed
container in the
refrigerator for up to
5 days.

Prep time 10 minutes | **Cook time** 50 minutes
Calorie count 385 calories per portion

Preheat the oven to 170°C/150°C fan/325°F/Gas mark 3. Spray a quiche dish or medium-sized baking dish with low-calorie cooking spray.

Put the bacon into a frying pan (skillet) sprayed with low-calorie cooking spray and cook for 4 minutes over a medium heat.

Add the garlic and mixed herbs to the bacon and fry for about 3 minutes. Add the broccoli to the pan and fry for a further 5 minutes until the broccoli has softened. Transfer all of this to the prepared baking dish.

Whisk up the eggs in a bowl and add the mascarpone and whisk together. Pour the egg mixture over the bacon and broccoli, then scatter the feta cheese on top.

Bake for 40–45 minutes, or until the quiche is golden and cooked all the way through.

Serve immediately or divide into 4 portions, then allow to cool completely before refrigerating.

MAKE IT VEGGIE
Use a meat-free alternative to bacon, or leave it out completely.

cheese and onion triangles

These little filo parcel triangles are like samosas, but with a delicious cheese and onion filling. They're perfect for packed lunches and are tasty served on their own, or as part of a larger lunch.

MAKES 6 TRIANGLES

1 large potato, peeled and chopped into cubes

150g (5oz) low-fat Cheddar cheese, grated

2 spring onions (scallions), finely chopped

1 tablespoon reduced-fat cream cheese

½ teaspoon English mustard

2 sheets of ready-made filo (phyllo) pastry

Low-calorie cooking spray

Prep time 10 minutes | **Cook time** 20 minutes
Calorie count 217 calories per triangle

Preheat the oven to 180°C/160°C fan/350°F/Gas mark 4.

Put the potatoes into a saucepan of boiling water and cook for 10 minutes until cooked all the way through. Drain the potatoes and then mash them until smooth.

Add the cheese, spring onions, cream cheese and mustard and mix together until the cheeses have melted.

Spray a sheet of filo with low-calorie cooking spray and cut it lengthways into 3 strips.

Put 2 tablespoons of the filling at the top of each strip and fold each diagonally to make a small triangle, then continue to fold over down the length of the pastry so that the filling is enclosed. Repeat this process with the remaining filling and pastry.

Arrange the parcels on a baking sheet and spray them with some more low-calorie cooking spray. Bake for 18–20 minutes, or until they're golden brown and cooked through.

Note Wrap and keep in the refrigerator for up to 5 days.

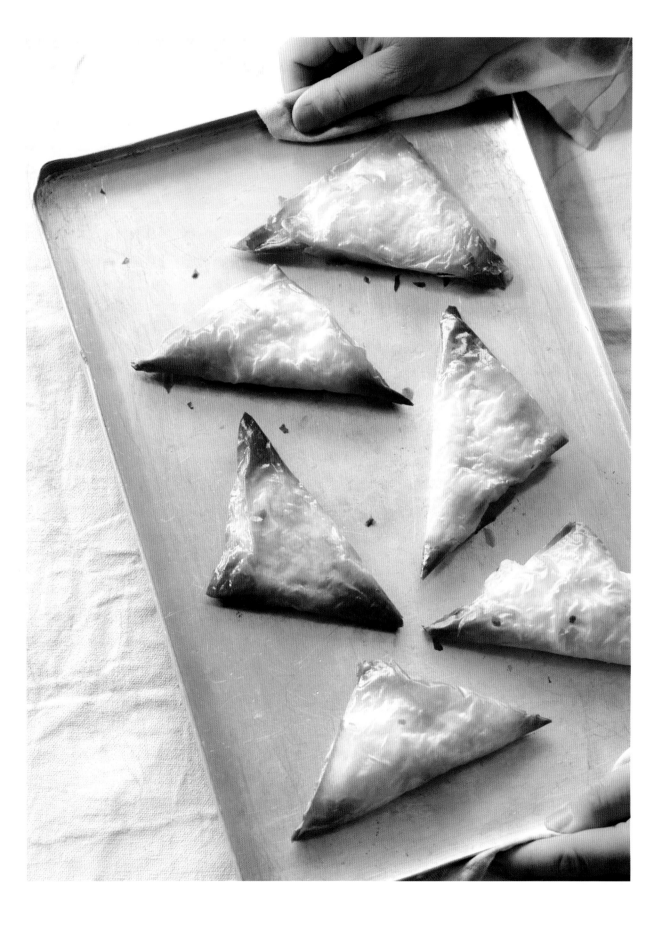

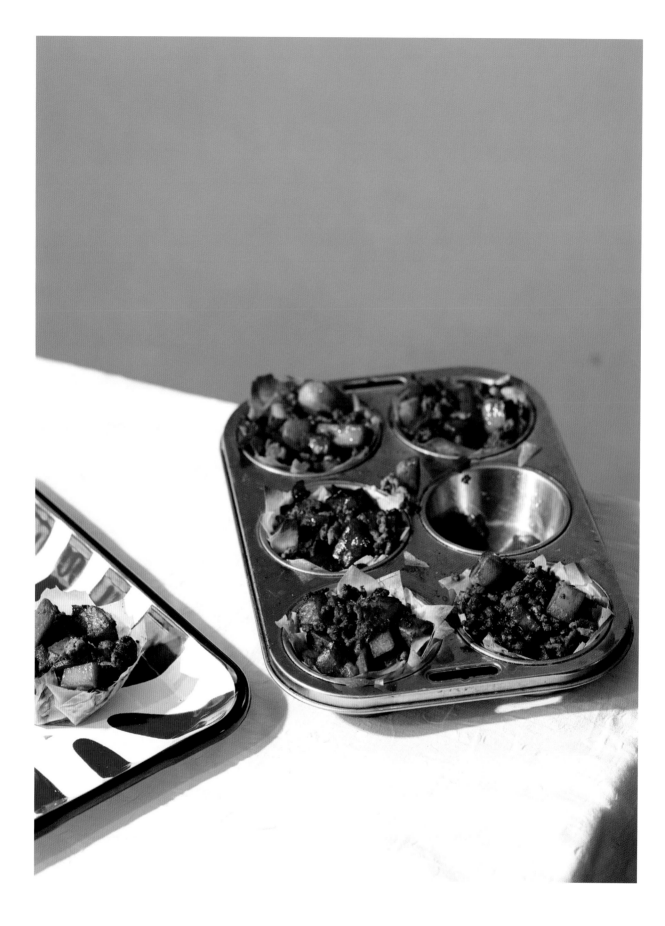

filo pastry pasty parcels

As a West Country girl, it would be rude of me to not include my take on a pasty! Now, I know this may not be a traditional pasty variety, but it is my favourite way to prepare one. These are delicious both hot and cold and are perfect to pack in a lunchbox.

MAKES 6 PARCELS

1 large onion, finely diced
1 garlic clove, finely diced
1 carrot, finely diced
1 large potato, peeled and cut into small chunks
250g (9oz) extra lean minced (ground) beef
1 tablespoon Worcestershire sauce
100ml (3½fl oz/⅓ cup) beef stock
2 sheets of ready-made filo (phyllo) pastry
Low-calorie cooking spray
Sea salt and freshly ground black pepper

Prep time 10 minutes | **Cook time** 40 minutes
Calorie count 271 calories per parcel

Preheat the oven to 180°C/160°C fan/350°F/Gas mark 4.

Spray a large frying pan (skillet) with low-calorie cooking spray. Add the onion and cook for 4 minutes until it softens.

Add the garlic, carrot and potato and fry for 3 minutes. The potato and carrot should have softened before moving into the next step.

Add the beef mince and cook for 7 minutes until browned. Add the Worcestershire sauce and beef stock. Season with a pinch of salt and pepper. Reduce the heat and let it simmer for 25 minutes.

Meanwhile, prepare the cases by cutting the filo pastry into roughly 5cm (2in) squares. Stack 3 squares on top of each other at odd angles so that the corners don't align – it should make a rough star shape.

Spray a muffin tin with low-calorie cooking spray and press one stack of filo pastry in each muffin hole. Spray with some more low-calorie cooking spray, then bake for 5 minutes to crisp up.

Once the filling has finished cooking, add a spoonful of mixture into each filo pastry case and bake for 15 minutes. Keep an eye on the filo to make sure it doesn't burn.

mini frittatas

The great thing about a frittata is that you can pretty much throw anything that you have in the house into the mix, and add as many vegetables as you like. You can prepare these at the weekend so you have them ready for lunches all week.

MAKES 8 MINI FRITTATAS (2 PER SERVING)

1 potato, peeled and thinly sliced
6 eggs
8 spring onions (scallions), sliced
2 garlic cloves, finely diced
1 red chilli, deseeded and diced
Handful of spinach
1 x 198g (7oz) tin of sweetcorn, drained
200g (7oz/1½ cups) frozen peas
Low-calorie cooking spray
Sea salt and freshly ground black pepper

Prep time 10 minutes | **Cook time** 40 minutes
Calorie count 120 calories per mini frittata

Preheat the oven to 180°C/160°C fan/350°F/Gas mark 4.

Put the potato slices into a saucepan of boiling water and cook for 5 minutes until softened, then drain.

Spray a muffin tin with low-calorie cooking spray. Place a couple of potato slices at the bottom of each muffin tin and set the rest aside.

Whisk the eggs in a mixing bowl, then add all the remaining ingredients and mix to combine, including any leftover potato slices. Season well and pour into the muffin tin holes.

Bake for 35 minutes, or until the eggs have set and the frittata is golden brown.

Once cooled slightly, you should be able to tip the muffin tin over to remove the frittatas.

Note Leave to cool completely and keep in the refrigerator in a sealable container for 5 days.

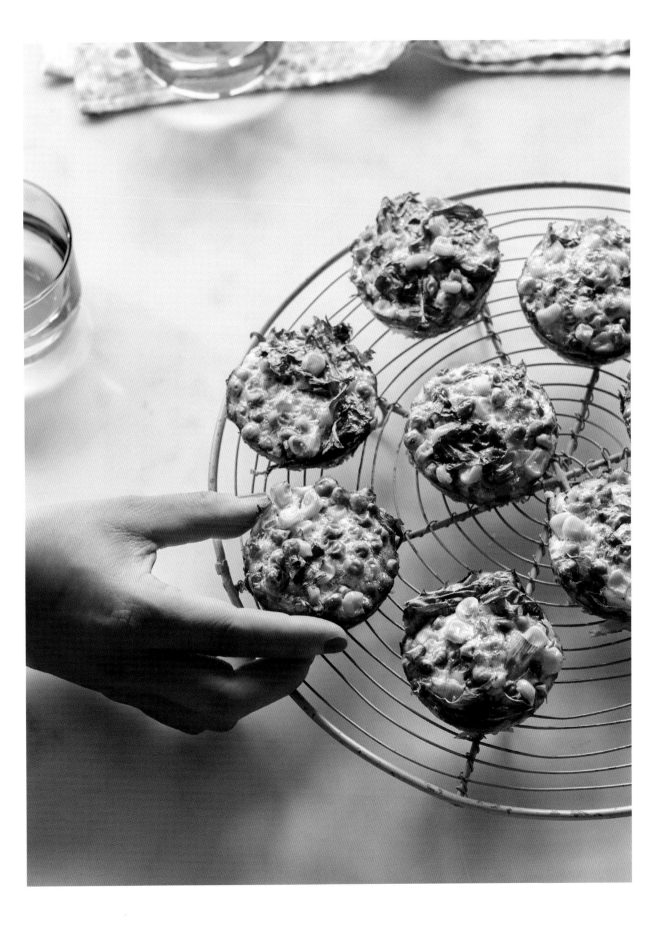

turkey club pinwheels

These mini turkey club sandwich bites are super moreish. Eating these mouth-sized tortilla wrap wheels makes grabbing lunch on the go even easier. They have all the flavours of an American turkey club sandwich – turkey, bacon, cheese and tomato – and are easy to make ahead the night before.

MAKES 1 PORTION

2 bacon medallions, all fat
   removed
1 tablespoon low-fat
   mayonnaise
¼ teaspoon garlic powder
¼ teaspoon onion powder
1 large tortilla wrap
3 large slices of lean
   turkey or turkey ham
4 slices of low-fat Cheddar
   cheese
2 large lettuce leaves,
   washed and dried
2 tomatoes, thinly sliced
Sea salt and freshly ground
   black pepper
Carrot sticks, to serve
   (optional)

Prep time 10 minutes | **Cook time** 10 minutes
Calorie count 408 calories per portion

Cook the bacon medallions in a frying pan (skillet) until crispy.

In a small bowl, mix together the mayonnaise, garlic powder, onion powder and some salt and pepper.

Place the tortilla wrap on your worktop, then spread the mayo mixture over the surface. Lay out the turkey slices to cover the whole wrap.

Add the slices of cheese and cover as much of the area as possible. Layer on the lettuce leaves, tomato slices and bacon evenly across the middle of the tortilla, covering as much area as you can.

Roll the tortilla up as tightly as possible in the opposite direction that you laid out the lettuce and bacon so that there is an even filling throughout. You should be left with a tortilla wrap sausage.

Cut off any excess edges. Slice the wrap in half, then slice those halves in half, and continue until you're left with 8 wheels.

You can hold them together with a cocktail stick, or by using any excess mayo to press any loose edges in place.

Serve with some carrot sticks or other prepared vegetables, if you like.

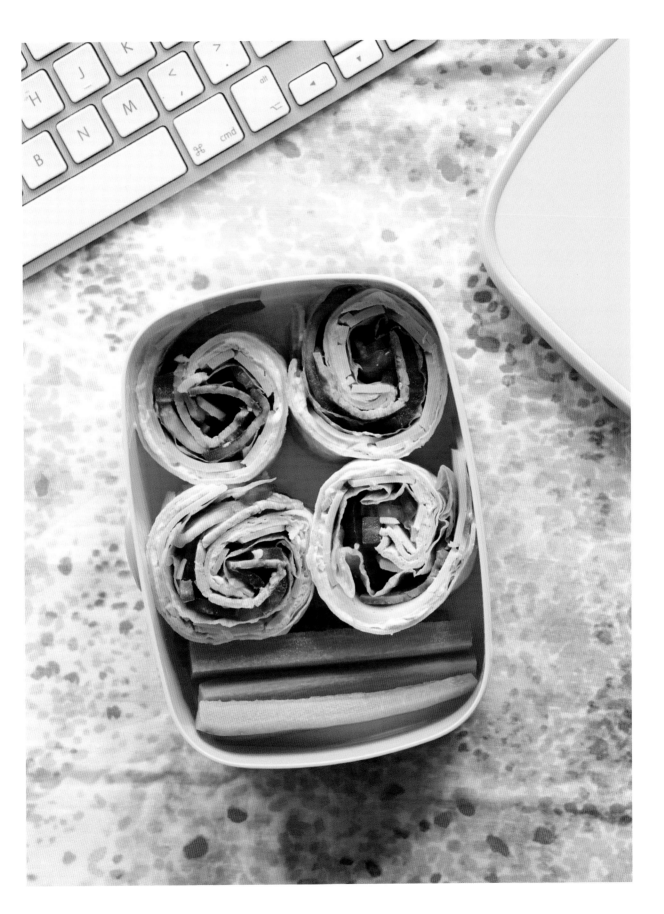

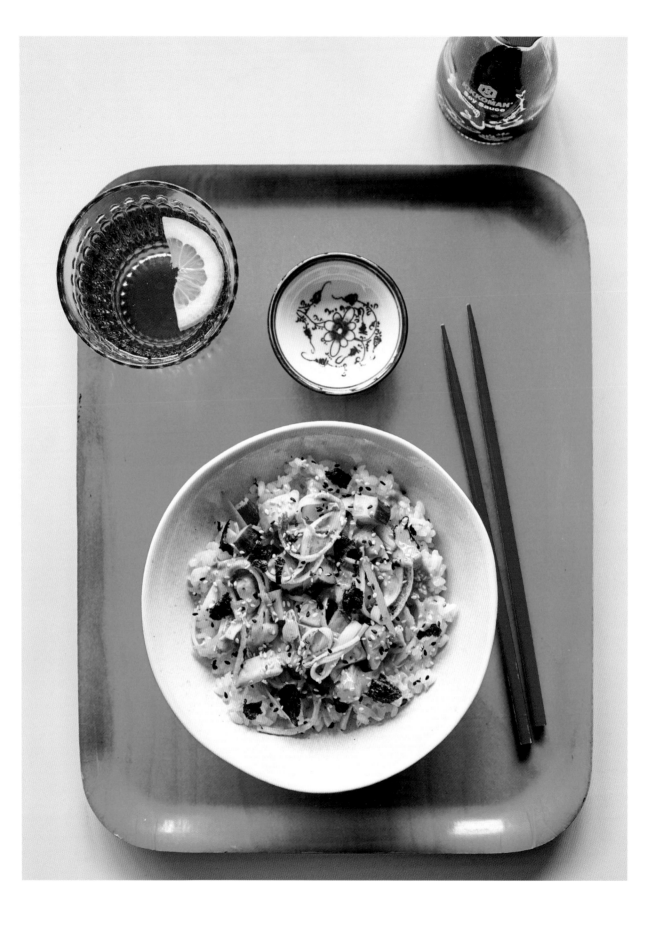

sushi roll in a bowl

This recipe has all my favourite flavours of a California roll sushi, but in a bowl instead. Making sushi is great, but can be super fiddly with the rolling. This recipe lets you enjoy it with half the effort.

MAKES 2 PORTIONS

100g (3½oz/½ cup) sushi rice

4 tablespoons rice vinegar

1 teaspoon granulated sweetener

250g (9oz) seafood sticks (or swap for tuna or smoked salmon)

½ cucumber, cut into cubes

1 avocado, peeled, stoned (pitted) and cubed

½ carrot, grated

1 nori seaweed sheet

2 tablespoons low-fat mayonnaise

1 tablespoon sriracha

2 tablespoons soy sauce (optional)

Black and toasted sesame seeds, to garnish

Notes If you don't like seafood sticks they can easily be replaced with tuna or smoked salmon. Store leftovers in a sealed container in the refrigerator for up to 3 days.

Prep time 5 minutes | **Cook time** 30 minutes
Calorie count 465 calories per portion

To cook the sushi rice, put the rice in a sieve and rinse with water until the water runs clear. Shake off the rice to remove any excess water, then put the rice into a saucepan and cover with cold water until it is about a centimetre higher than the rice in the pan.

Bring the water to the boil, then reduce the heat to low, cover with a lid and let it simmer for 15 minutes. Once cooked, remove from the heat and leave the rice in the pan with the lid on for a further 15 minutes.

Mix the rice vinegar together with the sweetener, then pour this over the rice (once it has stood for 15 minutes) and mix well.

In a separate bowl, crumble up the seafood sticks and mix with the cucumber, avocado and grated carrot.

Add the rice to a serving bowl, top with the seafood stick mixture, then rip the nori sheet into pieces and sprinkle over the top.

Mix the mayonnaise and sriracha together in a small bowl to make a sauce and drizzle this over the top of the rice salad. Add the soy sauce, if using, and sprinkle over some sesame seeds to garnish.

MAKE IT VEGGIE
Omit the seafood sticks and either replace them with tofu or add extra carrot, cucumber and avocado.

chicken and avocado pesto pasta

Pesto and avocado is a great flavour combination, which you can enjoy in this light, quick-to-prepare pasta. Perfect to prepare ahead for lunches, and even better for picnics. This is great just on its own, or with a side salad.

MAKES 4 PORTIONS

130g (4½oz) dried pasta of your choice

1 avocado, peeled, stoned (pitted) and chopped

2 cooked skinless and boneless chicken breasts, pulled apart with two forks

Sea salt and freshly ground black pepper

For the pesto

30g (1oz) basil leaves

½ tablespoon olive oil

2 tablespoons pine nuts

1 garlic clove

1 tablespoon grated Parmesan

Prep time 5 minutes | **Cook time** 10 minutes
Calorie count 398 calories per portion

Put all of the ingredients for the pesto into a food processor or blender along with a pinch of salt and pepper. Blitz until smooth, adding 1 teaspoon water at a time to make a smoother consistency. You shouldn't need any more than 3 teaspoons water, but add as required to get a pesto-like texture.

Cook the pasta in a saucepan of salted boiling water according to the packet instructions, then drain and run it under a cold tap to cool completely.

Mix the drained pasta with the avocado and chicken as well as the pesto in a mixing bowl and serve immediately. Alternatively, separate into portions and refrigerate for up to 5 days.

MAKE IT VEGGIE
Omit the chicken, or replace it with tofu or a meat-free alternative.

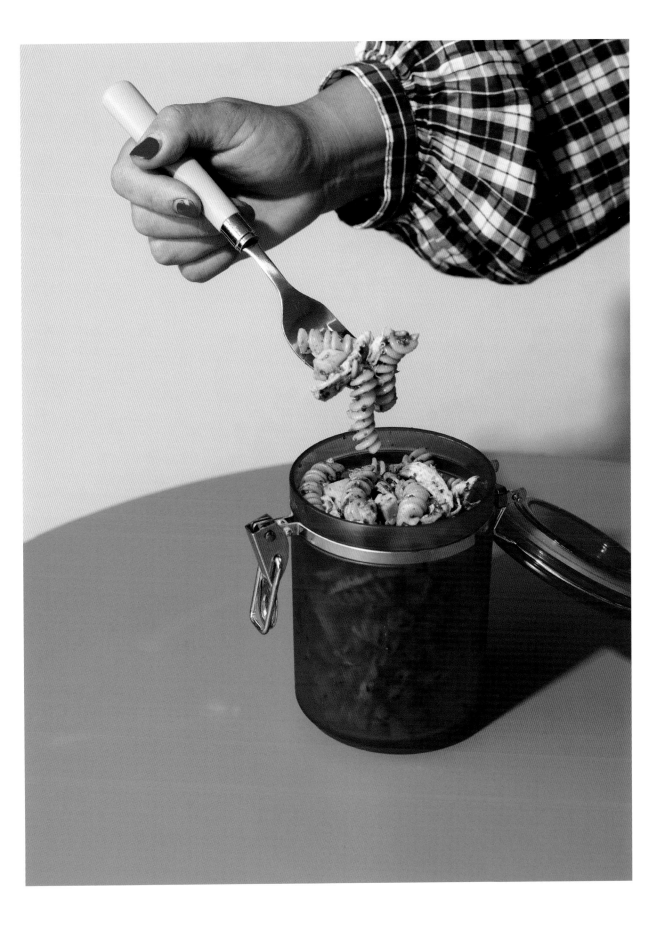

chicken and bacon ranch potato salad

This low-fat ranch dressing is amazing, and can be used for so many dishes as a dressing, or even just as a dip. This is another amazing lunchbox recipe and can be served immediately or separated out into lunchbox portions.

MAKES 5 PORTIONS

1kg (2lb 4oz) new potatoes, halved

2 skinless and boneless chicken breasts

5 bacon medallions, all fat removed

½ cucumber, cubed

½ head of iceberg lettuce, shredded

Low-calorie cooking spray

For the ranch dressing

1 tablespoon dried parsley

½ teaspoon garlic powder

½ teaspoon onion powder

1 tablespoon snipped chives

230g (8oz/generous 1 cup) fat-free Greek yoghurt

1 teaspoon Dijon mustard

1 teaspoon lemon juice

Sea salt and freshly ground black pepper

Prep time 10 minutes | **Cook time** 30 minutes
Calorie count 340 calories per portion

Preheat the oven to 200°C/180°C fan/400°F/Gas mark 6.

Put the new potatoes into a saucepan of boiling water and boil for 10 minutes until the potatoes are cooked through. Drain and set aside.

Put the chicken breasts and bacon into an ovenproof dish, spray with low-calorie cooking spray and bake for 25 minutes until the bacon is crispy and the chicken is cooked all the way through. Shred up the chicken breasts with two forks and cut the bacon into small strips.

For the dressing, mix all of the ingredients together in a bowl or jar until it forms a smooth sauce.

Put the drained potatoes, shredded chicken and bacon in a large bowl along with the cucumber and lettuce. Drizzle over the ranch dressing and mix everything together well. Serve immediately or portion up and store in the refrigerator.

Note Keep in a sealed container in the refrigerator for 5 days.

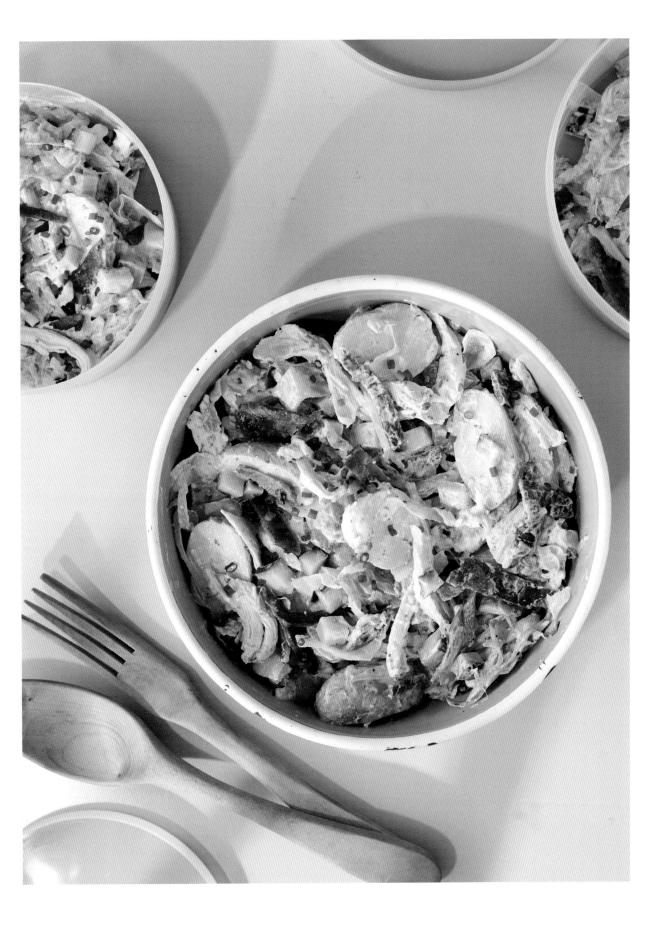

greek orzo

This recipe is perfect to prepare ahead of time to create a week's worth of 'take-to-work lunches'. You can literally throw this pasta salad together on a Sunday night to set yourself up for the rest of the working week. I love orzo, but this recipe would also work really well with any other pasta shape or even rice.

MAKES 5 PORTIONS

190g (6½oz) orzo
1 cucumber, cut into cubes
300g (10½oz) cherry
  tomatoes, sliced
1 red onion, finely diced
200g (7oz/2 cups) stoned
  (pitted) black olives,
  sliced
200g (7oz) feta cheese, cut
  into cubes

For the dressing

3 tablespoons balsamic
  vinegar
1 garlic clove, crushed
½ teaspoon dried oregano
¼ teaspoon Dijon mustard
¼ teaspoon sea salt
¼ teaspoon freshly ground
  black pepper
Juice of 1 lemon

Notes Keep in a
sealed container in
the refrigerator for up
to 5 days.

Prep time 10 minutes | **Cook time** 8 minutes
Calorie count 330 calories per portion

Bring a large saucepan of salted water to the boil, add the orzo and cook for 10 minutes, or until al dente.

Prepare the dressing by mixing all of the ingredients together in a bowl or jar.

Drain the cooked orzo and allow to cool, then transfer it to a mixing bowl. Add all the vegetables and the dressing and mix well to combine.

You can either serve straight away or separate into portions in sealable containers and refrigerate for up to 5 days.

MAKE IT VEGAN
This dish can be adapted to be vegan by swapping the feta cheese for a vegan alternative.

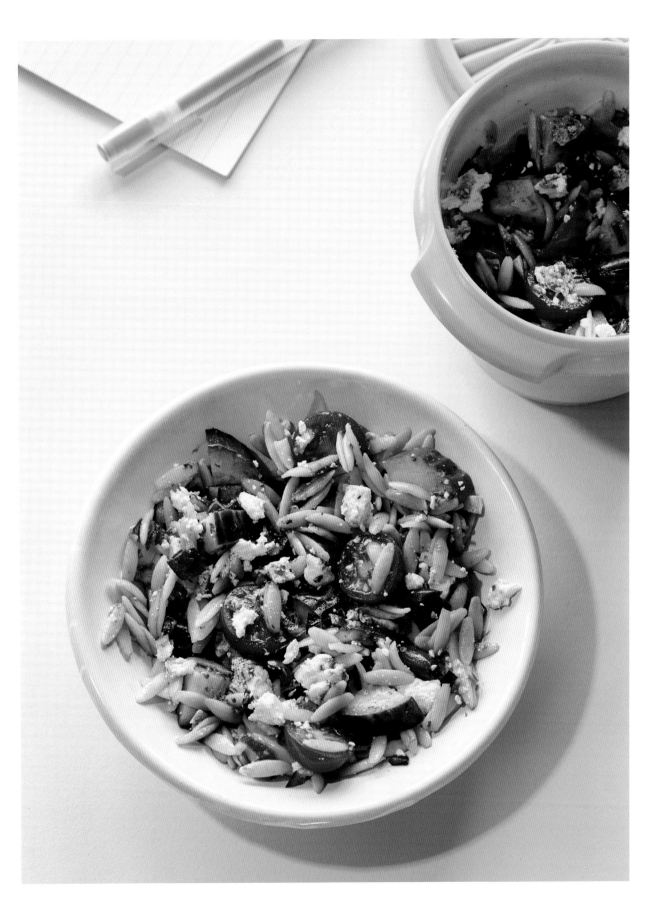

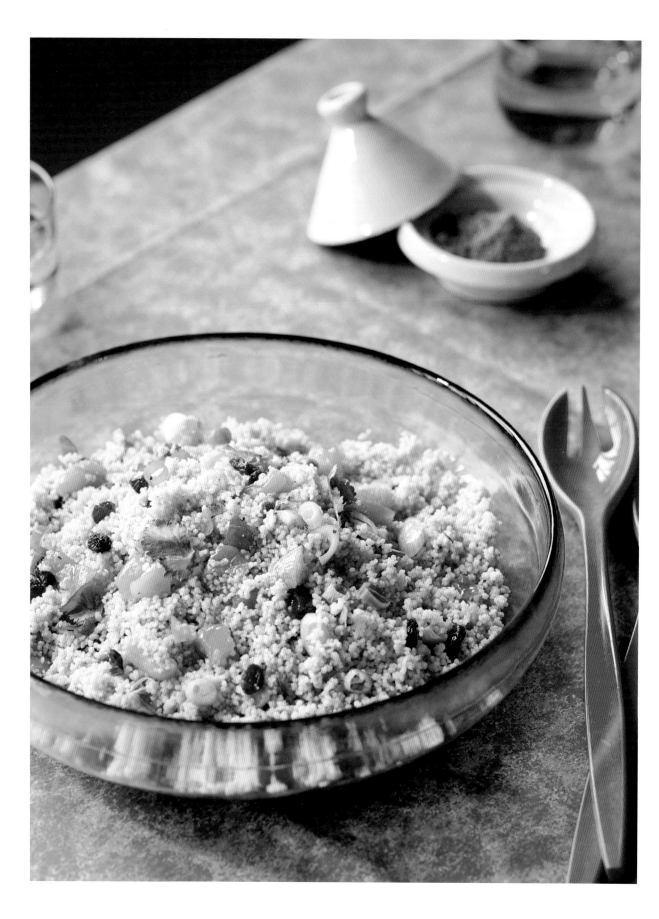

moroccan-style fruity couscous

I think couscous gets a bad reputation. It's so versatile that you can pretty much use it to go with anything. This is my favourite way to serve it, with a fruity, zesty and delicious flavour. This is a great stand-alone lunch and is also a perfect side dish for lamb.

MAKES 4 PORTIONS

150g (5oz) couscous
230ml (8fl oz/1 cup)
   vegetable stock, boiling
1 teaspoon ground cumin
½ teaspoon paprika
50g (1¾oz/⅓ cup) raisins
100g (3½oz/⅔ cup) dried
   apricots, chopped
1 spring onion (scallion),
   sliced
Small handful of coriander
   (cilantro) leaves
Juice from ½ lemon
Sea salt and freshly ground
   black pepper

Prep time 5 minutes | **Cook time** 10 minutes
Calorie count 230 calories per portion

Pour the couscous into a bowl and pour the hot stock over it. Leave for 10 minutes to allow the couscous to soak it all up.

Add the cumin and paprika and some salt and pepper to the couscous, then fluff it up with a fork.

Add the raisins, apricots, spring onion and coriander to the couscous, then squeeze over the lemon juice and mix well.

Note Can be eaten straight away or separated into portions in sealed containers and refrigerated for up to 5 days.

LEISURELY

LUNCHES

Quick and easy lunches are great, but sometimes you need a little more sustenance on days off. These flavour-packed lunches are the perfect partnership with my lazy weekend brunches. They're designed for cooking at home on a day off and can be shared with your partner or family. They require a bit of prepping and cooking, but I promise that they are totally worth the effort!

It's nice to have a bit of variety with lunch. These recipes are created to be enjoyed when you have the time and energy to get in the kitchen and create something delicious.

I have kept these recipes light, flavourful and easy to prepare, with plenty of vegetarian options. You could also save any leftovers to be enjoyed the next day or even to take them to work with you during the following week.

Food for me is a love language, and being able to make tasty treats for the people I love is something that I hold very dear. With these recipes, partnered up with the recipes in the rest of my book, you can treat the ones you love.

roasted mediterranean vegetable wraps with homemade hummus

This recipe can be prepared ahead by roasting the vegetables and making the hummus in advance, then just loading the filling onto a wrap when you're ready.

MAKES 4 WRAPS
(1 WRAP PER SERVING)

1 courgette (zucchini), cut in half lengthways, then sliced
1 red (bell) pepper, sliced
1 yellow (bell) pepper, sliced
1 green (bell) pepper, sliced
10 cherry tomatoes, halved
2 small red onions, finely diced
1 garlic clove, finely diced
½ teaspoon dried parsley
1 teaspoon dried basil
½ teaspoon sea salt
½ teaspoon dried oregano
Low-calorie cooking spray
4 tortilla wraps, to serve

For the hummus
1 x 240g (8½oz) tin of chickpeas, drained
Juice of 1 lemon
1 tablespoon olive oil
60ml (2fl oz) tahini
1 garlic clove
½ teaspoon paprika
½ teaspoon ground cumin
Sea salt

Prep time 10 minutes | **Cook time** 20 minutes
Calorie count 425 calories per portion

Preheat the oven to 220°C/210°C fan/425°F/Gas mark 7. Spray a large ovenproof dish or roasting tin with low-calorie cooking spray.

Put the courgette, peppers, cherry tomatoes, red onion and garlic into the ovenproof dish. Sprinkle with the parsley, basil, salt and oregano and then spray with some more low-calorie cooking spray. Give everything a good mix so that it is evenly coated in the seasonings.

Bake for 20 minutes, or until the veggies are cooked through.

To make the hummus, put all of the ingredients into a food processor or blender. Blitz until smooth, adding 1 tablespoon of water at a time to get a smooth consistency.

When ready to serve, load your tortilla wraps up with the roasted veggies and hummus.

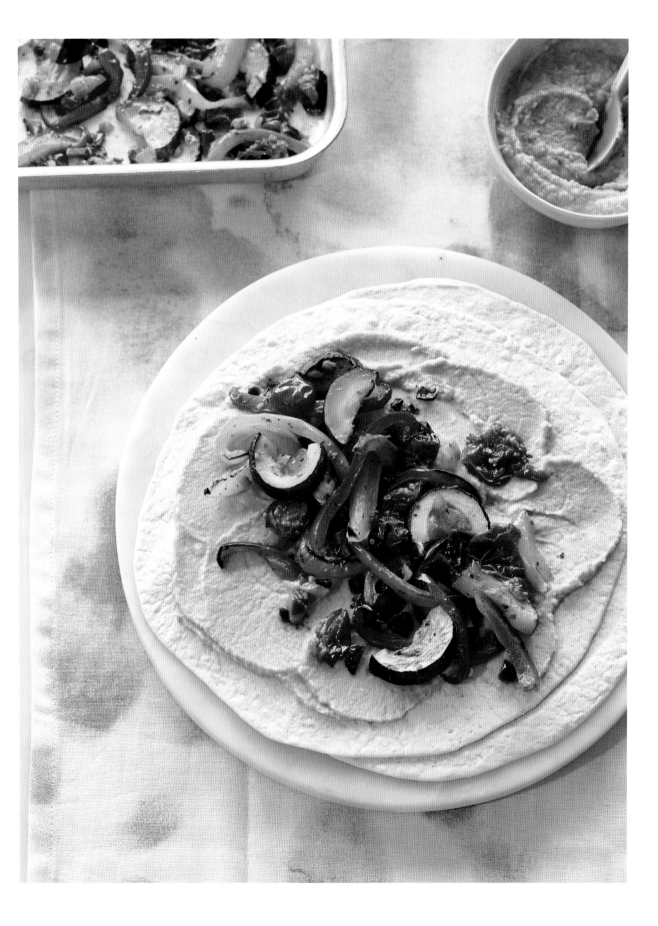

tomato bruschetta with balsamic glaze

When I was younger I used to go to the local village pub and order a tomato bruschetta, thinking I was being super fancy. I love these tomatoes on a slice of ciabatta bread. I used to buy balsamic glaze but you can recreate it yourself by literally reducing balsamic vinegar down in a saucepan; it's even better!

MAKES 2 PORTIONS

100ml (3⅓fl oz/⅓ cup) balsamic vinegar
10 cherry tomatoes, quartered
60g (2oz) reduced-fat mozzarella
2 garlic cloves, finely diced
Handful of basil leaves
1 ciabatta roll
Sea salt and freshly ground black pepper

Prep time 10 minutes | **Cook time** 30 minutes
Calorie count 300 calories per portion

Heat the balsamic vinegar in a saucepan over a medium heat. Bring to a gentle boil, then reduce the heat to low and let it simmer, stirring occasionally for about 20 minutes until it has reduced down to a sticky consistency.

In a mixing bowl, mix the tomatoes, mozzarella, garlic, basil and a pinch of salt and pepper.

Slice the ciabatta and place it under a hot grill (broiler) for a few minutes to warm.

Top each ciabatta slice with the tomato mixture. Put it back under the grill for a few minutes until the cheese has melted.

Drizzle with the balsamic glaze to serve.

grilled sweet potato pizza toasts

An amazing, lower carb pizza recipe! Sweet potato makes the perfect base, and you can load each pizza toast with as many toppings as you like, adjusting the calories as you go. I make this all the time when I need to get my pizza fix because it's so easy to do.

MAKES 2 PORTIONS

1 large sweet potato
2 tablespoons tomato purée (paste)
1 teaspoon dried basil
125g (4½oz) mozzarella, sliced or grated
Low-calorie cooking spray
Sea salt and freshly ground black pepper

Notes These pizza toasts are delicious both hot and cold! You can add vegetables or meat toppings, too, such as ham or pepperoni.

Prep time 5 minutes | **Cook time** 20 minutes
Calorie count 298 calories per portion

Preheat the grill (broiler) to 250°C/475°F.

Cut the sweet potato lengthways into 4 slices and spray each side with low-calorie cooking spray.

Spray some aluminium foil on a baking tray (sheet) with low-calorie cooking spray and lay out the sweet potato slices.

Grill for 10 minutes, then flip them over and grill the other side for 7 minutes. Remove the baking tray from the grill to add the toppings.

Spread the tomato purée over each potato slice, then sprinkle with the dried basil and a pinch of salt and pepper. Top with the mozzarella.

Grill for a further 5 minutes, or until the cheese is bubbling.

MAKE IT VEGAN
Replace the mozzarella with a vegan cheese alternative.

summer rolls and peanut sauce

Summer rolls were always my 'go to' order when eating out in my local Vietnamese restaurant until I figured out how easy they are to make yourself at home. You can pick up the rice paper sheets from any Asian food shop and most big supermarkets.

MAKES 4 SUMMER ROLLS

100g (3½oz) vermicelli rice noodles

1 teaspoon sesame oil

3 iceberg lettuce leaves, sliced into thin strips

3 cabbage leaves, sliced into thin strips

1 large carrot, grated

1 cucumber, sliced into thin strips

A few coriander (cilantro) leaves

A few mint leaves

6 round rice paper wrappers

Sea salt and freshly ground black pepper

For the peanut sauce

2 tablespoons smooth peanut butter

2 tablespoons rice vinegar

2 tablespoons reduced-sodium soy sauce

2 tablespoons honey

1 tablespoon sesame oil

1 garlic clove, crushed

Prep time 10 minutes | **Cook time** 10 minutes
Calorie count 180 calories per summer roll

Boil the noodles according to the packet instructions, then drain and rinse under cold water. Add the sesame oil and some salt and pepper, stir and set aside.

Put the lettuce, cabbage, carrot and cucumber in a bowl and sprinkle over the coriander and mint.

Fill a large bowl with tepid water and dip one of the rice paper wrappers in. Wait until it is softened, but not completely floppy – this should be about 30 seconds.

Lay the soaked wrapper on a chopping board and layer up the middle of the sheet with some noodles, vegetables and herbs. Fold the lower edge of the rice paper up over the filling. Fold over the short sides, then roll it up so that the filling is enclosed. Repeat with the remaining wrappers and filling.

Mix all of the ingredients for the peanut sauce together in a bowl or jar and whisk to mix. Add water to get the desired consistency.

Serve the summer rolls with the peanut sauce on the side, for dipping or drizzling.

Notes These are veggie but would also be great with some shredded chicken or prawns.

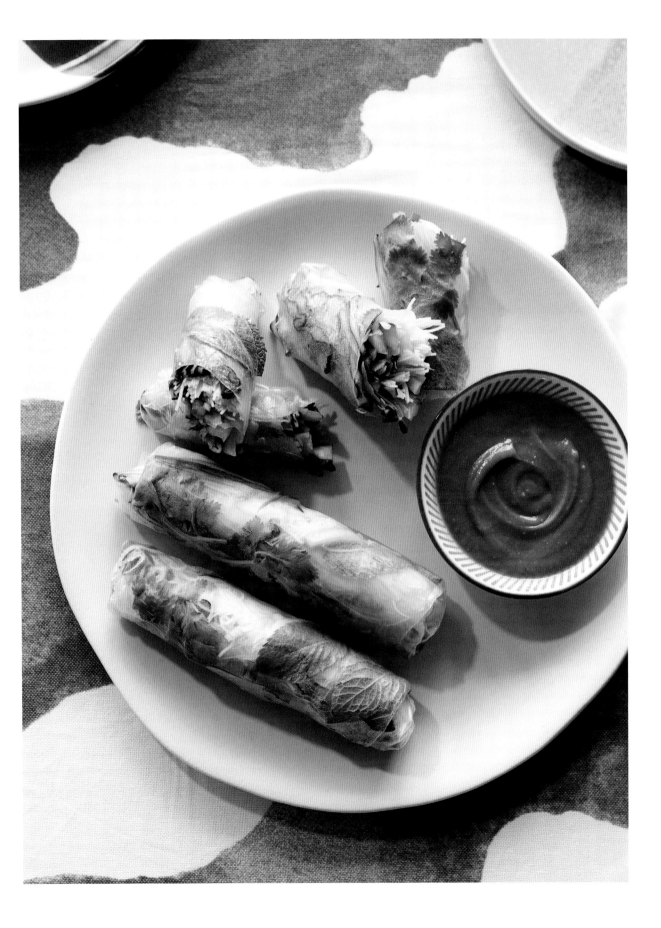

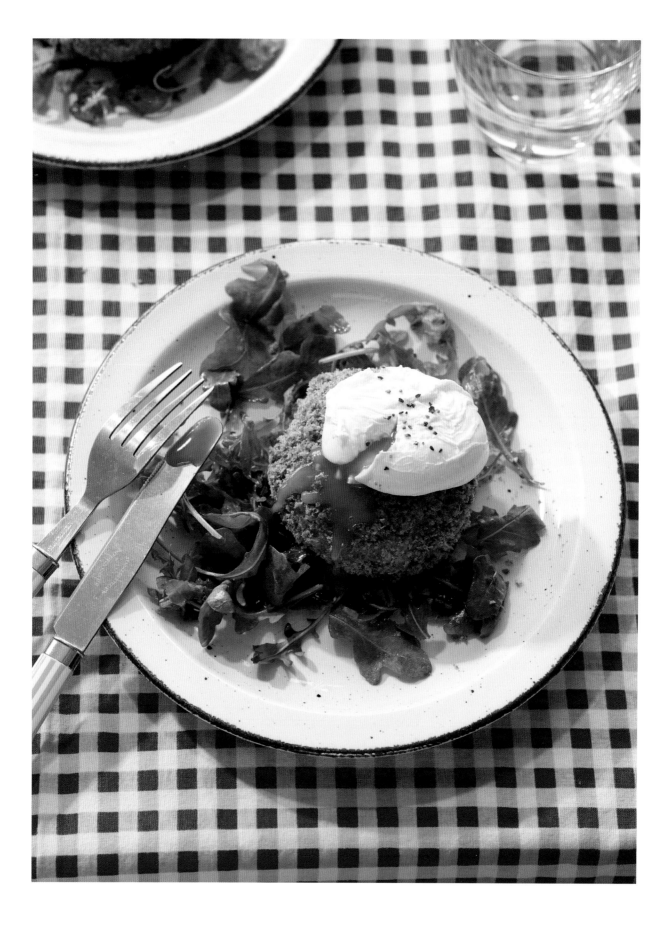

tuna fishcakes

These fishcakes are easy to prepare and are perfect for people who aren't keen on strong fish flavours. They can be put together with ingredients that you most likely already have in the house too. I love to eat them on their own, or with a runny poached egg on top – just remember to adjust the calories.

**MAKES 4 LARGE FISHCAKES
(OR 6 SMALLER FISHCAKES)**

2 medium potatoes, peeled
    and roughly chopped into
    chunks
2 slices of wholemeal bread
1½ tablespoons low-fat
    mayonnaise
Juice of ½ lemon
2 spring onions (scallions),
    finely chopped
1 x 150g (5oz) tin of tuna,
    drained
1 egg, lightly beaten
3 tablespoons plain (all-
    purpose) flour
Low-calorie cooking spray
Sea salt and freshly ground
    black pepper
Poached eggs and salad
    leaves, to serve
    (optional)

Prep time 10 minutes | **Cook time** 10 minutes
Calorie count 180 calories per large fishcake

Preheat the oven to 200°C/180°C fan/400°F/Gas mark 6. Line a baking tray (sheet) with baking paper or aluminium foil and spray with low-calorie cooking spray.

Put the potatoes into a saucepan of boiling water and simmer for 20 minutes until the potatoes are cooked through.

Put the slices of bread in a food processor and blitz until you have breadcrumbs.

Once the potatoes have cooked, drain and add the mayonnaise, lemon juice, spring onions and some salt and pepper and mash until smooth. Add the drained tuna to the mashed potato and mix it all together.

Shape the mixture into 4 large fishcakes, or 6 smaller fishcakes.

Put the egg in a small shallow dish and pour the breadcrumbs into another dish.

Dip the fishcakes in the egg first and then into the breadcrumbs. Repeat this process twice.

Place the fishcakes on the prepared baking tray and bake for 20 minutes until the fishcakes are crisp and golden.

Serve with poached eggs and salad leaves, if you like.

~~~~~~

Notes When breadcrumbing anything, use one hand for the wet bowl and the other hand for the dry breadcrumbs – that way you won't get the breadcrumbs stuck to your fingers.

refried bean and feta tostadas with coriander slaw

I like to think of tostadas as being kind of like a 'Mexican Pizza'. Your choice of toppings are loaded onto a baked tortilla wrap, and you can load as much or as little on as you like. This recipe is vegetarian, but you can easily adjust it to include cooked shredded chicken or minced beef.

MAKES 2 PORTIONS

2 large tortilla wraps
½ x 435g (15½oz) tin of refried beans
1 large ripe avocado, peeled and stoned (pitted)
Juice of 1 lime
100g (3½oz) cherry tomatoes, halved
100g (3½oz) feta cheese, crumbled
Low-calorie cooking spray

For the slaw

80g (3oz) white cabbage, shredded
90g (3¼oz) coriander (cilantro) leaves, chopped
Juice of 1 lime
½ teaspoon ground cumin
½ teaspoon chilli powder
Sea salt and freshly ground black pepper

Prep time 10 minutes | **Cook time** 8 minutes
Calorie count 450 calories per portion

Preheat the oven to 200°C/180°C fan/400°F/Gas mark 6. Line a baking tray (sheet) with baking paper.

First make the slaw. Combine the cabbage, coriander, lime juice, cumin and chilli powder in a bowl. Season with salt and pepper to taste, mix well and set aside.

Spray both sides of each tortilla with low-calorie cooking spray. Season with salt and place the wraps on the baking tray. Bake for 4 minutes, then flip and bake for a further 4 minutes, or until the tortillas are crisp and hold their shape.

Heat the refried beans in a saucepan over a medium heat until warmed through.

Mash the avocado in a small bowl with a fork until smooth and then stir in the lime juice.

Add a layer of refried beans to the baked tortillas, then spread some of the avocado over the top and finally layer with the slaw, cherry tomatoes and feta cheese.

MAKE IT VEGAN
Remove the feta or swap it for a vegan alternative.

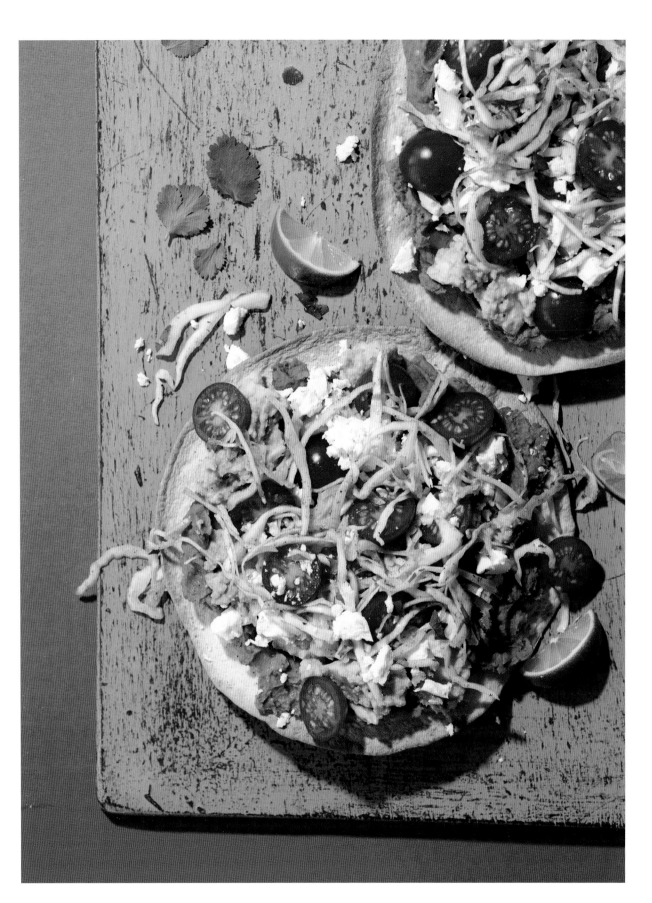

pulled beef bagels

I absolutely love salt beef, but to make the real thing you need to leave it for 7 days in a salt solution to brine, and I just don't have the time, patience or energy! So this is a salt beef-inspired dish, which you can prepare ahead at the weekend and serve on bagels or in a salad throughout the week.

MAKES 4 PORTIONS
1kg (2lb 4oz) beef topside
100ml (3½fl oz/⅓ cup) beef
   stock
2 tablespoons Worcestershire
   sauce
1 tablespoon balsamic
   vinegar
1 teaspoon English mustard
Sea salt and freshly ground
   black pepper

To serve
4 bagels
English mustard
Pickled gherkins

Prep time 5 minutes | **Cook time** 6 hours
Calorie count 550 calories per portion (including bagel)

Put the beef joint into the bowl of a slow cooker along with the stock, Worcestershire sauce, balsamic vinegar and some salt and pepper. Spread the mustard over the joint.

Cook on low for 6 hours. Once cooked, remove the beef joint and shred the meat with 2 forks.

Serve in a toasted bagel with mustard and pickled gherkins.

Note The beef can be kept in a sealable container for up to 5 days in the refrigerator.

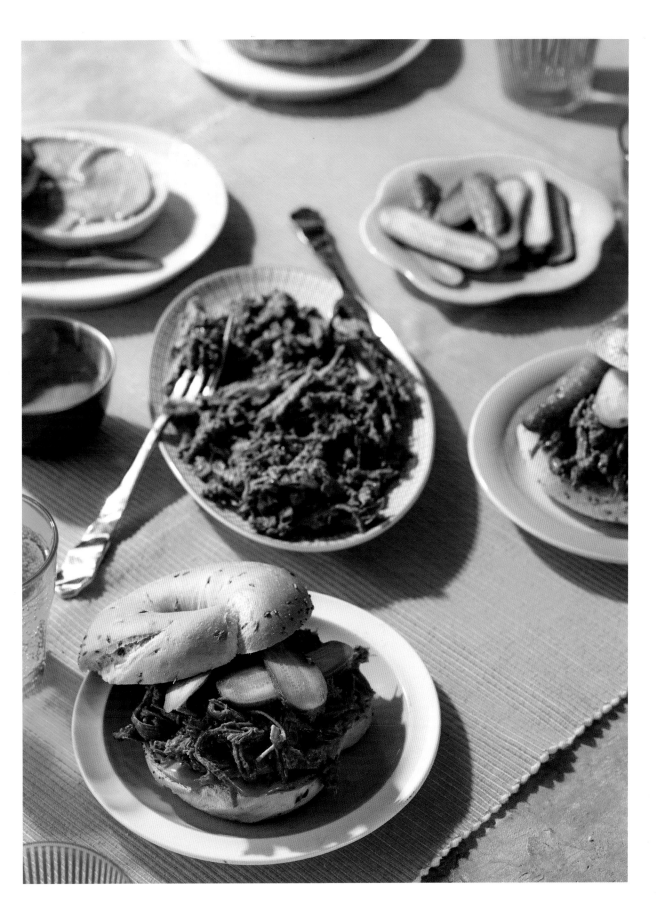

balsamic pork bowl

Sticky sweet balsamic pork with pickled cucumber, crispy sweet potato cubes and salad. Such a simple concept, but so incredibly tasty. Great to prep ahead and portion up for meal prepping or take-to-work lunches.

Prep time 10 minutes | **Cook time** 55 minutes
Calorie count 530 calories per portion

MAKES 2 PORTIONS

½ cucumber, sliced

2 tablespoons white wine vinegar

1 small sweet potato, peeled and finely cubed

Smoked paprika, to taste

1 x 400g (14oz) tin of black beans, drained

½ x 198g (7oz) tin of sweetcorn, drained

Handful of green beans

175g (6oz) cooked brown rice

1 tomato, chopped

½ avocado (optional)

Dried chilli flakes, to taste (optional)

Low-calorie cooking spray

Sea salt and freshly ground black pepper

Sesame seeds, to garnish

For the pork

1 red chilli, deseeded and finely chopped

2 garlic cloves, finely chopped

50ml (1¾fl oz/scant ¼ cup) balsamic vinegar

1 teaspoon sweetener

500g (1lb 2oz) extra lean minced (ground) pork

Preheat the oven to 200°C/180°C fan/400°F/Gas mark 6.

First, get the cucumber pickling. Put the cucumber slices into a small bowl with the white wine vinegar.

Put the sweet potato in an ovenproof dish. Spray with low-calorie cooking spray and sprinkle with a generous amount of salt, pepper and smoked paprika.

Bake for 25 minutes, or until they start to look crispy. They will crisp up a little more once you remove them from the oven.

Next, make the pork. Mix together the chilli, garlic, balsamic vinegar and sweetener in a small bowl.

Spray a frying pan (skillet) with low-calorie cooking spray and fry the pork mince over a medium heat until browned. Once browned, add the balsamic sauce and cook to reduce slightly over a low heat. Leave to simmer for 10 minutes.

Heat the black beans and sweetcorn according to the tins instructions, and boil the green beans in some boiling water for 10 minutes.

Drain the cucumber, then layer up the bowl with the pork, rice and all of your veggies to serve.

〰〰

Notes Add as many different vegetables as you like. Can be prepped ahead and eaten cold.

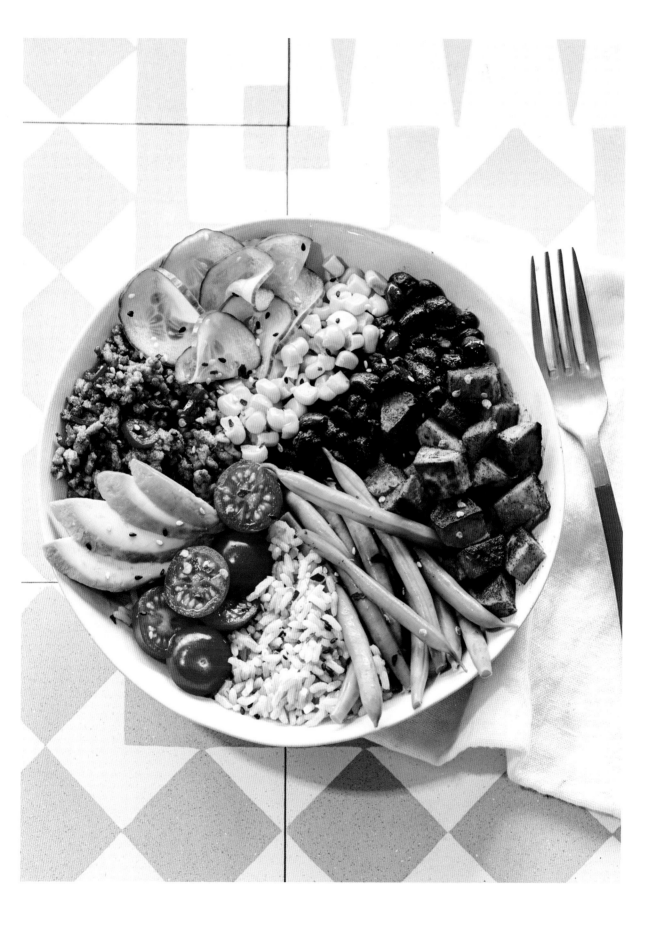

pulled paprika chicken jacket potato

This pulled paprika chicken is so versatile: you can serve it in a sandwich, a wrap, on a jacket potato, or even just with a salad. You can literally throw all of the ingredients into your slow cooker at the weekend so that you have a big batch ready for the week.

MAKES 4 PORTIONS

4 large skinless and
  boneless chicken breasts
1 red onion, finely sliced
1 garlic clove, diced
500g (1lb 2oz) carton of
  passata (sieved tomatoes)
2 tablespoons smoked paprika
1 tablespoon Worcestershire
  sauce
Sea salt and freshly ground
  black pepper

To serve

4 baked potatoes
Fat-free yoghurt
Chopped chives

Prep time 5 minutes | **Cook time** 4 or 6 hours – depending on what temp you use | **Calorie count** 300 calories per portion

Add all of the ingredients to a slow cooker and stir so that the chicken is covered in the sauce.

Heat on low for 6 hours or high for 4 hours. If you don't have a slow cooker, cook in a cast-iron casserole dish in an oven preheated to 140°C/120°C fan/275°F/Gas mark 1 for 2 hours.

Once cooked, remove the chicken and use 2 forks to pull it apart and shred it. Return the shredded chicken to the sauce and stir.

Leave to cool fully before serving with the baked potatoes, or separating into portions and storing in the refrigerator.

To serve, top with a dollop of yoghurt and a sprinkling of chives.

Note Keeps for up to 5 days in a sealable container.

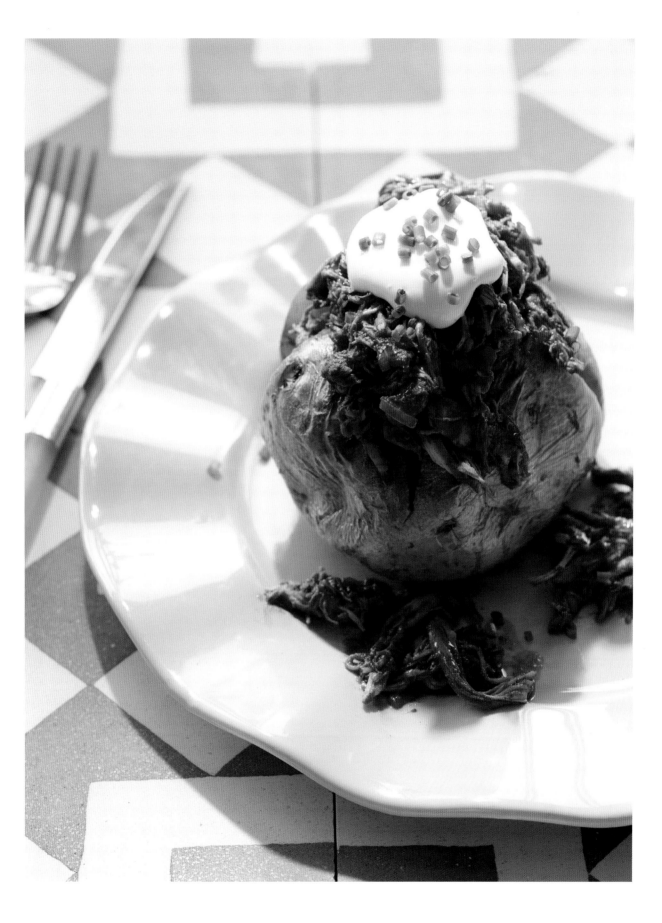

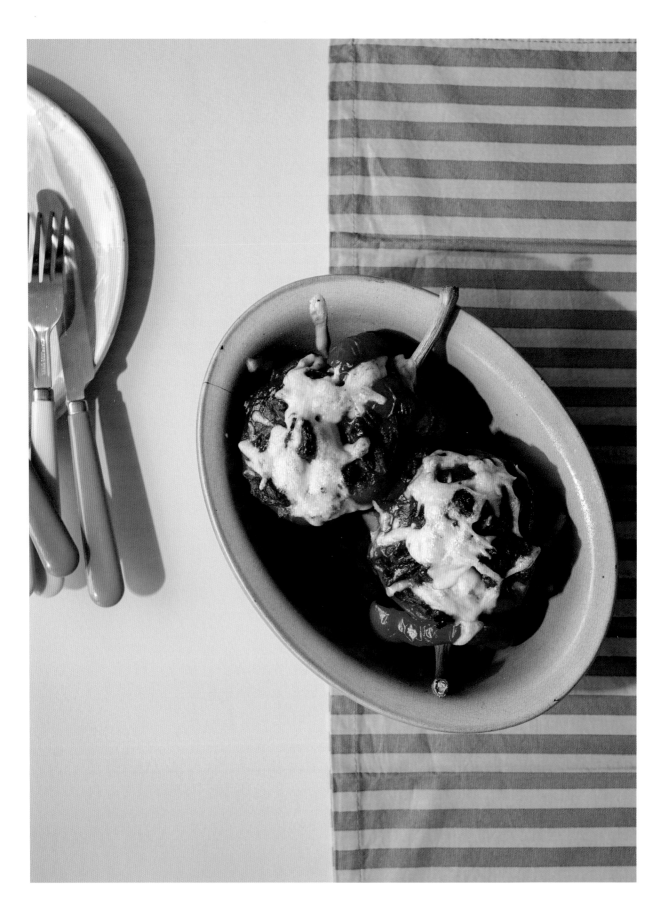

cheesy bolognese stuffed peppers

These cheesy stuffed peppers are a delight. They taste best when served hot, but are also great cold. You can prep these ahead of time and cook, grill or bake them in the oven when ready to eat. The cheese and speedy bolognese combination is one of my favourites!

**MAKES 2 PORTIONS
(2 STUFFED PEPPER HALVES
PER PORTION)**

1 onion, finely diced

2 garlic cloves, finely
   diced

250g (9oz) extra lean minced
   (ground) beef

1 beef stock cube

1 tablespoon tomato purée
   (paste)

500g (1lb 2oz) tomato
   passata (sieved tomatoes)

1 teaspoon dried basil

1 teaspoon smoked paprika

1 tablespoon balsamic
   vinegar

3 teaspoons Worcestershire
   sauce

2 red (bell) peppers

120g (4¼oz) reduced-fat
   Cheddar cheese

Low-calorie cooking spray

Sea salt and freshly ground
   black pepper

Note You can store the
mince and the pepper slices
separately if prepping
ahead.

Prep time 5 minutes | **Cook time** 30 minutes
Calorie count 365 calories per portion

Preheat the oven to 180°C/160°C fan/350°F/Gas mark 4.

Spray a large frying pan (skillet) with low-calorie cooking spray and set over a medium heat. Add the onion and garlic and fry for 5 minutes until the onions have softened.

Add the beef mince and beef stock cube and fry for 10 minutes until the meat has browned.

Add the remaining ingredients, except the peppers and cheese, and then leave to simmer over a low heat for 20 minutes, stirring regularly. Once the bolognese has reduced, season to taste and set it aside.

Slice the peppers in half from top to bottom. Alternatively, you can leave them whole, slice the tops off and fill them that way.

Stuff each halved pepper with bolognese, then add some cheese on top.

Bake for 7 minutes, or until the cheese has melted.

MAKE IT VEGGIE
Swap the beef mince for a meat-free alternative, or replace it with vegetables.

HEARTY

DINNERS

This chapter serves exactly what it says in the title: hearty dinners that are delicious, healthy and easy to prepare, and that the whole family will love.

Dinner recipes are where it all started for me on my blog. I remember posting my very first recipe - of course I had no followers then other than friends and family, but I was excited to be able to save a recipe I had created for another day.

It was these kinds of recipes that I first started creating and sharing, and they are what I am most passionate about recipe developing today. I will never forget the first time someone tagged me in a post saying that they had cooked something that I had created.

There is so much variety and so many flavour combinations that you can create when making an evening meal, and sitting around the table with your household to share food is very special.

This chapter contains a few of my most popular dinner recipes from my website, which have been updated for this book, and lots of fabulous brand-new recipes.

The dinners are either two or four portions, but if you're not feeding a whole family, leftovers can be kept for lunch the next day or frozen for another date. Lots of these recipes can be adapted to be gluten-free, veggie or vegan, just check the notes on each specific recipe.

peri-peri sweet potato gnocchi

I think the combination of spices and sweet potato is amazing, which is why I created this recipe. The light and fluffy gnocchi and creamy spicy sauce are perfect partners. Of course, if you're not a fan of spice you can adjust this to suit your taste.

MAKES 4 PORTIONS

2 large sweet potatoes
180g (6¼oz/1⅓ cups) plain (all-purpose) flour, plus extra for dusting
Sea salt and freshly ground black pepper

For the peri-peri sauce

2 red chillies (adjust according to how much you like spice!)
1 red (bell) pepper, roughly chopped
1 red onion, roughly chopped
1 tablespoon smoked paprika
2 teaspoons sea salt
1 teaspoon freshly ground black pepper
1 tablespoon dried oregano
½ teaspoon red chilli powder
4 garlic cloves
4 tablespoons malt vinegar
8 cherry tomatoes
Juice of 1 lemon
Juice of ½ lime

Note The gnocchi can be frozen after boiling. Leave to dry and cool completely before transferring to a sealable container and refrigerating.

Prep time 15 minutes | **Cook time** 1¼ hours
Calorie count 360 calories per portion

Preheat the oven to 180°C/160°C fan/350°F/Gas mark 4.

Use a fork to prick the sweet potatoes all over. Place them on a baking tray (sheet) and bake for 30 minutes. Remove from the oven, turn the potatoes over and bake for another 30 minutes.

Meanwhile, add all of the ingredients for the sauce to a food processor or blender and add 50ml (1¾fl oz/scant ¼ cup) water. Blitz to a smooth paste. You may need to add a little more water if it starts to look too thick.

Remove the sweet potatoes from the oven and leave to cool for 10 minutes, then peel off the skin, place the sweet potato flesh in a bowl and mash with a fork. Season with some salt and pepper.

Add the flour to the mashed potato and stir. It should start to come together and form a dough-like consistency.

Sprinkle some flour on the worktop and turn out the sweet potato dough. Gently knead the dough with your hands. If it starts to get too sticky, add a little more flour.

Roll the dough into a ball, then cut it into 4 smaller balls. Roll each ball into a long thin sausage, then slice it into small chunks. Using your hands, form each chunk into a gnocchi-shaped ball.

Bring a large saucepan of water to the boil and add the gnocchi. Once they start to float up from the bottom of the pan, they are ready. Drain on paper towels to remove any excess moisture.

Spoon the peri-peri sauce into a saucepan set over a medium heat and bring to the boil. Once boiling, reduce the heat and simmer for 5 minutes over a low heat. Add the gnocchi to the sauce, give it a stir to coat, then serve.

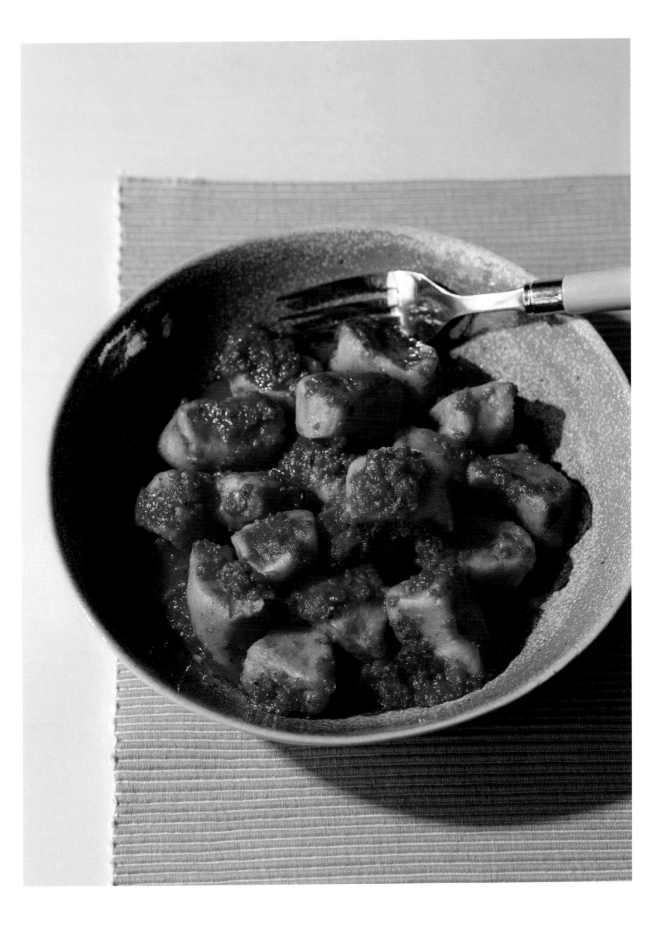

veggie chilli with coconut rice

Chilli is such a classic comfort food and this vegan version is just as delicious. It's also super versatile and can be served with rice, on a jacket potato or even on some nachos with cheese. Sweet potato is the base of this dish, which is beautiful once roasted in spices.

MAKES 4 PORTIONS

2 large sweet potatoes, peeled and cut into small chunks
1 teaspoon cayenne pepper, plus a pinch for the chilli
2 teaspoons smoked paprika
1 large red onion, finely diced
2 garlic cloves, crushed and chopped
2 red (bell) peppers, sliced
2 fresh chillies, deseeded and chopped
2 teaspoons ground cumin
1 teaspoon ground coriander
1 x 400g (14oz) tin of red kidney beans (no need to drain)
2 x 400g (14oz) tins of chopped tomatoes
Squeeze of lime juice
Low-calorie cooking spray
Sea salt and freshly ground black pepper
Chopped coriander (cilantro) leaves, to serve

For the rice

150g (5oz) jasmine rice
1 tablespoon desiccated coconut
Juice of 1 lime
Small handful of fresh coriander (cilantro), roughly chopped

Prep time 10 minutes | **Cook time** 1 hour
Calorie count 300 calories per portion

Preheat the oven to 200°C/180°C fan/400°F/Gas mark 6.

Lay the sweet potatoes out on a roasting dish and season with salt, pepper, the cayenne pepper and 1 teaspoon of the smoked paprika.

Spray with low-calorie cooking spray and bake for 45–60 minutes until golden and soft all the way through.

Meanwhile, prepare the chilli by spraying a large saucepan or cast-iron dish with low-calorie cooking spray and add the onion, garlic and peppers. Fry over a medium heat for 3 minutes until softened.

Add the chillies, cumin, ground coriander, the other teaspoon of smoked paprika and a pinch of cayenne pepper and cook for 5 minutes, stirring regularly.

Add the kidney beans with their liquid, and the tins of tomatoes. Bring to the boil, then reduce the heat to medium-low and leave to simmer while the sweet potatoes are roasting.

Bring a large saucepan of water to the boil and cook the rice according to the packet instructions. Add the coconut about 5 minutes before the end of the cooking time. Drain the rice, then stir in the lime juice and fresh coriander.

Once the sweet potato is ready, add it to the chilli with a squeeze of lime juice and some fresh coriander.

Notes Leftovers can be stored in the refrigerator for up to 5 days in a sealable cover. Can also be frozen for up to 6 months; defrost and reheat thoroughly to serve.

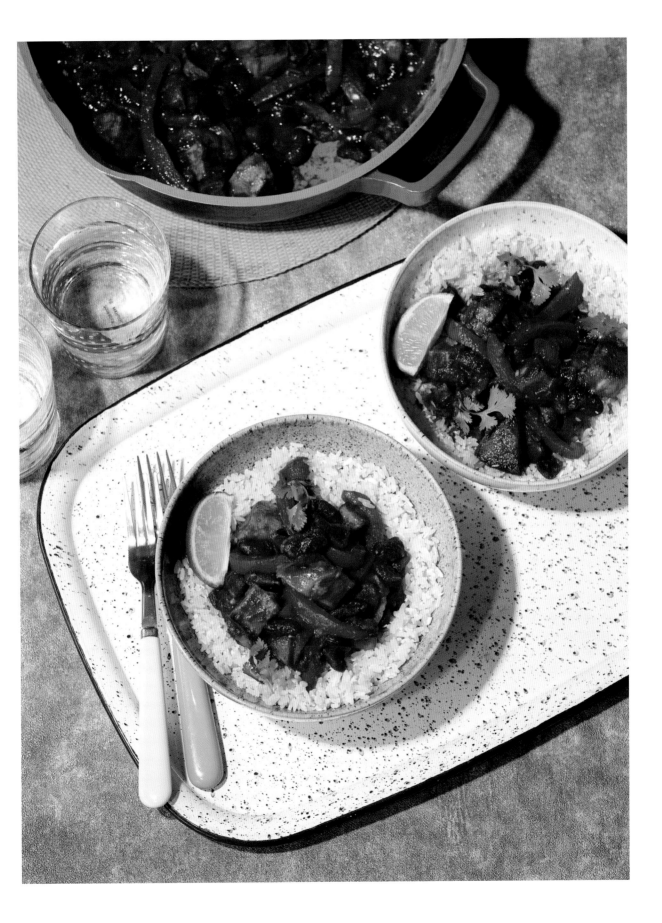

spinach, chickpea and halloumi curry

I have recently become a big fan of vegetarian curries. They're cheaper to make and can be whipped up in no time at all. The key to all good curries is to make an amazing curry paste to start with.

MAKES 2 PORTIONS

225g (8oz) halloumi cheese, cut into chunks
1 x 400g (14oz) tin of chickpeas, drained
1 x 400g (14oz) tin of chopped tomatoes
120g (4¼oz/⅔ cup) basmati rice
250g (9oz) spinach
1 tablespoon fat-free Greek yoghurt

For the curry paste

½ onion, diced
½ red (bell) pepper, diced
½ teaspoon fresh or dried chilli, to taste
½ tablespoon ground coriander
1 tablespoon ground cumin
½ tablespoon garam masala
Low-calorie cooking spray

Note This makes 2 large portions, but it could also be made into 4 smaller portions for half the calories.

Prep time 10 minutes | **Cook time** 30 minutes
Calorie count 489 calories per portion

Make the curry paste by blitzing the onion, pepper, chilli and ground spices in a food processor or by using a pestle and mortar.

Put a tablespoon of the paste in a bowl and set the rest aside. Add the halloumi and mix well.

Spray a frying pan (skillet) with low-calorie cooking spray and set over a medium heat. Add the halloumi and cook on each side for 3 minutes until browned. Remove and set aside.

Add the remaining curry paste to the pan and stir. Add the chickpeas and chopped tomatoes and mix it all together. Cover and simmer for 20 minutes. This helps the flavours develop.

Meanwhile, bring a large saucepan of water to the boil and cook the rice according to the packet instructions.

Add the spinach and halloumi to the curry and stir until the spinach has wilted into the curry.

Just before serving, stir through the yoghurt for a creamy curry. Serve with the basmati rice.

MAKE IT VEGAN
Omit the halloumi, or use a vegan alternative.

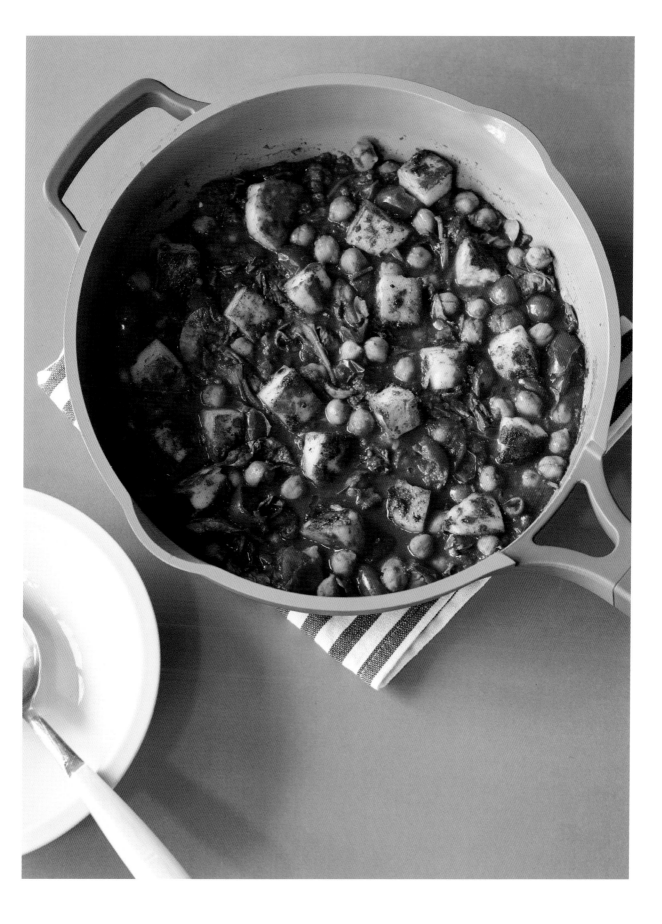

coconut prawns

This is a super speedy weeknight recipe. It just uses one pan and is as simple as throwing some bits together, but is really flavourful. I really enjoy the mild curry flavour with the creaminess of the coconut combined.

MAKES 4 PORTIONS

1 red onion, diced
1 garlic clove, diced
1 courgette (zucchini), chopped
3 tablespoons tikka curry paste
½ teaspoon lazy ginger (or 1 teaspoon grated ginger)
200g (7oz) mangetout
200ml (7oz/generous ¾ cup) light coconut milk
180g (6½oz) peeled raw king prawns
Low-calorie cooking spray
Sea salt and freshly ground black pepper

Prep time 5 minutes | **Cook time** 15 minutes
Calorie count 385 calories per portion

Spray a frying pan (skillet) with low-calorie cooking spray and set over a medium heat. Add the onion and fry for 2–3 minutes until it has softened.

Add the garlic, courgette, curry paste and ginger and cook for a further 3 minutes. Add the mangetout and coconut milk and cook for 3 minutes.

Season with salt and pepper, then add the prawns and cook for 4 minutes until the prawns are pink and cooked all the way through.

Note This is delicious served with rice, just adjust the calorie count accordingly.

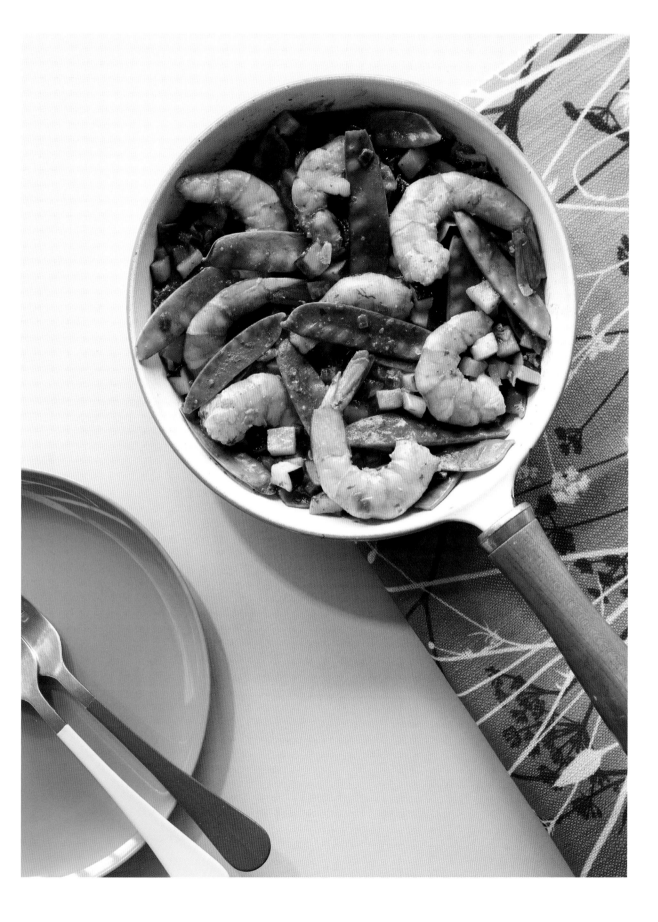

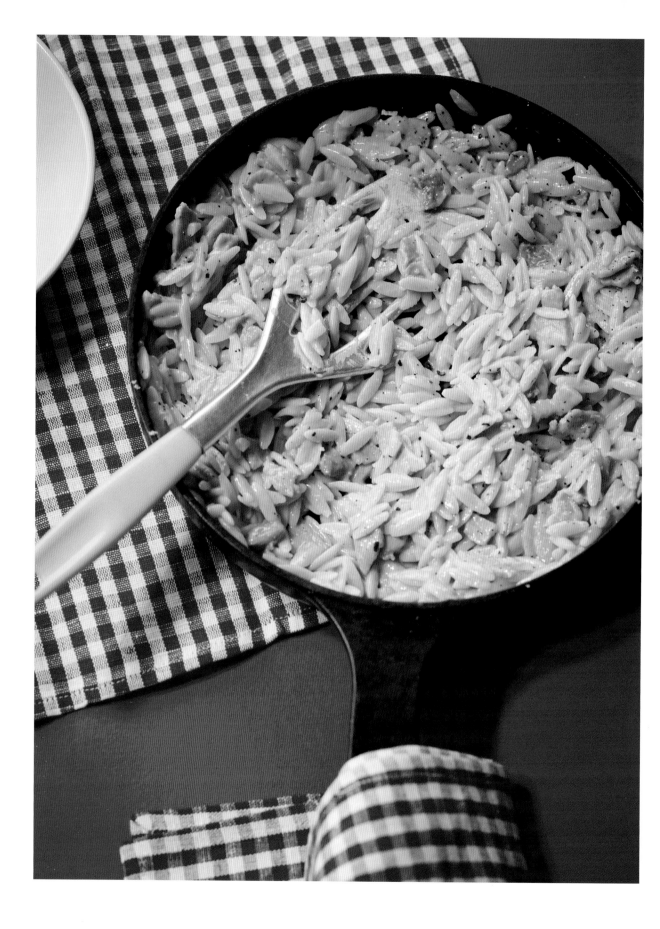

orzo carbonara

Orzo is something that I have only discovered recently. If you haven't tried it before, the best way I can describe it is 'pasta rice'. It is pasta that looks like rice, but I find it easier to cook and lighter to eat. If you're using cream in your carbonara, you're doing it wrong! A proper carbonara sauce simply requires eggs, Parmesan and pasta water, and absolutely no cream!

MAKES 4 PORTIONS

3 large egg yolks

40g (1½oz) grated Parmesan

1 teaspoon extra virgin olive oil (can be substituted for low-calorie cooking spray, but a little bit of oil works best)

1 garlic clove, lightly crushed but still whole

6 bacon medallions, all fat removed and cut into small cubes

200g (7oz) orzo

Sea salt and freshly ground black pepper

Prep time 10 minutes | **Cook time** 15 minutes
Calorie count 430 calories per portion

Place the egg yolks in a mixing bowl and add the Parmesan with a pinch of salt and pepper. Whisk together until it forms a smooth paste.

Heat the olive oil in a saucepan over a medium heat and add the garlic clove. Cook for 2 minutes, then remove the garlic.

Add the bacon to the pan and cook for 3 minutes until slightly crispy.

Cook the orzo according to the packet instructions, reserving some of the cooking water as you drain the cooked orzo.

Add the drained orzo to the bacon and mix well, then remove the pan from the heat.

Add a tablespoon of the pasta water to the orzo and bacon and give it a stir, then pour over the egg yolk and Parmesan paste. Give it a stir, then add another 1–2 tablespoons of the pasta water to help the sauce become smooth and glossy. The sauce shouldn't be lumpy as long as you keep the pan off the heat. Enjoy straight away.

MAKE IT VEGGIE
Omit the bacon completely, or use a meat-free alternative.

sticky BBQ dirty rice

Don't be put off by the name 'dirty rice'. It gets its name because the rice changes colour with all the flavours of this dish, meaning extra flavour! I first created a dirty rice recipe on my website about four years ago, and people went crazy for it. This is a slightly different flavour, as it is actually meat-free, but it would also work really well with bacon or chicken.

MAKES 4 PORTIONS

100g (3½oz/½ cup) rice of
  your choice
1 red onion, finely diced
1 red (bell) pepper, finely
  diced
1 yellow (bell) pepper,
  finely diced
2 tablespoons Worcestershire
  sauce
2 teaspoons balsamic vinegar
2 garlic cloves, finely
  diced
1 teaspoon mustard powder
2 teaspoons smoked paprika
Handful of frozen peas
½ x 198g tin of sweetcorn,
  drained
1 celery stick, sliced
1 vegetable stock cube,
  dissolved in 125ml (4½fl
  oz/½ cup) boiling water
¼ teaspoon chilli powder
Low-calorie cooking spray

Prep time 10 minutes | **Cook time** 20 minutes
Calorie count 250 calories per portion

Bring a large saucepan of water to the boil and cook the rice according to the packet instructions.

Spray a large frying pan (skillet) with low-calorie cooking spray and set over a medium heat. Fry the onion and peppers for 5–10 minutes. Add the Worcestershire sauce and balsamic vinegar, stir and cook for another minute.

Add the garlic, mustard powder, smoked paprika, peas, sweetcorn and celery and fry for a few minutes. Add the stock and chilli powder and cook for a further 2 minutes.

Stir in the cooked rice, mixing well to ensure it is fully coated in the flavours. Leave to cook for 5 minutes until the rice has changed colour and has a slightly sticky consistency.

MAKE IT VEGGIE
Leave out the Worcestershire sauce.

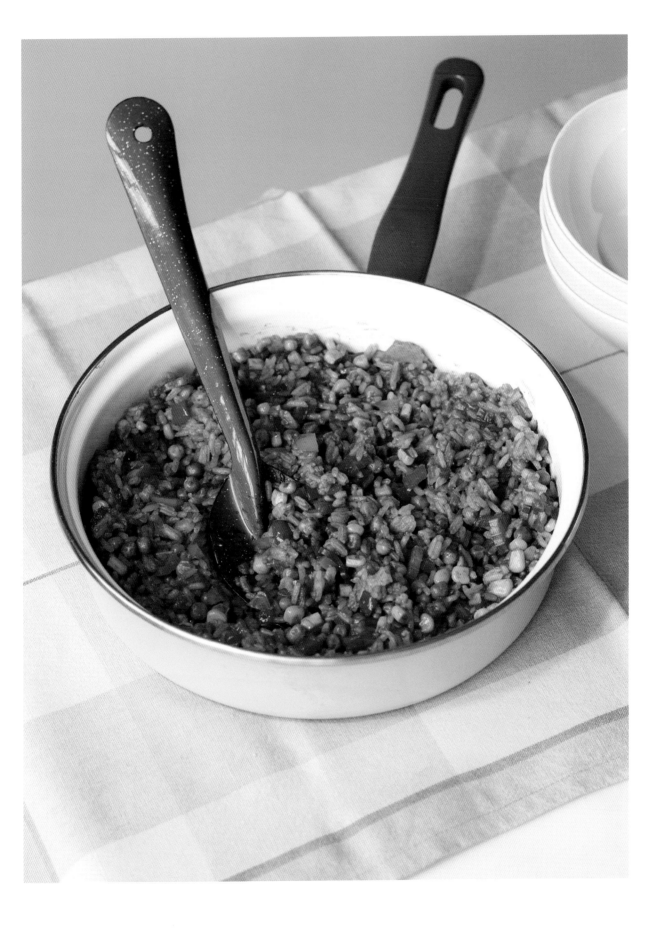

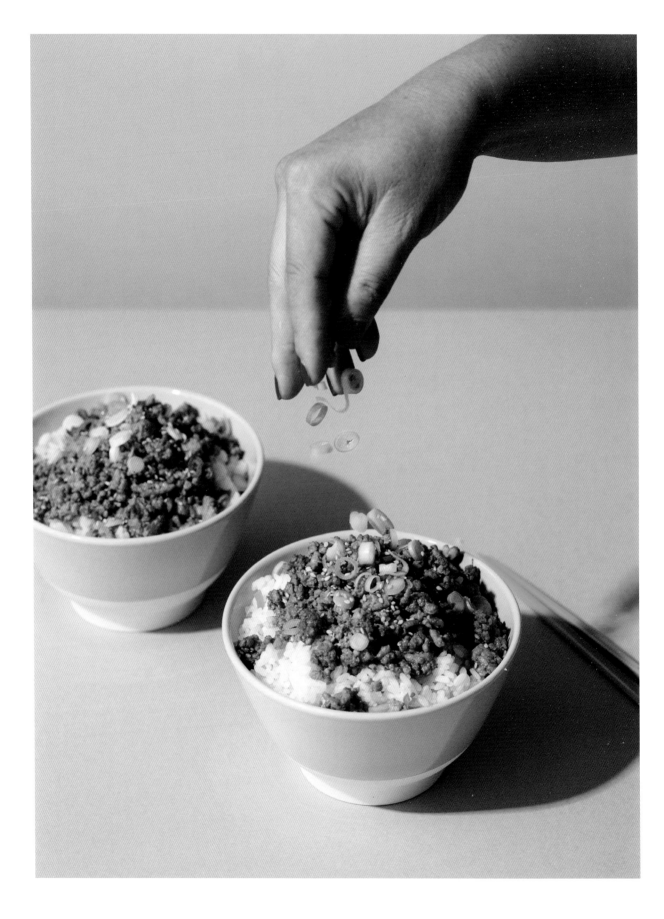

teriyaki turkey rice bowl

Turkey is such a versatile and naturally low-fat meat. A lot of people will only make something like turkey burgers using turkey mince, but it can be used in a variety of ways. This is one of my favourite ways to use turkey mince for a dinner recipe. The sticky teriyaki sauce is delicious!

MAKES 2 PORTIONS

500g (1lb 2oz) lean minced (ground) turkey
100ml (3½fl oz/scant ½ cup) soy sauce (I prefer using low-sodium soy sauce)
100ml (3½fl oz/scant ½ cup) rice vinegar
3 tablespoons honey
1 teaspoon brown sugar
1 garlic clove, crushed
1 teaspoon crushed or grated fresh ginger
Low-calorie cooking spray

To serve

200g (7oz) cooked rice or noodles
Sesame seeds, for sprinkling
1 spring onion (scallion), chopped

Prep time 5 minutes | **Cook time** 20 minutes
Calorie count 464 calories per portion

Spray a frying pan (skillet) with low-calorie cooking spray and set over a medium heat. Add the turkey and cook for 5 minutes until the turkey has browned. Remove from the pan and set aside.

Mix together the soy sauce, rice vinegar, honey, sugar, garlic and ginger in a mixing bowl. Pour the sauce into the pan you used to cook the turkey. Bring the sauce to the boil until it starts to thicken, then reduce the heat and return the turkey to the pan.

Leave to cook for 4–5 minutes until the sauce is sticky and coats the turkey mince.

Divide the rice between serving bowls, top with the turkey and sprinkle with sesame seeds and spring onion.

jerk-spiced chicken alfredo

This recipe is a bit of a melting pot of dishes, but I think the creaminess of the pasta with the spicy kick of the jerk-style chicken is the perfect partnership. While 'jerk' in Caribbean cuisine refers to how the chicken is cooked over a fire or wood grill, this recipe is inspired by the jerk seasoning flavours that are used when cooking. I added some spinach to this recipe, too, as I think it works really well with the spice.

MAKES 2 PORTIONS

2 large skinless and boneless chicken breasts

150g (5oz) dried pasta of your choice

1 garlic clove, finely diced

50g (1¾oz) mushrooms, sliced

1 small red onion, finely diced

120g (4¼oz) low-fat cream cheese

100g (3½oz) spinach

Low-calorie cooking spray

For the jerk marinade

½ onion

2 teaspoons dried thyme

1 teaspoon lazy ginger

5 garlic cloves

1 tablespoon ground cinnamon

1 teaspoon ground allspice

1 tablespoon ground white pepper

1 tablespoon granulated sweetener

1 tablespoon chicken gravy granules

1 tablespoon honey

1 teaspoon smoked paprika

2 tablespoons soy sauce

1 red chilli pepper, deseeded

Prep time 10 minutes, plus 30 minutes marinating

Cook time 35 minutes | **Calorie count** 481 calories per portion

Preheat the oven to 180°C/160°C fan/350°F/Gas mark 4.

To make the jerk marinade, blitz all of the ingredients together in a food processor or blender until smooth.

Pour this mixture over the chicken breasts, cover and leave to marinate for at least 30 minutes.

Transfer the marinated chicken to an ovenproof dish and bake for 35 minutes.

Meanwhile, cook the pasta according to the packet instructions, retaining some of the pasta water.

Spray a frying pan (skillet) with low-calorie cooking spray and add the garlic, mushrooms and onion. Cook over a medium heat for about 5 minutes until softened.

Add the cream cheese and stir until the cheese has melted. Add a couple of spoonfuls of the reserved pasta water to help thicken the sauce. Stir well, adding more water if you need to, to create a thick and creamy sauce. Add the spinach, reduce the heat to low and cook for 3 minutes until it has wilted.

Once the pasta is cooked, drain the rest of the water, add the pasta to the sauce and stir well.

Slice the chicken breast and serve on top of the pasta, drizzling any excess jerk seasoning over the top.

stuffed chicken breasts wrapped in parma ham with potato dauphinoise

This is a dish that is very close to my heart. When I was 18, having just started to take an interest in cooking, I invited all of my friends over for a dinner party, and this was the dish that I cooked. It is a little basic, but basic doesn't always have to be bad! The potato Dauphinoise is made with both sweet and normal potatoes.

MAKES 2 PORTIONS

130g (4½oz) spinach

3 tablespoons low-fat cream cheese

2 garlic cloves, finely chopped

2 large skinless and boneless chicken breasts

100g (3½oz) Parma ham or Prosciutto

Sea salt and freshly ground black pepper

Vegetables of your choice, to serve

For the potatoes Dauphinoise

250g (9oz) potatoes, peeled and sliced

250g (9oz) sweet potatoes, peeled and sliced

2 teaspoons cornflour (cornstarch)

250g (9oz) tub of quark (or low-fat cream cheese)

1 garlic clove, finely chopped

1 teaspoon mustard powder

80g (3oz) low-fat mature Cheddar, grated

Prep time 15 minutes | **Cook time** 30 minutes
Calorie count 580 calories per portion

Make the chicken filling by combining the spinach, cream cheese, garlic and a pinch of salt and pepper together in a bowl.

Lay out some cling film (plastic wrap) on the worktop, then place the chicken breasts on top. Fold the cling film over it, then use a rolling pin to bash the breasts out a little flatter, but not completely flat.

Remove the breasts from the cling film and place them on a baking tray (sheet). Make an incision along the side. Stuff each breast with the spinach and cream cheese mix.

Wrap the Parma ham around each breast, making sure you cover the incision you made for the stuffing. Set them aside in the refrigerator while you prepare the potato Dauphinoise.

Place the potato slices in a pan of cold water and bring to the boil. Cook for 8 minutes until the potatoes have softened. Once cooked, remove the potatoes and drain them of any water.

Add the cornflour and a teaspoon of water to a saucepan and mix to a paste. Add the quark, garlic, mustard powder and plenty of salt and pepper. Add the cooked potatoes and stir.

Pour the potato mixture into an ovenproof dish and top with the grated cheese.

Put the potatoes and chicken into the oven and cook for 25 minutes, or until the chicken is cooked through and the potatoes are golden.

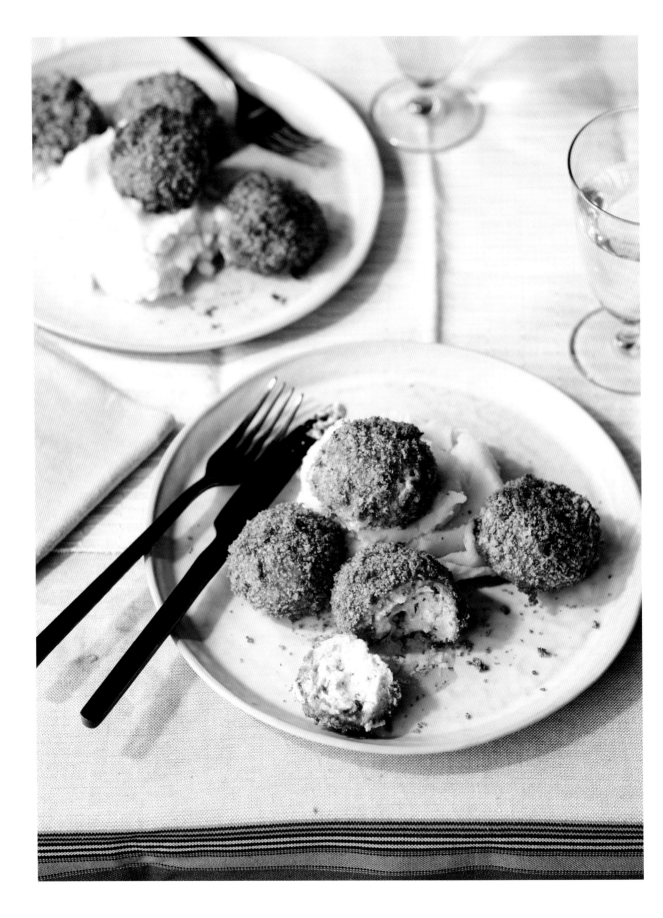

mini chicken kyivs with creamy mash

This was one of my favourite treats as a child! I just love a Kyiv, and these mini ones are delicious. The mash is super creamy, without needing to add extra butter, cream or milk. The trick is all in using a whisk.

MAKES 2 PORTIONS

500g (1lb 2oz) lean minced (ground) chicken

2 slices of wholemeal bread

1 teaspoon smoked paprika

1 egg, beaten

3 large potatoes, peeled and cubed

Low-calorie cooking spray

Sea salt and freshly ground black pepper

For the Kyiv filling

2 tablespoons low-fat butter spread

4 tablespoons low-fat cream cheese

2 tablespoons flat-leaf parsley, chopped

3 garlic cloves, finely diced

Prep time 15 minutes, plus 20 minutes freezing
Cook time 30 minutes | **Calorie count** 570 calories per portion

Preheat the oven to 200°C/180°C fan/400°F/Gas mark 6.

To make the filling, mix all the ingredients together in a bowl until combined. Divide into 12 equal-sized balls, place on a baking tray (sheet), then transfer to the freezer for about 20 minutes until solid.

Use your hands to split the chicken mince into 12 portions, then roll each into a ball. Press down in the middle of the ball to make a dent, then press a frozen garlic butter ball into the middle. Use your hands to mould the chicken around the garlic butter, making sure it is fully covered.

Blitz the wholemeal bread in a food processor or blender until you have breadcrumbs and place in a bowl with the paprika and a pinch of salt and pepper.

Put the egg into a separate bowl. The key to breadcrumbing is to make sure you use a different hand for the wet ingredients then you do for the dry ingredients. So use one hand to pick up the chicken ball and put it in the egg, the same hand to take it out of the egg and drop it into the breadcrumbs, then use the other hand to take it out of the breadcrumbs. This prevents you from breadcrumbing your fingers! Repeat this process twice so that the balls are evenly coated in the breadcrumbs.

Lay the balls out on a baking tray (sheet), spray with low-calorie cooking spray and bake for 25 minutes until crisp and golden.

Bring the potatoes to the boil in a saucepan of salted water and cook for 15 minutes. Drain, then return them to the pan. Use a potato masher to crush and mash the potatoes. Then use a whisk to whisk and whip the potatoes until they are completely smooth in texture. Add a pinch of salt and pepper to taste, then serve with the Kyivs.

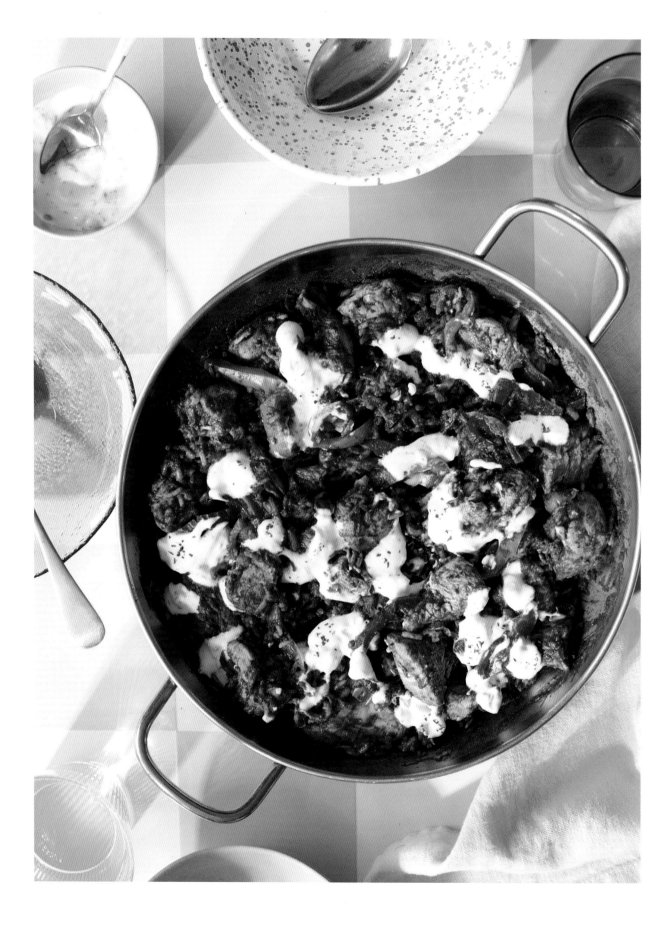

chicken tikka rice with yoghurt and mint drizzle

This is one of the most popular recipes on my blog, but with an added twist of a delicious yoghurt, garlic and mint drizzle. It reminds me of a takeaway curry raita, but with fewer calories and less sugar!

MAKES 4 PORTIONS

6 tablespoons tikka curry powder

2 tablespoons fat-free natural yoghurt

500g (1lb 2oz) skinless and boneless chicken breasts, diced

80g (3oz/scant ½ cup) long-grain rice

1 red onion, sliced

1 red (bell) pepper, sliced

1 yellow (bell) pepper, sliced

1 garlic clove, finely diced

2 teaspoons smoked paprika

1 chicken stock cube

125ml (4½fl oz/½ cup) boiling water

3 tablespoons tomato purée (paste)

Juice of 1 lime

Low-calorie cooking spray

For the drizzle

1 garlic clove, finely chopped

1 teaspoon dried mint

5 tablespoons fat-free Greek yoghurt

Prep time 15 minutes, plus 20 minutes marinating (or overnight) | **Cook time** 40 minutes
Calorie count 420 calories per portion

Mix half the tikka curry powder with the natural yoghurt in a large bowl. Add the diced chicken and mix until coated. Cover and refrigerate for at least 20 minutes, or overnight if you can.

Meanwhile, bring a large saucepan of water to the boil and cook the rice according to the packet instructions.

Once the chicken has marinated, spray a large frying pan (skillet) set over a medium heat with low-calorie cooking spray. Fry the onion and peppers for 5–10 minutes, or until softened.

Add the garlic, smoked paprika, the remaining curry powder and the marinated chicken. Stir well to mix everything together and cook for 10 minutes until the chicken is cooked all the way through.

Dissolve the stock cube in the boiling water and add to the pan along with the rice, tomato purée and lime juice. Mix well and leave to simmer until the stock has soaked into the rice, stirring occasionally to prevent it from sticking at the bottom.

Prepare the drizzle by mixing all the ingredients together in a small bowl, then drizzle over the top of the rice when ready to serve.

Note Leave the chicken to marinate as long as you possibly can before cooking.

MAKE IT VEGGIE
Replace the chicken with tofu, or swap for extra peppers and vegetables.

smoky chicken and pancetta pie

This special recipe is one of the reasons I started a food blog in the first place. I first created a (not in any way healthy!) version of this pie in 2013, and wrote out the recipe to send to some friends after I cooked it for them and they said it was 'the best pie I've ever eaten'. They all loved it so much that they encouraged me to keep writing down recipes. So this is my new, improved and much more slimming-friendly version. The filo (phyllo) pastry topping provides a lighter alternative to heavy pastry.

MAKES 4 PORTIONS

1 onion, finely diced
1 garlic clove, finely diced
70g (2¾oz) pancetta
150g (5oz) mushrooms, sliced
500g (1lb 2oz) skinless and boneless chicken breast, diced
2 teaspoons smoked paprika
1 teaspoon wholegrain mustard
200ml (7fl oz/scant 1 cup) chicken stock
120g (4¼oz) low-fat cream cheese
4 sheets of ready-made filo (phyllo) pastry
Low-calorie cooking spray
Sea salt and freshly ground black pepper

Prep time 25 minutes | **Cook time** 1 hour
Calorie count 526 calories per portion

Preheat the oven to 200°C/180°C fan/400°F/Gas mark 6.

Spray a large frying pan (skillet) with low-calorie cooking spray and add the onion and garlic. Fry for 4 minutes over a medium heat, or until the onion has softened.

Add the pancetta and cook for 5 minutes until browned and crispy. Add the mushrooms and cook for 3 minutes. Add the diced chicken and cook for 10 minutes until cooked all the way through.

Add the smoked paprika and wholegrain mustard and season with salt and pepper.

Add the chicken stock and cream cheese to the pan and stir until the cheese has melted into the stock.

Transfer the chicken mixture to a large ovenproof dish or pie dish.

Crumple up the filo pastry sheets and roughly place them on top of the pie mixture. This doesn't need to be exact, but do make sure that the pie filling is fully covered by pastry. Spray with some low-calorie cooking spray and bake for 25 minutes.

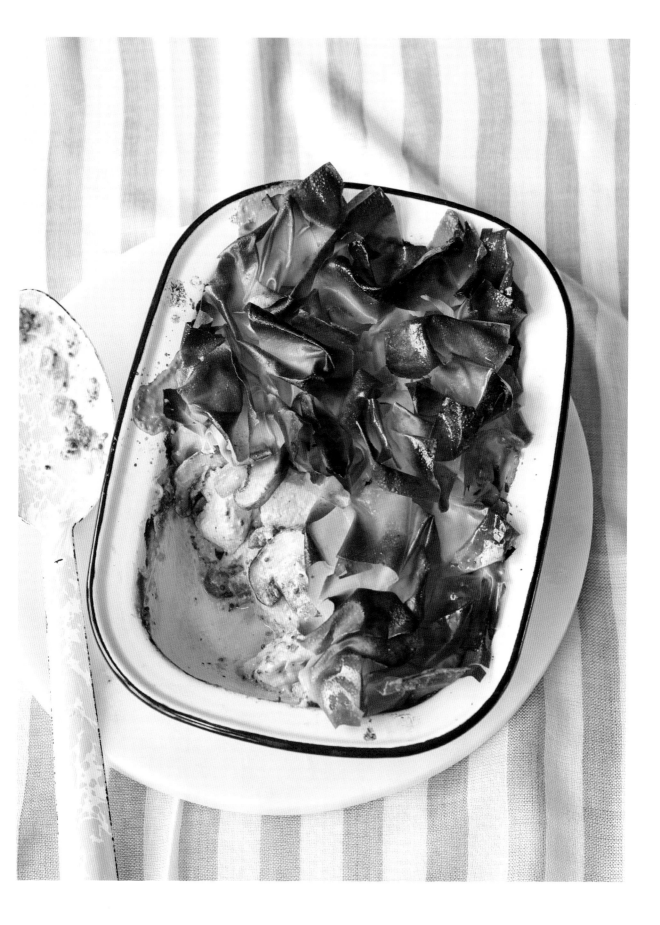

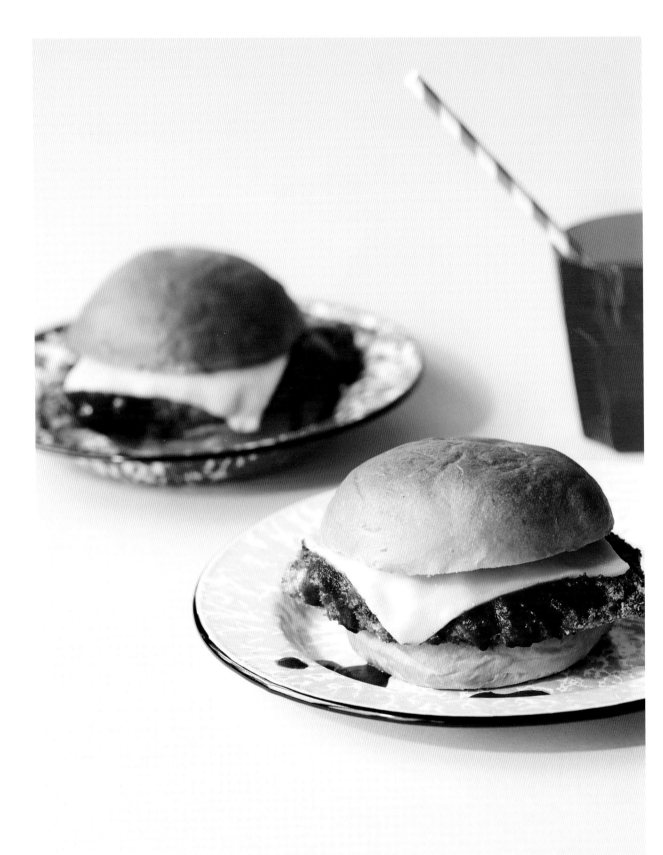

crispy BBQ glazed chicken burgers

I have been developing my BBQ sauce for years, and have so many followers tell me that they adore it, too. I used my classic BBQ sauce in this recipe to make the glaze for this crispy chicken burger.

MAKES 2 PORTIONS

2 skinless and boneless chicken breasts
2 slices of wholemeal bread
1 egg
2 reduced-fat Cheddar cheese slices
2 burger buns, to serve
Low-calorie cooking spray

For the BBQ glaze

5 tablespoons Worcestershire sauce
2 teaspoons mustard powder
250g (9oz) passata (sieved tomatoes)
3 tablespoons balsamic vinegar
2 garlic cloves, finely diced
3 tablespoons sweetener
2 teaspoons smoked paprika
300ml (¾ pint/1¼ cups) sugar-free cola
Sea salt and freshly ground black pepper

Prep time 10 minutes | **Cook time** 45 minutes
Calorie count 594 calories per portion

Preheat the oven to 200°C/180°C fan/400°F/Gas mark 6.

Place all of the ingredients for the BBQ glaze into a saucepan. Bring to the boil, then reduce the heat to low and leave to simmer and reduce for 10–15 minutes.

Wrap each chicken breast in cling film (plastic wrap), then use a rolling pin to hit the breast until you have evened it out so that it is thinner and flatter all over.

Blitz the bread in a food processor to make breadcrumbs, then add them to a shallow dish.

Beat the egg in a separate shallow bowl.

The key to breadcrumbing is to make sure you use a different hand for the wet ingredients than you do for the dry ingredients. So use one hand to pick up the breast and put it in the egg, the same hand to take it out the egg and drop it into the breadcrumbs, then use the other hand to take it out of the breadcrumbs. This prevents you from breadcrumbing your fingers! Repeat this process twice so that the breasts are evenly coated in the breadcrumbs.

Spray a baking tray (sheet) with low-calorie cooking spray and place the chicken on this. Give them another spray with low-calorie cooking spray and bake for 35 minutes, or until crispy and the chicken is cooked all the way through.

Once cooked, remove from the oven. Pour some of the BBQ sauce on each burger, top with a slice of cheese, then return to the oven until the cheese is melted and bubbling. Serve in burger buns.

~~~~~

Note If you want to save some calories, serve without the bun; this can save up to 200 calories.

creamy chicken casserole with dumplings

Casserole has to be one of the most comforting dishes that you can prepare, especially when it's cold outside. Dumplings are traditionally made using a fat such as suet or butter, but these are made with low fat yoghurt instead.

MAKES 4 PORTIONS

500g (1lb 2oz) skinless and
    boneless chicken breast,
    diced
6 bacon medallions, all fat
    removed, then sliced
350ml (12fl oz/1½ cups)
    chicken stock
1 red (bell) pepper, diced
1 x 198g (7oz) tin of
    sweetcorn
1 onion, finely diced
250g (9oz) mushrooms, sliced
1 garlic clove, crushed
2 teaspoons Italian herb mix
120g (4¼oz) low-fat cream
    cheese (or quark)
Low-calorie cooking spray
Sea salt and freshly ground
    black pepper

For the dumplings

5 tablespoons fat-free Greek
    yoghurt
6 tablespoons self-raising
    (self-rising) flour
½ teaspoon baking powder
½ teaspoon dried basil
½ teaspoon dried oregano

Prep time 10 minutes | **Cook time** 55 minutes
Calorie count 400 calories per portion

Preheat the oven to 150°C/130°C fan/300°F/Gas mark 2.

Spray a frying pan (skillet) with low-calorie cooking spray and set over a medium heat. Add the chicken and cook for 5–7 minutes until the chicken has browned. Add the bacon and cook for a further 5 minutes.

Remove the chicken and bacon and add to a large casserole dish. Add the stock, pepper, sweetcorn, onion, mushrooms and garlic to the dish. Season with salt, pepper and the Italian herb mix. Cover the dish and bake for 40 minutes.

Meanwhile, prepare the dumplings by mixing all the ingredients together in a bowl. You may need to add more flour or yoghurt to make a dough-like consistency. Keep stirring until it comes together. Roll the dough out into balls and leave it in the refrigerator until ready to use.

Add the cream cheese to the casserole and stir it in until it has melted. Add the dumplings and return to the oven to cook for a further 15 minutes until the dumplings have plumped up and are cooked.

Note Leftovers can be kept in the refrigerator in a sealed container for up to 5 days. Reheat fully before serving.

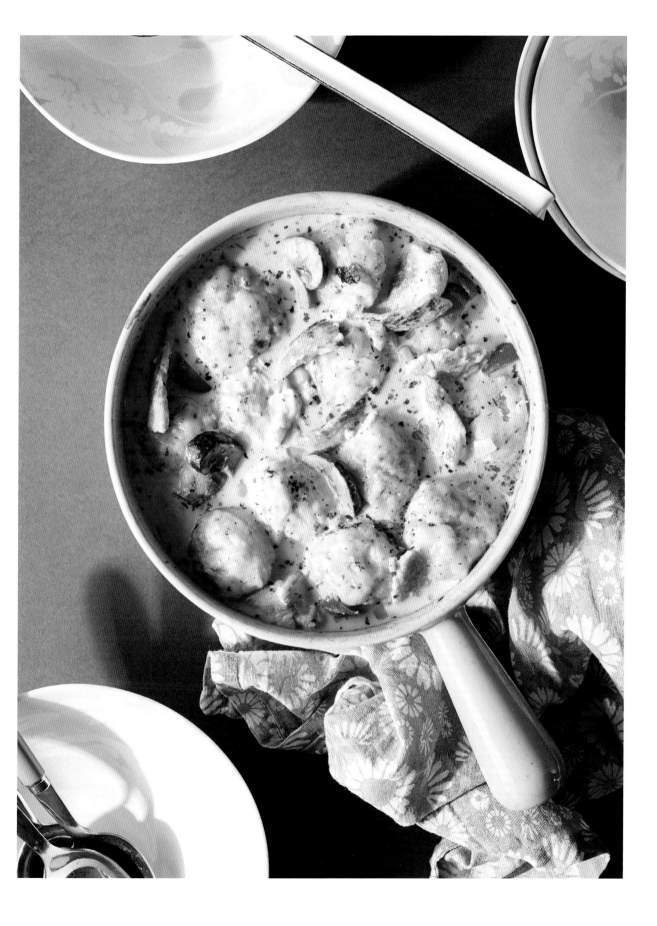

jambalaya

Jambalaya is a Cajun rice dish that I love to make all the time. It is a simple one-pan recipe, too, as the rice cooks together with the other ingredients.

MAKES 4 PORTIONS

2 large skinless and
   boneless chicken breasts,
   diced
1 red onion, diced
3 garlic cloves, crushed
1 red (bell) pepper, sliced
1 green (bell) pepper,
   sliced
1 yellow (bell) pepper,
   sliced
1 courgette (zucchini),
   chopped
2 tablespoons dried thyme
2 tablespoons chopped
   parsley
1 teaspoon smoked paprika
1 teaspoon cayenne pepper
1 x 400g (14oz) tin of
   chopped tomatoes
250g (9oz/1⅓ cups) long-
   grain rice
350ml (12fl oz/1½ cups)
   chicken stock
Low-calorie cooking spray
Sea salt and freshly ground
   black pepper

Prep time 10 minutes | **Cook time** 45 minutes
Calorie count 508 calories per portion

Spray a large frying pan (skillet) with low-calorie cooking spray and set over a medium heat. Add the diced chicken breasts and cook for 10–15 minutes until the chicken is cooked all the way through. Once cooked, remove the chicken from the pan and set it aside.

Give the pan another spray with low-calorie cooking spray and add the onion, garlic, peppers and courgette and cook for 2–3 minutes. Add the thyme, parsley, smoked paprika and cayenne, stir and cook for 2 minutes.

Return the chicken to the pan, along with the tomatoes, rice and stock and season with salt and pepper. Cover and leave to simmer over a low heat for 20–25 minutes until the rice is cooked and tender.

Note You will need a large, flat-bottomed frying pan (skillet) for this dish.

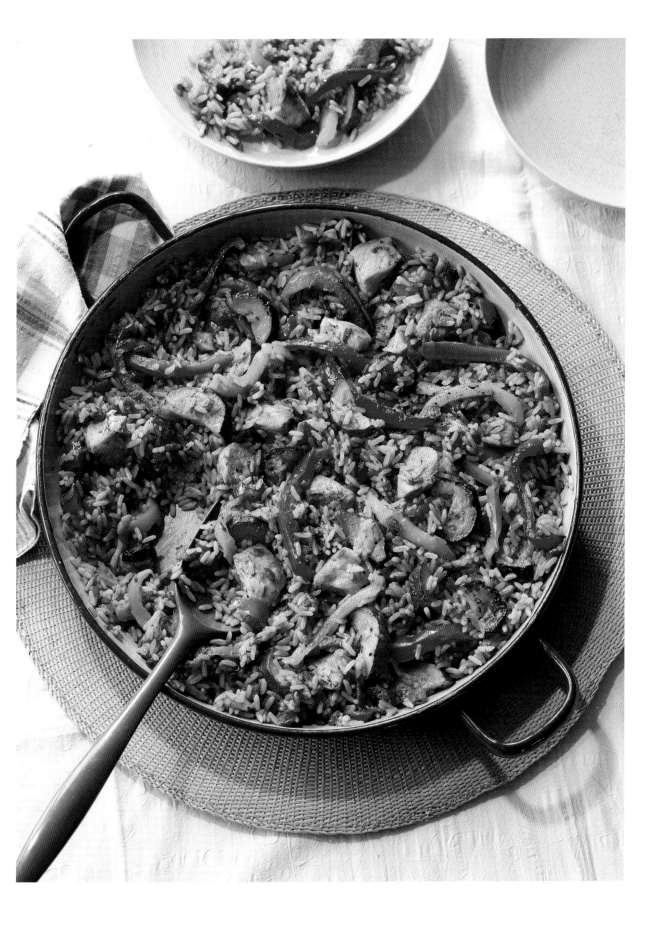

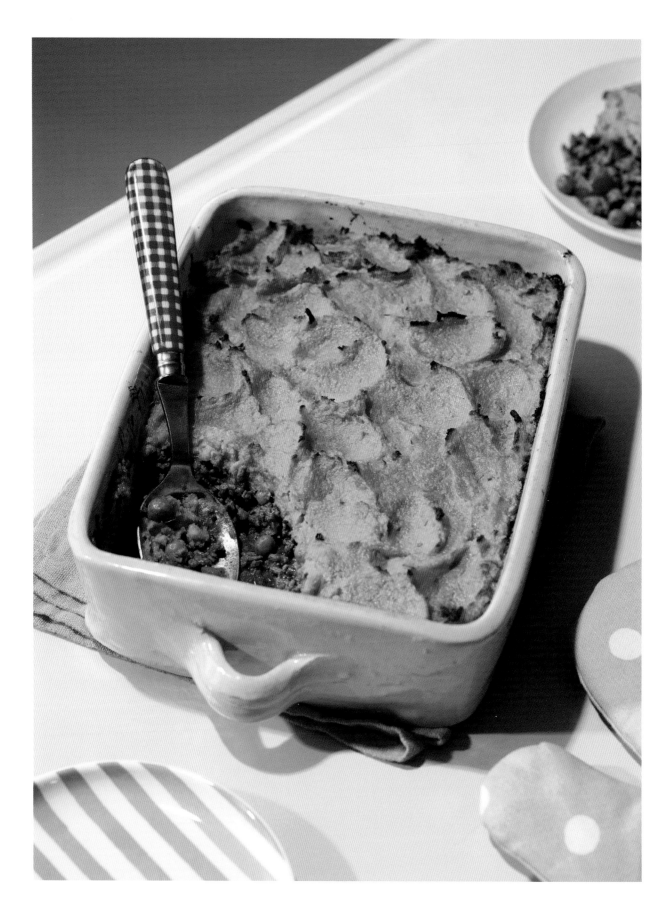

sweet potato cottage pie

Cottage pie is a good old classic British dish, and with this sweet potato topping, it makes a lighter and welcome change. I like to pack as many vegetables as I can into the cottage pie filling. To get the tastiest cottage pie, let the sauce reduce down and thicken.

MAKES 4 PORTIONS

1 onion, finely chopped
2 garlic cloves, minced
1 carrot, finely chopped
1 celery stick, finely
  chopped
1 red (bell) pepper, chopped
80g (3oz/⅔ cup) frozen peas
500g (1lb 2oz) 5% fat lean
  minced (ground) beef
2 tablespoons Worcestershire
  sauce
250ml (9fl oz/1 cup) beef
  stock
2 tablespoons tomato purée
  (paste)
1 teaspoon dried thyme
3 large sweet potatoes,
  peeled and chopped into
  chunks
Low-calorie cooking spray
Sea salt and freshly ground
  black pepper

Note Great for freezing.
Allow extra portions to cool
before freezing and reheat
fully when serving.

Prep time 15 minutes | **Cook time** 45 minutes
Calorie count 353 calories per portion

Spray a large frying pan (skillet) with low-calorie cooking spray and set over a medium heat. Add the onion and cook for 3 minutes until it softens.

Add the garlic, carrot, celery, red pepper and peas and cook for 3 minutes until everything starts to soften.

Add the beef mince, then splash over the Worcestershire sauce and cook for 5 minutes until the beef has browned.

Add the stock, tomato purée and thyme and season with a big pinch of salt and pepper. Reduce the heat and let it simmer for 20 minutes to reduce.

To make the topping, boil the sweet potatoes in a saucepan of boiling water and cook for 10 minutes, or until the sweet potato is soft. Drain, then mash with a potato masher, and use a whisk to make it extra creamy.

Spoon the filling into a large pie dish, then layer the sweet potato mash on top. Bake for 25 minutes until nicely browned on top.

MAKE IT VEGGIE
Remove the beef mince, use vegetable stock, and increase the number of vegetables you include. Alternatively, use a meat-free mince such as soya.

beef and broccoli noodles

A speedy, tasty, easy, Chinese-inspired recipe that's perfect for weeknight cooking and ready in less than half an hour.

MAKES 2 PORTIONS

120g (4¼oz) dried egg
    noodles
1 head of broccoli, chopped
    into small florets
1 carrot, cut into thin
    strips
400g (14oz) beef frying
    steaks, fat removed and
    cut into strips
150g (5oz) beansprouts
Low-calorie cooking spray
Sliced spring onions
    (scallions), to garnish

For the sauce

3 tablespoons soy sauce
2 tablespoons oyster sauce
1 tablespoon tomato ketchup
1 garlic clove, finely
    chopped
1 teaspoon of lazy garlic
    (or a thumbnail-sized
    piece of fresh ginger,
    grated)
1 tablespoon white wine
    vinegar
½ teaspoon Chinese five-
    spice

Prep time 10 minutes | **Cook time** 15 minutes
Calorie count 482 calories per portion

Prepare the sauce by mixing all of the ingredients together in a small bowl or jar and set aside until needed.

Bring a saucepan of water to the boil and add the egg noodles. Cook for 5 minutes, then add the broccoli and carrot and cook until just softened.

Meanwhile, spray a frying pan (skillet) with low-calorie cooking spray and set over a medium heat. Add the beef and beansprouts and cook for 3 minutes until the beef has browned. Add the sauce and cook for a further 3 minutes.

Drain the noodles, carrots and broccoli, then add this to the pan with the beef and sauce. Serve garnished with spring onions.

beef stroganoff pasta

This is a twist on one of the most popular recipes on my blog. My followers go mad for this tasty lower-calorie stroganoff recipe, and this pasta version will be a new favourite, too! It's so simple to make, light and creamy.

MAKES 4 PORTIONS

500g (1lb 2oz) beef frying steaks, cut into strips
1 teaspoon white wine vinegar
2 teaspoons Worcestershire sauce
1 large onion, finely diced
250g (9oz) button mushrooms, sliced
1 garlic clove, finely diced
1 teaspoon mustard powder
500ml (18fl oz/2 cups) beef stock
250g (7oz) dried pasta of your choice
200g (7oz) lightest cream cheese
Low-calorie cooking spray
Sea salt and freshly ground black pepper

Prep time 10 minutes | **Cook time** 25 minutes
Calorie count 450 calories per portion

Spray a large frying pan (skillet) with low-calorie cooking spray and place over a medium heat.

Season the beef strips with salt and pepper and add them to the pan. Sear the beef, keeping it moving around the pan – you just want to seal the outside of the meat at this stage, rather than cook it all the way through. Remove the beef from the pan and set it aside.

Add the white wine vinegar and Worcestershire sauce to the pan, then add the onion, mushrooms and garlic and cook over a medium heat for 5–10 minutes until softened.

Add the mustard powder and stock to the pan, reduce the heat and simmer for 15 minutes. Keep an eye on it to make sure it doesn't overheat or reduce down too much. Add more stock if needed. You want the consistency to become slightly thicker and the onions to be soft.

Meanwhile, cook the pasta according to the packet instructions. Drain, making sure you retain some of the water you used to cook the pasta in.

Stir the cream cheese into the mushrooms and onions in the frying pan and reduce the heat to low. Add a couple of tablespoons of the reserved pasta water and mix until it forms a smooth sauce.

Add the beef to the pan and stir well. Cook over a low heat for 3 minutes, then add the cooked pasta and stir again. Serve immediately.

Note Make it gluten free by swapping the pasta for gluten-free pasta

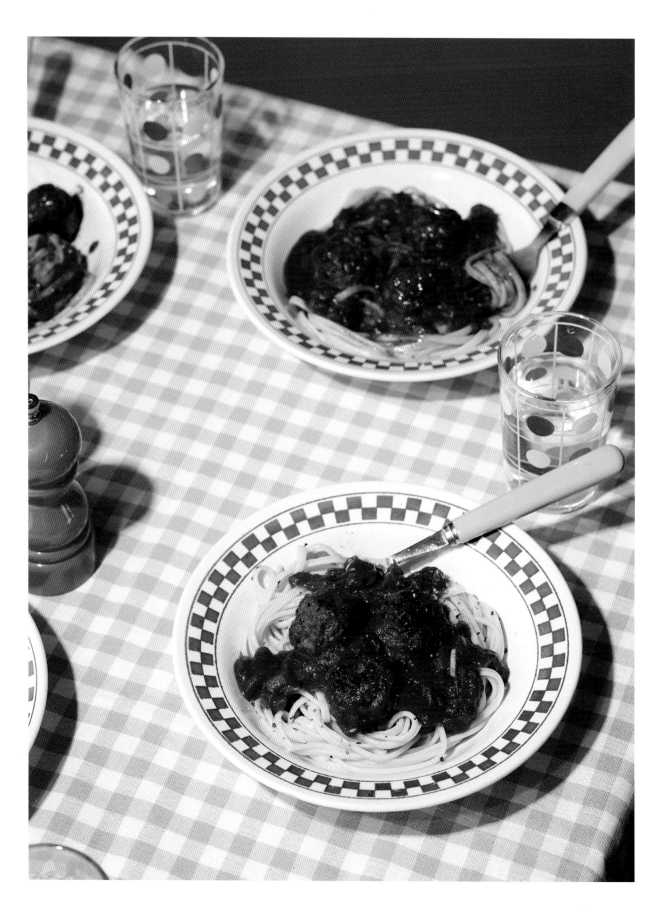

spicy sriracha meatballs with pasta

I am totally sriracha obsessed and would have it on most meals if I could! I think it provides the perfect amount of spice and flavour combined. These meatballs have a little sriracha kick to them and are so easy to prepare.

MAKES 4 PORTIONS

500g (1lb 2oz) 5% fat lean minced (ground) beef

2 garlic cloves, finely diced

2 tablespoons sriracha sauce

1 red onion, finely chopped

1 red (bell) pepper, finely chopped

1 teaspoon mixed Italian herbs

500g (1lb 2oz) passata (sieved tomatoes)

1 beef stock cube, crumbled

1 tablespoon balsamic vinegar

2 tablespoons Worcestershire sauce

1 tablespoon tomato purée (paste)

Low-calorie cooking spray

Sea salt and freshly ground black pepper

180g (6½oz) cooked pasta of your choice, to serve

Prep time 10 minutes | **Cook time** 35 minutes
Calorie count 481 calories per portion

In a large bowl, mix the beef mince, half of the garlic, half of the sriracha and a pinch of salt and pepper. Use your hands to mix everything together well and roll into 12 equal-sized meatballs.

Spray a frying pan (skillet) with low-calorie cooking spray and set over a medium heat. Fry the meatballs for 5–10 minutes until they are browned on the outside and sealed, turning them regularly. Remove the meatballs from the pan and set them aside.

Give the pan another spray with low-calorie cooking spray, add the remaining garlic, the onion and the pepper and fry for 5 minutes until the onion has softened.

Add all of the remaining ingredients to the pan, then reduce the heat to low and leave to simmer for 15 minutes. Add the meatballs back into the pan and simmer for a further 5 minutes.

Serve with the cooked pasta.

Notes If you don't like spice, use less sriracha. Leftovers can be kept in the refrigerator in a sealed container for up to 5 days. Reheat fully before serving.

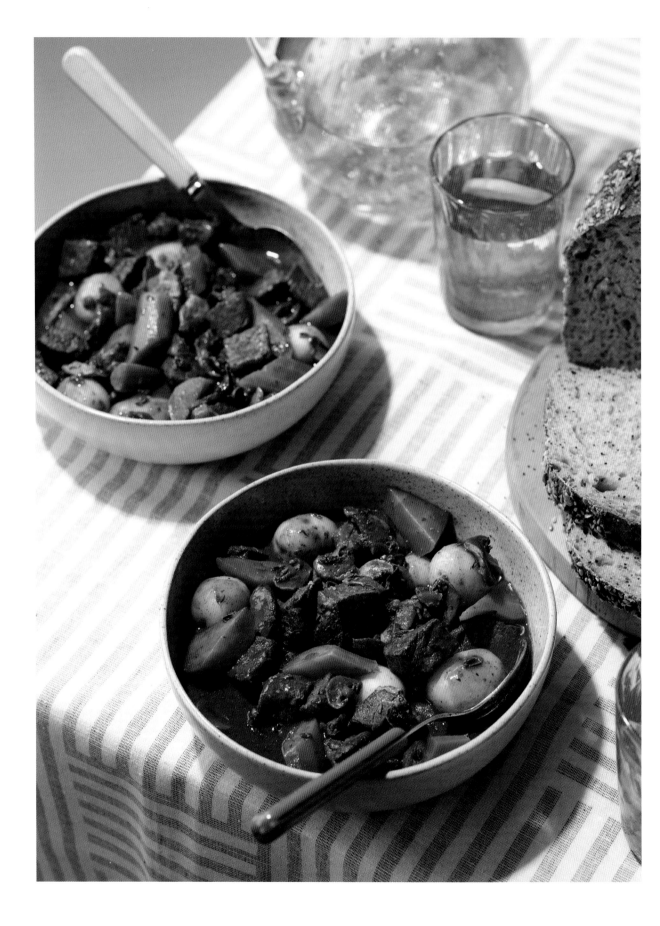

boozy beef bourguignon

This beef bourguignon is simple to prepare with a lovely, deep, rich, red wine sauce. As soon as there is the slightest chill in the air outside I just have to start preparing casseroles, stews and this beef bourguignon. It's proper winter warming comfort food!

MAKES 4 PORTIONS

500g (1lb 2oz) diced beef
    stewing steak
6 bacon medallions, all
    fat removed and cut into
    small chunks
250ml (9fl oz/1 generous
    cup) red wine
500ml (18fl oz/2 generous
    cups) beef stock
2 tablespoons tomato purée
    (paste)
4 tablespoons soy sauce
30g (1oz/2 tablespoons)
    plain (all-purpose) flour
2 garlic cloves, finely
    diced
2 tablespoons thyme, finely
    chopped
5 medium carrots, sliced
200g (7oz) baby potatoes
200g (7oz) button mushrooms,
    sliced
Low-calorie cooking spray
Sea salt and freshly ground
    black black pepper

Prep time 10 minutes | **Cook time** 1¼ hours
Calorie count 300 calories per portion

Spray a cast-iron casserole dish with low-calorie cooking spray and set over a medium heat. Add the beef and sear for a few minutes on each side. Once seared, remove from the pan.

Add the bacon and cook for 6 minutes until the bacon is crispy.

Add the red wine and turn the heat down to low, then add the beef stock, tomato purée and soy sauce. Whisk in the flour and stir until it forms a sauce.

Add the remaining ingredients to the dish, then cover with a lid. Cook over a low heat for 45 minutes, then remove the lid and cook for a further 15 minutes.

This is perfect served on its own, or with some bread for dipping – but remember to adjust the calories.

Notes Leave to cool completely before refrigerating in a sealable container. Can be kept for up to 5 days.

SIMPLE
AND TASTY

TRAYBAKES

You may be forgiven for thinking that baking trays are only good for baking brownies or flapjacks, but there is a whole world of savoury dinners that you can create with a tray.

A few years ago, I created my first traybake video recipe on my social media channels, and it absolutely blew up, with millions of views and followers begging me for more traybake ideas.

The concept of a traybake is that that it is an easy dinner that you can prepare by literally throwing everything into a tray and letting the oven do all the hard work for you. It's amazing what fabulous dinners you can create with just one tray and a small amount of ingredient preparation, such as peeling and chopping some vegetables.

Traybakes are super simple to prepare, so they are perfect for weeknight cooking when you may not have the energy to prepare a whole meal from scratch. Full-on flavour with as little effort as possible is what I am all about!

I use a shallow enamel baking tray for all my traybakes, but any tray will do. The trick to getting the best results from a traybake is to give the food room to breathe. Don't overfill the tray or the flavours won't be able to flow throughout, and you may find that areas of the tray won't cook as well.

Once you get into traybake cooking, you will try to cook all meals this way!

garlic bread pasta bake

Garlic bread has to be one of the ultimate side dishes, but with this pasta recipe, you can make the garlic bread flavour the star of the show! A creamy, cheesy pasta bake that packs a garlic punch.

MAKES 4 PORTIONS

400g (14oz) dried pasta of your choice

1 tablespoon low-fat butter spread

3 garlic cloves, finely chopped (add more if you like it garlicky!)

120g (4¼oz) low-fat cream cheese

½ teaspoon mustard powder

250g (9oz) low-fat grated mozzarella cheese

1 teaspoon dried parsley

Sea salt and freshly ground black pepper

Prep time 10 minutes | **Cook time** 30 minutes
Calorie count 560 calories per portion

Preheat the oven to 180°C/160°C fan/350°F/Gas mark 4.

Cook the pasta in a saucepan of boiling water according to the packet instructions. Drain, retaining some of the cooking water to use later.

Put the low-fat butter spread and garlic in a frying pan (skillet) over a low heat and fry for a couple of minutes, being careful not to burn the garlic. Add the cream cheese and stir until melted.

Once the pasta has cooked, add a few tablespoons of the reserved cooking water to the frying pan and stir until the sauce thickens. Add the mustard powder and some salt and pepper.

Add a pinch of the mozzarella to the sauce as well, then stir until it has melted and thickened the sauce.

Mix the cooked and drained pasta with the sauce, then put all of it in an ovenproof dish. Top with the rest of the mozzarella, then sprinkle the dried parsley over the top. Bake for 20 minutes, or until the cheese is melted and bubbling.

Notes This dish would also work with added vegetables like onion and peppers, just make sure to adjust the calories accordingly. Leftovers can be kept in a sealed container in the refrigerator for up to 3 days

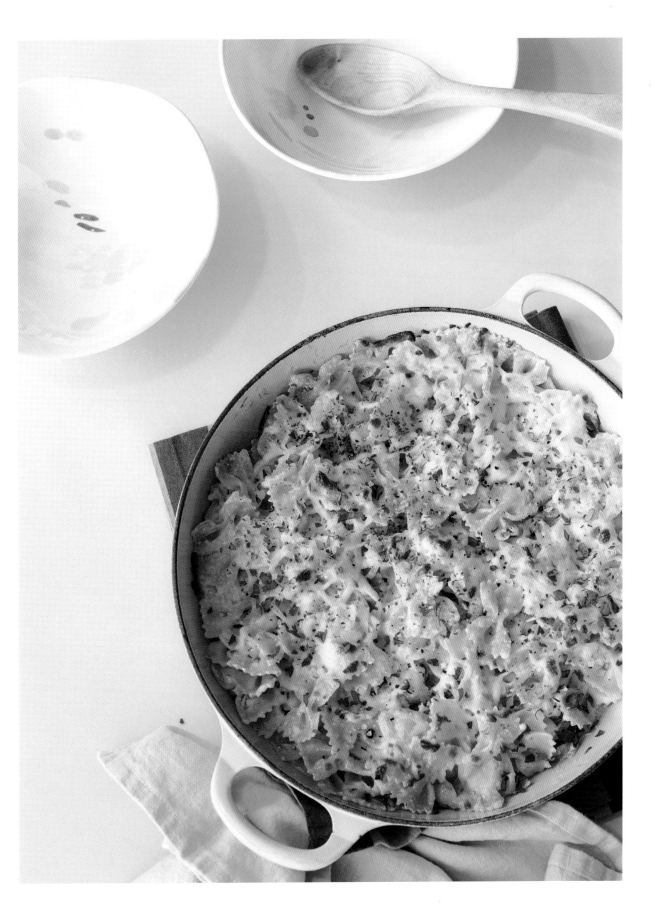

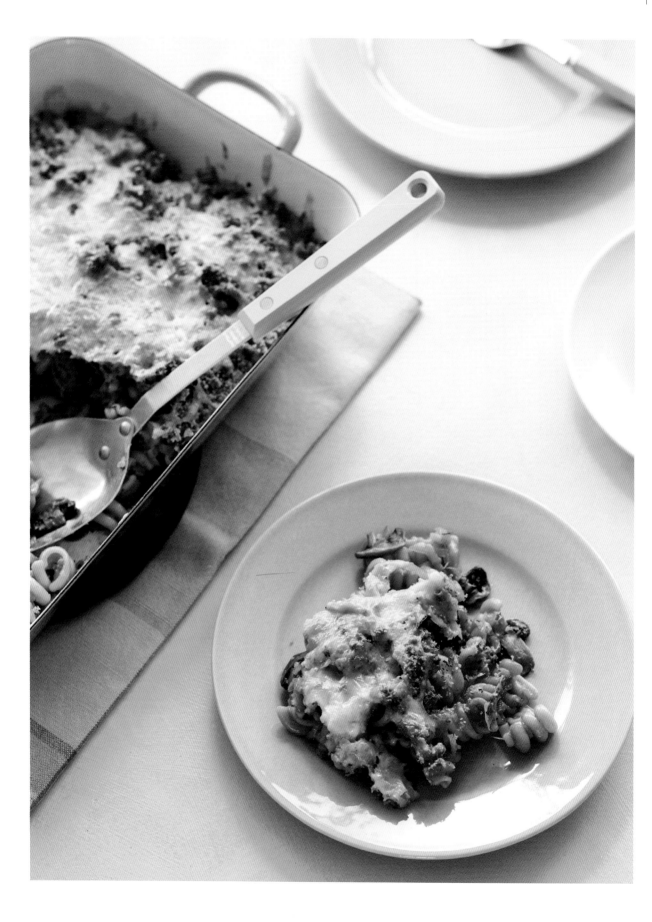

french onion soup pasta bake

French onion soup is incredible, but perhaps not a main meal in itself. This recipe has all the best bits of a French onion soup but with pasta, and less fat. It is topped with garlic and herb breadcrumbs and cheese, so you can still enjoy the cheesy crouton vibes from the traditional recipe. The key to this dish is caramelizing the onions slowly so they take on a deep, rich sweetness.

MAKES 4 PORTIONS

2 tablespoons low-fat butter spread
3 large onions, finely sliced
2 teaspoons honey
3 tablespoons red wine vinegar
100g (3½oz) button mushrooms, sliced
2 large garlic cloves, finely chopped
2 teaspoons dried thyme
2 bay leaves
¼ teaspoon cayenne pepper
700ml (24fl oz/3 cups) beef stock
1 tablespoon Worcestershire sauce (or vegetarian Worcestershire sauce or soy sauce)
400g (14oz) dried pasta of your choice
Sea salt and freshly ground black pepper

For the cheese and crumb topping

2 wholemeal bread slices
1 teaspoon garlic powder
1 teaspoon dried mixed herbs
240g (8½oz) low-fat Cheddar, grated

Note If you want to save on calories further you can omit the garlic breadcrumbs.

Prep time 10 minutes | **Cook time** 45 minutes
Calorie count 541 calories per portion

Preheat the oven to 180°C/160°C fan/350°F/Gas mark 4.

Put the low-fat butter spread, onions and honey in a large saucepan set over a medium heat. Stir together and cook for 5 minutes until the onions are a deep golden brown.

Add the red wine vinegar, 1 tablespoon at a time. Keep stirring and allow the vinegar to cook into the onions. This should take 5 minutes or so, and the onions should be caramelized and dark in colour.

Add the mushrooms and garlic, along with the thyme, bay leaves, cayenne pepper, stock, Worcestershire sauce, dried pasta and some salt and pepper. Mix everything together, bring this to the boil and keep stirring for about 8–10 minutes while the pasta cooks.

Meanwhile, blitz the wholemeal bread in a food processor or blender to make the topping. Mix the breadcrumbs with the garlic powder and dried herbs in a small bowl.

Transfer the pasta and sauce to an ovenproof dish. Sprinkle the breadcrumbs over the top, then grate the cheese on top of that. Bake for 20 minutes, or until the cheese is bubbling.

MAKE IT VEGGIE/VEGAN
While this dish doesn't have any meat in itself, beef stock cubes are used in the base. To make this vegetarian, use vegetable stock instead, and to make it vegan, swap in maple syrup for the honey.

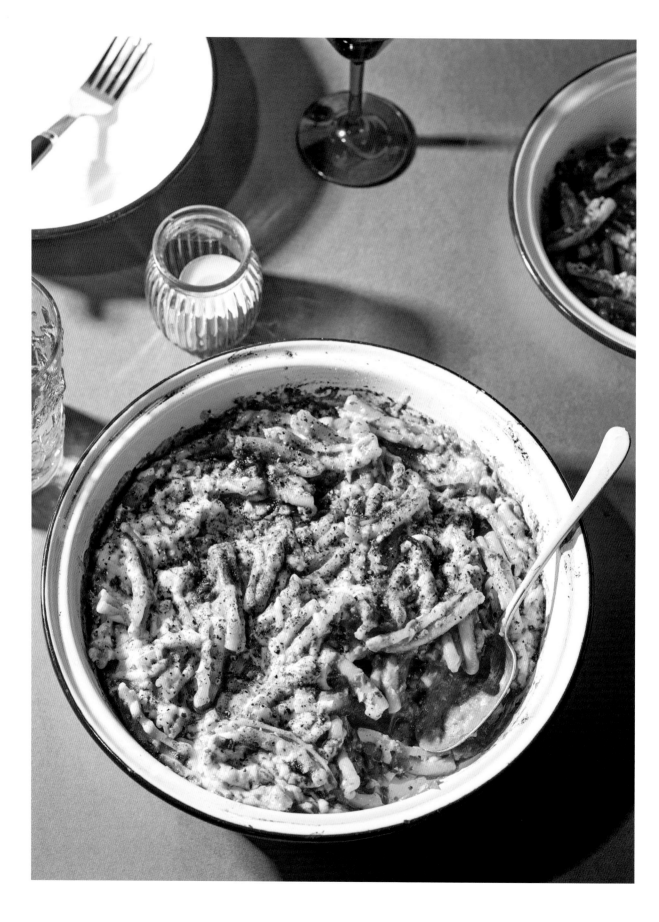

roasted red pepper and tomato pasta

This is a tasty, easy-to-throw-together vegetarian pasta dish that I absolutely love. I love making a big batch of this at the start of the week and feasting on it for my lunches.

MAKES 4 PORTIONS

400g (14oz) bunch of vine
    tomatoes

2 red (bell) peppers, sliced

1 red onion, sliced

1 large garlic clove

200g (7oz) dried pasta of
    your choice

1 tablespoon balsamic
    vinegar

1 tablespoon light cream
    cheese

Sea salt and freshly ground
    black pepper

To top

240g (8½oz) extra light
    Cheddar, grated

1 teaspoon smoked paprika

Pinch of dried parsley

Prep time 10 minutes | **Cook time** 50 minutes
Calorie count 380 calories per portion

Preheat the oven to 200°C/180°C fan/400°F/Gas mark 6.

Place the tomatoes, peppers, onion and garlic onto a baking tray (sheet) and bake in the oven for 40 minutes, or until the tomatoes are softened and roasted.

Meanwhile, parboil the pasta in a pan of boiling water according to the packet instructions. Drain, reserving some of the pasta water for the sauce.

Remove the tray from the oven and take the tomatoes off the vine. Add a dash of water, and then transfer everything to a food processor or blender and blitz until smooth.

Transfer the sauce to a large ovenproof dish and add the balsamic vinegar and cream cheese. Mix again until the cheese melts into the sauce. Add some of the pasta water, then the cooked pasta and mix well.

Top with the cheese and sprinkle over the smoked paprika and dried parsley.

Return to the oven for 10 minutes, or until the cheese is melted and bubbling.

Note Store leftovers in a sealed container in the refrigerator for up to 5 days.

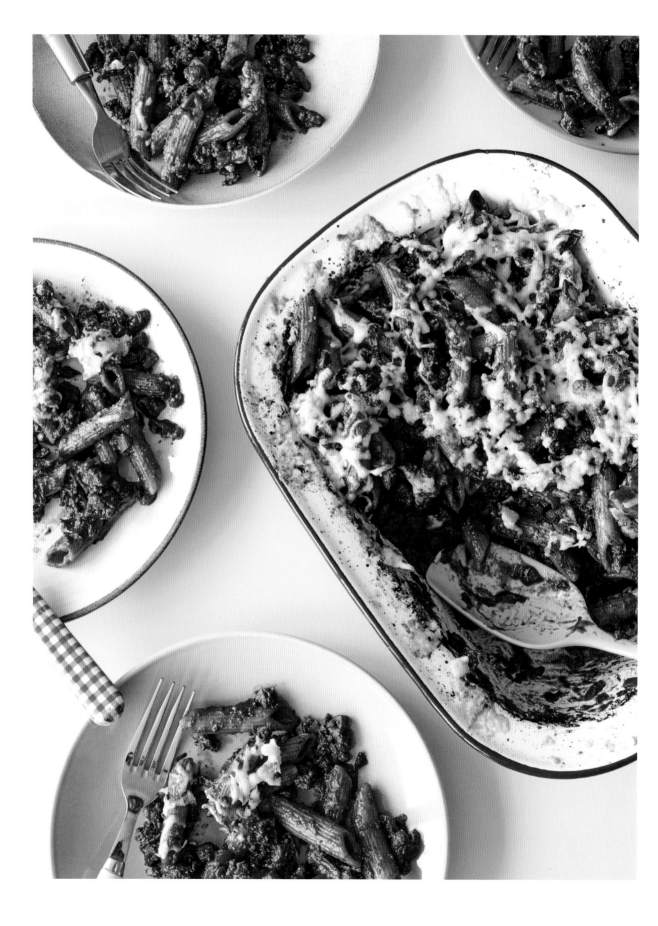

BBQ bolognese pasta bake

BBQ sauce in a bolognese? Trust me, this is incredible. Just when you think a classic spag bol couldn't get any better, this recipe comes along to prove you wrong! The key to making this recipe as delicious as possible is to cook the bolognese 'low and slow', so over a low heat for as long as possible.

MAKES 4 PORTIONS

1 red (bell) pepper, finely chopped

1 yellow (bell) pepper, finely chopped

1 red onion, finely chopped

1 carrot, grated

500g (1lb 2oz) extra lean minced (ground) beef

250g (9oz) dried pasta of your choice

160g (5½oz) low-fat Cheddar

Low-calorie cooking spray

For the BBQ Bolognese sauce

500g (1lb 2oz) passata (sieved tomatoes)

1 x 400g (14oz) tin of chopped tomatoes

5 tablespoons Worcestershire sauce

1 teaspoon mustard powder

3 tablespoons balsamic vinegar

3 garlic cloves, finely chopped

2 tablespoons sweetener

1 teaspoon onion powder

2 teaspoons smoked paprika

150ml (5fl oz/⅔ cup) sugar-free cola

1 beef stock cube

Sea salt and freshly ground black pepper

Prep time 15 minutes | **Cook time** 1 hour
Calorie count 577 calories per portion

Make the sauce by mixing the ingredients together in a bowl and stirring well. Set aside until needed.

Spray a large frying pan (skillet) or saucepan with low-calorie cooking spray and set over a medium heat. Add the peppers, onion and carrot and fry for 3–5 minutes until the onion has softened. Add the beef mince and fry for a further 5 minutes until the mince has browned.

Add the mixed BBQ sauce, stir well, then leave to simmer over a low heat for 25 minutes, stirring occasionally to prevent it from sticking at the bottom.

Preheat the oven to 220°C/200° fan/425°F/Gas mark 7.

Meanwhile, cook the pasta according to the packet instructions. Drain, reserving some of the pasta water, then add the pasta to the bolognese along with 2 tablespoons of the reserved pasta water.

Transfer the bolognese and pasta to an ovenproof dish and top with the cheese. Bake in the oven for 15 minutes, or until the cheese is melted and bubbling

honey marinated halloumi and vegetable traybake

Halloumi is so versatile, and can be the star of the show in any veggie dish. This recipe has a lovely balance of sweet and spice, is easy to make and very filling. I love eating this dish both hot and cold.

MAKES 4 PORTIONS

225g (8oz) block of
  halloumi, sliced
2 tablespoons honey
Juice of 1 lime
½ teaspoon dried chilli
  flakes
2 courgettes (zucchini),
  sliced
1 red onion, sliced
1 yellow (bell) pepper,
  sliced
1 red (bell) pepper, sliced
100g (3½oz) plum tomatoes,
  halved
2 garlic cloves, finely
  chopped
80g (3oz/½ cup) brown rice
60g (2oz) spinach
Low-calorie cooking spray
Sea salt and freshly ground
  black pepper

Prep time 10 minutes, plus 30 minutes marinating
Cook time 40 minutes | **Calorie count** 504 calories per portion

Preheat the oven to 200°C/180°C fan/400°F/Gas mark 6.

Put the halloumi slices into a large bowl and pour over the honey, lime juice and chilli flakes and give it a good stir. Leave to marinate for at least 30 minutes, or as long as possible.

Put the courgettes, onion, peppers, plum tomatoes and garlic in a large roasting tin. Give it a generous spray of low-calorie cooking spray and bake for 25 minutes until the vegetables have softened.

Meanwhile, bring a large saucepan of water to the boil and cook the rice according to the packet instructions.

Remove the halloumi from the honey, lime and chilli mixture and set it aside for a few moments.

Pour the leftover honey, lime and chilli mixture onto the roasted vegetables, add the cooked rice and the spinach and give everything a good mix.

Lay the halloumi slices on top of the rice and vegetable mixture and return to the oven for 15 minutes, or until the halloumi is golden.

Note Use a bread knife to slice the halloumi as it creates a serrated edge, making it more crispy.

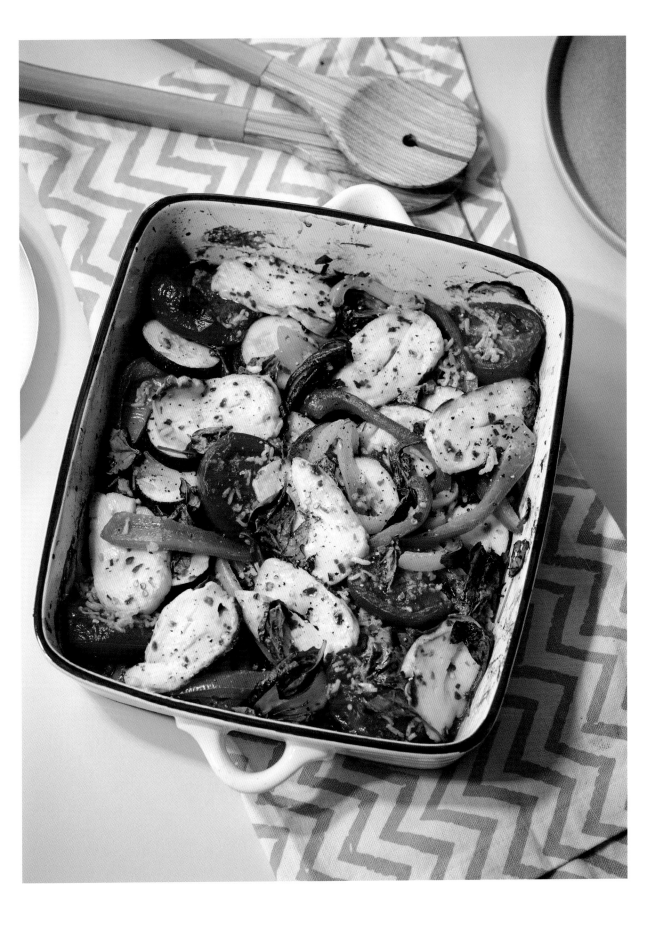

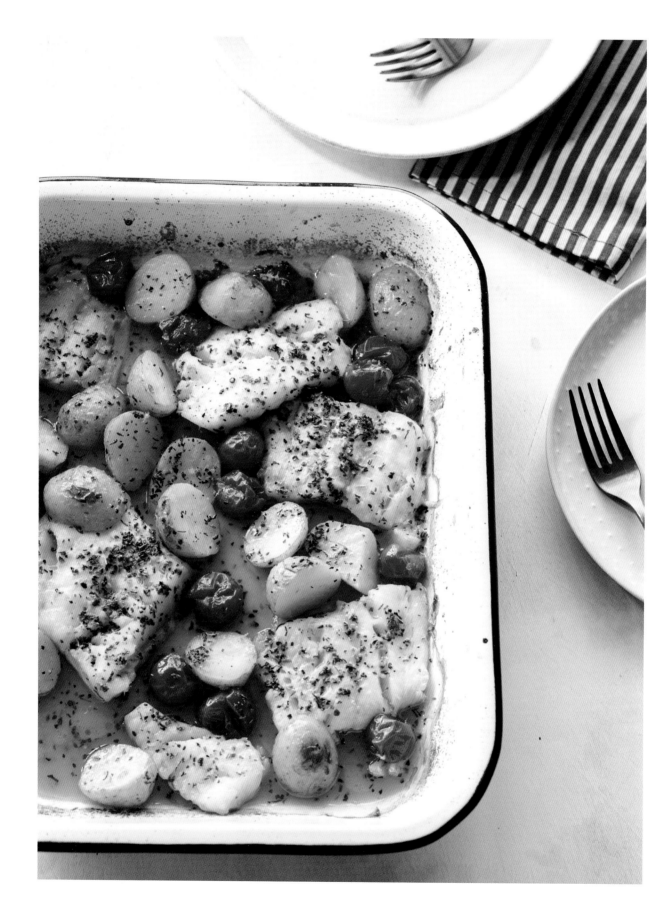

lemon baked cod with new potatoes

I am always trying to find ways to eat more fish as it is so good for you. I wanted to create a way of cooking cod that I would love (without the batter and chips!) and this dish is the one! Lemon and cod is such a perfect combination, and you can cook all the ingredients in one tray.

MAKES 4 PORTIONS

60g (2oz) low-fat butter
  spread
Grated zest and juice of
  1 lemon
1 garlic clove, finely
  chopped
1 teaspoon dried basil
1 teaspoon dried dill
1 teaspoon dried parsley
250g (9oz) new potatoes,
  halved
500g (1lb 2oz) cod fillets
120g (4¼oz) cherry tomatoes,
  halved

Prep time 5 minutes | **Cook time** 30 minutes
Calorie count 426 calories per portion

Preheat the oven to 200°C/180°C fan/400°F/Gas mark 6.

In a small mixing bowl, whisk the spread, lemon zest and juice, garlic, basil, dill, and parsley together until combined.

Put the potatoes into a saucepan of boiling water and bring to the boil. Boil for 6 minutes, then remove and drain the potatoes.

Add the cod to an ovenproof dish and add the tomatoes and parboiled potatoes.

Put some of the butter mix on each piece of cod, then add the rest around the fish in the bottom of the dish.

Bake for 10 minutes, then remove from the oven and baste the cod by pouring the melted butter back over the top.

Return to the oven to bake for a further 15 minutes until the cod is white and flakey.

creamy salmon and chorizo bake

I absolutely love the smokiness of the paprika and chorizo with the salmon in this dish. It is a super comforting salmon casserole, which is perfect for dipping bread into – just remember to adjust the calories.

MAKES 4 PORTIONS

1 red onion, sliced
1 garlic clove, finely
  chopped
1 yellow (bell) pepper,
  sliced
1 teaspoon smoked paprika
½ teaspoon dried chilli
  flakes
80g (3oz) sliced chorizo,
  halved
150g (5oz) plum tomatoes,
  halved
1 x 400g (14oz) tin of
  chopped tomatoes
100g (3½oz) new potatoes,
  cut into small chunks
1 tablespoon low-fat cream
  cheese
2 skinless salmon fillets
  (about 250g/9oz)
Sea salt and freshly ground
  black pepper
Roughly chopped flat-leaf
  parsley, to serve

Prep time 10 minutes | **Cook time** 40 minutes
Calorie count 380 calories per portion

Preheat the oven to 180°C/160°C fan/350°F/Gas mark 4.

Put the onion, garlic, yellow pepper, smoked paprika, chilli flakes, chorizo, plum tomatoes, chopped tomatoes and new potatoes into an ovenproof dish and mix everything together. Bake for 15 minutes.

Remove the dish from the oven and give everything a good stir. Add the cream cheese and stir well until it has melted throughout.

You can either add the whole salmon steaks on top or the roasted mixture or cut the salmon into smaller chunks and scatter them over the top.

Cover the dish with a layer of foil, then return to the oven for 25 minutes. When the salmon flakes easily with a fork, it's ready to serve. Sprinkle with a little parsley and enjoy.

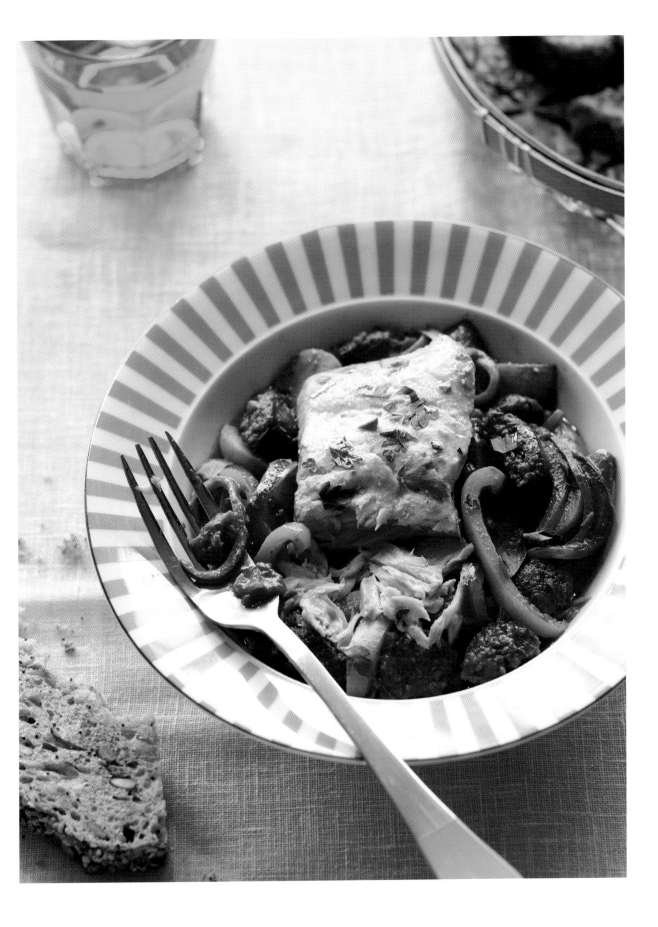

boursin chicken pasta traybake

I posted a video of a dish very similar to this one on my Facebook page, and it got over a million hits in a few days! This is a further adaptation of this dish, which I believe is better than ever. The creamy Boursin is baked in the oven and is the base of a delicious sauce.

MAKES 4 PORTIONS

1 x 150g (5½oz) pack of Boursin cheese (or garlic and herb cream cheese)
120g (4¼oz) cherry tomatoes
100g (3½oz) chestnut mushrooms, sliced
150g (5oz) spinach
500g (1lb 2oz) skinless diced chicken breast
4 smoked bacon medallions, all fat removed, cut into small strips
Drizzle of balsamic vinegar
180g (6½oz) dried pasta of your choice
Low-calorie cooking spray
Sea salt and freshly ground black pepper

Notes Boursin can be replaced with garlic and herb cream cheese. Leftovers can be kept in a sealed container in the refrigerator for up to 3 days.

Prep time 10 minutes | **Cook time** 35 minutes
Calorie count 450 calories per portion

Preheat the oven to 180°C/160°C fan/350°F/Gas mark 4.

Put the Boursin or cream cheese in the centre of baking tray (sheet), then scatter the cherry tomatoes, mushrooms and spinach around the cheese.

Add the diced chicken and bacon and sprinkle over a pinch of salt and pepper. Drizzle with a little balsamic vinegar and spray with low-calorie cooking spray.

Bake for 35 minutes, or until the tomatoes have cooked and are soft.

Meanwhile, cook the pasta in a saucepan of boiling water according to the packet instructions. Drain, retaining some of the cooking water to use later.

Remove the tray from the oven and mix everything together, breaking up the cheese. Make sure the chicken is cooked through at this point. Add a couple of tablespoons of the reserved pasta water to help create a smooth sauce.

Add the cooked and drained pasta, mix up with the rest of the dish and serve.

MAKE IT VEGGIE
This dish is also delicious without the chicken.

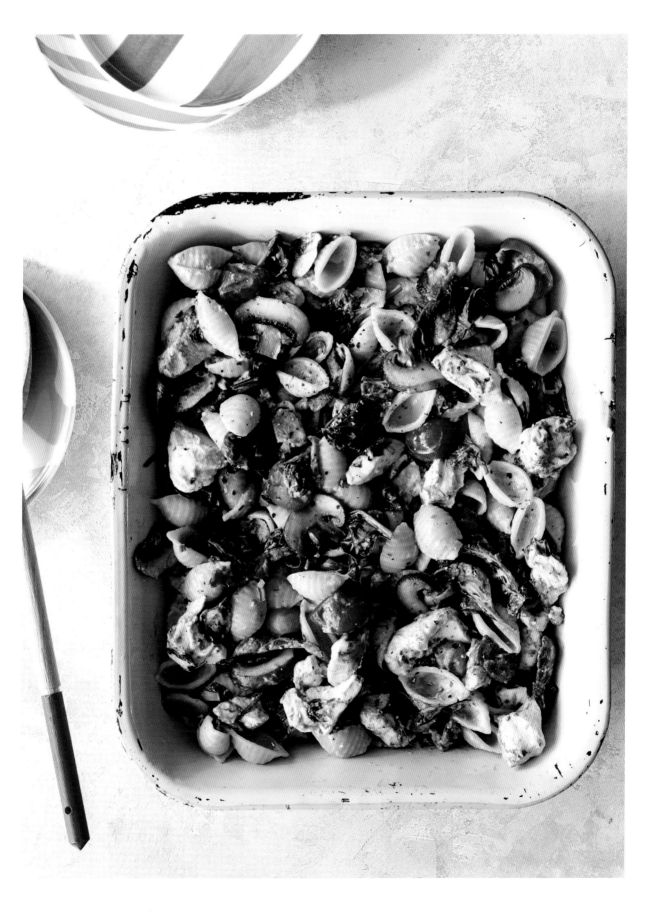

chicken, sweet potato and spinach bake

I am not exaggerating when I say that this is one of my favourite new meals that I have created. It is just so tasty! It's really easy to throw together and makes 4 good portions.

MAKES 4 PORTIONS

2 sweet potatoes, peeled and chopped into small chunks

1 tablespoon garlic powder

1 tablespoon onion powder

1 tablespoon smoked paprika

1 chicken stock cube, crumbled

2 large skinless and boneless chicken breasts, diced

1 red onion, finely chopped

10 mushrooms, sliced

2 garlic cloves, finely chopped

100ml (3½fl oz/scant ½ cup) chicken stock

100g (3½oz) low-fat cream cheese

Large handful of baby spinach

Low-calorie cooking spray

Sea salt and freshly ground black pepper

Note You can skip the parboiling of the sweet potatoes if you cut them into small enough chunks.

Prep time 15 minutes | **Cook time** 25 minutes
Calorie count 400 calories per portion

Parboil the sweet potatoes for 6 minutes in a saucepan of boiling water.

In a bowl, mix the garlic powder, onion powder, paprika, crumbled chicken stock cube and a large pinch of salt and pepper. Sprinkle this mixture over the diced chicken breasts in a mixing bowl and mix well.

Spray a frying pan (skillet) with low-calorie cooking spray and set over a medium heat. Add the chicken and cook for 2–3 minutes on each side. Once done, transfer the chicken to a baking dish.

Add the sweet potatoes to the pan you used to cook the chicken and fry for 3 minutes. Add the onion, mushrooms and garlic and cook for another 2–3 minutes. Turn off the heat, then add the stock and cream cheese and mix until the cheese has melted. Add more stock if it looks too thick, or more cream cheese if it looks too thin.

Pour this mix over the chicken in the baking dish and bake for 18–20 minutes, adding the spinach on top for the last 10 minutes of cooking time. Mix well and serve.

MAKE IT VEGGIE
Swap the chicken for tofu or a meat-free alternative, or omit and add extra vegetables instead.

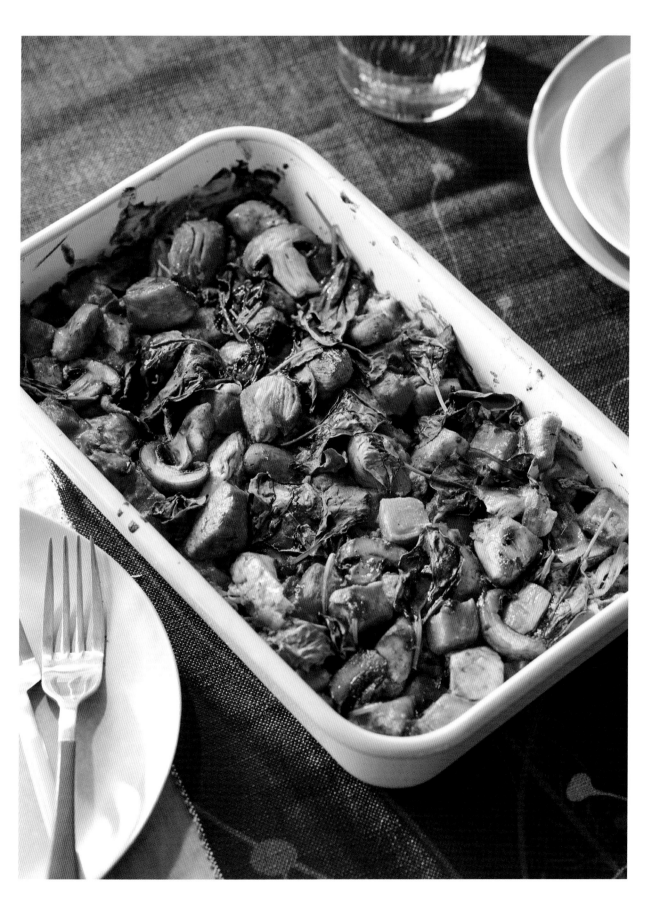

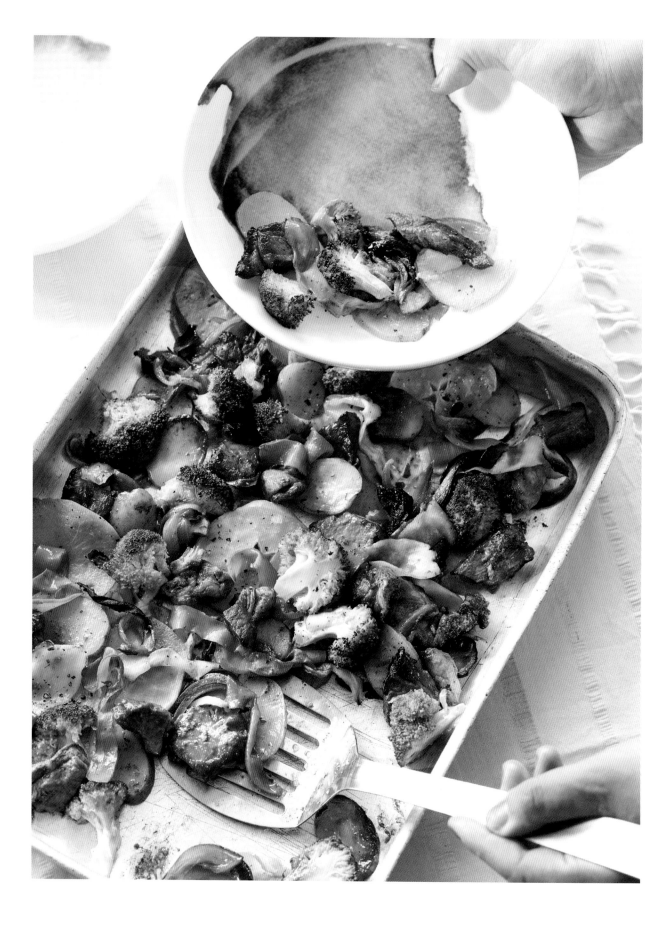

pork and apple traybake with honey and garlic

This is another recipe that is perfect for weeknight cooking. I love the sweet honey, apple and garlic flavours with the pork. The whole dish can be cooked in the tray, so there is minimal washing up to do.

MAKES 4 PORTIONS

2 tablespoons honey

2 garlic cloves, finely chopped

1 tablespoon balsamic vinegar

500g (1lb 2oz) diced pork (shoulder or leg)

1 red onion, sliced

1 carrot, peeled and sliced into thin strips

1 parsnip, peeled and sliced into thin strips

1 apple, skin on and sliced

1 head of broccoli, cut into small florets

150g (5oz) new potatoes, sliced into small chunks (make sure they're small or it won't cook through)

1 teaspoon dried parsley

Low-calorie cooking spray

Sea salt and freshly ground black pepper

Prep time 10 minutes, plus 30 minutes marinating
Cook time 50 minutes | **Calorie count** 320 calories per portion

Preheat the oven to 180°C/160°C fan/350°F/Gas mark 4.

Mix together the honey, garlic and balsamic vinegar in a small bowl. Place the pork in a large bowl and pour over the marinade. Leave for 30 minutes to marinate in the refrigerator.

Meanwhile, put the onion, carrot, parsnip, apple, broccoli and new potatoes in an ovenproof dish. Sprinkle over the parsley and some salt and pepper. Spray it with low-calorie cooking spray, then bake for 10 minutes.

Remove from the oven, then add the marinated pork to the dish. Pour over the excess honey and garlic mixture, then give everything in the dish a good mix around so that the flavours are evenly distributed.

Return to the oven for 40 minutes, or until the veggies and pork are fully cooked through

Notes I used diced pork in this recipe as it is my preferred cut, but this recipe would also work really well with pork chops, just adjust the calories. Leftovers can be kept in a sealed container in the refrigerator for up to 3 days. Reheat fully before serving.

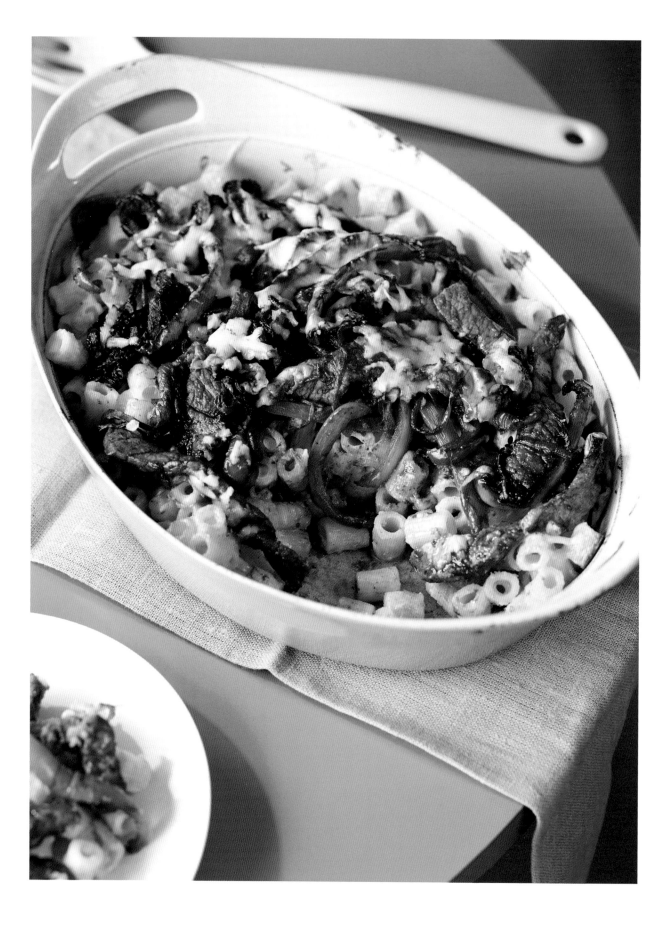

philly mac and cheesesteak

When I came up with the title of this recipe, I was so chuffed with myself. As the it suggests, this is two dishes fused together – Philadelphia cheesesteak and mac and cheese. If you're not familiar with Philadelphia Cheesesteak, it's an American dish with strips of steak and peppers with cheese in a baguette.

MAKES 4 PORTIONS

250g (9oz) dried pasta of your choice
1 green (bell) pepper, sliced
1 yellow (bell) pepper, sliced
1 large red onion, sliced
1 garlic clove, finely chopped
1 tablespoon balsamic vinegar
1 tablespoon Worcestershire sauce
1 teaspoon cayenne pepper
1 teaspoon smoked paprika
½ beef stock cube, crumbled
350g (12oz) thin beef steaks, cut into strips (often called minute steaks or sizzler steaks)
165g (5½oz) extra light cream cheese
160g (5½oz) extra light Cheddar
½ teaspoon mustard powder
Low-calorie cooking spray
Sea salt and freshly ground black pepper

Prep time 15 minutes | **Cook time** 25 minutes
Calorie count 445 calories per portion

Preheat the oven to 180°C/160°C fan/350°F/Gas mark 4.

Cook the pasta in a saucepan of boiling water according to the packet instructions. Drain, retaining some of the pasta water for use later.

Spray a frying pan (skillet) with low-caloric cooking spray and set over a medium heat. Add the peppers, onion and garlic and cook for about 3 minutes, or until the veg has softened.

Add the balsamic vinegar, Worcestershire sauce, cayenne pepper and smoked paprika and the crumbled up stock cube and season with salt and pepper.

Add the beef strips and cook for 2 minutes, turning them constantly and mixing them in with the sauce you've just created. After 2 minutes, remove from the heat and set the pan aside.

Put the cream cheese in a saucepan set over a low heat and stir until it has melted, careful not to let it overheat. Add half the Cheddar and the mustard powder, along with 3 tablespoons of the reserved pasta water.

Add the cooked pasta to the cheesy sauce, then pour the pasta into an ovenproof dish. Top with the steak, pepper and onion mixture and then the rest of the Cheddar and bake for 15 minutes, or until the cheese has completely melted.

tuscan sausage traybake

Sausages are so versatile, and they deserve so much more than being served with just breakfast or mash. This dish has so many tasty flavours all together in one.

MAKES 4 PORTIONS

8 lean chicken sausages
   (or lean pork sausages)
1 red onion, sliced
1 red (bell) pepper, sliced
1 yellow (bell) pepper,
   sliced
1 courgette (zucchini),
   sliced
1 garlic clove, finely
   chopped
350g (12oz) cherry tomatoes,
   halved
60g (2oz) stoned (pitted)
   black olives, halved
150ml (5fl oz/⅔ cup)
   vegetable stock
1 x 400g (14oz) tin of
   butter beans, drained
1 tablespoon cider vinegar
A few basil leaves
Low-calorie cooking spray
Sea salt and black pepper

Notes I really like this dish on its own, but it would also work well with some boiled new potatoes. Leftovers can be kept in a sealed container in the refrigerator for up to 3 days.

Prep time 10 minutes | **Cook time** 40 minutes
Calorie count 350 calories per portion (depending on the sausages used!)

Preheat the oven to 220°C/200°C fan/425°F/Gas mark 7.

Spray a roasting tin with low-calorie cooking spray and add the sausages. Bake for 15 minutes until the sausages have browned.

Add the onion, peppers, courgette, garlic, tomatoes and olives to the roasting tin and sprinkle with salt and pepper. Return to the oven for 10 minutes, turning the sausages halfway through.

Pour over the vegetable stock, butter beans and cider vinegar. Return to the oven for a final 15 minutes, or until the sausages are cooked through and the vegetables have softened. Serve sprinkled with the basil.

MAKE IT GLUTEN-FREE
Use gluten-free sausages to make the dish gluten-free.

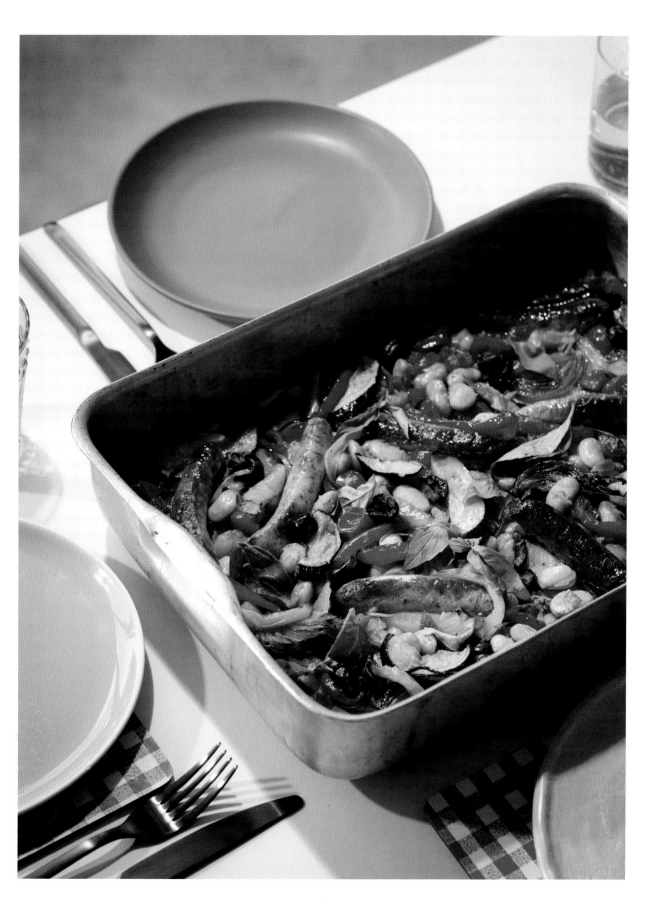

FABULOUS

FAKEAWAYS

One of my proudest moments, other than creating this book, was when I was dubbed the 'Queen of the Fakeaways' in the press.

I remember when I created my first fakeaway. It wasn't all that 'healthy', but making it myself meant it was much healthier than if I had ordered the takeaway itself. I made a pizza fakeaway with chicken strips, dough balls and mozzarella sticks. The feeling of accomplishment that I felt after making it, knowing that I had not only saved money, but had saved some calories too, was amazing.

Creating a Friday and Saturday night fakeaway became a weekly tradition for me. I would research different cuisines to try to recreate each time. Fakeaways don't just have to be a replication of certain brands or restaurant chains, but also different cuisines that you might get from a local takeaway, such as Chinese, Indian or Greek.

My fakeaway recipes have always been extremely popular, but they really went viral during the first lockdown when everything shut, including huge fast-food chains. People started searching how to recreate the food that they literally could no longer get hold of, meaning the concept of a fakeaway was even more important than ever. I was interviewed by television and radio about my recipes, which opened up my website to a whole host of new eyes.

This chapter contains a few of my classics, but also plenty of delicious new ideas to add to your repertoire.

loaded dirty fries

How do you make a portion of chips better? By loading them up with loads of toppings, of course! These chips are perfect for air frying (see note below), but also come out great if oven cooking.

MAKES 2 PORTIONS

450g (1lb) potatoes, cut into chips (no need to peel)

2 teaspoons Worcestershire sauce

2 teaspoons Cajun seasoning

1 red (bell) pepper, finely chopped

1 red onion, finely diced

4 smoked bacon medallions, fat removed, cut into strips

30g (1oz) low-fat red Leicester, grated

30g (1oz) low-fat Cheddar, grated

2 spring onions (scallions), thinly sliced

Low-calorie cooking spray

Sea salt and freshly ground black pepper

For the sriracha mayo

1 tablespoon sriracha

1 tablespoon mayonnaise

Note If you are using an air fryer for the chips, add them straight to the air fryer without par boiling, just sprinkle with 1 teaspoon Cajun seasoning, Worcestershire sauce, salt and pepper and give them a good spray with low-calorie cooking spray.

Prep time 10 minutes | **Cook time** 45 minutes
Calorie count 476 calories per portion

Preheat the oven to 200°C/180°C fan/400°F/Gas mark 6.

Make the sriracha mayo by mixing the ingredients together in a small bowl and set aside until needed.

Place the potatoes into a saucepan of boiling water and bring to the boil. Cook for 6 minutes until the chips start to soften. Drain, then shake them up in the saucepan to give them a fluffy edge.

Lay the chips out on a baking tray (sheet) and spray them with low-calorie cooking spray and sprinkle over half the Cajun seasoning and the Worcestershire sauce. Bake for 25 minutes until the chips start to crisp up and be golden. The cooking time will depend on how thin the chips have been cut, so keep an eye on them.

Meanwhile, prepare the topping. Spray a frying pan (skillet) with low-calorie cooking spray and set over a medium heat. Add the pepper and onion and fry for 3 minutes until the onion has softened. Add the bacon and cook for 5 minutes until the bacon has browned. Add the remaining Cajun seasoning and stir well.

Once the chips have cooked, remove them from the oven. I serve them on the same baking tray I used to cook them, but move the chips closer together into the middle of the tray.

Load the bacon, onion and pepper mix on top of the chips. Sprinkle the cheeses on top, then return the tray to the oven for 10 minutes, or until the cheese has melted.

Sprinkle over the spring onions and drizzle with the sriracha mayo to serve.

MAKE IT VEGGIE
Remove the bacon and Worcestershire sauce.

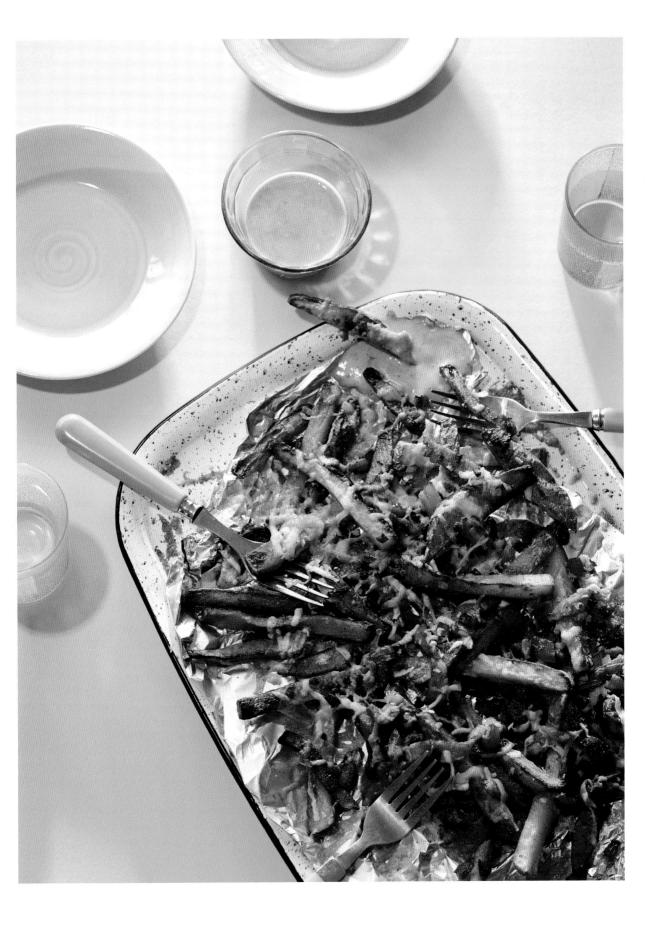

salt and pepper chilli chicken nuggets and chips

This is a twist on the Chinese takeaway classic salt and pepper chicken and salt and pepper chips. I breadcrumb the chicken so that it is more chicken nugget-like. The nuggets can be prepared ahead of time and refrigerated until ready to serve.

MAKES 2 PORTIONS

½ teaspoon Chinese five-spice
1 teaspoon sea salt
1 teaspoon ground black pepper
½ teaspoon dried chilli flakes
2 wholemeal bread slices, blitzed in a food processor to form breadcrumbs
1 egg
250g (9oz) skinless and boneless chicken breast, cut into chunks

For the chips

3 large potatoes, cut into chunky chips or wedges
½ teaspoon Chinese five-spice
½ teaspoon sweetener
1 teaspoon sea salt
1 teaspoon ground black pepper
½ teaspoon chilli flakes
1 onion, finely chopped
1 red (bell) pepper, finely chopped
1 green (bell) pepper, finely chopped
2 garlic cloves, sliced
1 red chilli, finely sliced
3 spring onions (scallions), finely sliced
Low-calorie cooking spray

Prep time 10 minutes | **Cook time** 35 minutes
Calorie count 589 calories per portion

Preheat the oven to 200°C/180°C fan/400°F/Gas mark 6.

Bring a saucepan of water to the boil, add the chips and simmer for 7 minutes.

Meanwhile, mix the Chinese five-spice, salt, pepper and chilli flakes for the chicken together with the breadcrumbs in a bowl.

Beat the egg in a separate bowl. Use one hand to dip the chicken pieces into the egg and drop them into the breadcrumbs, then use the other hand to take them out of the breadcrumbs. Repeat this process twice so that the chicken pieces are evenly coated in the breadcrumbs.

Drain the potatoes and give them a good shake in the saucepan so they get fluffy on the outside to help with the crispiness.

Mix the Chinese five-spice, sweetener, salt, pepper and chilli flakes for the chips together in a small bowl, then sprinkle this over the chips and give them a good stir.

Spread the chips out on a baking sheet and spray generously with low-calorie cooking spray. Bake for 20–25 minutes.

Lay the chicken nuggets out on a separate baking tray, spray with low-calorie cooking spray and bake for 25 minutes until the chicken is cooked all the way through in the middle.

Meanwhile, spray a frying pan (skillet) with low-calorie cooking spray and set over a low heat. Add the onion, peppers, garlic and chilli and fry for 5 minutes until the onions turn golden.

Remove the chips from the oven and tip them into a serving dish. Top with the fried onion and pepper mixture and the spring onions and serve with the chicken nuggets.

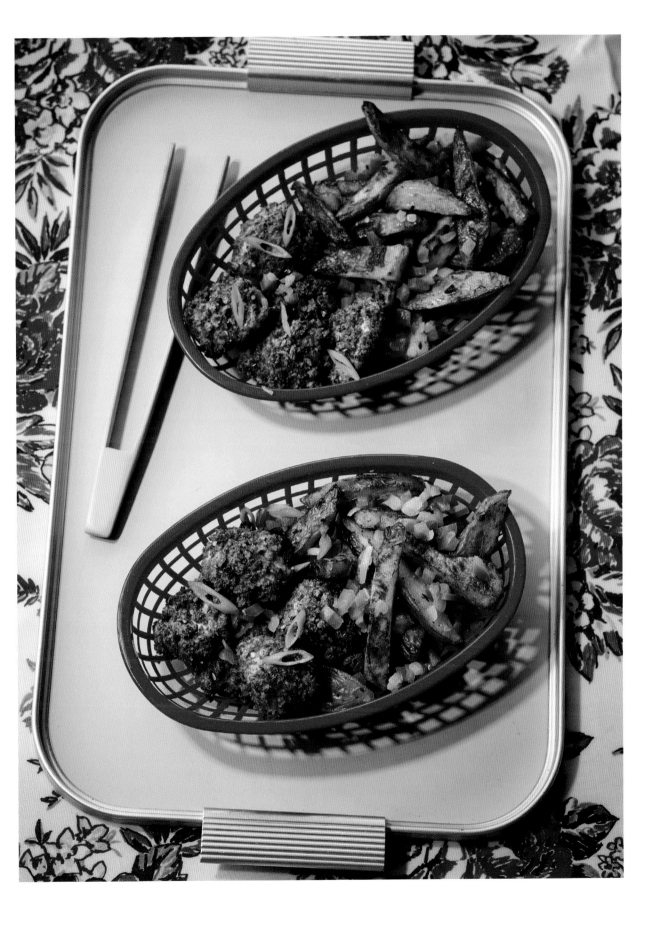

greek nachos

What are Greek nachos, I hear you ask? Well, it is my take on a Greek-Mexican fusion, with pitta bread nachos and a Greek salad salsa! This is makes a great sharing plate to have with friends.

MAKES 2 PORTIONS

2 large skinless and
    boneless chicken breasts
Juice of 1 lemon
3 garlic cloves, crushed
2 teaspoons red wine vinegar
2 tablespoons fat-free Greek
    yoghurt
2 teaspoons dried oregano
1 teaspoon dried sage
1 teaspoon dried oregano
½ small red onion

For the pitta nachos

4 wholemeal pitta breads,
    cut into small triangles
1 teaspoon dried oregano
Low-calorie cooking spray
Sea salt and freshly ground
    black pepper

For the Greek salsa

100g (3½oz) cherry tomatoes,
    chopped
½ red onion, finely chopped
30g (1oz) stoned (pitted)
    black olives, chopped
½ cucumber, chopped
½ teaspoon dried oregano
100g (3½oz) reduced-fat feta
    cheese, cubed

For the tzatziki

½ cucumber, chopped into
    small cubes
100g (3½oz) fat-free Greek
    yoghurt
1 small garlic clove, finely
    chopped
½ teaspoon dried mint

Prep time 10 minutes | **Cook time** 3/6 hours depending on slow cooker setting | **Calorie count** 400 calories per portion

Add the chicken, lemon juice, garlic, vinegar, yoghurt, dried herbs and onion into the slow cooker and cook on low for 6 hours or high for 3 hours.

Once the chicken has cooked, use two forks to shred it all apart then leave it in the slow cooker to keep warm while you prepare the rest of the dish.

Preheat the oven to 220°C/200°C fan/425°F/Gas mark 7.

To make the nachos, lay the pitta triangles out on a baking tray (sheet). Season with salt, pepper and the oregano and spray with low-calorie cooking spray. Bake for 10 minutes until they start to go golden and crispy.

Mix all the ingredients together for the salsa in a bowl.

Prepare the tzatziki by mixing all the ingredients together in another bowl.

Put the crisp nachos in a serving dish and layer the chicken, salsa and tzatziki on top.

Note This recipe uses a slow cooker to cook the chicken, but you could also cook it in a cast-iron casserole dish in an oven preheated to 160°C/140°C fan/325°F/Gas mark 3 for 1½ hours.

188

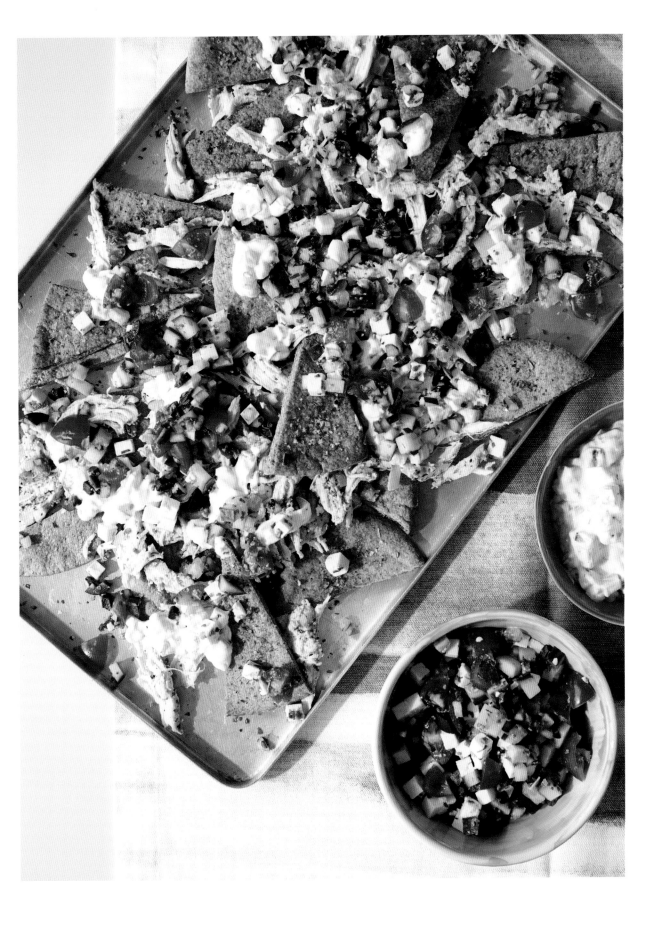

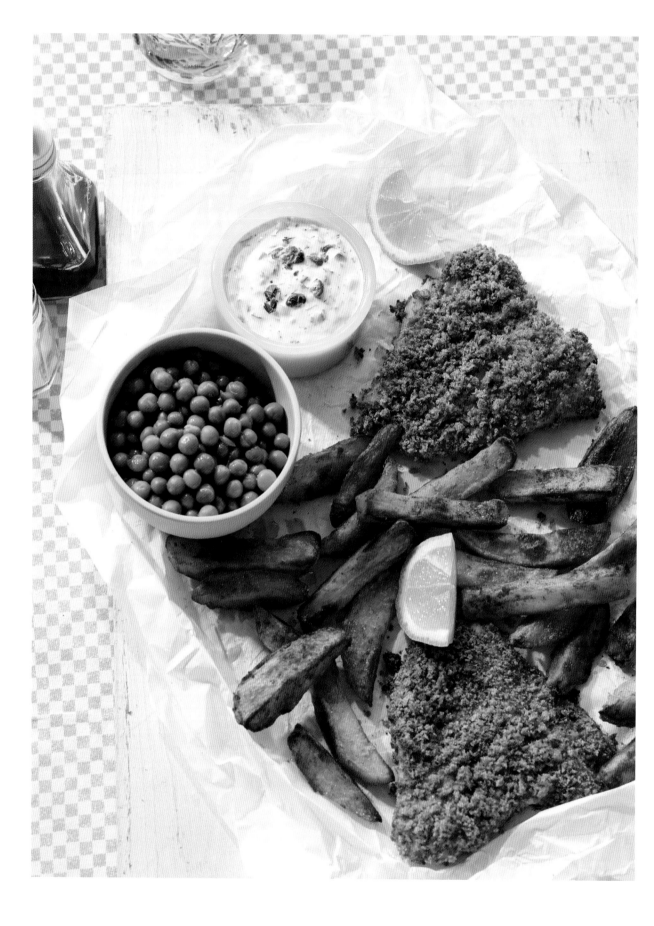

baked fish and chips with tartare sauce

All the flavours of the seaside, without any of the deep-frying. Simple to recreate at home with tasty oven-baked fish and chips and homemade tartare sauce. I absolutely LOVE tartare sauce – I think it's because of the pickled gherkins in it.

MAKES 2 PORTIONS

2 x 150g (5oz) skinless cod or haddock fillets

2 wholemeal bread slices, blitzed in the food processor to make breadcrumbs

1 egg, beaten

300g (2½ cups) frozen or tinned peas

Lemon wedges, to serve

Sea salt and freshly ground black pepper

For the chips

2 large potatoes, peeled and cut into chips

½ teaspoon smoked paprika

Low-calorie cooking spray

For the tartare sauce

4 tablespoons low-fat mayonnaise

1 tablespoon capers, drained and chopped

2 tablespoons gherkins, drained and chopped

1 small shallot, finely chopped

Juice of ½ lemon

1 tablespoon chopped parsley

Prep time 10 minutes | **Cook time** 40 minutes
Calorie count 560 calories per portion

Preheat the oven to 200°C/180°C fan/400°F/Gas mark 6.

Bring a saucepan of water to the boil and add the chips. Reduce the heat to a simmer and cook for 7 minutes. Drain the chips and give them a good shake in the pan so they get fluffy on the outside to help with the crispiness. Season the chips in the pan with salt, pepper and smoked paprika.

Spread the chips out on a baking tray (sheet) and give them a good spray of low-calorie cooking spray. Bake for 15 minutes.

Meanwhile, prepare the fish. Put the breadcrumbs and the beaten egg in separate bowls. The key to breadcrumbing is to make sure you use a different hand for the wet ingredients than you do for the dry ingredients. So use one hand to pick up the fish and put it in the egg, the same hand to take it out of the egg and drop it into the breadcrumbs, then use the other hand to take it out of the breadcrumbs. This prevents you from breadcrumbing your fingers! Repeat this process twice so that the fish is evenly coated in the breadcrumbs.

Lay the fish out on a baking tray, and after the chips have been in for 15 minutes, add the fish on the shelf below. Allow the fish and chips to cook for a further 15 minutes until the fish is cooked through and flakey.

Prepare the tartare sauce by mixing all the ingredients together in a bowl.

Warm the peas in a small pan or the microwave.

Serve the fish and chips with the peas, tartare sauce and lemon wedges for squeezing.

greek turkey meatball wraps

I love Greek flavours, and this is such a great use of turkey mince. Serving meatballs in warm pitta is my favourite way to eat them. Tzatziki is really easy to make and packs loads of flavour, too.

Meatballs are Gluten Free, just serve with a Gluten-free pitta or wrap

MAKES 2 PORTIONS

250g (9oz) extra lean minced (ground) turkey

25g (1oz) spinach, chopped

½ red onion, finely diced

3 garlic cloves, crushed

100g (3½oz) reduced-fat feta cheese, crumbled

2 tablespoons chopped parsley

1 teaspoon dried oregano

Sea salt and freshly ground black pepper

For the salad

100g (3½oz) cherry tomatoes, chopped

½ red onion, finely chopped

30g (1oz) stoned (pitted) black olives, chopped

½ cucumber, chopped into small cubes

½ teaspoon dried oregano

To serve

Wholemeal pitta bread (use gluten-free if needed)

Tzatziki (see page 188)

Prep time 10 minutes | **Cook time** 25 minutes
Calorie count 530 calories per portion

Preheat the oven to 220°C/200°C fan /425°F/Gas mark 7.

Line a baking tray (sheet) with baking paper.

Combine the turkey mince, spinach, red onion, garlic, feta, parsley, oregano and some salt and pepper in a large bowl. Use your hands to split the mixture into equal-sized chunks, then use the palms of your hands to roll them into even balls.

Lay the meatballs out on the lined baking tray and bake for 25 minutes until they are cooked through.

Prepare the salad by mixing all of the ingredients together in a large bowl.

Heat up a wholemeal pitta bread and layer on the meatballs, salad and tzatziki and serve.

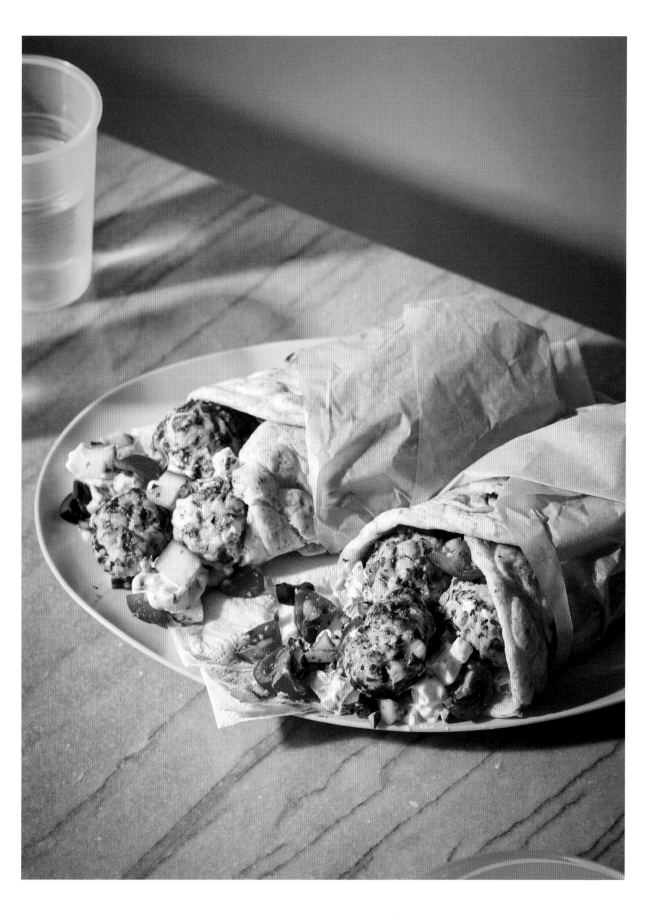

big double cheeseburger

This is my favourite dish on the popular burger chains' menu, but once I cracked the code of the delicious burger sauce, I make them at home all the time. It's the burger sauce that makes this dish – it tastes just like the sauce we all know and love!

MAKES 2 BURGERS

250g (9oz) extra lean minced (ground) beef
1 tablespoon tomato ketchup
½ teaspoon English mustard
Low-calorie cooking spray
Sea salt and freshly ground black pepper

For the burger sauce

2 tablespoons low-fat mayonnaise
2 small gherkins, finely chopped
1 teaspoon white vinegar
Pinch of white pepper
1 teaspoon English mustard
½ teaspoon onion powder
½ teaspoon garlic powder
½ teaspoon smoked paprika
1 teaspoon pickle juice

To serve

3 burger buns
Iceberg lettuce, shredded
Low-fat cheese slices

Prep time 10 minutes | **Cook time** 10 minutes
Calorie count 475 calories per portion

Make the burgers by mixing the beef mince with the ketchup, mustard and a generous pinch of salt and pepper in a mixing bowl. Give it a good stir, then split it into 4 equal-sized balls and set them aside.

Prepare the burger sauce by mixing all of the ingredients together in a small bowl.

Spray a frying pan (skillet) with low-calorie cooking spray and set over a medium heat. Add 2 of the burgers and use the back of a spatula to press the ball out as flat as possible to create a burger. I like mine thin, so press down as much as you can. Fry on each side for 4 minutes, or until the middle is no longer pink. Repeat this with the other 2 balls.

To assemble the burger as authentically as possible, start with the base of the burger bun. Then add the lettuce, burger sauce and a cheese slice. Then add one of the burgers, then the other base of the bun, more sauce and lettuce, the second burger and then the top of the bun.

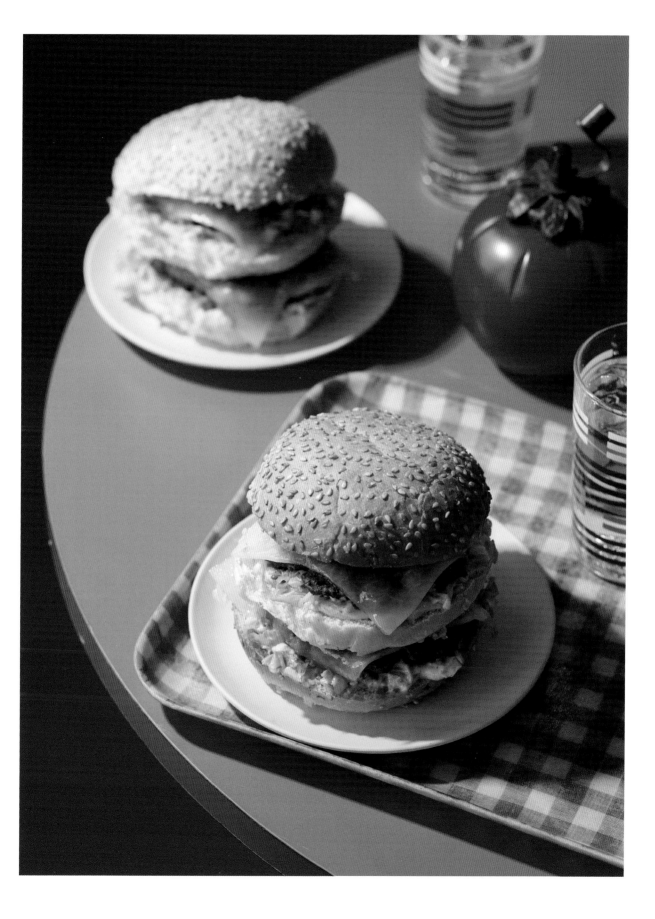

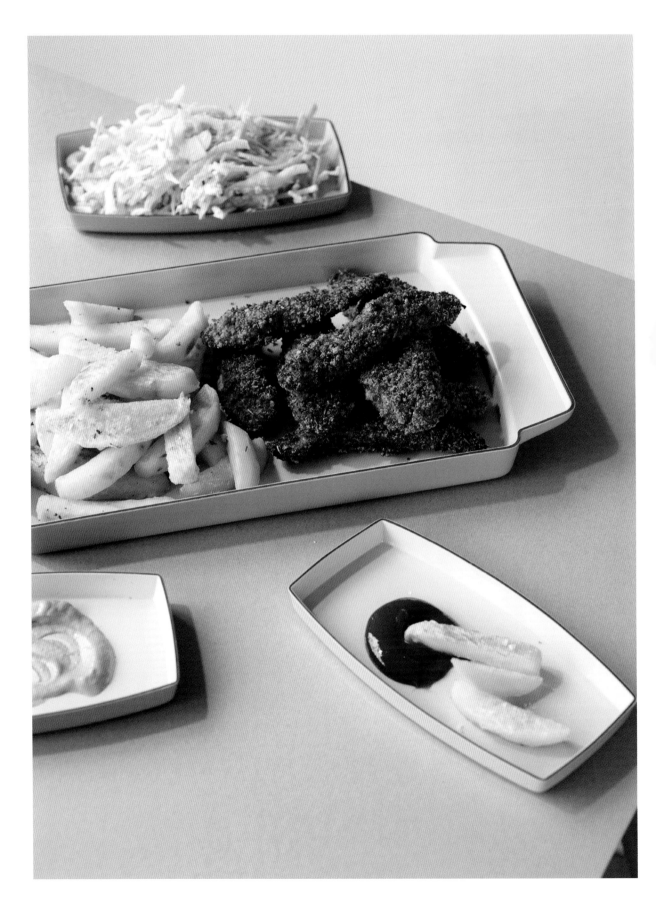

southern 'fried' chicken feast

I have been making this fakeaway dish for years, and it still remains one of the oldest and most popular recipes on my blog. It's so simple to prepare and the classic coleslaw and chips are the perfect accompaniment for this fakeaway feast.

MAKES 2 PORTIONS

4 wholemeal bread slices, blitzed in a food processor to breadcrumbs
1 teaspoon dried oregano
1 teaspoon chilli powder
1 teaspoon dried sage
1 teaspoon dried basil
1 teaspoon freshly ground black pepper
2 teaspoons sea salt
2 teaspoons paprika
1 teaspoon garlic powder
1 teaspoon garlic salt
1 egg, beaten
2 large skinless or boneless chicken breasts, cut into smaller strips or chunks

For the chips
2 large potatoes, cut into thin chips
Low-calorie cooking spray

For the coleslaw
2 carrots, grated
½ head of white cabbage, shredded
1 apple, peeled and grated
½ onion, grated
3 tablespoons fat-free Greek yoghurt
1 tablespoon low-fat mayonnaise

Prep time 15 minutes | **Cook time** 40 minutes
Calorie count 590 calories per portion

Preheat the oven to 200°C/180°C fan/400°F/Gas mark 6.

Bring a saucepan of water to the boil and add the chips. Reduce the heat to a simmer and cook for 7 minutes.

Meanwhile, mix the breadcrumbs with the all of the seasonings in a bowl and mix until combined.

Beat the egg in a separate bowl. The key to breadcrumbing is to make sure you use a different hand for the wet ingredients than you do for the dry ingredients. So use one hand to pick up the chicken pieces and put it in the egg, the same hand to take it out of the egg and drop it into the breadcrumbs, then use the other hand to take it out of the breadcrumbs. This prevents you from breadcrumbing your fingers! Repeat this process twice so that the chicken pieces are all evenly coated in the breadcrumbs.

Place the chicken pieces on a baking tray (sheet).

Drain the chips, then give them a good shake in the pan so they get fluffy on the outside to help with the crispiness. Season with salt and pepper, give them a good spray of low-calorie cooking spray and spread out on a baking tray (sheet).

Bake the chicken and the chips for 20–25 minutes until the chicken is cooked through and the chips are crispy.

To make the coleslaw, mix all the ingredients together in a bowl.

Serve the chicken with the crispy chips and creamy coleslaw.

Note I like to use boneless chicken breasts, but this also works with chicken on the bone, such as drumsticks.

speedy cheesy pizza with roasted cherry tomato sauce

I absolutely adore pizza, but making pizza from scratch can be time-consuming, and I am far too impatient to wait for the cheesy goodness! This pizza base is very similar to a flatbread, made with Greek yoghurt and self-raising (self-rising) flour. This means you don't need to use yeast or wait around for the base to rise, and the cherry tomato sauce can roast itself while you make the base. Once you get this recipe down, you can let your creativity go wild and add all your favourite toppings.

**MAKES 2 PORTIONS
(2 SMALL PIZZAS OR 1
LARGE PIZZA TO SHARE)**

110g (4oz/generous ¾ cup)
    self-raising (self-
    rising) flour, plus extra
    for dusting
125g (4½oz) fat-free Greek
    yoghurt
80g (3oz) reduced-fat
    Cheddar
120g (4¼oz) reduced-fat
    fresh mozzarella
Low-calorie cooking spray

For the sauce
170g (6oz) cherry tomatoes,
    halved
1 large garlic clove
1 tablespoon balsamic
    vinegar
1 teaspoon dried oregano
1 teaspoon dried basil
Sea salt and freshly ground
    black pepper

Note Any leftover pizza
sauce is perfect to use as
a dip.

Prep time 15 minutes | **Cook time** 25 minutes
Calorie count 473 calories per serving

Preheat the oven to 220°C/200°C fan/425°F/Gas mark 7.

Put all of the sauce ingredients into an ovenproof dish and bake for 15 minutes.

Meanwhile, prepare the base. Mix the flour and yoghurt together in a large bowl until combined and starts to form a dough. If it looks a little too wet or sticky, add a tiny bit more flour (adjust the calories though if you do!)

Sprinkle some flour on the worktop and turn the dough out. Knead the dough for about 10 minutes, or until it looks like a proper dough and is springy to the touch.

Spray a pizza dish or large baking tray (sheet) with some low-calorie cooking spray. Press the pizza dough onto the tray, forming 2 small pizzas or 1 large sharing pizza.

Remove the sauce from the oven, the tomatoes should now be soft enough to mash up with a fork. If you like a smoother sauce, blitz it up in a food processor or blender until smooth. Otherwise, use a fork to mash it all together.

Spread the sauce on the pizza base, then top with grated Cheddar. Rip the mozzarella into small chunks and spread out evenly on top of the Cheddar.

Place the pizza in the oven on a high shelf and bake for 15 minutes until the crust is golden and the cheese is bubbling.

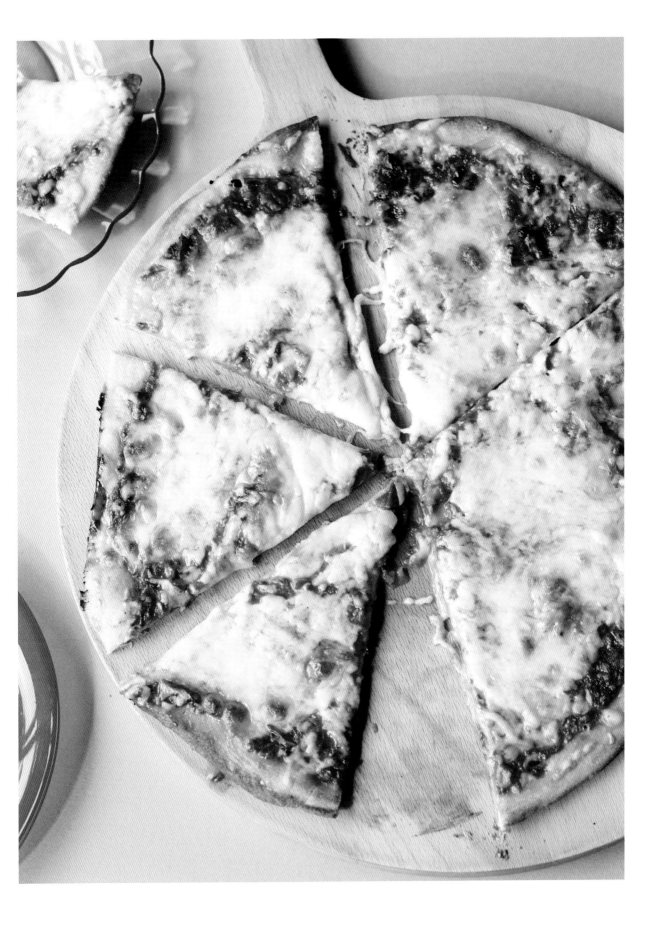

beef burritos

I love Mexican food. Growing up in the UK, I think many of us started learning how to make Mexican food from those kits you can get in the supermarket. But, once you get the hang of making it without those kits, you'll realize just how easy (and how much cheaper, healthier and tastier) it is to do it from scratch yourself.

MAKES 2 PORTIONS

1 onion, finely chopped

3 garlic cloves, very finely chopped

1 tablespoon ground cumin

1 tablespoon ground coriander

Small pinch of cayenne pepper (adjust according to your taste)

1 teaspoon dried oregano

1 beef stock cube, crumbled

500g (1lb 2oz) extra lean minced (ground) beef

1 tablespoon red wine vinegar

1 x 400g (14oz) tin of chopped tomatoes

1 x 400g (14oz) tin of black beans or kidney beans

60g (2oz) long-grain rice

2 tortilla wraps

Low-calorie cooking spray

To serve

½ avocado, peeled, stoned (pitted) and sliced

2 tablespoons reduced-fat sour cream

½ head of iceberg lettuce

120g (4¼oz) grated Cheddar

Sliced jalapeños

Chopped cherry tomatoes

Prep time 15 minutes | **Cook time** 40 minutes
Calorie count 440 calories per portion

Spray a frying pan (skillet) with low-calorie cooking spray and set over a medium heat. Add the onion and fry for 5 minutes until softened.

Add the garlic, cumin, coriander, cayenne, oregano and crumbled stock cube and cook for 1 minute.

Add the beef mince and fry for 5 minutes, then add the red wine vinegar and chopped tomatoes. Leave to simmer for 10 minutes over a low heat, then add the black beans or kidney beans with the water from the tin. Leave the beef to simmer for 20 minutes until the sauce has reduced down.

Meanwhile, bring a large saucepan of water to the boil and cook the rice according to the packet instructions. Drain.

To assemble the burrito, heat up the tortilla wraps, then add some rice, the beef mixture and then the toppings of your choice. Keep the filling in the middle, then fold up the edges and roll up the wrap to enclose all of the fillings.

Note The beef filling can be kept in the refrigerator for 2 days and reheated with a splash of water.

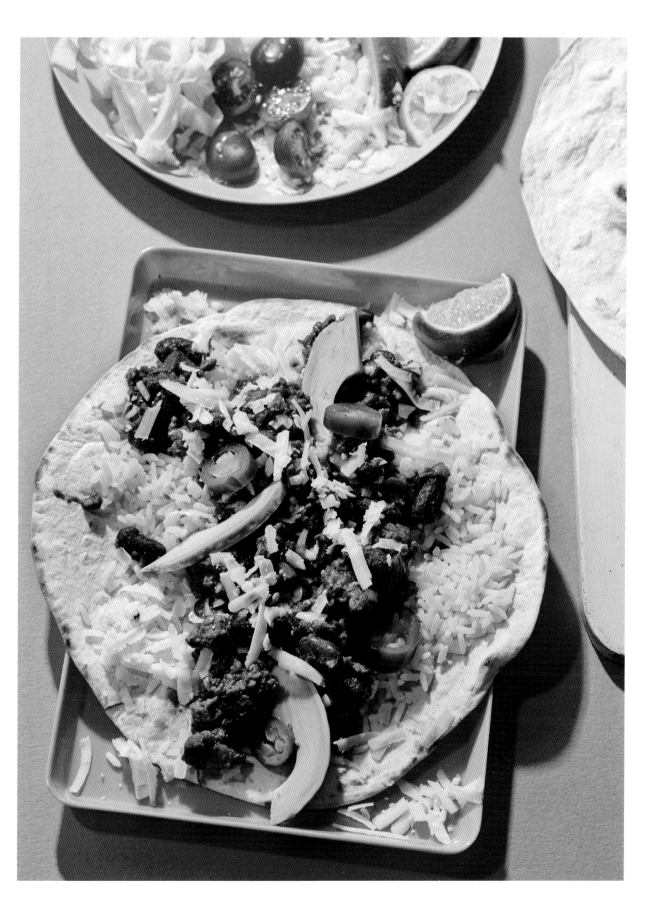

cheesy chilli chicken enchiladas

I absolutely LOVE enchiladas. They're probably one of the first things I started to regularly cook from scratch when I first left home. No need for a kit, because they are so easy to prepare yourself.

MAKES 4 PORTIONS

4 skinless and boneless
   chicken breasts
4 teaspoons ground cumin
4 teaspoons garlic powder
4 teaspoons smoked paprika
2 x 500g (1lb 2oz) cartons
   of passata (sieved
   tomatoes)
2 garlic cloves, crushed
1 green chilli, deseeded and
   finely chopped (leave out
   if you don't want spice!)
1 teaspoon granulated
   sweetener
1 large red (bell) pepper,
   chopped
1 red onion, finely chopped

To assemble

8 tortilla wraps
160g (5¾oz) extra-light
   Cheddar
Low-calorie cooking spray

Prep time 10 minutes | **Cook time** 55 minutes
Calorie count 550 calories per portion

Preheat the oven to 200°C/180°C fan/400°F/Gas mark 6.

Put all the ingredients into a large ovenproof dish and give everything a good mix. Bake for 40 minutes.

Remove the chicken breasts from the dish and use 2 forks to shred the meat. Return the shredded chicken back to the dish and mix well. This is the enchilada filling.

Spray a separate ovenproof dish with low-calorie cooking spray.

Spoon a couple of tablespoons of the chicken filling onto a wrap, then fold the edges over to enclose the filling. Place the folded wrap in the ovenproof dish, seam side down. Repeat until the wraps have been used, reserving some of the filling for topping.

Pour the remaining filling over the top of the enchiladas in the dish, then top with the cheese.

Bake for 15 minutes until the cheese has melted and is bubbling.

Note Leftovers can be kept in a sealed container in the refrigerator for up to 3 days. Reheat fully before serving.

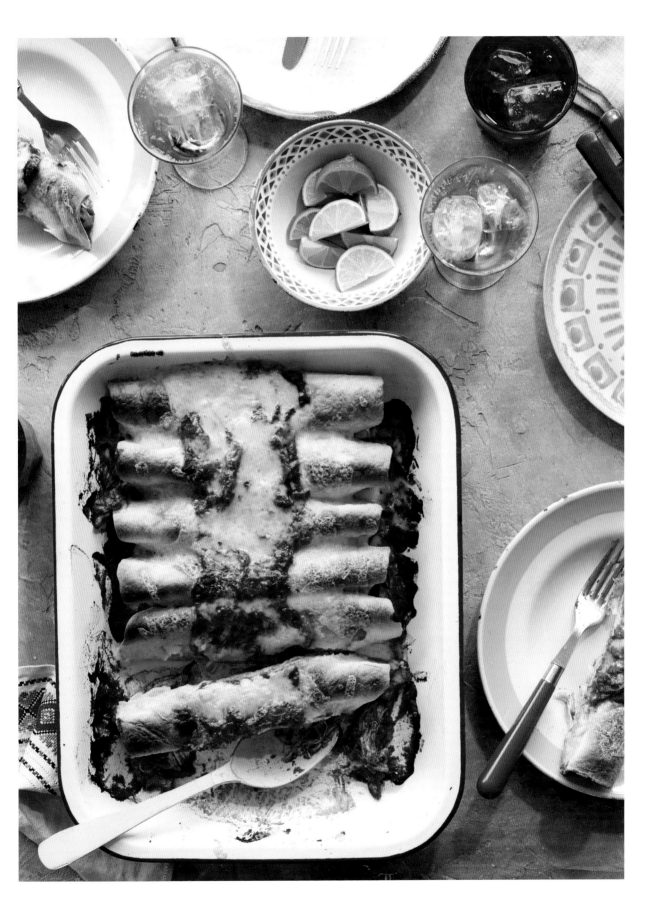

creamy swedish-style meatballs

No trip to the Swedish home superstore would be complete without some meatballs at the end! This is a super easy take on their classic dish. The original is made with lots of cream and butter, which I have swapped for low-fat cream cheese.

MAKES 2 PORTIONS

400g (14oz) lean minced
(ground) pork
1 egg
Sea salt and freshly ground
black pepper

For the sauce

1 onion, finely chopped
1 garlic clove, crushed
120g (4¼oz) mushrooms,
chopped
150g (5oz) low-fat cream
cheese
100ml (3½fl oz/scant ½ cup)
beef stock
1 tablespoon chopped dill,
plus extra to serve
1 teaspoon beef gravy
granules
Low-calorie cooking spray

Prep time 10 minutes | **Cook time** 15 minutes
Calorie count 536 calories per portion

Prepare the meatballs by mixing the the pork mince with the egg in a large bowl. Season well. Use your hands to form about 12 small, equal-sized meatballs.

Spray a large frying pan (skillet) with low-calorie cooking spray and set over a medium heat. Fry the onion, garlic and mushrooms for a few minutes to soften. Add the meatballs and cook until browned on all sides. Use a slotted spoon to remove the meatballs and set aside.

Add the cream cheese and beef stock to the pan and stir into the cooking juices. Stir in the dill and gravy granules and cook for 10 minutes. Add the meatballs back to the pan to heat through and mix with the sauce. Taste and season.

Serve the meatballs with mashed potato (remembering to add the calories) and some dill sprinkled on top.

~~~~~

Notes Delicious with pasta, rice or mashed potatoes - just adjust the calories accordingly. Leftovers can be kept in a sealed container in the refrigerator for up to 5 days.

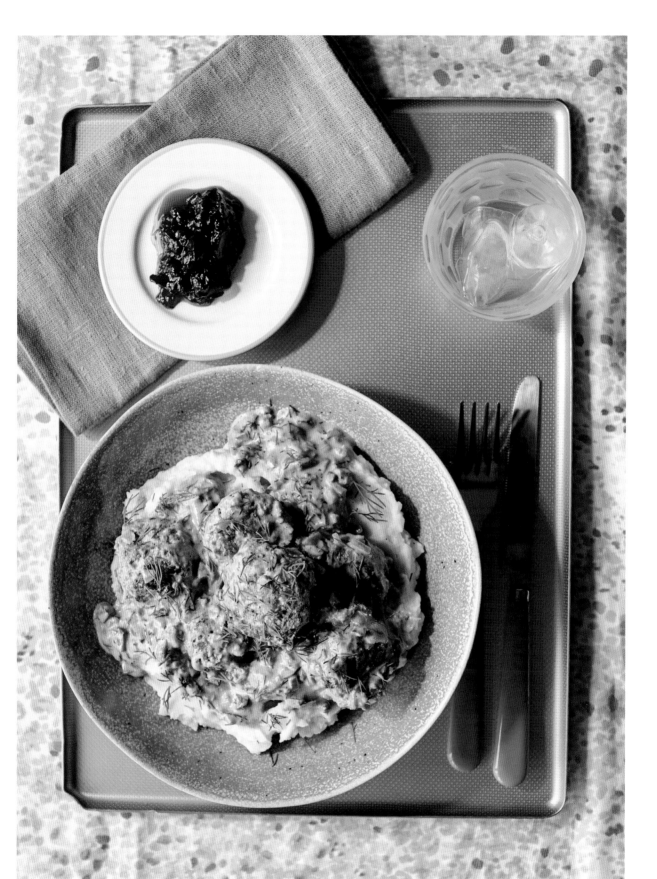

chicken katsu curry burger

This is my take on a high street burger chain katsu burger with a pickled slaw and curry sauce. Any excuse for a bit of katsu curry! Did you know that the base of a katsu curry sauce is made from carrots? You do now!

MAKES 2 PORTIONS

2 skinless and boneless chicken breasts
50g (1¾oz) panko breadcrumbs
1 egg, beaten
2 burger buns, to serve

For the katsu curry sauce

4 garlic cloves, crushed
1 teaspoon fresh grated ginger
1 large onion, chopped
1 courgette (zucchini), chopped
2 carrots, chopped
1 teaspoon ground turmeric
2 teaspoons ground cumin
2 teaspoons ground coriander
1 teaspoon chilli powder
1 tablespoon sweetener
1 tablespoon soy sauce
250ml (9fl oz/1 cup) chicken stock
1 bay leaf
Low-calorie cooking spray

For the pickled slaw

120ml (4½fl oz/½ cup) rice vinegar
½ teaspoon sea salt
½ head of white cabbage, shredded
2 carrots, grated
3 radishes, grated

Prep time 15 minutes | **Cook time** 40 minutes
Calorie count 540 calories per portion

Preheat the oven to 200°C/180°C fan/400°F/Gas mark 6.

First, prepare the slaw by mixing together all the ingredients in a bowl. Leave to pickle while you prepare the rest of the dish.

Place each chicken breast in some cling film (plastic wrap) and flatten with a rolling pin or meat tenderizer to get a flatter breast. This helps with the cooking. Once flattened, remove from the cling film.

Put the breadcrumbs and beaten egg in separate shallow bowls. Use one hand to pick up the chicken, dip it in the egg, then drop it into the breadcrumbs, then use the other hand to take it out of the breadcrumbs. Repeat this process twice so that the chicken is evenly coated in the breadcrumbs.

Place the breasts on a baking tray (sheet) and bake for 25 minutes until crisp and golden and cooked through.

Meanwhile, make the sauce. Spray a saucepan with low-calorie cooking spray and set over a medium heat. Add the onion, garlic and ginger and cook for 3 minutes until the onion is softened. Add the courgette and carrots and lightly fry for a further 4–5 minutes.

Add the turmeric, cumin, coriander, chilli powder, sweetener, soy sauce, stock and bay leaf and bring to the boil. Reduce the heat and simmer for 20 minutes.

Remove the bay leaf from the sauce and pour the contents into a food processor or blender. Blitz to a thick, smooth sauce.

Drain any excess vinegar off the pickled slaw.

Prepare your burger by spooning some pickled slaw on the burger base, top with the chicken and spoon over some curry sauce, then add the top bun.

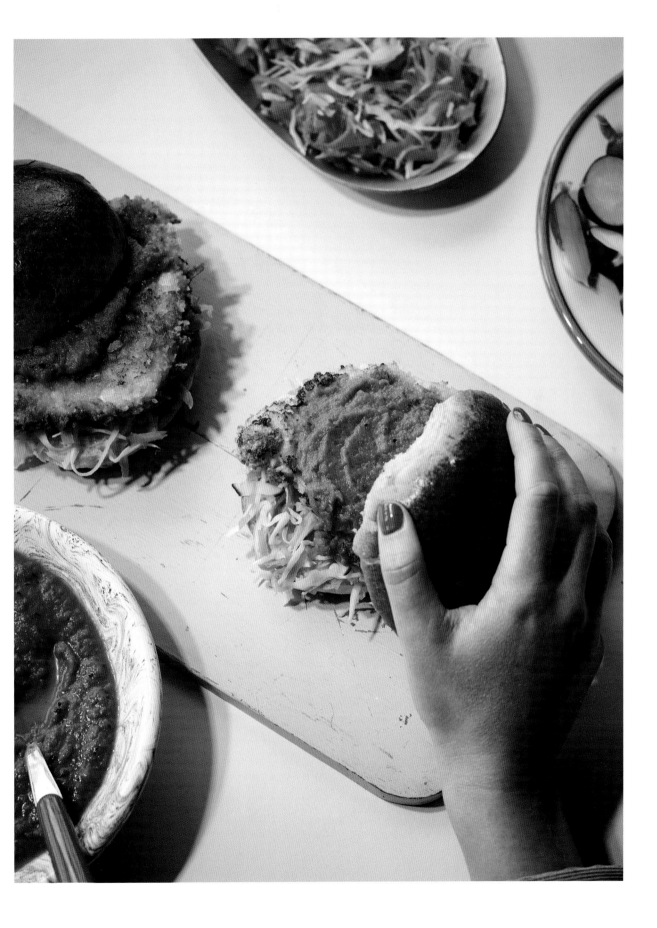

tandoori chicken kebabs with flatbreads

This dish is inspired by Tandoori flavours, with marinated chicken in yoghurt, lemon and spices. Unfortunately, I don't own a tandoor – the clay oven used to make authentic tandoori chicken – but this is the next best way to recreate those flavours at home.

**MAKES 2 PORTIONS
(2 KEBABS)**

4 tablespoons fat-free Greek yoghurt
2 teaspoons chilli powder (adjust according to taste)
½ teaspoon garam masala
½ teaspoon ground coriander
½ teaspoon ground cumin
1 teaspoon ground turmeric
½ teaspoon ground cardamom
¼ teaspoon ground cinnamon
¼ teaspoon ground nutmeg
1 teaspoon grated fresh ginger
1 garlic clove, grated
Juice of 1 lemon
2 skinless and boneless chicken breasts, cut into chunks
Low-calorie cooking spray
Lettuce and tomatoes, to serve

For the flatbreads

75g (2¾oz/generous ½ cup) self-raising (self-rising) flour, plus a little extra for dusting
½ teaspoon baking powder
75g (2¾oz) natural yoghurt
Pinch of crushed garlic
Sea salt

Note The longer you can marinate the chicken, the better.

Prep time 10 minutes, plus 1 hour marinating
Cook time 20 minutes | **Calorie count** 400 calories per portion

Make the chicken marinade by mixing the yoghurt, chilli powder, garam masala, ground spices, ginger, garlic and lemon juice together in a large bowl. Taste it at this point to make sure it isn't too spicy; if it is, add a little more yoghurt and lemon to reduce the spice levels.

Add the chicken and mix well to make sure the chicken is well coated. Cover and leave to marinate for 1 hour.

Put all the ingredients for the flatbreads into a bowl, mix with a spoon, then use your hands to bring everything together into a dough.

Sprinkle the worktop with a little flour. Turn the dough out and knead for a minute or so to bring it all together. It won't need as much kneading as traditional bread.

Split the dough into 2 portions, then pat and flatten the each piece. Use a rolling pin to roll each piece into a 12cm (4¾in) round, about 2–3mm (⅛in) thick.

Spray a griddle pan with low-calorie cooking spray and heat over a medium-high heat. Add each flatbread, one at a time, and heat for 2 minutes on each side until it has slightly puffed up and has griddle lines.

Thread the chicken pieces onto a metal kebab stick (if using wooden sticks, soak them in water for 30 minutes first).

Preheat the grill (broiler) to high and grill (broil) the kebabs for 7 minutes on each side until the chicken is cooked all the way through.

Serve the chicken in the flatbreads with salad.

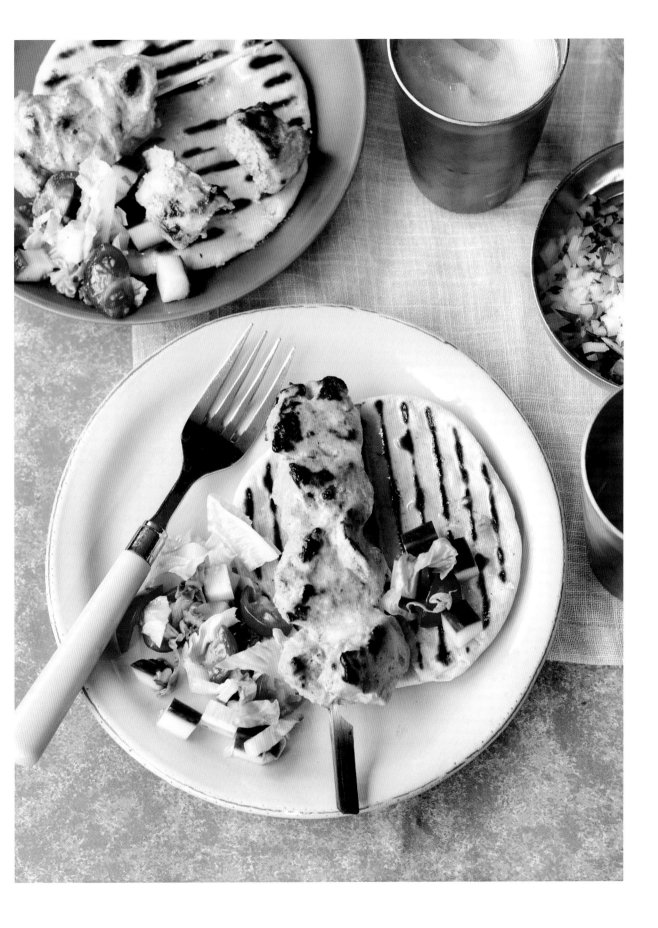

lamb bhuna

My favourite way to cook lamb curry is in the slow cooker as it helps the lamb to just melt in the mouth when you eat it. Slow cooking a curry also helps the flavours to develop. Above all else, it's super easy to just pop in the slow cooker after a little prep work and leave it to do its thing! I love serving with this rice – just remember to adjust the calories.

MAKES 4 PORTIONS

600g (1lb 5oz) diced lamb leg, extra fat trimmed off

2 onions, finely chopped

10 curry leaves

1 fresh red chilli, deseeded and finely chopped

1 teaspoon cumin seeds

1 teaspoon mustard seeds

1 teaspoon ground coriander

½ teaspoon ground fenugreek

1 tablespoon tomato purée (paste)

1 x 400g (14oz) tin of chopped tomatoes

1 teaspoon garam masala

Low-calorie cooking spray

For the marinade

6 garlic cloves, finely chopped

1 teaspoon of lazy ginger (or a small thumb-sized piece of ginger, grated)

2 tablespoons malt vinegar

½ teaspoon ground cinnamon

Prep time 15 minutes, plus 1 hour marinating
Cook time 3½ hours | **Calorie count** 350 calories per portion

Mix all the ingredients for the marinade together in a small bowl and pour over the lamb. Cover and leave to marinate for 1 hour.

Meanwhile, start preparing the curry. Spray a large frying pan (skillet) with low-calorie cooking spray and set over a medium heat. Add the onions and cook for 5 minutes until they are golden and softened.

Add the curry leaves and chopped chilli and cook for a minute, then add the cumin seeds, mustard seeds, ground coriander and ground fenugreek. Stir and allow the spices to fry and become aromatic for a 1–2 minutes.

Add the marinated lamb and any excess marinade and cook for 5 minutes until the lamb has browned on each side.

At this point, pour the contents of the pan into the slow cooker Add the tomato purée, chopped tomatoes and garam masala, stir and cover. Cook on high for 3 hours.

Alternatively, cook in a cast-iron casserole dish for 2 hours in an oven preheated to 140°C/120°C fan/275°F/Gas mark 1.

Note Will keep in a sealed container in the refrigerator for up to 3 days. Reheat fully before serving.

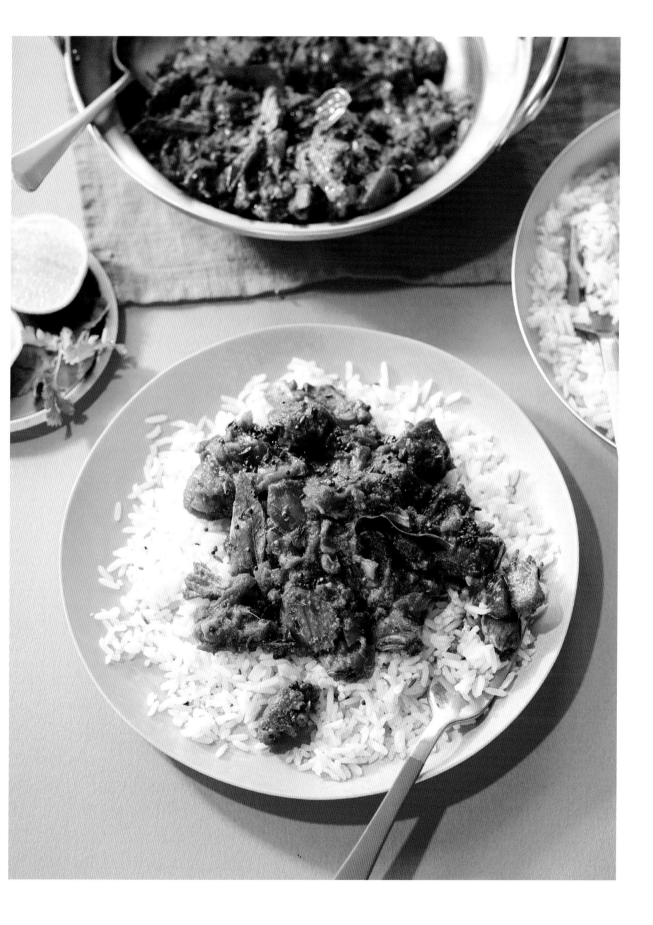

sugar pink special fried rice

You may think of fried rice as being a side dish, but I truly believe that it is good enough to be the star of the show! This recipe works best if using a little oil in the pan or wok.

MAKES 2 PORTIONS

85g (3oz/½ cup) long-grain rice (or 225g/8oz/scant 2 cups leftover cooked rice)

1 tablespoon vegetable oil

1 garlic clove, chopped

1 tablespoon fresh grated ginger

2 eggs, beaten

100g (3½oz/generous ¾ cup) frozen peas, thawed and drained

100g (3½oz) cooked chicken, diced

285g (10oz) cooked small prawns

2 tablespoons soy sauce

3 spring onions (scallions), finely chopped

Sea salt and freshly ground black pepper

Prep time 10 minutes | **Cook time** 15 minutes
Calorie count 559 calories per portion

First, bring a large saucepan of water to the boil and cook the rice according to the packet instructions. Once cooked, drain and chill the rice.

Heat the vegetable oil in a wok or frying pan (skillet) over a medium heat. Add the garlic and ginger to the pan and cook for 2 minutes.

Add the cooked and chilled rice, season with salt and pepper and stir-fry for about 5 minutes over a high heat.

Move the rice to one half of the pan/wok, then add the beaten eggs to the other.

Mix the eggs as they cook, then as they start to set, gradually mix parts of the rice in with the eggs.

Add the peas, chicken, prawns and soy sauce, mix well and allow to heat through. Season with salt and pepper.

Serve with chopped spring onions on top.

MAKE IT VEGGIE
Omit the prawns and chicken and replace them with vegetables.

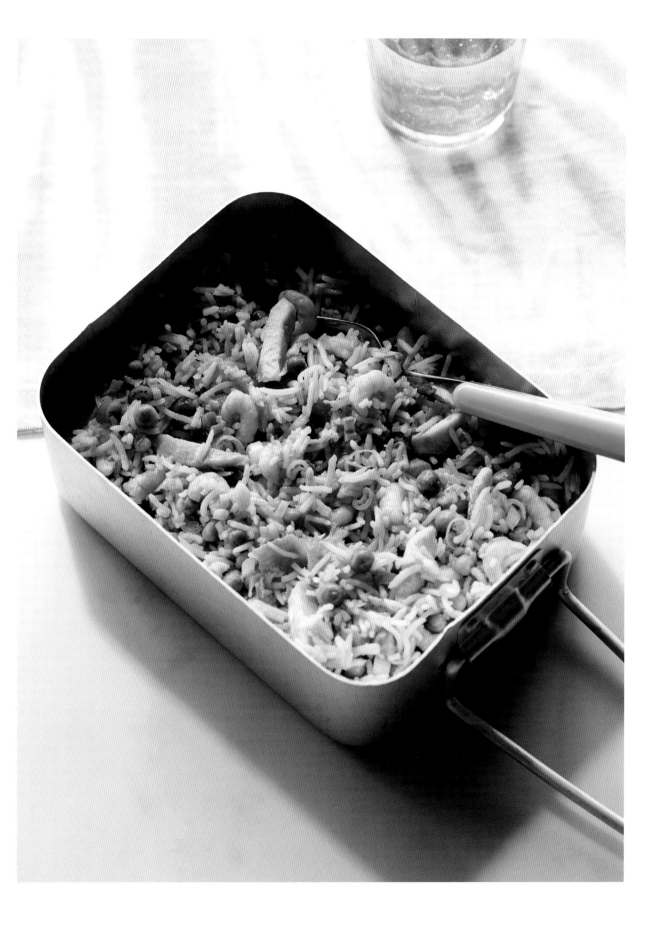

chinese crispy shredded chilli beef

I absolutely love crispy shredded beef from the Chinese takeaway, but since I worked out how to recreate a 'fakeaway' version instead, I've never looked back! It's much simpler than you may think, too.

MAKES 4 PORTIONS

500g (1lb 2oz) lean rump
    steak, any extra fat
    removed
2 tablespoons cornflour
    (cornstarch)
1 carrot, cut into
    matchsticks
½ onion, chopped
1 garlic clove, finely
    chopped
1 red (bell) pepper, sliced
½ teaspoon grated fresh
    ginger
2 tablespoons sweet chilli
    sauce
2 tablespoons tomato purée
    (paste)
2 tablespoons Worcestershire
    sauce
1 tablespoon clear honey
1 tablespoon lemon juice
1 teaspoon dried chilli
    flakes
200ml (7fl oz/generous
    ¾ cup) beef stock
5 spring onions (scallions),
    chopped
Low-calorie cooking spray
Sea salt and freshly ground
    black pepper

Prep time 10 minutes | **Cook time** 15 minutes
Calorie count 350 calories per portion

Preheat the oven to 200°C/180°C fan/400°F/Gas mark 6.

Flatten out the rump steak and cut it into thin strips. Season the meat, then coat each strip in cornflour and lay them out flat on a shallow baking tray (sheet). Bake for 10 minutes, turning the strips over halfway through.

Spray a frying pan (skillet) with low-calorie cooking spray and set over a low heat. Add the carrot, onion, garlic, red pepper and ginger and and fry for about 5 minutes.

In a bowl, mix together the sweet chilli sauce, tomato purée, Worcestershire sauce, honey, lemon juice, chilli flakes and enough of the stock to bring it together into a smooth sauce (you can discard any leftover stock). Add the sauce to the frying pan and cook for a few minutes until it thickens.

Add the cooked beef strips to the pan, mix well, then serve immediately so that they stay crispy.

Sprinkle the spring onions on top to serve.

Note The key to keeping the beef crispy is to very quickly mix it around in the sauce, and then serve straight away.

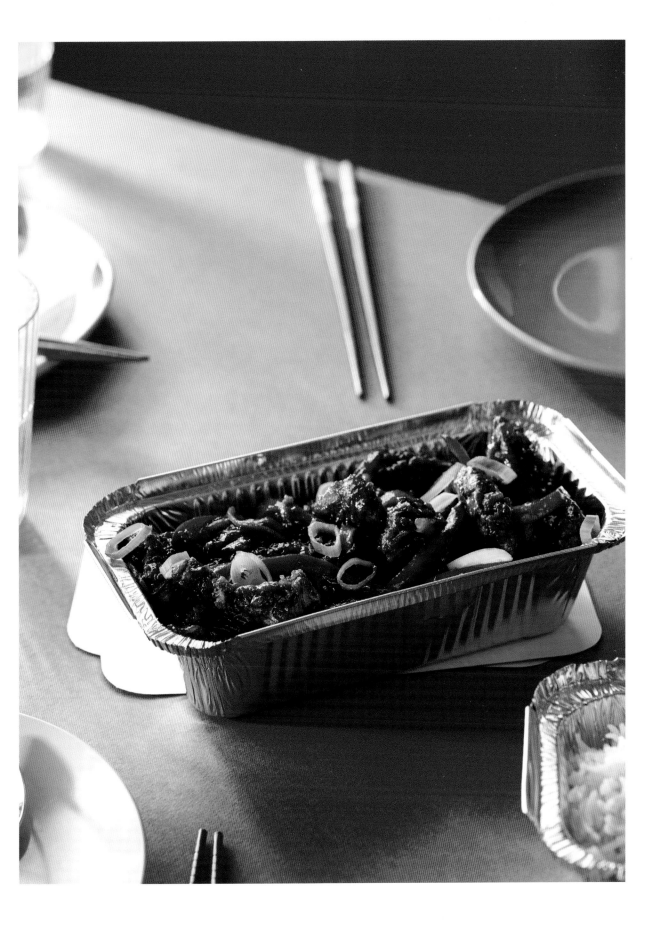

slow cooker chinese chicken curry noodles

Chinese curries are elite, and in my opinion, you can't beat a classic Chinese chicken curry! This is a super simple all-in-one slow cooker dish, making your fakeaway life even easier! I used coconut milk because it makes it extra creamy and delicious.

MAKES 4 PORTIONS

500g (1lb 2oz) skinless and
  boneless chicken breast,
  diced
1 onion, finely chopped
2 tablespoons tomato purée
  (paste)
1 x 400g (14oz) tin of light
  coconut milk
1 tablespoon ground turmeric
2 tablespoons curry powder
1 garlic clove, finely
  chopped
Thumb-sized piece of fresh
  ginger, grated
1 teaspoon chilli powder
½ teaspoon Chinese
  five-spice
1 teaspoon soy sauce
150g (5oz) dried egg noodles
100g (3½oz/¾ cup) frozen
  peas

Note If you don't have
a slow cooker, you can
cook this in a frying pan
(skillet). Just cook the
onion first, then the
chicken and then the rest of
the ingredients and cook for
15 minutes until the chicken
has cooked through.

Prep time 5 minutes | **Cook time** 5 hours
Calorie count 400 calories per portion

Place all of the ingredients, except the noodles and peas, into the bowl of a slow cooker and stir well. Set the slow cooker to high and leave for 4 hours.

Add the noodles and peas and stir together. Leave for another hour in the slow cooker, then serve.

MAKE IT VEGGIE
Swap the chicken for vegetables of your choice, or use a meat-free alternative.

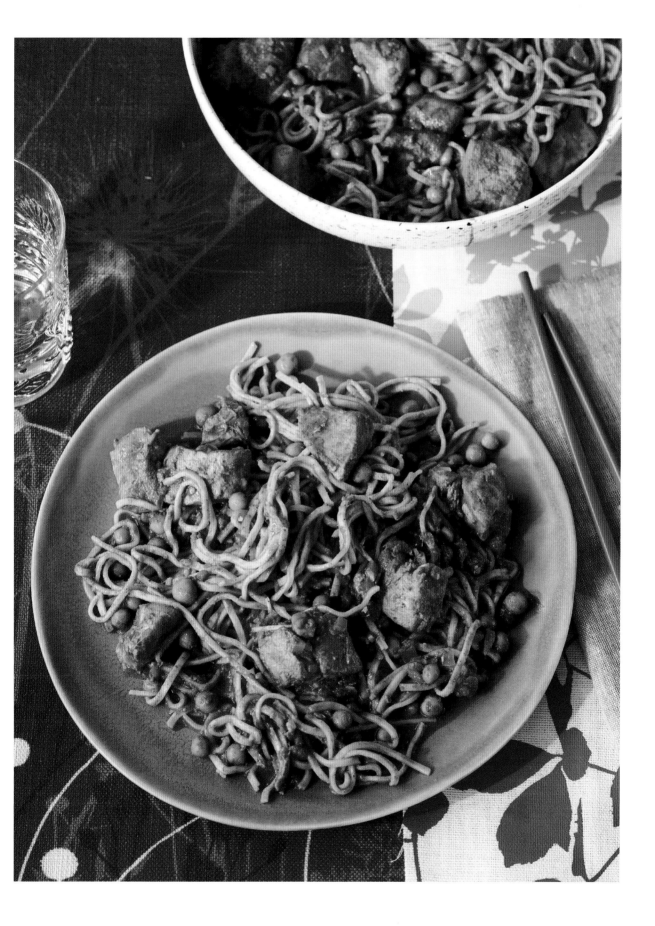

honey and chilli chicken

Honey and chilli are such a traditional and delicious combination; the spice and the sweet balance each other out perfectly. I like to use sriracha, but you could use any chilli sauce. I like mine pretty spicy, too, so adjust according to your taste.

Prep time 5 minutes, plus 30 minutes marinating
Cook time 25 minutes | **Calorie count** 450 calories per portion

MAKES 2 PORTIONS

2 large skinless and boneless chicken breasts
4 lime wedges

For the marinade

3 tablespoons honey
2 tablespoons sriracha (or chilli sauce)
3 garlic cloves, finely chopped
2 tablespoons rice wine vinegar
1 tablespoon low sodium soy sauce
1 tablespoon freshly squeezed lime juice

To serve

Cooked rice
Sliced spring onions (scallions)

Mix the ingredients of the marinade together in a bowl. Add the chicken breasts and stir to make sure the chicken is well covered with sauce. Leave to marinate for at least 30 minutes, or preferably for a few hours.

Preheat the oven to 200°C/180°C fan/400°F/Gas mark 6.

Lay the chicken out in an ovenproof dish and add the lime wedges on top. Bake for 25 minutes, basting the chicken with the sauce halfway through the cooking time. Check to make sure the breasts are fully cooked through before serving.

Serve with rice, sprinkling over some spring onions. Drizzle any leftover sauce on top.

MAKE IT VEGGIE
Swap the chicken for a meat-free alternative.

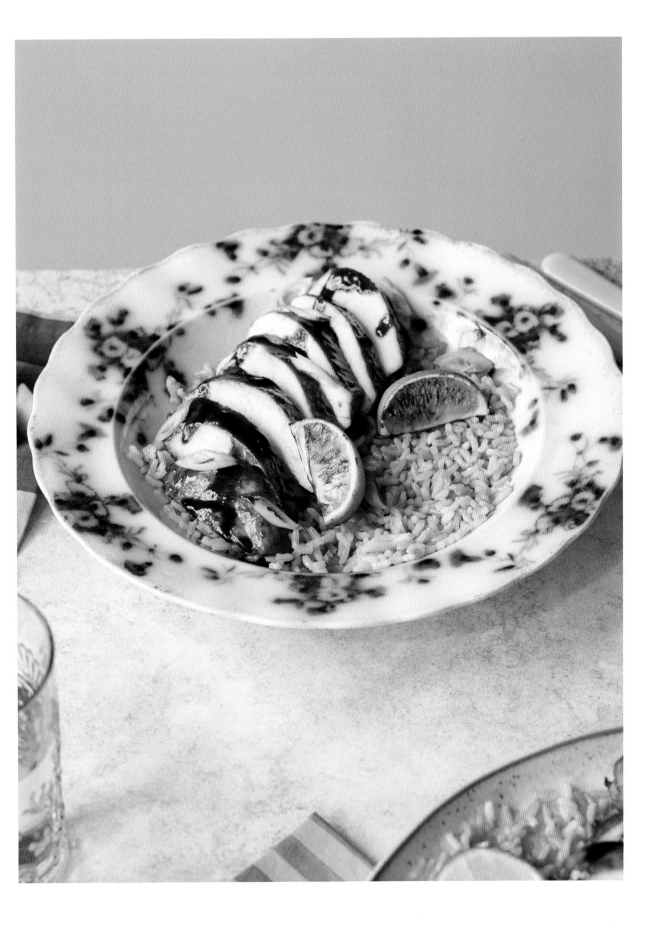

chicken satay with lime and chilli rice

I have paired this chicken in a delicious peanut sauce with a zingy chilli and lime rice. This dish is a peanut butter lover's dream, with succulent grilled chicken skewers in a tasty peanut marinade and tasty peanut dipping sauce.

MAKES 4 PORTIONS

2 teaspoons clear honey

2 tablespoons soy sauce

2 tablespoons mild curry powder

Small piece of fresh ginger, peeled and grated

3 garlic cloves, finely chopped

Juice of 1 lime

5 tablespoons smooth peanut butter

500g (1lb 2oz) skinless and boneless chicken breast fillets

165ml (5½fl oz/⅔ cup) tin of light coconut milk

For the rice

150g (5oz/¾ cup) jasmine rice

1 red chilli, deseeded and finely chopped

Juice of 1 lime

Fresh coriander (cilantro), roughly chopped

Note Leftover sauce can be kept in the refrigerator for up to 3 days in a sealed container.

Prep time 10 minutes, plus 30 minutes marinating
Cook time 20 minutes | **Calorie count** 479 calories per portion

Make the marinade for the chicken by combining the honey, soy sauce, curry powder, ginger, garlic, lime juice and peanut butter together in a bowl.

Place the diced chicken in a large bowl and add 2 tablespoons of the marinade. Mix well and leave to marinate for 30 minutes.

Thread the diced chicken onto kebab skewers.

Preheat the grill (broiler) to high, then cook the skewers for 7 minutes on each side until the chicken is cooked through.

Add the rest of the marinade to a saucepan set over a low heat and mix with the coconut milk. Keep stirring while you heat the sauce through.

Meanwhile, boil the rice according to the packet instructions. Add the chopped chilli about 5 minutes before the end of the cooking time.

Drain the rice, then stir through the lime juice and coriander.

Serve the chicken skewers on the rice and pour over the satay sauce, or leave on the side for dipping.

MAKE IT VEGGIE
Swap the chicken for a meat-free alternative.

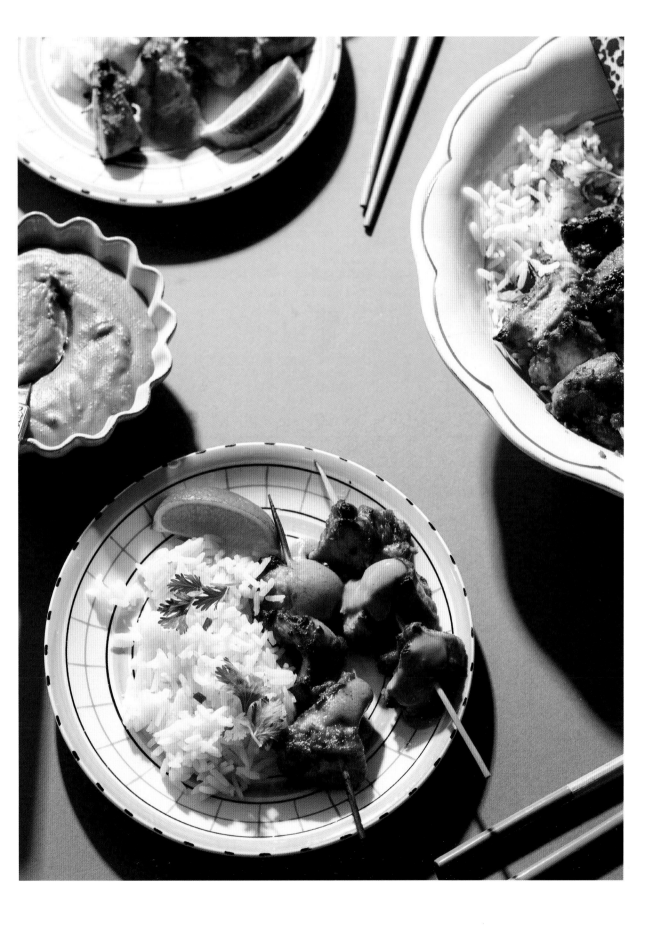

lo mein noodles

You may have heard of a chow mein, but this lo mein recipe could be your new favourite. The difference between the two is how the noodles are prepared. In a chow mein, the noodles are fried, whereas with a lo mein the cooked noodles are tossed in the sauce and veggies. This recipe has a bit of a kick to it, so don't forget to adjust the spice if you don't like it too hot. Sriracha is relatively spicy, so if you're not a fan of spice, only add half a tablespoon instead.

MAKES 2 PORTIONS

300g (10½oz) dried egg
    noodles
1 garlic clove, finely
    chopped
1 tablespoon fresh grated
    ginger (or 'lazy' ginger
    from a jar)
1 teaspoon dried chilli
    flakes
1 red (bell) pepper, sliced
½ head of broccoli, cut into
    small florets
Low-calorie cooking spray

For the sauce

2 tablespoons low salt soy
    sauce
1 tablespoon sriracha
1 tablespoon rice vinegar
1 teaspoon sesame oil
½ teaspoon sweetener
Sea salt and freshly ground
    black pepper

Note I love to eat this dish
cold as well as hot, so if
you have any leftovers, keep
them in a sealable container
in the refrigerator for up
to 5 days.

Prep time 10 minutes | **Cook time** 10 minutes
Calorie count 330 calories per portion

Bring a large saucepan of water to the boil and cook the noodles according to the packet instructions. Drain, then set aside.

Spray a large frying pan (skillet) or wok with low-calorie cooking spray, set over a medium-high heat and add the garlic, ginger and chilli flakes. Stir-fry for 2 minutes. Add the veggies and fry for 2 minutes.

Mix all the ingredients for the sauce together in a bowl with 2 tablespoons water.

Pour the sauce into the vegetables, and leave it to simmer for 3 minutes.

Add the cooked noodles to the sauce and stir well until everything is coated evenly.

MAKE IT VEGAN
Swap the egg noodles for rice noodles.

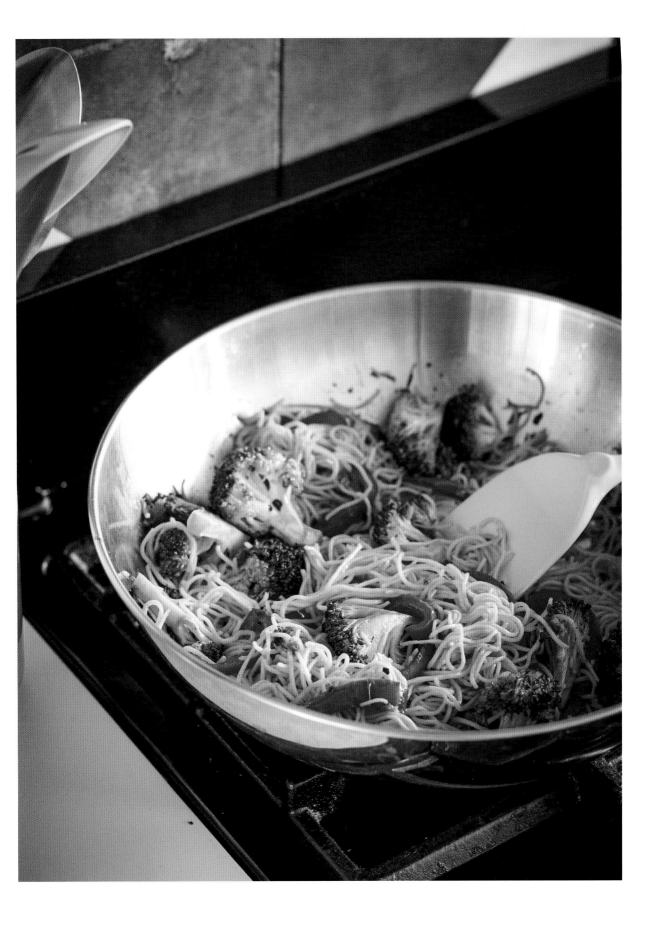

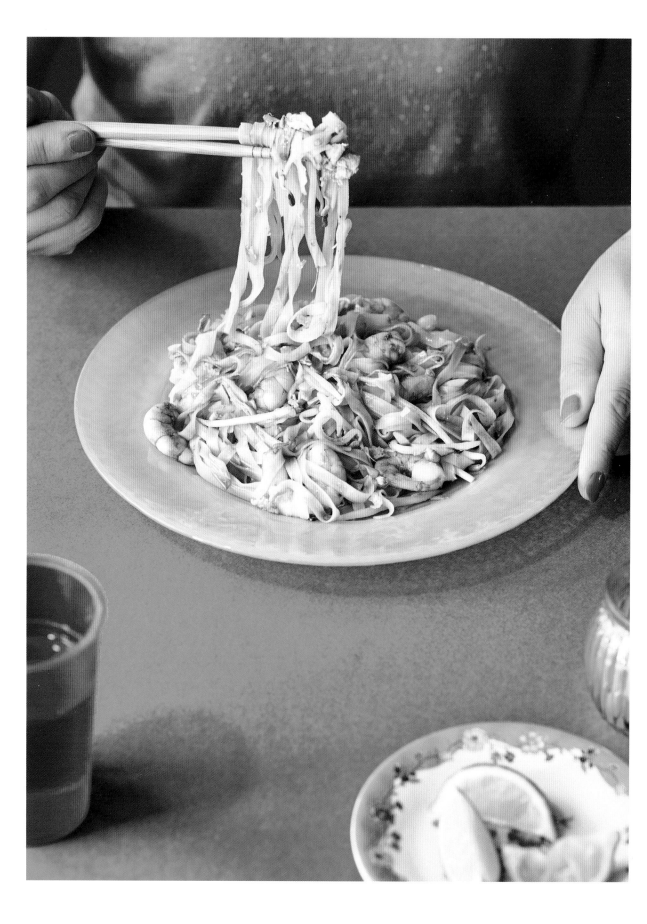

pad thai

Pad Thai is a street-food-style noodle dish from Thailand. It's so easy to whip up, and I find it a really light and tasty meal to enjoy in the evenings. You should be able to get tamarind paste from your local supermarket or Asian food shop.

MAKES 4 PORTIONS

250g (9oz) wide rice noodles
2 teaspoons tamarind paste
3 tablespoons fish sauce
1 teaspoon granulated
 sweetener
1 garlic clove, finely diced
3 spring onions (scallions),
 finely diced
1 egg
200g (7oz) large cooked
 prawns (shrimps)
75g (2¾oz) beansprouts
Low-calorie cooking spray
Lime wedges, to serve

Prep time 5 minutes | **Cook time** 10 minutes
Calorie count 359 calories per portion

Add the noodles to a bowl and pour over some boiling water. Leave to stand for 5 minutes, or until they are soft. Once softened, drain them well.

Mix the tamarind paste, fish sauce and sweetener together in a small bowl.

Heat a large frying pan (skillet) or wok over a high heat. Spray with low-calorie cooking spray and add the garlic and spring onions.

Push the vegetables to the sides of the wok, then crack the egg into the centre. Keep stirring the egg for 30 seconds until it begins to set.

Add the prawns and beansprouts, followed by the noodles, then pour over the fish sauce mixture. Mix everything together and heat through.

Note Leftovers can be kept in the refrigerator for up to 5 days

MEAL

PLANS

For years I have been sharing 'Meal Plan Monday' posts on my social media channels, where I share a seven-day meal plan with delicious, low-calorie breakfast, lunch and dinner recipes. Thousands of people interact with these posts, telling me how much they help them prepare for the week.

I find that having a meal plan in place not only helps keep me on track, but it saves a lot of effort in the evenings trying to decide what I can make for dinner or what ingredients I have left to use up before they go off. It is great for saving money on the food shop, too, as I only buy the ingredients that I need to make the meals in the plan.

This plan uses some of the delicious slimming and tasty meals from the book. If any don't take your fancy, they could easily be swapped out for others.

Snacks
Here are some snack suggestions to accompany all of the meal plans:
- fruit
- low-calorie crisps
- low-fat yoghurts
- fruit dipped in nut butter
- vegetable crisps
- protein bars
- breakfast bars

the working week meal plan

This is the meal plan for you if you are a busy worker who struggles to have the motivation to cook healthy meals for yourself.

The plan assumes that you are preparing breakfasts and lunch for yourself, and then cooking a shared evening meal. Of course, if you are not sharing your evening meal you can utilize the leftovers to have as your lunch instead.

Breakfast and lunch are both prep-ahead meals to make life easier, and the evening meals are simple and easy recipes. Of course, Friday and Saturday nights wouldn't be complete without a cheeky fakeaway!

This meal plan is based on 1500 calories per day. If you are not following a plan as strict as this, this leaves room for some low-calorie snacks.

If you do any exercise during the day, track the number of calories you burn as you will be able to have additional snacks or a larger portion size. Some meals are split into four portions, so if not all four portions are being eaten and you want to use some extra calories, you could have a larger portion.

	BREAKFAST	LUNCH	DINNER	TOTAL CALORIES
MONDAY	Sunny Breakfast Casserole (445 calories) See page 29	Greek Orzo (330 calories) See page 94	Boursin Chicken Pasta Traybake (450 calories) see page 172	**1,225** — Total left over for snacks: 275
TUESDAY	Sunny Breakfast Casserole (445 calories) see page 29	Greek Orzo (330 calories) see page 94	Lemon Baked Cod with New Potatoes (426 calories) see page 169	**1,201** — Total left over for snacks: 299
WEDNESDAY	Sunny Breakfast Casserole (445 calories) see page 29	Greek Orzo (330 calories) see page 94	Smoky Chicken and Pancetta Pie (526 calories) see page 140	**1,301** — Total left over for snacks: 199
THURSDAY	Sunny Breakfast Casserole (445 calories) see page 29	Greek Orzo (330 calories) see page 94	Creamy Salmon and Chorizo Bake (380 calories) see page 170	**1,155** — Total left over for snacks: 345
FRIDAY	Tiramisu Overnight Oats (309 calories) see page 22	Greek Orzo (330 calories) see page 94	Chinese Crispy Shredded Chilli Beef (350 calories) see page 214; plus 100g (3½oz) cooked rice (130 calories)	**1,119** — Total left over for snacks: 381
SATURDAY	Wholegrain Mustard Roasted Potatoes with Spinach and Feta (330 calories) see page 48	Roasted Mediterranean Vegetable Wraps with Hummus (425 calories) see page 100	Slow Cooker Chinese Chicken Curry Noodles (400 calories) see page 216	**1,155** — Total left over for snacks: 345
SUNDAY	Smoky Bacon Shakshuka (300 calories) see page 345	Slow Cooker Creamy Spicy Tomato and Vodka Soup (175 calories) See page 59) plus 100g (3½oz) bread for dipping (265 calories)	Creamy Chicken Casserole with Dumplings (400 calories) see page 144	**1,140** — Total left over for snacks: 360

the family meal plan

This meal plan is designed to suit those who are cooking meals from scratch for every meal, for the whole family (or friends!). If you are cooking for fewer people, you can easily portion up the recipes and use the leftovers for lunch or dinner the next day.

This meal plan is based on 1500 calories per day. If you are not following a plan as strict as this, this leaves room for some low-calorie snacks.

If you do any exercise during the day, track the number of calories you burn as you will be able to have additional snacks or a larger portion size.

Some meals are split into four portions, so if not all four portions are being eaten and you want to use some extra calories, you could have a larger portion. Also, you could utilize the spare calories for a portion of vegetables or salad with your main meal.

	BREAKFAST	LUNCH	DINNER	TOTAL CALORIES
MONDAY	Breakfast Quesadilla (480 calories) see page 31	Bumper BLT Pasta Salad (407 calories) see page 60	Jambalaya (508 calories) see page 146	**1,395** — *Total left over for snacks: 105*
TUESDAY	BBQ Bean and Cheese Bake (400 calories) see page 44	Slow Cooker Creamy Spicy Tomato and Vodka Soup (175 calories) See page 59) plus 100g (3½oz) bread for dipping (265 calories)	Coconut Prawns (385 calories) see page 126; plus 100g (3½oz) cooked rice (130 calories)	**1,355** — *Total left over for snacks: 145*
WEDNESDAY	Tiramisu Overnight Oats (309 calories) see page 22	Slow Cooker Creamy Spicy Tomato and Vodka Soup (175 calories) See page 59) plus 100g (3½oz) bread for dipping (265 calories)	Jerk-spiced Chicken Alfredo (481 calories) see page 134	**1,230** — *Total left over for snacks: 320*
THURSDAY	Perfect Pesto Eggs (424 calories) see page 43	Curried Chicken Salad (250 calories) see page 75	Smoky BBQ Bolognese Bake (577 calories) see page 165	**1,251** — *Total left over for snacks: 249*
FRIDAY	White Chocolate Summer Fruits Baked Crumpets (400 calories) see page 39	Slow Cooker Creamy Spicy Tomato and Vodka Soup (175 calories) See page 59) plus 100g (3½oz) bread for dipping (265 calories)	Greek Nachos (400 calories) see page 188	**1,240** — *Total leftover for snacks: 260*
SATURDAY	Bumper Breakfast Traybake (545 calories) see page 55	Grilled Sweet Potato Pizza Toasts (298 calories) see page 103	Lamb Bhuna (350 calories) see page 210; plus 100g (3½oz) cooked rice (130 calories)	**1,323** — *Total left over for snacks: 177*
SUNDAY	Cheesy Bacon Hash Brown Waffles (450 calories) see page 50	Rainbow Buddha Bowl (504 calories) see page 72	Sweet Potato Cottage Pie (353 calories) see page 149	**1,307** — *Total left over for snacks: 193*

Index

about the author

I'm Latoyah. I am the creator of the popular blog Sugar Pink Food, where I share my low-calorie, slimming-friendly recipes. I have spent my life living in beautiful Devon, in the south-west of England, and have lived in Devon's capital, Exeter, since I was 18.

I have always been passionate about creating delicious dishes with a healthy touch, feeding friends and family with tasty treats, and coming up with fabulous 'fakeaways'. I started my website as a place to store recipes as I could never seem to recreate the same dish twice, and it started to build a following via social media. The popularity of my website grew over the years, and has now received over 20 million views, creating a large and loyal social media following.

I was dubbed the 'Queen of the Fakeaway' by the national press after recreating low-calorie versions of the best-loved takeaway dishes at home, with my blog being featured in publications including the *Metro*, *Daily Mail*, *My London*, *Devon Live* and the *Daily Star*. I released my first book *Healthy Home Cooking* in January 2020 and in 2021 I appeared as a judge on Channel 4's *Beat the Chef*.

f @sugarpinkfood
@sugarpinkfood
Website: https://www.latoyah.co.uk/

acknowledgements

I would like to thank my friends, Emma, James, Jamie, Kirsty, Dawn, Troy and David, for being so supportive throughout this process. And 'The Seagull', for eating everything I put in front of him so enthusiastically and distracting me with Halo.

To Claire, for being there from the very first video call when we discussed the possibility of this book happening to the day of announcing the book publicly, for pulling me out of self-doubt every time, and for tasting the veggie dishes.

To my parents for always supporting me and to Nanny Jean and Grandad Brian for being my biggest fans, I hope I've made you all proud!

To everyone over the years who chose to follow me on social media – this wouldn't be happening without your ongoing support and interest in what I create, so thank you for being here.

To you, who are reading this, thank you for taking the time to read this book (or perhaps you just skipped to the end!). I hope you find a new favourite meal.

And to the teacher at school who told me that I would never amount to anything in life. Does this count?

First published in Great Britain in 2022 by Greenfinch
An imprint of Quercus Editions Ltd
Carmelite House
50 Victoria Embankment
London
EC4Y 0DZ

An Hachette UK company

A CIP catalogue record for this book is available from the British Library.

HB ISBN 978-1-52942-725-7

eBook ISBN 978-1-52942-726-4

10 9 8 7 6 5 4 3 2 1

Commissioned by Emily Arbis
Cover design by Sarah Pyke
Internal design by Sarah Pyke and Ginny Zeal
Photography by Uyen Luu
Food styling by Sam Dixon and Francesca Paling
Prop styling and project editing by Lucy Kingett

Printed and bound in Italy

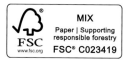

COLLEGE ALGEBRA

THOMAS W. HUNGERFORD
Cleveland State University

RICHARD MERCER
Wright State University

SAUNDERS COLLEGE PUBLISHING

Philadelphia   New York   Chicago
San Francisco   Montreal   Toronto
London   Sydney   Tokyo   Mexico City
Rio de Janeiro   Madrid

This book was set in Caledonia by York Graphic Services.
The editors were James Porterfield, Janis Moore, and Elaine Honig.
The art and design director was Richard L. Moore.
The new artwork was drawn by Linda Savalli.
The production manager was Tom O'Connor.
The printer was Fairfield Graphics.

COLLEGE ALGEBRA   ISBN 0-03-059521-5

Printed in the United States of America.
Library of Congress catalog card number 81-53087.

789-016-9876543

TO MY CHILDREN
Anne Elizabeth Hungerford
Thomas Joseph Hungerford

TO MY SISTER
Susan Aileen Mercer

Preface

This book is designed to provide the essentials of algebra for students who have had two years of high school mathematics. It can be effectively used both by students who are preparing for calculus and by those for whom college algebra may be a terminal mathematics course. It follows the traditional college algebra order, beginning with a full chapter of review material and a chapter on solving equations.

Except for the order of topics and the absence of trigonometry, our general approach here is the same one used in our other books, *Precalculus Mathematics* and *Algebra & Trigonometry*. Our classroom experience has led to two inescapable conclusions:

(i) It is not sufficient merely to present the necessary technical tools, without explaining both how and why they work *in language that the student understands*.

(ii) A large number of students taking a course such as this at the college level simply do *not* understand the terse "definition-example-theorem-proof" style of many mathematics texts. For whatever reasons, such an approach does not appear to them as reasonable and logical, but rather as an arbitrary, unreasonable, and often incomprehensible foreign language.

We have attempted to write a book that deals effectively with these facts, one that helps students to discover that mathematics can be both comprehensible and reasonable. As a first step toward this goal, the text is designed to be readable and understandable by an average student, with a minimal amount of outside assistance. This has been accomplished without any sacrifice of rigor. But excessive and unnecessary formalism has been omitted in both format and content. We have done our best to present sound mathematics in an informal manner that stresses

> detailed explanations of basic ideas, techniques and results;
>
> extensive use of pictures and diagrams;
>
> the fundamental reasons *why* a given technique works, as well as numerous examples showing *how* it is used;
>
> the origins of many concepts (especially functions) in the real world and the ways that the common features of such real-life situations are abstracted to obtain a mathematical definition.

There is, alas, no way to do this in a short space. Consequently, a given topic may well occupy more space here than in some other texts. But this length is misleading. We have found that

> **because of the detailed explanations and numerous examples, a typical student can usually read the longer discussion here more easily and with greater understanding than a terse, compact presentation elsewhere.**

v

So in the long run the extra length should cause no serious scheduling problems. Most important, it provides the added benefit of greater understanding.

Another reason for the length of the book is that it has been designed for the instructor's convenience. It is extremely flexible and adaptable to a wide variety of courses. In many cases entire chapters or sections within chapters may be omitted, shortened, or covered in several different orders, *without* impairing the book's readability by students.

> **A complete discussion of the possible ways of using this text, including**
>
> > **the interdependence of the various chapters,**
> > **the interdependence of the sections within each chapter,**
> > **section-by-section pedagogical comments,**
> > **numerous exam questions, and**
> > **answers to exercises**
>
> **is given in the Instructor's Manual. It is available on request from the publisher.**

Since calculators are now a fact of mathematical life, the book discusses both the uses and limitations of calculators in the study of functions. A student does not need to have a calculator to use the text, and exercises involving calculators are clearly labeled. But those students who do have one (the majority, in our experience) will benefit from seeing that calculators are not a substitute for learning the underlying theory, but can make that theory much easier to deal with in practical problems.

There are an unusually large number of exercises of widely varying types. The exercises labeled "A" are routine drill designed primarily to develop algebraic and manipulative skills. The "B" exercises are somewhat less mechanical and may occasionally require some careful thought. But any student who has read the text carefully should be able to do the majority of the "B" exercises. *The "C" label is used for exercises that are unusual* for one reason or another. Most of the time, "C" exercises are not difficult but are different from the sort of thing most students have seen before. A few of the "C" exercises are difficult mathematically. But most of them should be well within reach of most students.

Finally, there are scattered throughout the text sections labeled DO IT YOUR-SELF! Some of these include topics that are not absolutely essential, but which some instructors may want to include as a regular part of the course. Others provide interesting mathematical background or useful applications of the topics discussed in the text. Still others are needed by some students but not by others. Although they vary in level of difficulty, all of them can be read by students on their own.

Our earlier book, *Precalculus Mathematics*, contained almost half a page of acknowledgments. We are happy to thank all of those people once again. This book has benefited as much as the previous one from their contributions.

T. W. H.
R. E. M.

Cleveland, Ohio
Dayton, Ohio
August, 1981

Contents Overview

Contents

To the Student

Read this—or you will turn into a frog!

If you want to succeed in this course, remember that *mathematics is not a spectator sport.* You can't learn math simply by listening to your instructor lecture or work problems, by looking at examples in the text, by reading the answers in the back of the book, or by borrowing your neighbor's homework. You have to take an active role, using pencil and paper and working out many problems yourself. And you *can* do this—even if you haven't taken math for a while or if you're a bit afraid of math—by making wise use of your chief resources: your instructor and this book.

When it comes to math textbooks, many students make a serious mistake, they use their books only for finding out what the homework problems are. If they get stuck on a problem, they page back through the text until they find a similar example. If the example doesn't clarify things, they may try reading part of the text (as little as possible). On a really bad day they may end up reading most of the section—piecemeal, from back to front. Rarely, if ever, do such students read through an entire section (or subsection) from beginning to end.

If this description fits you, don't feel guilty. Some mathematics texts *are* unreadable. But don't use your bad past experiences as an excuse for not reading this book. It has been classroom tested for years by students like yourself. Some parts were rewritten several times to improve their clarity. Consequently we can assure you that this book is readable and understandable by an average student, with a minimal amount of outside assistance. So if you want to get the most out of this course, we strongly suggest that you follow these guidelines:

1. Read the pages assigned by your instructor from beginning to end *before* starting the homework problems.
2. You can't read a math book as you would read a newspaper or a novel, so go slowly and carefully. If you find calculations you don't understand, take pencil and paper and try to work them out. If you don't understand a particular statement, reread the preceding material to see if you missed something.
3. Don't get bogged down on the first reading. If you have spent a reasonable amount of time trying to figure something out, mark the place with a question mark and continue reading.
4. When you've read through the assigned material once, go back and reread the parts you marked with question marks. You will often find that you can now understand many of them. Plan to ask your instructor about the rest.
5. *Now* do the homework problems. You should be able to do all, or almost all, of the assigned problems. After you've worked at the homework for a reasonable amount of time and answered as many problems as you can, mark the exercises that are still causing trouble. Plan to ask your instructor about them.

If you follow these five guidelines, you will get the most out of this book. But no book can answer all your questions. That's why your instructor is there. Unfortunately, many students are afraid to ask questions in class for fear that the questions will seem "dumb." Such students should remember this:

> **If you have honestly followed the five guidelines above and still have unanswered questions, then there are *at least* six other students in your class who have the same questions.**

So it's not a dumb question. Furthermore, your instructor will welcome questions that arise from a serious effort on your part. In any case, your instructor is being paid (with your tuition money) to answer questions. So do yourself a favor and get your money's worth—*ask questions.*

Basic Algebra

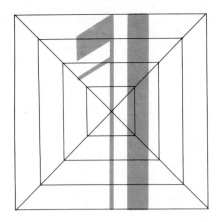

Since it may have been some time since you had any algebra, you may be a bit rusty. This chapter is designed to help you remove the rust and to refresh your algebraic and manipulative skills. Although some students may remember enough to skip much of this chapter, others will need to spend considerably more time on it. Simply reading statements and examples is *not* enough. You must be able to handle these algebraic manipulations quickly and efficiently. The *only* way to achieve this level of skill is to do a large number of exercises.

1. THE REAL NUMBER SYSTEM

In grade school and high school mathematics you were introduced to the system of real numbers. These are the numbers used in everyday life. The most familiar ones are the **integers** (or whole numbers), that is, the numbers $0, 1, -1, 2, -2, 3, -3, \ldots$, and so on. The numbers $1, 2, 3, 4, \ldots$ are called the natural numbers or the positive integers.

The real number system also includes all **rational numbers,** that is, all fractions r/s, where r and s are integers and $s \neq 0$. Each of the following is a rational number:

$$\frac{1}{2} \qquad \frac{-4}{3} \qquad \frac{99{,}642}{716} \qquad \frac{-1400}{2} = \frac{-700}{1} = -700 \qquad 3\frac{5}{16} = \frac{53}{16} = 3.3125$$

The word "rational" in this context has no psychological implications. It refers to the ratio or quotient of two integers.

A crucial fact is that

some real numbers are *not* rational numbers

1

For example, consider a right triangle° with two equal sides of length 1, as shown in Figure 1-1.

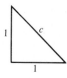

Figure 1-1

According to the Pythagorean Theorem,° the length of the hypotenuse° is a real number c that satisfies the equation $c^2 = 1^2 + 1^2 = 2$. (The number c is called the square root of 2 and is denoted $\sqrt{2}$.) We claim that

$$c = \sqrt{2} \text{ is } \textit{not} \text{ a rational number}$$

In other words, it is not possible to find integers a and b such that $(a/b)^2 = 2$.

A proof of this claim is given in Exercise C.1 on page 94. For now you can convince yourself of its *plausibility* by trying to find a rational number whose square is 2 (of course, you won't succeed). For example, if we square $\frac{1414}{1000}$ ($= 1.414$), we obtain 1.999396, which is *close* to 2, but is not exactly *equal* to 2. It doesn't take much of this to convince most people that no matter what rational number they square, the answer will never be *exactly* 2.† In other words, $\sqrt{2}$ cannot be a rational number.

A real number that is *not* a rational number (such as $\sqrt{2}$) is called an **irrational number** (ir-rational = not rational = not a ratio). Another well-known irrational number is the number π, which is used to calculate the area of a circle. In grade school you probably used $\frac{22}{7}$ or 3.1416 as the number π. But these rational numbers are just *approximations* of π (close to, but not quite *equal* to π).

Although only two irrational numbers have been mentioned, there are in fact infinitely many of them. Rationals and irrationals are further discussed in the DO IT YOURSELF! segment at the end of this section.

THE NUMBER LINE

The real number system can be pictured geometrically by using the real **number line** (or **coordinate line**). Take a straight line and choose a point on it; label this point 0 and call it the **origin**. Now choose some unit of measurement and label the point that is one unit to the *right* of 0 by the number 1. Using this unit length over and over, label the point one unit to the right of 1 as 2, the point one unit to the right of 2 as 3, and so on, as shown in Figure 1-2. Then do the same to the left of the origin. The point one unit to the left of 0 is labeled -1, the point one unit to the left of -1 is labeled -2, and so on. By now the scheme should be clear: The point $1\frac{1}{2}$ units to the *right* of 0 is labeled $1\frac{1}{2} = \frac{3}{2}$, the point 5.78 units to the *left* of 0 is labeled -5.78, and so on (see Figure 1-2).

° The terms "right triangle," "Pythagorean Theorem," and "hypotenuse" are explained in the Geometry Review at the end of this book.
† A calculator may display $\sqrt{2}$ as a decimal (rational number), such as 1.414213562. It may even display the square of this number as 2. But this happens because the calculator rounds off long decimals. If you perform the squaring by hand, you will find that the answer is *not* 2.

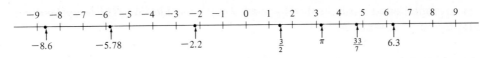

Figure 1-2

In the preceding construction of the number line, one fact is evident:

Every real number is the label of a unique point on the line.

We shall also assume the converse of this statement as a basic axiom:

Every point on the line has a unique real number label.

This correspondence between points on the line and real numbers will be used constantly. Strictly speaking, the number 3.6 and the point on the line labeled 3.6 are two different things. Nevertheless, we shall frequently use such phrases as "the point 3.6" or refer to a "number on the line." In context this usage will not cause any confusion. Indeed, the mental identification of real numbers with points on the line is often extremely helpful in understanding and solving various problems.

ORDER

The statement "a is less than b" (written $a < b$) and the statement "b is greater than a" (written $b > a$) mean exactly the same thing, namely, a lies to the *left* of b on the number line (or equivalently, b lies to the *right* of a on the number line).

EXAMPLE $-50 < 10$ and $10 < 30$ since on the number line -50 lies to the left of 10 and 10 lies to the left of 30 (see Figure 1-3).

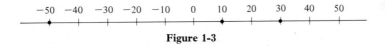

Figure 1-3

Often we shall write $a \leq b$ (or $b \geq a$), which means "a is less than or equal to b" (or "b is greater than or equal to a"). The statement $a \leq b \leq c$ means

$$a \leq b \quad and \quad b \leq c$$

Geometrically, the statement $a \leq b \leq c$ means that a lies to the left of c and b lies between a and c on the number line (and may possibly be equal to one or both of them). The preceding example shows that $-50 \leq 10 \leq 30$. Similarly, $a \leq b < c$ means $a \leq b$ and $b < c$ and so on.

The following facts are used frequently. For any real numbers a, b, and c

$a \leq a$;		
if $a \leq b$	*and*	$b \leq a$,	*then* $a = b$;
if $a \leq b$	*and*	$b \leq c$,	*then* $a \leq c$

These properties are easily verified by looking at the number line. The last property is also true if $\leq$ is replaced by $<$.

NEGATIVE NUMBERS AND NEGATIVES OF NUMBERS

The numbers to the right of 0 on the number line, that is,

$$\text{all numbers } a \text{ with } a > 0$$

are called **positive** numbers. The numbers to the left of 0, that is,

$$\text{all numbers } b \text{ with } b < 0$$

are called **negative** numbers. Finally, the **nonnegative** numbers are

$$\text{all numbers } a \text{ with } a \geq 0$$

Unfortunately for students, the word "negative" is used in two different ways in mathematics. As we just saw, a *negative* number is a number less than 0. The second usage of "negative" occurs in the phrase "*the negative of a* number":

The negative of a number *is the number obtained by changing the sign of the original number*°

For example, the negative of 3 is the number -3 and the negative of -7 is the number 7. It is customary to consider 0 to be its own negative since $0 = -0$. Naturally, the use of the same word to describe two different situations can be confusing. Unfortunately, however, the usage is so widespread that we are stuck with it.

Observe that you can *always* change the sign of a given number by inserting a minus sign in front of it. For instance, to change the sign of 3 we insert a minus sign and get -3. To change the sign of the number -7 we put a minus sign in front and obtain $-(-7) = 7$. Consequently, the following statement is always true:

> *The negative of the number* c *is the number* $-$c.

When you see a statement such as the one in the box above, it is important to remember that the number c may be either positive or negative or zero. As we have just seen, the negative of the positive number 3 is the negative number -3 and the negative of the negative number -7 is the positive number 7. Thus

> *If* c *is a positive number, then* $-$c *is a negative number.*
> *If* c *is a negative number, then* $-$c *is a positive number.*

° The negative of a number is sometimes called the additive inverse of the number.

ARITHMETIC

A summary of the important properties of addition, subtraction, multiplication, and division of real numbers is given below. You have been using these properties for years but may not have seen them stated in this manner. So if you don't understand a statement in one of the boxes, consult the numerical examples immediately after the box for clarification. Remember that the letters b, c, and d used in the boxes may represent positive or negative numbers or zero. Some of these properties (or "laws") have names. These names are convenient for reference purposes, but it is more important that you understand the meaning of each property and be able to use it.

NEGATIVES

(*i*) *The sum of a real number* c *and its negative is zero; that is,*
$$c + (-c) = 0.$$

(*ii*) $-(-c) = c;$

(*iii*) $(-1) \cdot c = -c$

If b *and* c *are any real numbers, then*

(*iv*) $b + (-c) = b - c;$

(*v*) $-(b + c) = -b - c;$

(*vi*) $b - (-c) = b + c$

EXAMPLE (i) Let $c = 5$; then $5 + (-5) = 0$. Let $c = -\frac{3}{4}$; then $(-\frac{3}{4}) + [-(-\frac{3}{4})] = 0$.

EXAMPLE (ii) Let $c = 4$; then $-(-4) = 4$.

EXAMPLE (iii) Let $c = 5$; then $(-1) \cdot 5 = -5$. Let $c = -6$; then $(-1)(-6) = 6 = -(-6)$.

EXAMPLE (iv) Let $b = 5$ and $c = 7$; then $5 + (-7) = 5 - 7 = -2$. Let $b = -2$ and $c = 3$; then $-2 + (-3) = -2 - 3 = -5$.

EXAMPLE (v) Let $b = -7$ and $c = 3$; then $-(-7 + 3) = -(-7) - 3 = 7 - 3 = 4$.

EXAMPLE (vi) Let $b = \frac{3}{4}$ and $c = \frac{19}{4}$; then $\frac{3}{4} - (-\frac{19}{4}) = \frac{3}{4} + \frac{19}{4} = \frac{22}{4} = \frac{11}{2}$.

SIGNS

If b *and* c *are any real numbers, then*

(i) $(-b)(-c) = bc;$

(ii) $(-b)c = b(-c) = -bc;$

(iii) $\dfrac{-b}{-c} = \dfrac{b}{c}$ $(c \neq 0);$

(iv) $\dfrac{-b}{c} = \dfrac{b}{-c} = -\dfrac{b}{c}$ $(c \neq 0)$

EXAMPLE (i) Let $b = 4$ and $c = 6$; then $(-4)(-6) = 24 = 4 \cdot 6$.

EXAMPLE (ii) Let $b = \frac{1}{2}$ and $c = \frac{3}{5}$; then $(-\frac{1}{2})(\frac{3}{5}) = \frac{1}{2}(-\frac{3}{5}) = -(\frac{1}{2} \cdot \frac{3}{5}) = -\frac{3}{10}$.

EXAMPLE (iii) Let $b = \pi$ and $c = 2$; then $\dfrac{-\pi}{-2} = \dfrac{\pi}{2}$.

EXAMPLE (iv) Let $b = 2$ and $c = 7$; then $\dfrac{-2}{7} = \dfrac{2}{-7} = -\dfrac{2}{7}$.

COMMUTATIVE LAWS

If b *and* c *are real numbers, then*

$b + c = c + b$ *and* $bc = cb$

EXAMPLE Let $b = -7$ and $c = 6$; then $-7 + 6 = -1 = 6 + (-7)$ and $(-7)6 = -42 = 6(-7)$.

There is no commutative law for subtraction because order *does* make a difference in subtraction. For instance, $5 - 2 = 3$, but $2 - 5 = -3$.

ASSOCIATIVE LAWS

If b, c, *and* d *are real numbers, then*

$b + (c + d) = (b + c) + d$ *and* $b(cd) = (bc)d$

EXAMPLE Let $b = 3$, $c = 5$, and $d = 7$; then $3 + (5 + 7) = 3 + 12 = 15$, and $(3 + 5) + 7 = 8 + 7 = 15$ so that $3 + (5 + 7) = (3 + 5) + 7$. Similarly, $3(5 \cdot 7) = (3 \cdot 5)7$ since $3(5 \cdot 7) = 3(35) = 105$ and $(3 \cdot 5)7 = (15)7 = 105$.

DISTRIBUTIVE LAWS

If b, c, *and* d *are real numbers, then*

$$b(c + d) = bc + bd \quad and \quad (c + d)b = cb + db$$
$$b(c - d) = bc - bd \quad and \quad (c - d)b = cb - db$$

It really isn't necessary to state four versions of the distributive law. The first version includes all the others as special cases since $b(c + d) = (c + d)b$ by commutativity and $c + (-d) = c - d$.

EXAMPLE Let $b = 3$, $c = -7$, and $d = 6$; then $3(-7 + 6) = 3(-1) = -3$ and $3(-7) + 3 \cdot 6 = -21 + 18 = -3$ so that $3(-7 + 6) = 3(-7) + 3 \cdot 6$.

IDENTITIES

For every real number c

$$c + 0 = c \quad and \quad c \cdot 1 = c$$

EXAMPLE Let $c = -5$; then $-5 + 0 = -5$ and $(-5) \cdot 1 = -5$.

ZERO PRODUCTS

(*i*) *For every real number* b,

$$b \cdot 0 = 0 = 0 \cdot b$$

(*ii*) *If a product is zero, then at least one of the factors is zero; in other words,*

if cd = 0, *then* c = 0 *or* d = 0 *(or both).*

An immediate consequence of statement (ii) is that:

A product of nonzero factors is nonzero; that is,

if c ≠ 0 *and* d ≠ 0, *then* cd ≠ 0

Finally, you should remember that the quotient of two real numbers c/d is defined only when $d \neq 0$. Expressions such as $1/0$, $\pi/0$, $0/0$, $-3/0$, and so on, have no meaning; they are *not* real numbers. In other words,

$$\boxed{\text{division by 0 is not defined}}$$

There are good reasons for excluding division by zero, some of which are considered in Exercise C.1.

PRIORITY OF OPERATIONS AND PARENTHESES

A common source of arithmetic mistakes is the fact that an expression such as $4 + 3 \cdot 2$ can be interpreted in two ways. It could mean:

Add 4 and 3, then multiply the result by 2, so that
the final answer is $7 \cdot 2 = 14$.

But it could also mean:

Multiply 3 times 2, then add 4 to the result, so that
the final answer is $4 + 6 = 10$.

So performing the operations in one order (addition first) gives the answer 14, while performing them in another order (multiplication first), gives the answer 10. Obviously this will cause great confusion unless we have a consistent plan for performing arithmetic operations. Mathematicians have agreed to adopt this convention

$$\boxed{\begin{array}{c} \textit{Multiplication and division are performed first;} \\ \textit{addition and subtraction are performed last.} \end{array}}$$

According to this convention, there is only one correct way to interpret the expression $4 + 3 \cdot 2$: it means $4 + 6$ (multiplication first) so that the final answer is 10.

EXAMPLE To evaluate $2 \cdot 6 + \frac{5}{2}$, we first perform the multiplication and division, obtaining $12 + 2.5$. Then we perform the addition: $12 + 2.5 = 14.5$.

Calculator Warning Some calculators automatically follow the convention in the box above, but others do not. A calculator with "algebraic hierarchy of operations" *does* follow the convention. With such a calculator you can compute $2 \cdot 6 + \frac{5}{2}$ by performing this sequence of key strokes:

| 2 | × | 6 | + | 5 | ÷ | 2 | = |

The calculator will display the correct answer 14.5 just as in the preceding example. But if your calculator has "left-to-right sequencing of operations", then it may *not* follow the convention above. If you perform the same sequence of key strokes on such a calculator, namely:

$$\boxed{2} \quad \boxed{\times} \quad \boxed{6} \quad \boxed{+} \quad \boxed{5} \quad \boxed{\div} \quad \boxed{2} \quad \boxed{=}$$

the result will be the incorrect answer 8.5. The reason is that such a calculator interprets this key stroke sequence as meaning "first multiply 2 times 6, then add 5 (producing 17), and then divide by 2 (producing 8.5)." Since such a calculator does *not* follow the convention that all multiplication and division be done first, you must use a different sequence of key strokes in order to obtain the correct answer here. For instance, you could first do the multiplication (6×2) and store or remember the answer 12; then do the division ($5 \div 2$); finally add the division answer 2.5 to the stored number 12 to obtain the final correct answer 14.5.

The moral here is: Find out what priority of operations is built into your calculator and (if necessary) adjust your key stroke sequences so that your computations follow the convention in the second box on page 8.

The convention does not eliminate all ambiguity. For instance, it does not tell us how to interpret the expression $9 - 2 + 4$. In such cases we use parentheses to indicate the intended interpretation. If you intend to say: "first subtract 2 from 9 and then add 4 to the result", you write $(9 - 2) + 4$. On the other hand if you intend to say "subtract $2 + 4$ from 9", then you write $9 - (2 + 4)$. The parentheses are essential here since

$$(9 - 2) + 4 = 7 + 4 = 11, \quad \text{while} \quad 9 - (4 + 2) = 9 - 6 = 3.$$

The first basic rule when dealing with parentheses is:

> *Do all computations inside the parentheses before doing any computations outside the parentheses.*

EXAMPLE To compute $(7 - 4)(5 + 1)$ we first do the subtraction $7 - 4 = 3$ and the addition $5 + 1 = 6$, and then do the multiplication:

$$(7 - 4)(5 + 1) = 3 \cdot 6 = 18.$$

The second rule for parentheses is:

> *When dealing with parentheses within parentheses, work from the inside out.*

EXAMPLE To calculate $7 + (11 - (6 \div 3))$, we first work on the innermost set of parentheses and compute $6 \div 3 = 2$. Then we do the outer set of parentheses $(11 - (6 \div 3)) = (11 - 2) = 9$. Finally, we add 7 to the result:

$$7 + (11 - (6 \div 3)) = 7 + (11 - 2) = 7 + 9 = 16.$$

ORDER AND ARITHMETIC

The interaction of the order relation and the operations of arithmetic sometimes causes confusion. So be sure you understand each of the following statements.

Let a, b, *and* c *be real numbers.*

(*i*) If $a \leq b$,   then $a + c \leq b + c$;

(*ii*) If $a \leq b$, and $c > 0$,   then $ac \leq bc$;

(*iii*) If $a \leq b$ and $c < 0$,   then $ac \geq bc$ (*note direction of inequality*);

(*iv*) If $0 < a \leq b$,   then $\dfrac{1}{a} \geq \dfrac{1}{b}$ (*note direction of inequality*)

EXAMPLES (i), (ii) Suppose $a = -6$, $b = 2$, and $c = 5$. Then we have:

$$
\begin{array}{ccc}
a \leq b & a + c \leq b + c & ac \leq bc \\
-6 \leq 2 & -6 + 5 \leq 2 + 5 & (-6)5 \leq (2)5 \\
 & -1 \leq 7 & -30 \leq 10
\end{array}
$$

EXAMPLES (iii), (iv) Suppose $a = 3$, $b = 7$, and $c = -4$. Then we have:

$$
\begin{array}{ccc}
a \leq b & ac \geq bc & \dfrac{1}{a} \geq \dfrac{1}{b} \\
\\
3 \leq 7 & 3(-4) \geq 7(-4) & \dfrac{1}{3} \geq \dfrac{1}{7} \\
\\
 & -12 \geq -28 &
\end{array}
$$

The various rules that you have learned about the products of positive and negative numbers are special cases of the properties listed in the last box above. For example, the fact that $(-3)(-4) = +12$ reflects the fact that multiplying both sides of the inequality $-3 < 0$ by -4 reverses the direction of the inequality: $(-3)(-4) > 0$.

EXERCISES

A.1. Draw a number line and mark the location of each of these numbers: 0, -7, $\frac{8}{3}$, 10, -1, -4.75, $\frac{1}{2}$, -5, and 2.25.

A.2. Express each of the following statements in symbols:
   (a) 7 is greater than 5
   (b) -4 is greater than -8
   (c) x is nonnegative
   (d) y is positive
   (e) z lies strictly between -3 and -2
   (f) x is positive, but not more than 7
   (g) c is less than 4 and d is at least 4

A.3. Find the negative of each of these numbers:

(a) 0

(b) 1

(c) $-\pi$

(d) -67.43

(e) $[4 + (-6)]$

(f) $[-(37 - 2)]$

(g) $[7.53 - (6 - 2.13)]$

(h) $[17.77 + (-7.7 + .7)]$

(i) $2\pi(7 - \pi)$

A.4. Express each of the following numbers as a single integer:

(a) $14 - 10 + 3$

(b) $2 - (3 - 5) + 3 - (-7)$

(c) $(1 - 8 + 7) - (3 - 5 + 8(2 - 5))$

(d) $(-5)8$

(e) $7(-2)(-5)$

(f) $(-1)(-2)(-3)(-4)(-5)$

(g) $(-6)(5 - 1 + 4) - 3.25 + 1.25$

(h) $\dfrac{-15}{2 - 7}$

(i) $\dfrac{-266}{-12 - (-26)}$

A.5. Express each of the following numbers as a single integer:

(a) $\dfrac{17 + 3}{4} - 5$

(b) $(-6)\left(\dfrac{9 + 3}{9 - 3} - 2\right)$

(c) $\dfrac{\dfrac{5 + 7}{5 - 7} + 10}{\dfrac{18 - 3}{5(-3)} - 3}$

(d) $\dfrac{(2 \cdot 3) + 4(2 - 11)}{2(-2) + 1}$

(e) $\dfrac{(-2)\left(\dfrac{2 + 1}{3 - 5}\right) + 6}{-2 + 8\left(\dfrac{8 + 2}{7 + 9}\right)}$

B.1. (a) Use one of the irrational numbers mentioned in the text to show that the product of an irrational number with itself may be a rational number.

(b) Is the product of two rational numbers always a rational number? (This wasn't discussed in the text, but you should be able to answer it.)

B.2. (a) Find a rational number that is strictly between $\frac{2}{7}$ and $\frac{5}{8}$ on the number line.

(b) Let r/s and a/b be rational numbers with $r/s < a/b$. Find a rational number that is strictly between r/s and a/b on the number line.

B.3. Let h be a nonzero real number. Illustrate the truth of each of the following statements by three examples (that is, choose three different numbers that suggest the truth of the statement).

(a) If h is a large positive number, then $1/h$ is a small positive number.

(b) If h is a very small positive number, then $1/h$ is a very large positive number.

(c) If h is a very small negative number, then $1/h$ is very close to zero.

(d) If h is a negative number that is very close to 0, then $1/h$ is a very small negative number.

[*Hint:* Remember that as you move to the *right* on the number line, the numbers get larger and larger; but as you move to the *left*, the numbers get smaller and smaller.]

B.4. In each of the following statements, insert either $\leq$ or $\geq$ in the blank so as to make a *true* statement *and then* give an example of the statement, using specific numbers. For instance, in the statement

$$\text{if } 0 < a \leq b, \qquad \text{then } \frac{1}{a} \underline{\quad} \frac{1}{b}$$

insert $\geq$; example: $0 < 2 \leq 3$ and $\frac{1}{2} \geq \frac{1}{3}$.

(a) if $a \leq b < 0$, then $1/a \underline{\quad} 1/b$ (d) if $a \leq b \leq 0$, then $a^2 \underline{\quad} b^2$

(b) if $a < 0 < b$, then $1/a \underline{\quad} 1/b$ (e) if $a \leq 0 \leq b$, then $a^3 \underline{\quad} b^3$

(c) if $0 \leq a \leq b$, then $a^2 \underline{\quad} b^2$ (f) (sneaky) if $a \leq 0 \leq b$,

                                                   then $a^2 \underline{\quad} b^2$

B.5. Fill the blanks in the following table, which shows the equivalence of arithmetic statements about real numbers and geometric statements about the corresponding points on the number line.

Arithmetic Statement	**Geometric Statement**
(a) a is negative	The point a lies to the left of the point 0.
(b) $a \geq b$	_____
(c) _____	a lies c units to the right of b
(d) _____	a lies between b and c
(e) $a - b > 0$	_____
(f) a is positive	_____
(g) _____	a lies strictly to the left of b

C.1. Suppose that division by zero *was* defined. Then $\frac{1}{0}$ would be a real number. Hence $\frac{1}{0}$ would either be a nonzero number or $\frac{1}{0}$ would be 0. This exercise shows that the first of these possibilities leads to a logical contradiction and that the second is highly unreasonable, if we want division by zero to "behave" like division by other numbers. Consequently, it is better to leave division by zero undefined.

(a) Assuming that division by zero obeys the usual rules of arithmetic of fractions, show that $\dfrac{1}{\frac{1}{0}} = 0$. [*Remember:* $\frac{0}{1}$ is defined and $\frac{0}{1} = 0$.]

(b) Suppose $\frac{1}{0}$ is a nonzero number, say, $\frac{1}{0} = c$ with $c \neq 0$. Use part (a) to show that $1/c = 0$. Consequently,

$$c\left(\frac{1}{c}\right) = c \cdot 0$$
$$1 = 0$$

This is a logical contradiction. Therefore $\frac{1}{0}$ cannot be a nonzero number.

(c) Suppose that $\frac{1}{0} = 0$. If division by 0 behaves like division by other numbers, then all four of the following statements *should* be true:

(i) Whenever a is very close to 5, then $1/a$ is very close to $\frac{1}{5} = .2$.

(ii)   Whenever a is very close to 2, then $1/a$ is very close to $\frac{1}{2} = .5$.

(iii)   Whenever a is very close to 1, then $1/a$ is very close to $\frac{1}{1} = 1.0$.

(iv)   Whenever a is very close to 0, then $1/a$ is very close to $\frac{1}{0} = 0$.

Use an electronic calculator (if necessary) to verify that the first three statements are true but that *the last statement is false.* For example, $a = 4.999$ and $a = 5.0001$ are very close to 5 and $\dfrac{1}{4.999} = .2000040$ and $\dfrac{1}{5.00001} = .1999996$ are very close to $\frac{1}{5} = .2$. Since statement (iv) is false, we conclude that $\frac{1}{0} = 0$ is an unreasonable definition if we want division by 0 to behave like division by other numbers.

DO IT YOURSELF!

DECIMAL REPRESENTATION

We take it for granted that you are familiar with decimal notation for rational numbers whose denominators can be expressed as a power of ten, such as:

$$\tfrac{1}{10} = .1, \qquad -\tfrac{4}{1000} = -.004, \qquad 2\tfrac{3}{4} = 2.75 = \tfrac{275}{100}, \qquad -\tfrac{745}{100} = -7.45$$

Terminating decimals, such as these, are usually easier to compute with than are the corresponding fractions. Of course, some rational numbers cannot be expressed as terminating decimals. Nevertheless, such rational numbers can be expressed as repeating decimals, as the following example illustrates.

EXAMPLE   In order to express $\frac{4359}{925}$ as a decimal, we divide the numerator (top) by the denominator (bottom) and obtain:

```
                4.7124324
        925 ) 4359.0000000
              3700
               659 0
               647 5
                11 50
                 9 25
               → 2 250
                 1 850
                  4000
                  3700
                  3000
                  2775
               → 2250
                 1850        repeats as above
                 4000
                 3700
                   ⋮
```

Since the remainder at the third step (namely, 225) occurs again at the sixth step, it is clear that the division process goes on forever, with the three-digit block "243" repeating over and over in the quotient: $\frac{4359}{925} = 4.71243243243\cdots$. Similarly, division shows that $\frac{1}{12} = .083333\cdots$, with the 3's continually repeating.

It is easy to see that the method used in the preceding example (namely, divide the top by the bottom) can be used to express any rational number (fraction) as a decimal. If at some stage of the long division process, you obtain a remainder of 0, then the process stops and the result is a terminating decimal. Otherwise, some nonzero remainder *necessarily* repeats during the division process° and you obtain a repeating decimal.

When convenient we shall consider a terminating decimal as a repeating decimal ending in zeros (for instance, $.75 = .75000\cdots$). There is also a simple method for converting a repeating decimal into a rational number (see Exercise C.1.). Consequently, we conclude that

> Every rational number can be expressed as a terminating or repeating decimal and every such decimal represents a rational number.

Although we shall not prove it here, irrational numbers can also be expressed as decimals. Of course, a decimal that represents an *irrational* number is necessarily nonterminating and *nonrepeating* (that is, no block of digits repeats forever). If you learned a method for finding square roots in grade school, you have already seen one example of this. That method (whose details need not concern us here) shows that $\sqrt{2} = 1.414213562373095\cdots$. As usual,. the three dots indicate that the decimal goes on forever. But this time there is no block of digits that repeats forever. The only way to find out what digit comes next is to carry out the computation that far. Another irrational number is π, whose decimal expansion begins $3.14159265358979\cdots$; this expansion has been carried out to over one million decimal places by computer.

Conversely, every nonrepeating decimal represents an irrational real number (no proof to be given here). Consequently, we can summarize the preceding discussion as follows.

> (i) *Every real number can be expressed as a decimal.*
> (ii) *Every such decimal represents a real number.*
> (iii) *The repeating decimals are precisely the rational numbers.*
> (iv) *The nonrepeating decimals are precisely the irrational numbers.*

EXERCISES

A.1. Express each of the following rational numbers as a repeating decimal.
   (a) $\frac{7}{9}$;   (b) $\frac{2}{13}$;   (c) $\frac{23}{14}$;   (d) $\frac{19}{88}$;   (e) $\frac{1}{19}$ (long);   (f) $\frac{9}{11}$.

° For instance, if you divide a number by 23, the only possible remainders at each step are the numbers 0, 1, 2, 3, ..., 22. Hence after *at most* 23 steps, some remainder must occur for a second time.

B.1. If two real numbers have the same decimal expansion through three decimal places, how far apart can they be on the number line?

C.1. Here is a method for expressing a repeating decimal as a rational number (fraction). For example, let $d = 52.31272727\cdots$. Assuming that the usual laws of arithmetic hold, we see that

$$10,000d = 523127.272727\cdots \qquad \text{and} \qquad 100d = 5231.272727\cdots$$

Now subtract $100d$ from $10,000d$:

$$
\begin{aligned}
10,000d &= 523127.272727\cdots \\
-\ 100d &= -5231.272727\cdots \\
\hline
9,900d &= 517896.
\end{aligned}
$$

Dividing both sides of this last equation by 9900 yields $d = \frac{517896}{9900}$. The idea here is to subtract two *suitable* multiples of d, so as to eliminate the repeating part of the decimal. Here is a second example. If $c = .272727\cdots$, then verify that $100c - c = 27$. Hence $99c = 27$, so that $c = \frac{27}{99} = \frac{3}{11}$. Express each of the following repeating decimals as rational numbers.

(a) $.373737\cdots$;　　(c) $76.63424242\cdots$;　　(e) $.135135135\cdots$;

(b) $.929292\cdots$;　　(d) $13.513513\cdots$;　　(f) $.33030303\cdots$.

C.2. Use the methods in Exercise C.1 to show that both $.75000\cdots$ and $.749999\cdots$ are decimal expansions of $\frac{3}{4}$. [In general it is true that every terminating decimal (that is, a repeating decimal ending in zeros) can also be expressed as a decimal ending in repeated 9's. It can be proved that these are the only real numbers with more than one decimal expansion.]

2. INTEGRAL EXPONENTS AND ROOTS

Exponents provide a convenient shorthand notation for certain products. If c is a real number, then c^2 denotes the product cc and c^3 denotes the product ccc. More generally:

If c *is a real number and* n *is a positive integer, then*

c^n *denotes the product* $ccc\cdots c$　(n *factors*).

In this notation c^1 is just c, so we usually omit the exponent 1.

EXAMPLE $3^4 = 3\cdot3\cdot3\cdot3 = 81$ and $0^6 = 0\cdot0\cdot0\cdot0\cdot0\cdot0 = 0$.

EXAMPLE $(-2)^5 = (-2)(-2)(-2)(-2)(-2) = -32$ and $(-2)^4 = (-2)(-2)(-2)(-2) = 16$.

EXAMPLE If a and b are real numbers, then $a^3b^7 = aaabbbbbbb$.

Because exponents are just shorthand, the rules they obey are easy to determine. For example, the product of c^3 and c^5 is

$$c^3 c^5 = (ccc)(ccccc) = c^8$$

Since $8 = 3 + 5$, we see that $c^3 c^5 = c^{3+5}$. A similar argument applies to any two exponents. Thus to *multiply c^m by c^n, add the exponents*: $c^m c^n = c^{m+n}$.

EXAMPLE $\quad 4^2 \cdot 4^3 = 4^{2+3} = 4^5 \quad$ and $\quad 7^2 \cdot 3^2 \cdot 7^6 \cdot 3^8 = 7^2 \cdot 7^6 \cdot 3^2 \cdot 3^8 = (7^{2+6})(3^{2+8}) = 7^8 \cdot 3^{10}$.

If you divide c^7 by c^4 (with $c \neq 0$, of course), you obtain:

$$\frac{c^7}{c^4} = \frac{ccccccc}{cccc} = \frac{\cancel{cccc}ccc}{\cancel{cccc}} = ccc = c^3$$

Since $3 = 7 - 4$, we see that $c^7/c^4 = c^{7-4}$. The same argument applies in the general case. So to *divide c^m by c^n, subtract the exponents*: $c^m/c^n = c^{m-n}$.

EXAMPLE $\quad 2^6/2^3 = 2^{6-3} = 2^3$; that is, $\frac{64}{8} = 8$.

If c is a nonzero real number, we would like to extend this exponent notation so that c^n will have a meaning when $n = 0, -1, -2, -3$, and so on. We would like to do this in such a way that the exponent laws $c^m c^n = c^{m+n}$ and $c^m/c^n = c^{m-n}$ remain true, even when m and n are zero or negative integers. In particular, we want statements such as

$$c^5 c^0 = c^{5+0} = c^5 \quad \text{and} \quad \frac{c^7}{c^0} = c^{7-0} = c^7$$

to be true. Since $c^5 \cdot 1 = c^5$ and $c^7/1 = c^7$, it seems natural to *define c^0 to be the number 1.*

> If c *is a nonzero real number, then* c^0 *is defined to be the number 1.*

Note that 0^0 is *not* defined.

EXAMPLE $\quad 3^0 = 1$; $(-\frac{17}{4})^0 = 1$; $\pi^0 = 1$; $a^0 = 1 \quad (a \neq 0)$.

In order to define c^{-1}, c^{-2}, c^{-3}, and so on in such a way that the exponent law for multiplication remains true, we should have:

$$c^{-1} c^1 = c^{-1+1} = c^0 = 1 \qquad c^{-2} c^2 = c^{-2+2} = c^0 = 1 \qquad \text{and so on}$$

But for $c \neq 0$ we *already* have:

$$\frac{1}{c} \cdot c = 1 \qquad \frac{1}{c^2} \cdot c^2 = 1 \qquad \frac{1}{c^3} \cdot c^3 = 1 \qquad \text{and so on}$$

These facts suggest that we should define c^{-1} to be the number $1/c$, define c^{-2} to be the number $1/c^2$, and more generally:

> *For any nonzero real number* c *and positive integer* n,
>
> c^{-n} *is defined to be the number* $\dfrac{1}{c^n}$.

EXAMPLE $6^{-3} = \dfrac{1}{6^3} = \dfrac{1}{216}; \, (-2)^{-5} = \dfrac{1}{(-2)^5} = -\dfrac{1}{32}; \, \left(\dfrac{1}{3}\right)^{-4} = \dfrac{1}{(\frac{1}{3})^4} = \dfrac{1}{\frac{1}{81}} = 81.$

Note that negative powers of 0 are not defined since 0^{-1} would be $\frac{1}{0}$, which is *not* a real number.

LAWS OF EXPONENTS

Exponents obey several other laws, in addition to the two mentioned above. Here is a list of the important ones, each illustrated by examples. Note that in these statements *m* and *n* can be *any* integers, positive or negative or zero.

> *If* c *and* d *are nonzero real numbers and* m, n *are integers, then*
>
> *(i)* $c^m c^n = c^{m+n}$ *(iv)* $(cd)^n = c^n d^n$
>
> *(ii)* $\dfrac{c^m}{c^n} = c^{m-n}$ *(v)* $\left(\dfrac{c}{d}\right)^n = \dfrac{c^n}{d^n}$
>
> *(iii)* $(c^m)^n = c^{mn}$ *(vi)* $\dfrac{1}{c^{-n}} = c^n$

EXAMPLE (i) $\pi^{-5}\pi^2 = \pi^{-5+2} = \pi^{-3}$ since $\pi^{-5}\pi^2 = \dfrac{1}{\pi^5}\pi^2 = \dfrac{\cancel{\pi}\cancel{\pi}}{\cancel{\pi}\cancel{\pi}\pi\pi\pi} = \dfrac{1}{\pi^3} = \pi^{-3}$.
Similarly, $2^{-3} \cdot 2^{-4} = 2^{-3-4} = 2^{-7}$.

EXAMPLE (ii) $\dfrac{(-3)^2}{(-3)^4} = (-3)^{2-4} = (-3)^{-2}$ since $\dfrac{(-3)^2}{(-3)^4} = \dfrac{\cancel{(-3)}\cancel{(-3)}}{\cancel{(-3)}\cancel{(-3)}(-3)(-3)} =$
$\dfrac{1}{(-3)^2} = (-3)^{-2}$. Similarly, $\dfrac{6^{-3}}{6^{-5}} = 6^{-3-(-5)} = 6^{-3+5} = 6^2 = 36$.

EXAMPLE (iii) $(5^{-3})^2 = (5^{-3})(5^{-3}) = 5^{-6} = 5^{(-3)2}$ and $[(\frac{3}{2})^4]^{13} = (\frac{3}{2})^{4\cdot13} = (\frac{3}{2})^{52}$.

EXAMPLE (iv) If x is a real number, then $(2x)^5 = 2^5 x^5 = 32x^5$.

EXAMPLE (v) If r is a real number, then $\left(\dfrac{r}{-3}\right)^4 = \dfrac{r^4}{(-3)^4} = \dfrac{r^4}{81}$.

EXAMPLE (vi) $\dfrac{1}{5^{-3}} = \dfrac{1}{\frac{1}{5^3}} = 5^3$.

These exponent laws can often be used to simplify complicated expressions.

EXAMPLE To evaluate $\dfrac{2^4 \cdot 5^6}{125 \cdot 10^3}$, we first rewrite and then use the exponent laws:

$$\frac{2^4 \cdot 5^6}{125 \cdot 10^3} = \underset{\underset{\text{Law (iv)}}{\uparrow}}{\frac{2^4 \cdot 5^6}{5^3(5 \cdot 2)^3}} = \underset{\underset{\text{Law (i)}}{\uparrow}}{\frac{2^4 \cdot 5^6}{5^3(5^3 \cdot 2^3)}} = \underset{\underset{\text{Law (ii)}}{\uparrow}}{\frac{2^4 \cdot 5^6}{5^6 \cdot 2^3}} = 2^{4-3}5^{6-6} = 2^1 5^0 = 2 \cdot 1 = 2$$

EXAMPLE If x, y, and z are fixed real numbers, then

$$(2x^3y^4)(5xy^2z) = \underset{\underset{\substack{\text{Commutative}\\\text{Law}}}{\uparrow}}{2 \cdot 5 \cdot x^3 x y^4 y^2 z} = \underset{\underset{\text{Law (i)}}{\uparrow}}{10x^{3+1}y^{4+2}z} = 10x^4y^6z$$

EXAMPLE Simplify $\dfrac{x^5(y^2)^3}{(x^2y)^2}$ (where x and y are some fixed nonzero real numbers):

$$\frac{x^5(y^2)^3}{(x^2y)^2} = \underset{\underset{\text{Law (iii)}}{\uparrow}}{\frac{x^5y^6}{(x^2y)^2}} = \underset{\underset{\text{Law (iv)}}{\uparrow}}{\frac{x^5y^6}{(x^2)^2y^2}} = \underset{\underset{\text{Law (iii)}}{\uparrow}}{\frac{x^5y^6}{x^4y^2}} = \underset{\underset{\text{Law (ii)}}{\uparrow}}{x^{5-4}y^{6-2}} = xy^4$$

EXAMPLE Simplify and express without negative exponents $\dfrac{a^{-2}(b^2c^3)^{-2}}{(a^{-3}b^{-5})^2c}$ (where a, b, c are nonzero real numbers):

$$\frac{a^{-2}(b^2c^3)^{-2}}{(a^{-3}b^{-5})^2c} = \underset{\underset{\text{Law (iv)}}{\uparrow}}{\frac{a^{-2}(b^2)^{-2}(c^3)^{-2}}{(a^{-3})^2(b^{-5})^2c}} = \underset{\underset{\text{Law (iii)}}{\uparrow}}{\frac{a^{-2}b^{-4}c^{-6}}{a^{-6}b^{-10}c}} = \underset{\underset{\text{Law (ii)}}{\uparrow}}{a^{-2-(-6)}b^{-4-(-10)}c^{-6-1}} = a^4b^6c^{-7} = \frac{a^4b^6}{c^7}$$

SCIENTIFIC NOTATION

Every positive real number can be written as a product of some power of 10 and a number between 1 and 10. For example,

$$356 = 3.56 \times 100 = 3.56 \times 10^2;$$

$$1{,}563{,}627 = 1.563627 \times 1{,}000{,}000 = 1.563627 \times 10^6;$$

$$.072 = 7.2 \times \frac{1}{100} = 7.2 \times 10^{-2};$$

$$.000862 = 8.62 \times \frac{1}{10{,}000} = 8.62 \times 10^{-4}$$

When a number is written in this form it is said to be written in **scientific notation**.

Scientific notation is useful for writing and calculating with certain very large or very small numbers.

EXAMPLE

$$\frac{(50,000,000)^3(.000002)^5}{(.000008)} = \frac{(5 \times 10^7)^3(2 \times 10^{-6})^5}{8 \times 10^{-6}} = \frac{(5^3 \cdot 10^{21})(2^5 \cdot 10^{-30})}{8 \cdot 10^{-6}}$$

$$= \frac{125 \cdot 32 \cdot 10^{21-30}}{8 \cdot 10^{-6}} = 125 \cdot 4 \cdot 10^{21-30+6} = 500 \cdot 10^{-3} = \frac{500}{1000} = \frac{1}{2}.$$

Some calculators are equipped with scientific notation. Usually, they have a key labeled EE (for enter exponent). If you enter the number 7.235, press the EE key and then enter the number -12, the calculator display will read: $\boxed{7.235 \quad -12.}$ This indicates the number $7.235 \times 10^{-12} = .000000000007235$. Notice that this number cannot even be entered on a ten-digit calculator that does not have scientific notation capability.

SQUARE ROOTS

Since $(-5)^2 = 25$ and $5^2 = 25$, there are two real numbers whose square is 25. But only *one* of them is nonnegative. More generally:

> *If* d *is a nonnegative real number, then there is one and only one nonnegative real number* c *such that* $c^2 = d$. *This number* c *is called the square root of* d *and is denoted* $\sqrt{d}$.°

Thus we write $\sqrt{25} = 5$. Similarly, $\sqrt{\frac{9}{4}} = \frac{3}{2}$ since $\frac{3}{2}$ is the one and only *nonnegative* number whose square is $\frac{9}{4}$. The square root of a *rational* number need not be a rational number. For example, we saw in Section 1 that the real number $\sqrt{2}$ is not a rational number.

Warning In high school you may have considered both 5 and -5 as square roots of 25 and written $\sqrt{25} = \pm 5$. But here, as in most advanced texts, the term **square root** and the symbol $\sqrt{}$ always **denote a nonnegative number.** If we want to express -5 in terms of square roots, we write $-5 = -\sqrt{25}$.

OTHER ROOTS

The square root of 64 is defined to be 8 since $8^2 = 64$. Since $4^3 = 64$ we might say that 4 is the *cube root* of 64. Similarly, since $2^6 = 64$ we could say that 2 is the *sixth root* of 64. A reasonable question now might be: Is there a number c such that $c^5 = 64$? In other words, does 64 have a fifth root? Although it is not obvious, the answer is yes. In fact, even more is true and we shall assume without proof this important property of the real number system:

° The symbol $\sqrt{}$ is called a **radical.**

If d *is a nonnegative real number and* n *is a positive integer, then
there is one and only one nonnegative real number* c *such that*
$c^n = d$. *This number* c *is called the **nth root** of* d *and is denoted*
$\sqrt[n]{d}$.

In other words, $\sqrt[n]{d}$ is the unique *nonnegative* number such that $(\sqrt[n]{d})^n = d$.

EXAMPLE Suppose $n = 3$. Then $\sqrt[3]{8} = 2$ since $2^3 = 8$ and $\sqrt[3]{125} = 5$ since $5^3 = 125$. When $n = 3$, we usually use the term cube root instead of the *n*th root or third root.

EXAMPLE $\sqrt[4]{81} = 3$ since $3^4 = 81$. It is also true that $(-3)^4 = 81$. But $\sqrt[4]{81}$ is defined to be a *nonnegative* number. So $-3 \neq \sqrt[4]{81}$. As with square roots, however, we can say $-3 = -\sqrt[4]{81}$.

EXAMPLE $\sqrt[5]{.00032} = .2$ since $(.2)^5 = .00032$ and $\sqrt[6]{\frac{729}{64}} = \frac{3}{2}$ since $(\frac{3}{2})^6 = 3^6/2^6 = \frac{729}{64}$.

EXAMPLE If $n = 2$, then the *n*th root (or 2nd root) of a nonnegative number d is just the square root of d since $(\sqrt{d})^2 = d$. We shall continue to write $\sqrt{d}$ rather than $\sqrt[2]{d}$.

Despite these examples, the *n*th root of a rational number need *not* be rational. For instance, it can be shown that $\sqrt[3]{2}$ and $\sqrt[11]{225}$ are irrational numbers. In such cases a suitably equipped calculator will provide a decimal (rational) *approximation* for the desired *n*th root. Such a calculator shows, for example, that $\sqrt[3]{2} \approx 1.25992105$.* If you use the calculator to cube this last number, it will probably round off the answer and display 2. If you cube this number by hand, you will find that the answer is very close, but not exactly equal, to 2. If you must carry a number such as $\sqrt[3]{2}$ through a series of calculations by hand, it is almost always better to leave it in the form $\sqrt[3]{2}$ rather than to use a decimal approximation. If necessary, you can insert the approximation at the end of the calculation.

Here is a list of the important properties of roots, followed by some examples.

If c *and* d *are nonnegative real numbers and* m *and* n *are positive
integers, then*

(i) $(\sqrt[n]{d})^n = d$ \qquad (iv) $\sqrt[n]{cd} = \sqrt[n]{c}\sqrt[n]{d}$

(ii) $\sqrt[n]{d^n} = d$ \qquad (v) $\sqrt[n]{\dfrac{c}{d}} = \dfrac{\sqrt[n]{c}}{\sqrt[n]{d}}$ \quad $(d \neq 0)$

(iii) $\sqrt[m]{\sqrt[n]{d}} = \sqrt[mn]{d}$

---

* The symbol $\approx$ means "is approximately equal to."

EXAMPLE $(3 + 5\sqrt{2})(7 - \sqrt{2}) = 3 \cdot 7 + (5\sqrt{2})7 - 3\sqrt{2} - 5\sqrt{2}\sqrt{2}$
$$= 21 + 35\sqrt{2} - 3\sqrt{2} - (5 \cdot 2)$$
$$= 11 + 32\sqrt{2}.$$

EXAMPLE Using property (iv) we see that $\sqrt{2025} = \sqrt{25 \cdot 81} = \sqrt{25}\sqrt{81} = 5 \cdot 9 = 45$ and $\sqrt{48} = \sqrt{16 \cdot 3} = \sqrt{16}\sqrt{3} = 4\sqrt{3}$.

EXAMPLE If x, y, and z are nonnegative real numbers, then properties (ii) and (iv) show that

$$\sqrt[3]{54x^3y^6z} = \sqrt[3]{27 \cdot 2x^3y^6z} = \sqrt[3]{27}\sqrt[3]{2}\sqrt[3]{x^3}\sqrt[3]{y^6}\sqrt[3]{z} = 3\sqrt[3]{2}x\sqrt[3]{(y^2)^3}\sqrt[3]{z}$$
$$= 3\sqrt[3]{2}xy^2\sqrt[3]{z}.$$

EXAMPLE If x is a positive real number and y a nonnegative one, then $\dfrac{\sqrt{6xy^2}}{\sqrt{3x^5}}$ can be simplified as follows:

$$\underset{\substack{\uparrow \\ \text{Property: (v)}}}{\frac{\sqrt{6xy^2}}{\sqrt{3x^5}}} = \sqrt{\frac{6xy^2}{3x^5}} = \underset{\substack{\uparrow \\ \text{(v)}}}{\sqrt{\frac{2y^2}{x^4}}} = \underset{\substack{\uparrow \\ \text{(iv)}}}{\frac{\sqrt{2y^2}}{\sqrt{x^4}}} = \underset{\substack{\uparrow \\ \text{(ii)}}}{\frac{\sqrt{2}\sqrt{y^2}}{\sqrt{(x^2)^2}}} = \frac{\sqrt{2}y}{x^2}$$

EXAMPLE Since $\sqrt[3]{\sqrt[2]{64}} = \sqrt[3]{8} = 2$ and $\sqrt[6]{64} = 2$, we see that $\sqrt[3]{\sqrt[2]{64}} = \sqrt[3 \cdot 2]{64}$ as stated in Property (iii).

Warning If c and d are nonnegative real numbers, then $\sqrt[n]{c + d}$ is *not* the same as $\sqrt[n]{c} + \sqrt[n]{d}$ in most cases. For example, $\sqrt{9 + 16} = \sqrt{25} = 5$, but $\sqrt{9} + \sqrt{16} = 3 + 4 = 7$, so $\sqrt{9 + 16}$ is *not equal* to $\sqrt{9} + \sqrt{16}$.

ROOTS OF NEGATIVE NUMBERS

The nth root of a negative number can be defined when n is *odd* ($n = 1, 3, 5, 7$, etc.). For example, we say that

$$\sqrt[3]{-125} = -5 \quad \text{since} \quad (-5)^3 = -125$$
$$\sqrt[9]{-512} = -2 \quad \text{since} \quad (-2)^9 = -512$$

But when n is *even* ($n = 2, 4, 6$, etc.), it is impossible to define the nth root of a negative number. The reason is that the nth root of a given number is a number c whose nth *power* is the given number. But when n is even, c^n is nonnegative for *every* number c. For instance,

$$(-12)^2 = 144 \qquad (-2)^6 = 64 \qquad 5^4 = 625 \qquad (-10)^8 = 100,000,000$$

Consequently, when n is even, c^n is *never* negative no matter what number c is. So *no* real number can be the nth root of a negative number when n is even. Thus expressions such as $\sqrt{-3}$, $\sqrt{-64}$, $\sqrt[4]{-17}$, $\sqrt[20]{-673}$, and so on are meaningless in the real number system.°

Since the nth root $\sqrt[n]{d}$ is not always defined when d is negative, we shall deal only with nth roots of nonnegative numbers hereafter, unless stated otherwise.

EXERCISES

A.1. Evaluate:

(a) $(-6)^2$

(b) -6^2

(c) $5 + 4(3^2 + 2^3)$

(d) $\dfrac{(-3)^2 + (-2)^4}{-2^2 - 1}$

(e) $(-3)2^2 + 4^2 - 1$

(f) $\dfrac{(-4)^2 + 2}{(-4)^2 - 7} + 1$

(g) $\left(\dfrac{-5}{4}\right)^3$

(h) $-\left(\dfrac{7}{4} + \dfrac{3}{4}\right)^2$

(i) $\left(\dfrac{1}{3}\right)^3 + \left(\dfrac{2}{3}\right)^3$

(j) $\left(\dfrac{5}{7}\right)^2 + \left(\dfrac{2}{7}\right)^2$

A.2. Compute carefully:

(a) $2^4 - 2^7 = ?$

(b) $3^3 - 3^{-7} = ?$

(c) $(2^{-2} + 2)^2 = ?$

(d) $2^2 \cdot 3^{-3} - 3^2 \cdot 2^{-3} = ?$

(e) $\dfrac{1}{2^3} + \dfrac{1}{2^{-4}} = ?$

(f) $3^2\left(\dfrac{1}{3} + \dfrac{1}{3^{-2}}\right) = ?$

A.3. Simplify the following expressions. Each letter represents a nonzero real number and should appear at most once in your answer.

(a) $x \cdot x^2 \cdot x^5$

(b) $(.03)y^2 \cdot y^7$

(c) $(2x^2)^3 3x$

(d) $(3x^2y)^2$

(e) $(1.3)z^2(\sqrt{10y})^2$

(f) $(a^2)(7a)(-3a^3)$

(g) $(2w)^3(3w)(4w)^2$

(h) $(\sqrt[3]{11}x^2y)^3(xy)^2$

(i) $(\sqrt{6uv})^4(\sqrt{6uv})^2$

A.4. Simplify (as in Exercise A.3):

(a) $\dfrac{x^4(x^2)^3}{x^3}$

(b) $\left(\dfrac{z^2}{t^3}\right)^4 \cdot \left(\dfrac{z^3}{t}\right)^5$

(c) $\left(\dfrac{e^6}{c^4}\right)^2 \cdot \left(\dfrac{c^3}{e}\right)^3$

(d) $\left(\dfrac{x^7}{y^6}\right)^2 \cdot \left(\dfrac{y^2}{x}\right)^4$

(e) $\left(\dfrac{ab^2c^3d^4}{abc^2d}\right)^2$

(f) $\dfrac{(3x)^2(y^2)^3x^2}{(2xy^2)^3}$

A.5. Simplify and express each of the following without negative exponents. Assume r, s, and t are positive integers and a, b, and c are positive real numbers.

(a) $\dfrac{3^{-r}}{3^{-s}}$

(d) $\dfrac{4^{-(t+1)}}{9r^{-2}}$

(g) $\dfrac{r^{-t}}{(6s)^{-s}}$

° There is a larger number system, called the complex numbers, in which negative real numbers *do* have square roots, fourth roots, sixth roots, and so on. But these roots are not real numbers and our discussion here is confined to real numbers. Complex numbers will be discussed in Chapter 7.

    (b) $a^{-2}b^3$ (e) $a^2(a^{-1} + a^{-3})$ (h) $(a^{-2}/b^{-2}) + (b^2/a^2)$

    (c) $(a^2 a^{-5} a^4)^{-3}$ (f) $\dfrac{a^{-2}(b^2 c^3)^{-3}}{(a^{-5} b^{-4})^2 c^{-7}}$ (i) $\left(\dfrac{a^6}{b^{-4}}\right)^t$

A.6. Evaluate:

    (a) $\sqrt{11^2}$ (c) $\sqrt[17]{0}$ (e) $\sqrt[3]{54 \cdot 2^2}$ (g) $(\sqrt[3]{13})^{-3}$

    (b) $\sqrt[4]{9^2}$ (d) $\sqrt{(-12)^2}$ (f) $\sqrt[4]{(-7)^4}$ (h) $(\sqrt[27]{8})^{-54}$

A.7. Find an equivalent expression involving at most one radical sign. Assume all letters represent positive real numbers.

    (a) $\sqrt{c}\sqrt{c^{10}}$ (d) $\sqrt[3]{\sqrt[4]{\sqrt{7xy}}}$

    (b) $\left(\sqrt[3]{\dfrac{16rs}{t}}\right)(\sqrt[3]{4s^2 t^7})$ (e) $(4 - \sqrt{3})(5 + 2\sqrt{3})$

    (c) $\sqrt[5]{2}\sqrt[5]{ab}\sqrt[5]{7cd}$ (f) $\sqrt[3]{40} + 2\sqrt[3]{135} - 4\sqrt[3]{320}$

A.8. Assume all letters represent positive real numbers and express without radicals:

    (a) $\sqrt[3]{8a^3 b^3}$ (e) $\sqrt{\sqrt[3]{a^6 b^{12}}}$ (i) $\dfrac{\sqrt[3]{64x^5 y^{14}}}{\sqrt[3]{8x^{-1} y^2}}$

    (b) $\sqrt[3]{27a^6 b^3}$ (f) $\sqrt{u^2 \sqrt{u^8}}$ (j) $\dfrac{\sqrt[3]{27c^4 d^{-3}}}{\sqrt[3]{8c^{-2} d^9}}$

    (c) $\sqrt[4]{81x^8 y^{16}}$ (g) $\sqrt{2}\sqrt{xy}\sqrt{8xy}$ (k) $\dfrac{(\sqrt{xy})^3 \sqrt{y}}{(\sqrt{x^2 y})^2 \sqrt{x}}$

    (d) $\sqrt[5]{32c^{10} d^{15}}$ (h) $\dfrac{\sqrt{6x}}{\sqrt{24x^5}}$

B.1. Express each of these numbers in scientific notation:

    (a)   79,327   (e)   5,963,000,000,000

    (b)   5,200,000   (f)   .00000000000035

    (c)   .002   (g) $\dfrac{.00032}{160,000,000}$

    (d)   .00000079   (h) $\dfrac{(1,000,000)^2 \cdot \sqrt{.00000004}}{\sqrt[3]{(8,000,000,000)^2}}$

B.2. Find the square roots of these numbers, without using a calculator or tables:

    (a)   2304   [*Hint:* Factor 2304 as a product of small integers.]

    (b)   2116   (c)   .1764   (d)   10.89   (e) $(1700 + 64)$ (f) $(2000 - 844)$

B.3. Express each of these numbers as a power of 2. For example, $(\tfrac{1}{8})^3 = (1/2^3)^3 = (2^{-3})^3 = 2^{-9}$.

    (a)   64   (c) $(\tfrac{1}{2})^{-8}(\tfrac{1}{4})^4(\tfrac{1}{16})^{-3}$ (e) $\sqrt[8]{(1024)^4}$

    (b) $(2^4 \cdot 16^{-2})^3$ (d) $\sqrt{\tfrac{128}{2048}}$ (f) $\sqrt[4]{(64)^2}$

B.4. Since $\sqrt{2} + \sqrt{3}$ is nonnegative and $(\sqrt{2} + \sqrt{3})^2 = 2 + 2\sqrt{2}\sqrt{3} + 3 =$

$5 + 2\sqrt{6}$, we conclude that $\sqrt{2} + \sqrt{3}$ must be the square root of $5 + 2\sqrt{6}$. Use similar methods to verify that:

(a) $\sqrt{9 - 2\sqrt{14}} = \sqrt{7} - \sqrt{2}$ (c) $\sqrt[3]{-17\sqrt{2} + 11\sqrt{5}} = \sqrt{5} - \sqrt{2}$

(b) $\sqrt{8 + 2\sqrt{15}} = \sqrt{3} + \sqrt{5}$ (d) $\sqrt[4]{49 + 20\sqrt{6}} = \sqrt{2} + \sqrt{3}$

B.5. **Errors to Avoid** In each part give an example to show that the given statement may be *false* for some numbers.

(a) $a^r + b^r = (a + b)^r$ (f) $\dfrac{c^r}{c^s} = c^{r/s}$

(b) $a^r a^s = a^{rs}$ (g) $\sqrt[3]{a + b} = \sqrt[3]{a} + \sqrt[3]{b}$

(c) $a^r b^s = (ab)^{r+s}$ (h) $\sqrt{c^2 + 1} = c + 1$

(d) $c^{1/k} = \dfrac{1}{c^k}$ (i) $\sqrt{8a} = 4\sqrt{a}$

(e) $c^{-r} = -c^r$

C.1. If c is *any* real number, then $c^2 \geq 0$. So $\sqrt{c^2}$ is defined for *every* real number c. Think carefully and answer this: $\sqrt{c^2} = ?$

3. SETS AND INTERVALS

The *language* of set theory is frequently convenient, so we introduce a small amount of it here. Indeed, all this section amounts to is a short list of names for various concepts with which you are already familiar.

Roughly speaking, a **set** is any collection of objects. In this book the objects will usually be numbers or other mathematical entities. For example, we have the set of integers, the set of positive real numbers, and the set of points on the number line that lie to the left of 3.

The objects in a set are called **elements** or **members** of the set. For instance, -6 is an element of the set of integers. But -7 is *not* an element of the set of all positive real numbers. The number $\sqrt{2}$ is a member of the set of irrational numbers.

Suppose a and b are real numbers with $a < b$. The word **interval** is used to describe the set of all real numbers between a and b. Actually, there are four such sets, depending on whether one, both, or neither of a and b are included:

$[a, b]$ denotes the set of all real numbers x such that $a \leq x \leq b$;
(a, b) denotes the set of all real numbers x such that $a < x < b$;
$[a, b)$ denotes the set of all real numbers x such that $a \leq x < b$;
$(a, b]$ denotes the set of all real numbers x such that $a < x \leq b$.

All four of these sets are called **intervals** from a to b. The numbers a and b are the **endpoints** of the interval. $[a, b]$ is called the **closed interval** from a to b (both endpoints included) and (a, b) is called the **open interval** from a to b (neither endpoint included).

If we think of the real numbers as the points on the number line, then an interval from a to b is just the line segment from a to b, which may or may not include these endpoints. Figure 1-4 shows some specific examples.

Interval	Picture on the number line*
$[-7, 2]$	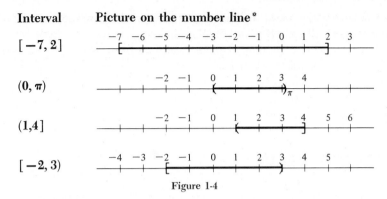
$(0, \pi)$	
$(1,4]$	
$[-2, 3)$	

Figure 1-4

There are other sets of real numbers which are also called intervals. Let b be a real number. Then

$(-\infty, b)$ denotes the set of all real numbers less than b;
$(-\infty, b]$ denotes the set of all real numbers less than or equal to b;
(b, ∞) denotes the set of all real numbers greater than b;
$[b, \infty)$ denotes the set of all real numbers greater than or equal to b.

If we think of the real numbers as the points on the number line, then these four intervals are simply the half-lines extending to the left or right of b, either including or not including b, as shown in Figure 1-5.

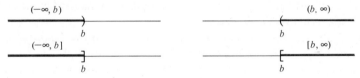

Figure 1-5

Note   The symbol ∞ is sometimes read "infinity" and one sometimes says, for example, that $[b, \infty)$ is the "interval from b to infinity." Don't be misled by this casual use of language. We have simply used the symbol ∞ and the word "infinity" as part of a convenient notation for certain *sets of real numbers*. In particular,

The concept of "infinity", whatever it may be, has *not* been defined here;
There is no real number called "infinity" or "minus infinity";
The symbols ∞ and $-\infty$ are *not* real numbers.

EXERCISES

A.1.   Draw a picture on the number line of each of the following intervals:
  (a) $(0, 8]$;   (b) $(0, \infty)$;   (c) $[-2, 1]$;   (d) $(-1, 1)$;   (e) $(-\infty, 0]$.

---

* In Figures 1-4 and 1-5, a round bracket, such as) or (, at the endpoint of an interval indicates that this endpoint is *not* included. A square bracket, such as] or [, indicates that the endpoint *is* included.

B.1. Let $\mathbf{Z}$ denote the set of all integers, $\mathbf{Q}$ the set of all rational numbers, A the interval $(-7, 12]$, and B the set of all rational numbers in the interval $[0, 4]$. The number 2, for instance, is an element of all four of these sets. Of which sets are the following numbers elements?

(a) $-\frac{3}{2}$ (c) -2 (e) π (g) $\pi - 2$
(b) 4.001 (d) -7 (f) -12 (h) $\sqrt{2}$

4. ABSOLUTE VALUE

On an *informal* level, many students think of absolute value as follows:

The absolute value of a nonnegative number is the number itself;
The absolute value of a negative number is obtained by "erasing the minus sign."

If $|c|$ denotes the absolute value of the number c, then, for example:

$$|7| = 7, \qquad |-3| = 3, \qquad \left|\frac{\pi}{7}\right| = \frac{\pi}{7}, \qquad \left|\frac{-37}{5}\right| = \frac{37}{5}, \qquad |0| = 0$$

But when asked to find the absolute value of the negative number $\pi - 6$, such students are often puzzled: what does "erase the minus sign" mean here?

Is $|\pi - 6| = \pi$ 6?   Is $|\pi - 6| = \pi + 6$?   or what?

This quandary suggests that a more formal and precise algebraic definition of absolute value is needed. The earlier examples, where things were clear, can guide us here.
   Since the absolute value of a nonnegative number is just the number itself, we have:

$$|c| = c \text{ whenever } c \geq 0$$

When c is a negative number, the informal idea of "erasing the minus sign" means, for example, that

$$|-4| = 4, \qquad |-3| = 3, \qquad |-\tfrac{37}{5}| = \tfrac{37}{5}$$

Observe that

$$|-4| = 4 = -(-4), \qquad |-3| = 3 = -(-3), \qquad |-\tfrac{37}{5}| = \tfrac{37}{5} = -(-\tfrac{37}{5})$$

These examples suggest that the absolute value of a *negative* number c is the *positive* number $-c$. In other words,

$$\text{If } c < 0, \text{ then } |c| = -c.$$

For instance,

$$\text{If } c = -7, \text{ then } |-7| = |c| = -c = -(-7) = 7;$$
$$\text{If } c = -12, \text{ then } |-12| = |c| = -c = -(-12) = 12.$$

The preceding discussion leads to this formal definition of absolute value:

> The **absolute value** of a real number c is denoted |c| and defined as follows:
>
> $$\text{if } c \geq 0, \text{ then } |c| = c$$
> $$\text{if } c < 0, \text{ then } |c| = -c$$

EXAMPLE   In order to find $|\pi - 6|$, we observe that $\pi - 6 < 0$, so that

$$|\pi - 6| = -(\pi - 6) = -\pi + 6 = 6 - \pi$$

EXAMPLE   Since $\pi - 3 > 0$, we have $|\pi - 3| = \pi - 3$.

BASIC PROPERTIES OF ABSOLUTE VALUES

We list below some frequently used facts about absolute values. You should be familiar with all of them and should be able to give numerical examples of each.

> **FACT** $|c| \geq 0$ and $|c| > 0$ when $c \neq 0$

EXAMPLES $|3| = 3 > 0;$ $|-7| = 7 > 0;$ $|0| = 0;$ $|-\frac{1}{3}| = \frac{1}{3} > 0.$

> **FACT** $|c| = |-c|$

EXAMPLES $|4| = 4 = |-4|;$ $|\pi| = \pi = |-\pi|;$ $|0| = 0 = |-0|;$
$|\frac{7}{2}| = \frac{7}{2} = |-\frac{7}{2}|.$

> **FACT** $|c|^2 = c^2 = |c^2|$

EXAMPLE   Let $c = -3$; then

$$c^2 = (-3)^2 = 9$$
$$|c^2| = |(-3)^2| = |9| = 9$$
$$|c|^2 = |-3|^2 = |-3||-3| = 3 \cdot 3 = 9$$

> **FACT** $\sqrt{c^2} = |c|$

EXAMPLES Let $c = -3$. Then

$$\sqrt{c^2} = \sqrt{(-3)^2} = \sqrt{9} = 3 = |-3| = |c|$$

Let $c = 7$; then

$$\sqrt{c^2} = \sqrt{7^2} = \sqrt{49} = 7 = |7| = |c|$$

FACT $|cd| = |c|\,|d|$ *and if* d $\neq 0$, $\left|\dfrac{c}{d}\right| = \dfrac{|c|}{|d|}.$

EXAMPLES Let $c = 6$ and $d = -2$; then

$$|cd| = |6(-2)| = |-12| = 12 \quad \text{and} \quad |c|\,|d| = |6|\,|-2| = 6 \cdot 2 = 12$$

Let $c = -7$ and $d = -\frac{1}{4}$; then

$$|cd| = |(-7)(-\tfrac{1}{4})| = |\tfrac{7}{4}| = \tfrac{7}{4} \quad \text{and} \quad |c|\,|d| = |-7|\,|-\tfrac{1}{4}| = 7(\tfrac{1}{4}) = \tfrac{7}{4}$$

Let $c = -\sqrt{3}$ and $d = \frac{7}{3}$; then

$$\left|\frac{c}{d}\right| = \left|\frac{-\sqrt{3}}{\frac{7}{3}}\right| = \left|\frac{-3\sqrt{3}}{7}\right| = \frac{3\sqrt{3}}{7} \quad \text{and} \quad \frac{|c|}{|d|} = \frac{|-\sqrt{3}|}{|\frac{7}{3}|} = \frac{\sqrt{3}}{\frac{7}{3}} = \frac{3\sqrt{3}}{7}$$

DISTANCE ON THE NUMBER LINE

We would like to have a formula for calculating the distance between any two numbers on the number line. We shall now see that such a formula can be obtained by using absolute values.

EXAMPLE In Figure 1-6 the distance between -6 and 0 on the number line is easily seen to be 6 units.

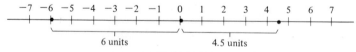

Figure 1-6

Observe that $|-6| = 6 =$ distance between -6 and 0. Figure 1-6 also shows that the distance between 4.5 and 0 on the number line is 4.5 units. Note that $|4.5| =$ distance between 4.5 and 0.

The preceding example is an illustration of this general fact:

$|c|$ *is the distance between* c *and* 0 *on the number line.*

This geometric interpretation of absolute value as a distance leads to another useful property of absolute values.

EXAMPLE How many real numbers have absolute value 3? Since absolute value can be interpreted as distance to 0, this question is the same as: how many real numbers are 3 units from 0 on the number line? For the answer, look at Figure 1-7.

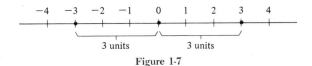

Figure 1-7

There are just two numbers whose distance to 0 is 3 units, namely, 3 and −3.

The argument used in the preceding example works in the general case as well, and proves this fact:

> *If* k *is a positive number, then the only numbers with absolute value* k *are* k *and* −k.

In order to determine the distance between two (possibly) nonzero numbers on the line, we consider another example.

EXAMPLE The distance between −5 and 3 on the number line is 8 units, as shown in Figure 1-8.

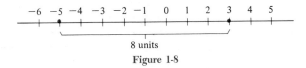

Figure 1-8

Note that $|-5 - 3| = 8 =$ distance between −5 and 3. It is also true that $|3 - (-5)| = |3 + 5| = 8 =$ distance between −5 and 3.

The preceding examples suggest that the distance between two numbers on the number line is always given by the absolute value of their difference. In other words,

> *The distance between the numbers* c *and* d *on the number line is the number* $|c - d|$.

As the examples illustrate, it doesn't matter in which order you take the difference—the same distance results in either order. The reason is that for any two numbers c and d,

$$-(c - d) = -c + d = d - c$$

Since any number and its negative have the same absolute value, we see that

$$|c - d| = |-(c - d)| = |d - c|$$

This is just an algebraic statement of the geometric fact that the distance from c to d is the same as the distance from d to c.

ALGEBRA AND GEOMETRY

We have already seen several examples of how absolute values may be interpreted either algebraically or geometrically. This close relationship between algebra and geometry often suggests two different ways of thinking about the same problem, which usually increases the chances of solving the problem.

EXAMPLE The geometric statement "the distance between t and 7 is $\frac{3}{2}$" can be expressed algebraically as $|t - 7| = \frac{3}{2}$.

EXAMPLE The inequality $|x - 3| < |z + 4|$ can be rewritten as $|x - 3| < |z - (-4)|$. This is just an algebraic way of saying,

The distance from x to 3 is less than the distance from z to -4,

or equivalently, x is closer to 3 than z is to -4.

EXAMPLE The solution of the equation $|x + 5| = 3$ can easily be found geometrically. If we rewrite the equation as $|x - (-5)| = 3$, it states that

The distance from x to -5 is 3 units.

On the number line in Figure 1-9, it's easy to see that there are only two numbers that are exactly 3 units from -5, namely, -8 and -2.

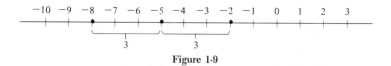

Figure 1-9

Thus $x = -8$ and $x = -2$ are the solutions of $|x + 5| = 3$.

EXAMPLE The solutions of the inequality $|x - 7| < 2.5$ are all numbers x such that

The distance from x to 7 is less than 2.5.

If we look at the number line in Figure 1-10,

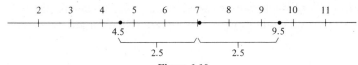

Figure 1-10

we see that any number x between 4.5 and 9.5 is *at most* 2.5 units from 7 and all other numbers are *more than* 2.5 units from 7. Thus the set of all solutions of $|x - 7| < 2.5$ is the interval $(4.5, 9.5)$.

EXERCISES

A.1. Compute:

(a) $-|-7|$

(b) $|3 - 14|$

(c) $|(-13)^2|$

(d) $||-7| - |-4||$

(e) $\dfrac{|-5|}{-5}$

(f) $|\sqrt{2} - 2|$

(g) $|\pi - \sqrt{2}|$

(h) $|(-2)(3)|$

A.2. Fill the blank with one of $<$, $=$, or $>$ so that the resulting statement is true.

(a) $|-2|$ _____ $|-5|$;

(b) 5 _____ $|-2|$;

(c) $|3|$ _____ $-|4|$.

(d) $|-3|$ _____ 0;

(e) -7 _____ $|-1|$;

(f) $-|-4|$ _____ 0;

(g) $|-4 + |-4||$ _____ 0;

A.3. In each of the following, find two pairs of numbers that make the statement true *and* two pairs that make it false. (For instance $|x| < |y|$ is true for 1,2 and $-1,7$ but is false for 3,1 and $-3, -2$.)

(a) $|x| + |y| = 1$

(b) $|y| - |x| < 0$

(c) $|x + y| = |x| + |y|$

(d) $|x + y| < |x| + |y|$

(e) $|x - y| = y - x$

(f) $|x - y| = |x| - |y|$

A.4. In each part, find the distance between the two given numbers.

(a) -7 and $\frac{15}{2}$

(b) $-\frac{3}{4}$ and -10

(c) 7 and 107

(d) π and 3

(e) π and -3

(f) $\sqrt{2}$ and $\sqrt{3}$

B.1. (a) Explain why the statement $|a| + |b| + |c| > 0$ is algebraic shorthand for "at least one of the numbers a,b,c is different from zero."

(b) Find an algebraic shorthand version of the statement "the numbers a,b,c are all different from zero."

B.2. Explain why each of the following is a true statement, no matter what the numbers c and d may be. (*Hint*: look back at the Facts about absolute values in the text.)

(a) $|c - d| = |d - c|$

(b) $|(c - d)^2| = c^2 - 2cd + d^2$

(c) $\sqrt{9c^2 - 18cd + 9d^2} = 3|c - d|$

B.3.   Fill the blanks in the following table.

Algebraic Statement	Equivalent Geometric Statement
(a) $\|x - c\| > 6$	x is more than 6 units from c.
(b) $\|x - 3\| < 2$	_____
(c) _____	c is closer to 0 than b is
(d) $\|b\| < \|c - 3\|$	_____
(e) $\|x + 7\| \leq 3$	_____
(f) _____	x is 5 units from c.
(g) _____	x is at most 17 units from -4.
(h) $\|c\| \geq 12$	_____

B.4.   Explain geometrically why each of the following statements is *always false*.
(a) $\|c - 1\| < 2$ and $\|c - 12\| < 3$.   (b) $\|d + 1\| > 3$ and $\|d - 1\| < 1$.

B.5.   For what values of x is each of the following statements true? For example, the statement $\|x\| = x$ is true for all nonnegative numbers x and the statement $\|x\| \geq 0$ is true for all real numbers x.
(a) $x \leq \|x\|$ (b) $\|x\| \leq x$ (c) $\|x\| \leq -x$ (d) $-\|x\| \leq x$

B.6.   Use the geometric approach explained in the text to solve these equations.
(a) $\|x\| = 1$ (c) $\|x - 2\| = 1$ (e) $\|x + \pi\| = 4$
(b) $\|x\| = \frac{3}{2}$ (d) $\|x + 3\| = 2$ (f) $\|x - \frac{3}{2}\| = 5$

B.7.   Suppose $\|x - 2\| = 3$. In this case $\|x - 1\| = ?$ $\|x + 1\| = ?$ $\|x\| = ?$ $\|x - 3\| = ?$

B.8.   Suppose $\|x + 1\| = 4$. In this case $\|x\| = ?$ $\|x - 2\| = ?$ $\|x - 4\| = ?$ $\|x + 4\| = ?$

B.9.   Use the geometric approach explained in the text to solve these inequalities:
(a) $\|x\| < 7$ (c) $\|x + 3\| < 1$ (e) $\|x\| \geq 5$
(b) $\|x - 5\| < 2$ (d) $\|x + \frac{1}{2}\| < 2$ (f) $\|x - 6\| > 2$

B.10.   Suppose $\|x - 2\| < 1$. In this case, what can you say about $\|x\|$ and $\|x - 3\|$?

5. ALGEBRAIC EXPRESSIONS AND POLYNOMIALS

The basic idea in algebra is to use letters or other symbols to represent numbers. For example, the statement

the sum of one number and 3 times the square of a second number is 12

can be written concisely by letting b denote the first number and c the second. Then the statement can be written: $b + 3c^2 = 12$. Similarly, the expression $\dfrac{x^2}{7\pi + y} + \sqrt{z}$

is shorthand for the number obtained by

dividing the square of the number x by the sum of 7π and the number y;
then adding the result to the square root of the number z

Expressions such as $b + 3c^2$ and $\dfrac{x^2}{7\pi + y} + \sqrt{z}$ and $3x^2 - 5x + 4$, and so on are
called **algebraic expressions.** Each expression represents a number that is obtained by
performing various algebraic operations (such as addition or division or taking roots)
on one or more numbers, some of which are denoted by letters. Unless stated otherwise, you should assume that every algebraic expression represents a well-defined *real*
number. For instance, in the expression $\dfrac{1}{c^3 - 5}$ we assume that the denominator
$c^3 - 5$ is not zero since $\frac{1}{0}$ is *not* a real number. Similarly, in the expression $\sqrt{z}$ we
assume that z is a nonnegative number so that $\sqrt{z}$ will be a real number.

ARITHMETIC WITH ALGEBRAIC EXPRESSIONS

Since algebraic expressions are just shorthand notations for certain real numbers, the
same rules of arithmetic presented earlier for numbers are also valid for algebraic
expressions. The only difference that occurs when doing arithmetic with algebraic
expressions is that the answer is often another algebraic expression instead of a single
number. It is customary to rearrange and collect similar terms so that the final answer
will be in as simple a form as possible.

EXAMPLE

$$
\begin{aligned}
(a^2b - 3\sqrt{c}) + (5ab + 7\sqrt{c}) + 7a^2b &= a^2b - 3\sqrt{c} + 5ab + 7\sqrt{c} + 7a^2b \\
&= a^2b + 7a^2b - 3\sqrt{c} + 7\sqrt{c} + 5ab \\
&= (1 + 7)a^2b + (-3 + 7)\sqrt{c} + 5ab \\
&= 8a^2b + 4\sqrt{c} + 5ab
\end{aligned}
$$

Be careful with minus signs and subtraction of terms in parentheses. For instance,
$-(b + 3) = -b - 3$ and *not* $-b + 3$. Also, $-(7 - y) = -7 - (-y) = -7 + y$.

EXAMPLE $(x^4 + 6x^2 + x - 11) - (3x^2 - 5x - 2)$

$$
\begin{aligned}
&= x^4 + 6x^2 + x - 11 - 3x^2 + 5x + 2 \\
&= x^4 + 6x^2 - 3x^2 + x + 5x - 11 + 2 \\
&= x^4 + (6 - 3)x^2 + (1 + 5)x - 11 + 2 \\
&= x^4 + 3x^2 + 6x - 9
\end{aligned}
$$

In actual practice, addition and subtraction of algebraic expressions is seldom written out in such detail. You usually do most of the intermediate steps in your head.

When multiplying algebraic expressions, the commutative laws (page 6) and the
exponent laws (page 17) are frequently used without explicit mention. For example,

$$(2x)(7x^5) = 14x^6 \quad \text{since} \quad (2x)(7x^5) = 2 \cdot 7 \cdot x \cdot x^5 = 14 \cdot x^{1+5} = 14x^6$$

The usual method of multiplying two sums is to use the distributive laws repeatedly, as
shown in the following examples. What this amounts to in practice is to

Multiply every term in the first expression by *every*
term in the second expression and add the results.

EXAMPLE $(3x + 2)(x + 5) = 3x(x + 5) + 2(x + 5) = 3x \cdot x + 3x \cdot 5 + 2 \cdot x + 2 \cdot 5$
$$= 3x^2 + 15x + 2x + 10 = 3x^2 + 17x + 10$$

EXAMPLE $(2x - 5y)(3x - 4y) = 2x(3x - 4y) - 5y(3x - 4y)$
$$= 2x(3x) + 2x(-4y) - 5y(3x) - 5y(-4y)$$
$$= 6x^2 - 8xy - 15xy + 20y^2 = 6x^2 - 23xy + 20y^2$$

EXAMPLE $(y - 2)(3y^2 - 7y + 4) = y(3y^2 - 7y + 4) - 2(3y^2 - 7y + 4)$
$$= 3y^3 - 7y^2 + 4y - 6y^2 + 14y - 8$$
$$= 3y^3 - 13y^2 + 18y - 8$$

Certain multiplication patterns appear so often that they should be memorized. One such pattern occurs with products of the form $(u + v)(u - v)$:

$$(u + v)(u - v) = u(u - v) + v(u - v) = u^2 - uv + uv - v^2 = u^2 - v^2$$

The pattern

$$\boxed{(u + v)(u - v) = u^2 - v^2}$$

can be used to compute the product of the sum and difference of any two quantities.

EXAMPLE   To compute $(2x + 5)(2x - 5)$ we substitute $2x$ for u and 5 for v in the pattern: $(2x + 5)(2x - 5) = (2x)^2 - 5^2 = 4x^2 - 25$. Similarly,

$$(\sqrt{c} + 7)(\sqrt{c} - 7) = (\sqrt{c})^2 - 7^2 = c - 49$$
$$(x^3 + y^5)(x^3 - y^5) = (x^3)^2 - (y^5)^2 = x^6 - y^{10}$$

Another common pattern occurs when the quantity $u + v$ is squared:

$$(u + v)^2 = (u + v)(u + v) = u(u + v) + v(u + v)$$
$$= u^2 + uv + uv + v^2 = u^2 + 2uv + v^2$$

The pattern

$$\boxed{(u + v)^2 = u^2 + 2uv + v^2}$$

can be used to square the sum of any two quantities.

EXAMPLE   To find $(y + 3)^2$ we substitute y for u and 3 for v in the pattern:

$$(y + 3)^2 = y^2 + 2 \cdot y \cdot 3 + 3^2 = y^2 + 6y + 9$$

Similarly,

$$(2x + \sqrt{7})^2 = (2x)^2 + 2 \cdot 2x \cdot \sqrt{7} + (\sqrt{7})^2 = 4x^2 + 4\sqrt{7}x + 7$$

EXAMPLE To find $(x - 3y)^2$, we write $x - 3y$ as $x + (-3y)$ and substitute x for u and $-3y$ for v of the square pattern:

$$(x - 3y)^2 = x^2 + 2 \cdot x(-3y) + (-3y)^2 = x^2 - 6xy + 9y^2$$

Warning Don't forget the middle term! $(u + v)^2$ is *not* equal to $u^2 + v^2$ but *is* equal to $u^2 + 2uv + v^2$.

POLYNOMIALS

Some kinds of algebraic expressions are given special names. A **polynomial** is an algebraic expression, such as

$$x^3 - 6x^2 + \sqrt{2}x - 7 \qquad\qquad 37y^{15} + 12y^9 + y^7 - 4 \qquad\qquad z + \tfrac{3}{5} \qquad\qquad 11$$

Notice that all the constants $(-6, \sqrt{2}, 37, \tfrac{3}{5},$ etc.$)$ are real numbers, that all the exponents are nonnegative integers, and that no roots, quotients, or negative powers of the letters x, y, and z appear. None of the following expressions are polynomials because they involve either roots, quotients, or negative powers of the letter x:

$$\sqrt{x^3 + 2x - 1} \qquad x^4 + 3\sqrt{x} - 4 \qquad \frac{1}{x^2} = x^{-2} \qquad 2x^4 - \frac{5}{x^3} + 7x^2 + \frac{3}{x} + 9$$

Although any letter may be used when writing polynomials, we shall generally use x in this discussion. A more formal definition of a polynomial is that a polynomial is an algebraic expression that can be written in the form:

$$a_n x^n + a_{n-1} x^{n-1} + a_{n-2} x^{n-2} + \cdots + a_3 x^3 + a_2 x^2 + a_1 x^1 + a_0$$

where $a_0, a_1, a_2, \ldots, a_{n-1}, a_n$ are fixed real numbers (constants) and n is a nonnegative integer. The numbers $a_0, a_1, \ldots, a_n$ are called **coefficients.**

EXAMPLE The expression $-7x^4 + x^3 + 4x - 5$ is a polynomial because it can be written as $(-7)x^4 + 1x^3 + 0x^2 + 4x^1 + (-5)$. Here we have $n = 4, n - 1 = 3$, and so on, and the coefficients are

$$a_4 = -7 \qquad a_3 = 1 \qquad a_2 = 0 \qquad a_1 = 4 \qquad a_0 = -5$$

Once you understand the formal definition, it is usually more convenient to write such a polynomial in its original shorter form: $-7x^4 + x^3 + 4x - 5$. In other words, we omit any term with zero coefficient (in this case, $0x^2$) and we don't write a coefficient or an exponent if it is the number 1 (in this case, x^3 instead of $1x^3$ and $4x$ instead of $4x^1$).

Because it is often inconvenient to keep writing an arbitrary polynomial as $a_n x^n + a_{n-1} x^{n-1} + \cdots + a_1 x + a_0$, we shall sometimes use symbols such as $f(x)$ or $h(x)$ to denote polynomials. For example, $f(x)$ might denote the polynomial $7x^5 - 6x^2 + 2x - 5$.

When a polynomial is written so that the powers of x appear in *descending* order, as in $6x^7 + 4x^3 + 5x^2 - 7x + 10$ or $x^4 + 2x^3 + 3x^2 + 4x + 5$, the *nonzero coefficient* of the highest power of x is called the **leading coefficient** and the last term (the one without a power of x) is the **constant term.** For example,

Polynomial	Leading Coefficient	Constant Term
$6x^7 + 4x^3 + 5x^2 - 7x + 10$	6	10
$-x^4 + 2x^3 + 3x^2 + 4x + 5$	-1	5
$0x^4 + 5x^3 - 6x^2 + 2x - 1$	5 (note well)	-1
$7x^5 - 3x^3 + x^2 + 4x$	7	0 (note well)
$2x^6 + 3x^7 + x^8 - 2x - 4 + 4x^2$	1 (be careful)	-4 (ditto)
$a_n x^n + a_{n-1} x^{n-1} + \cdots + a_2 x^2 + a_1 x + a_0 \ (a_n \neq 0)$	a_n	a_0

A polynomial that consists only of a constant term, such as 11 or -7 or 0, is called a **constant polynomial.**

The **degree** of a nonconstant polynomial is the highest *exponent* that occurs in the polynomial with a nonzero coefficient. For example, $6x^3 + 2x^2 - x + 5$ has degree 3 and $2x + 18$ has degree 1. But $0x^5 + 5x^4 - 7x + 3$ has degree 4 since 4 is the highest exponent that occurs with a *nonzero* coefficient. And $7x^3 + x^8 - 14x + 1$ has degree 8 since 8 is the *highest* (but not the first) exponent that occurs with a nonzero coefficient.

First-degree polynomials are often called **linear polynomials.** Second-degree polynomials are called **quadratics** and third-degree polynomials, **cubics.**

The degree of a *nonzero* constant polynomial, such as 11 or -7, is defined to be 0. This is a reasonable definition if you consider the constant term of a polynomial as being the coefficient of x^0 and assume that $x^0 = 1$. Then $11 = 11x^0$ has degree 0, the highest exponent that occurs with a nonzero coefficient.

The **zero polynomial** is the constant polynomial 0. The degree of the zero polynomial is *not defined* since no exponent occurs with a nonzero coefficient.

POLYNOMIAL ARITHMETIC

Earlier in this section we saw examples of addition, subtraction, and multiplication of polynomials. As you may recall from previous algebra courses, it is also possible to divide one polynomial by another. To review polynomial division, we shall begin by recalling how long division of numbers is carried out.

EXAMPLE To divide 4509 by 31 we proceed as follows:

$$
\begin{array}{r}
145 \\
31\overline{\smash{)}4509} \\
\underline{31} \quad \leftarrow 1 \cdot 31 \\
140 \quad \leftarrow \text{subtract} \\
\underline{124} \quad \leftarrow 4 \cdot 31 \\
169 \quad \leftarrow \text{subtract} \\
\underline{155} \quad \leftarrow 5 \cdot 31 \\
14 \quad \leftarrow \text{subtract}
\end{array}
$$

check:
$$
\begin{array}{r}
145 \leftarrow \text{quotient} \\
\times 31 \leftarrow \text{divisor} \\
\hline
145 \\
435 \\
\hline
4495 \\
+14 \leftarrow \text{remainder} \\
\hline
4509 \leftarrow \text{dividend}
\end{array}
$$

The number 4509 is the **dividend,** 31 is the **divisor,** 145 is the **quotient,** and 14 is the **remainder.** The division process stops when we reach a remainder (namely, 14) that is *less* than the divisor 31. The procedure shown above for checking the division may be summarized in one line by:

$$(31)(145) + 14 = 4509$$

or expressed in words:

$$(\text{Divisor})(\text{Quotient}) + (\text{Remainder}) = \text{Dividend}$$

Long division of polynomials is similar in many ways to long division of numbers, as shown in the following examples.

EXAMPLE To divide $2x^5 + 5x^4 - 4x^3 + 8x^2 + 1$ by $2x^2 - x + 1$, we first write:

$$2x^2 - x + 1 \overline{\smash{\big)}\, 2x^5 + 5x^4 - 4x^3 + 8x^2 + 1}$$

We call $2x^2 - x + 1$ the **divisor** and $2x^5 + 5x^4 - 4x^3 + 8x^2 + 1$ the **dividend.** The **quotient** of the division will be written above the horizontal line. We begin by dividing the first term of the divisor $(2x^2)$ into the first term of the dividend $(2x^5)$ and putting the result $\left(\text{namely, } \dfrac{2x^5}{2x^2} = x^3\right)$ on the top line, as shown below. Then multiply x^3 times the entire dividend, put the result on the third line, and subtract:

$$
\begin{array}{r}
x^3 \\
2x^2 - x + 1 \overline{\smash{\big)}\, 2x^5 + 5x^4 - 4x^3 + 8x^2 + 1} \\
\underline{2x^5 - x^4 + x^3} \qquad \leftarrow x^3 \cdot (2x^2 - x + 1) \\
6x^4 - 5x^3 + 8x^2 + 1 \leftarrow \text{subtract}^{\circ}
\end{array}
$$

Next, divide the first term of the divisor $(2x^2)$ into $6x^4$ and put the result $\left(\dfrac{6x^4}{2x^2} = 3x^2\right)$ on the top line, as shown below. Then multiply $3x^2$ times the entire dividend, put the result on the fifth line, and subtract. Continuing this procedure, we obtain:

$$
\begin{array}{r}
x^3 + 3x^2 - x + 2 \qquad\qquad \leftarrow \text{quotient} \\
2x^2 - x + 1 \overline{\smash{\big)}\, 2x^5 + 5x^4 - 4x^3 + 8x^2 + 1} \\
\underline{2x^5 - x^4 + x^3} \qquad\qquad \leftarrow x^3 \cdot (2x^2 - x + 1) \\
6x^4 - 5x^3 + 8x^2 + 1 \leftarrow \text{subtract} \\
\underline{6x^4 - 3x^3 + 3x^2} \qquad\qquad \leftarrow 3x^2 \cdot (2x^2 - x + 1) \\
-2x^3 + 5x^2 + 1 \leftarrow \text{subtract} \\
\underline{-2x^3 + x^2 - x + 1} \leftarrow (-x)(2x^2 - x + 1) \\
4x^2 + x + 1 \leftarrow \text{subtract} \\
\underline{4x^2 - 2x + 2} \leftarrow 2 \cdot (2x^2 - x + 1) \\
3x - 1 \leftarrow \text{subtract}
\end{array}
$$

The polynomial $3x - 1$ is called the **remainder.** The division process always stops when the remainder is zero or has *smaller degree* than the divisor (here the divisor $2x^2 - x + 1$ has degree 2 and the remainder $3x - 1$ has degree 1). We can check this

---

° If this subtraction is confusing, write it out horizontally and watch the signs carefully: $(2x^5 + 5x^4 - 4x^3 + 8x^2 + 1) - (2x^5 - x^4 + x^3) = 2x^5 + 5x^4 - 4x^3 + 8x^2 + 1 - 2x^5 + x^4 - x^3 = 6x^4 - 5x^3 + 8x^2 + 1$, as shown above in vertical fashion.

division by the same method used with numbers: Verify that the product of the divisor and the quotient is

$$(2x^2 - x + 1)(x^3 + 3x^2 - x + 2) = 2x^5 + 5x^4 - 4x^3 + 8x^2 - 3x + 2$$

Adding the remainder $3x - 1$ to this result yields the original dividend:

$$(2x^5 + 5x^4 - 4x^3 + 8x^2 - 3x + 2) + (3x - 1) = 2x^5 + 5x^4 - 4x^3 + 8x^2 + 1$$

So just as with division of numbers, we have:

$$(\text{Divisor})(\text{Quotient}) + (\text{Remainder}) = \text{Dividend}$$

When the divisor is a first-degree polynomial such as $x - 2$ or $x + 5$, there is a convenient shorthand method of performing polynomial division. It is called **synthetic division** and is explained in the DO IT YOURSELF! segment at the end of this section. Whatever method of division is used, the fact illustrated in the preceding example is always true: When the polynomial $f(x)$ is divided by the polynomial $h(x)$, the remainder is 0 or has smaller degree than the divisor and

$$(\text{Divisor})(\text{Quotient}) + (\text{Remainder}) = \text{Dividend}$$

Because this fact is so important, it is given a special name and a formal statement:

THE DIVISION ALGORITHM

If a polynomial f(x) *is divided by a nonzero polynomial* h(x), *then there is a quotient polynomial* q(x) *and a remainder polynomial* r(x) *such that*

$$h(x)q(x) + r(x) = f(x)$$

where either r(x) = 0 *or* r(x) *has degree less than the degree of the divisor* h(x).

The division algorithm can be used to determine whether a given polynomial $h(x)$ is a factor of another polynomial $f(x)$. (Recall that $h(x)$ is a factor of $f(x)$ if $f(x) = h(x)q(x)$ for some polynomial $q(x)$.)

EXAMPLE To determine if $h(x) = 2x^2 + 1$ is a factor of $f(x) = 6x^3 - 4x^2 + 3x - 2$, we divide $f(x)$ by $h(x)$:

$$
\begin{array}{r}
3x \quad - 2 \\
2x^2 + 1 \overline{\smash{\big)}\, 6x^3 - 4x^2 + 3x - 2} \\
\underline{6x^3 \qquad\quad + 3x} \\
-4x^2 \qquad\; - 2 \\
\underline{-4x^2 \qquad\; - 2} \\
0
\end{array}
$$

Since the remainder is 0, the division algorithm tells us that:

$$\text{Dividend} = (\text{Divisor})(\text{Quotient}) + (\text{Remainder})$$

$$6x^3 - 4x^2 + 3x - 2 = (2x^2 + 1)(3x - 2) + 0 = (2x^2 + 1)(3x - 2)$$

Therefore $2x^2 + 1$ *is* a factor of $6x^3 - 4x^2 + 3x - 2$ and the other factor $3x - 2$ is just the quotient of the division.

The argument used in the preceding example works in general and shows that:

The remainder in polynomial division is 0 *exactly when the divisor* h(x) *is a factor of the dividend* f(x). *In this case, the other factor is the quotient.*

EXERCISES

A.1. Perform the indicated addition or subtraction and simplify your answer:
  (a) $x + 7x$
  (b) $5w + 7w - 3w$
  (c) $6a^2b + (-8b)a^2$
  (d) $-6x^3\sqrt{t} + 7x^3\sqrt{t} - 15x^3\sqrt{t}$
  (e) $(x^2 + 2x + 1) - (x^3 - 3x^2 + 4)$

  (f) $\left(u^4 - (-3)u^3 + \dfrac{u}{2} + 1\right) + \left(u^4 - 2u^3 + 5 - \dfrac{u}{2}\right)$

  (g) $\left(u^4 - (-3)u^3 + \dfrac{u}{2} + 1\right) - \left(u^4 - 2u^3 + 5 - \dfrac{u}{2}\right)$

  (h) $(6a^2b + 3a\sqrt{c} - 5ab\sqrt{c}) + (-6ab^2 - 3ab + 6ab\sqrt{c})$
  (i) $(4z - 6z^2w - (-2)z^3w^2) + (8 - 6z^2w - zw^3 + 4z^3w^2)$
  (j) $(x^5y - 2x + 3xy^3) - (-2x - x^5y + 2xy^3)$
  (k) $(9x - x^3 + 1) - (2x^3 + (-6)x + (-7))$
  (l) $(x - \sqrt{y} - z) - (x + \sqrt{y} + z) - (\sqrt{y} + z - x)$
  (m) $(x^2 - 3xy) - (x + xy) - (x^2 + xy)$

A.2. Perform the indicated multiplication:
  (a) $2x(x^2 + 2)$ (f) $6z^3(2z + 5)$
  (b) $(-5y)(-3y^2 + 1)$ (g) $-3x^2(12x^6 - 7x^5)$
  (c) $x^2y(xy - 6xy^2)$ (h) $3ab(4a - 6b + 2a^2b)$
  (d) $3ax(4ax - 2a^2y + 2ay)$ (i) $(-3ay)(4ay - 5y)$
  (e) $2x(x^2 - 3xy + 2y^2)$

A.3. Perform the indicated multiplication and simplify your answer:
  (a) $(x + 1)(x - 2)$ (d) $(y - 6)(2y + 2)$
  (b) $(x + 2)(2x - 5)$ (e) $(y + 3)(y + 4)$
  (c) $(-2x + 4)(-x - 3)$ (f) $(w - 2)(3w + 1)$

      (g) $(3x + 7)(-2x + 5)$ **(i)** $(y - 3)(3y^2 + 4)$
      (h) $(ab + 1)(a - 2)$

A.4.   Use the multiplication patterns discussed in the text to compute these products:
      (a) $(y + 8)(y - 8)$ **(g)** $(2x + 3y)^2$
      (b) $(x + 4)(x - 4)$ **(h)** $(5x - b)^2$
      (c) $(3x - y)(3x + y)$ **(i)** $(2s^2 - 9y)(2s^2 + 9y)$
      (d) $(4a + 5b)(4a - 5b)$ **(j)** $(4x^3 - y^4)^2$
      (e) $(x + 6)^2$ **(k)** $(4x^3 - 5y^2)(4x^3 + 5y^2)$
      (f) $(y - 11)^2$ **(l)** $(-3x^2 + 2y^4)^2$

A.5.   Perform the indicated multiplication and simplify your answer:
      (a) $(c - 2)(2c^2 - 3c + 1)$ **(f)** $2x(3x + 1)(4x - 2)$
      (b) $(2y + 3)(y^2 + 3y - 1)$ **(g)** $3y(-y + 2)(3y + 1)$
      (c) $(x + 2y)(2x^2 - xy + y^2)$ **(h)** $(x - 1)(x - 2)(x - 3)$
      (d) $(5w + 6)(-3w^2 + 4w - 3)$ **(i)** $(y - 2)(3y + 2)(y + 2)$
      (e) $(5x - 2y)(x^2 - 2xy + 3y^2)$ **(j)** $(x + 4y)(2y - x)(3x - y)$

A.6.   Determine whether the given algebraic expression is a polynomial. If it is, list its leading coefficient, constant term, and degree.

      (a) $1 + x^3$ **(e)** $(x + \sqrt{3})(x - \sqrt{3})$

      (b) -7 **(f)** $4x^2 + 3\sqrt{x} + 5$

      (c) $(x - 1)(x^2 + 1)$ **(g)** $\dfrac{7}{x^2} + \dfrac{5}{x} - 15$

      (d) $7^x + 2x + 1$ **(h)** $(x - 1)^k$ (where k is
                                       a fixed positive integer)

A.7.   Divide the first polynomial by the second. Check your division by calculating (divisor)(quotient) + remainder.
      (a) $3x^4 + 2x^2 - 6x + 1$; $x + 1$
      (b) $x^5 - x^3 + x - 5$; $x - 2$
      (c) $x^5 + 2x^4 - 6x^3 + x^2 - 5x + 1$; $x^3 + 1$
      (d) $3x^4 - 3x^3 - 11x^2 + 6x - 1$; $x^3 + x^2 - 2$
      (e) $5x^4 + 5x^2 + 5$; $x^2 - x + 1$
      (f) $x^5 - 1$; $x - 1$

A.8.   Determine whether the first polynomial is a factor of the second:
      (a) $x^2 + 3x - 1$; $x^3 + 2x^2 - 5x - 6$
      (b) $x^2 + 9$; $x^5 + x^4 - 81x - 81$
      (c) $x^2 + 3x - 1$; $x^4 + 3x^3 - 2x^2 - 3x + 1$
      (d) $x^2 - 5x + 7$; $x^3 - 3x^2 - 3x + 9$

B.1.   Find the coefficient of x^2 in each of these products. Avoid doing any more multiplying than is necessary. *Example:* since $(x + 3)(x^2 + x) = x^3 + 4x^2 + 3x$ (verify!), the coefficient of x^2 is 4.
      (a) $(x^2 + 3x + 1)(2x - 3)$ **(f)** $(x^2 + x + 1)(x - 1)$
      (b) $(x^2 - 1)(x + 1)$ **(g)** $(x^2 + x + 1)(x^2 - x + 1)$

    (c) $(x^3 + 2x - 6)(x^2 + 1)$ **(h)** $(2x^2 + 1)(2x^2 - 1)$

    (d) $(\sqrt{3} + x)(\sqrt{3} - x)$ **(i)** $(2x - 1)(x^2 + 3x + 2)$

    (e) $(x + 2)^3$

B.2. Perform the indicated multiplication and simplify your answer if possible:

    (a) $(\sqrt{x} + 5)(\sqrt{x} - 5)$ **(d)** $(7w - \sqrt{2x})^2$

    (b) $(2\sqrt{x} + \sqrt{2y})(2\sqrt{x} - \sqrt{2y})$ **(e)** $(1 + \sqrt{3}x)(x + \sqrt{3})$

    (c) $(3 + \sqrt{y})^2$ **(f)** $(2y + \sqrt{3})(\sqrt{5}y - 1)$

B.3. Compute the product and arrange the terms of your answer according to decreasing powers of x, with each power of x appearing at most once. *Example:* $(ax + b)(4x - c) = 4ax^2 + (4b - ac)x - bc$.

    (a) $(ax + b)(3x + 2)$ **(d)** $rx(3rx + 1)(4x - r)$

    (b) $(4x - c)(dx + c)$ **(e)** $(x - a)(x - b)(x - c)$

    (c) $(ax + b)(bx + a)$ **(f)** $(2dx - c)(3cx + d)$

B.4. If $f(x)$ is a polynomial of degree m and $g(x)$ is a polynomial of degree n, what is the degree of the product polynomial $f(x)g(x)$? [*Hint:* The products computed in Exercises A.3–A.5 may give you a clue. Remember that the product of nonzero numbers is always nonzero.]

B.5. Assume that all exponents are nonnegative integers and find the product. *Example:* $2x^k(3x + x^{n+1}) = (2x^k)(3x) + (2x^k)(x^{n+1}) = 6x^{k+1} + 2x^{k+n+1}$.

    (a) $3^r 3^4 3^t$ **(d)** $(y^r + 1)(y^s - 4)$

    (b) $(2x^n)(8x^k)$ **(e)** $(2x^n - 5)(x^{3n} + 4x^n + 1)$

    (c) $(x^m + 2)(x^n - 3)$ **(f)** $(3y^{2k} + y^k + 1)(y^k - 3)$

B.6. **Errors to Avoid** Find a numerical example to show that the given statement is *false*. Then find the mistake in the statement and correct it. *Example:* the statement $-(b + 2) = -b + 2$ is false when $b = 5$, since $-(5 + 2) = -7$ but $-5 + 2 = -3$. The mistake is the sign on the 2. The correct statement is $-(b + 2) = -b - 2$.

    (a) $3(y + 2) = 3y + 2$ **(f)** $(x + y)^2 = x^2 + y^2$

    (b) $x - (3y + 4) = x - 3y + 4$ **(g)** $y + y + y = y^3$

    (c) $(x + y)^2 = x + y^2$ **(h)** $(a - b)^2 = a^2 - b^2$

    (d) $(2x)^3 = 2x^3$ **(i)** $(x - 3)(x - 2) = x^2 - 5x - 6$

    (e) $(7x)(7y) = 7xy$ **(j)** $(a + b)(a^2 + b^2) = a^3 + b^3$

C.1. Explain algebraically why each of these parlor tricks always works.

    (a) Write down a nonzero number. Add 1 to it and square the result. Subtract 1 from the original number and square the result. Subtract this second square from the first one. Divide by the number with which you started. The answer is 4.

    (b) Write down a number. Add 4 to it. Multiply the result by the original number. Add 4 to this result and then take the square root. Subtract the number with which you started. The answer is 2.

    (c) Invent a similar parlor trick in which the answer is always the number with which you started.

DO IT YOURSELF!

SYNTHETIC DIVISION

Synthetic division is a fast method of doing polynomial division when the divisor is a first-degree polynomial of the form $x - c$ for some real number c. We begin with an example of ordinary long division. We shall see that the calculations can be written in a brief shorthand notation. This shorthand version will then lead to the method of synthetic division.

The usual long division process for dividing $3x^4 - 8x^2 - 11x + 1$ by $x - 2$ goes like this:

$$
\begin{array}{r}
3x^3 + 6x^2 + 4x - 3 \quad \leftarrow \text{quotient} \\
\text{divisor} \rightarrow x - 2 \overline{)3x^4 - 8x^2 - 11x + 1} \quad \leftarrow \text{dividend} \\
\underline{3x^4 - 6x^3} \\
6x^3 - 8x^2 \\
\underline{6x^3 - 12x^2} \\
4x^2 - 11x \\
\underline{4x^2 - 8x} \\
- 3x + 1 \\
\underline{- 3x + 6} \\
- 5 \quad \leftarrow \text{remainder}
\end{array}
$$

This calculation obviously involves a lot of repetitions. If we keep the various powers of x aligned properly, we can eliminate many of these repetitions without causing any confusion:

$$
\begin{array}{r}
3x^3 + 6x^2 + 4x - 3 \quad \leftarrow \text{quotient} \\
\text{divisor} \rightarrow x - 2 \overline{)3x^4 - 8x^2 - 11x + 1} \quad \leftarrow \text{dividend} \\
\underline{- 6x^3} \\
6x^3 \\
\underline{- 12x^2} \\
4x^2 \\
\underline{- 8x} \\
- 3x \\
\underline{+ 6} \\
- 5 \quad \leftarrow \text{remainder}
\end{array}
$$

As long as we keep the coefficients in the proper columns, there is no need to keep writing out all the powers of x. But to avoid confusion here we must insert 0 coefficients for those terms that don't appear above, such as the x^3 term in the dividend:

$$
\begin{array}{r}
 3 \quad\; 6 \quad\;\; 4 \quad -3 \qquad\quad \leftarrow \text{quotient} \\
\text{divisor} \rightarrow 1-2\,\overline{)3 \quad\; 0 \quad -8 \quad -11 \quad\;\; 1} \;\; \leftarrow \text{dividend} \\
\underline{-6} \\
6 \\
\underline{-12} \\
4 \\
\underline{-8} \\
-3 \\
\underline{+6} \\
-5 \;\; \leftarrow \text{remainder}
\end{array}
$$

Since it's easy to remember that the coefficient of x in the divisor $x - 2$ is the number 1, there's really no need to write the 1 in this last calculation. Furthermore, we can save some space by moving the various numbers upward, thus obtaining this shorthand version of the calculation:

$$
\begin{array}{r}
 3 \quad\; 6 \quad\;\; 4 \quad -3 \qquad\quad \leftarrow \text{quotient} \\
\text{divisor} \rightarrow -2\,\overline{)3 \quad\; 0 \quad -8 \quad -11 \quad\;\; 1} \;\; \leftarrow \text{dividend} \\
\underline{-6 \quad -12 \quad -8 \quad\;\; 6} \\
6 \quad\;\; 4 \quad -3 \;\boxed{-5} \;\; \leftarrow \text{remainder}
\end{array}
$$

But there are still some repetitions: the last three entries in the quotient row are the same as the first three entries in the last row. By inserting a 3 at the beginning of the last row, we can omit the top row and still preserve all the essential information:

$$
\begin{array}{r}
\text{divisor} \rightarrow -2\,\overline{)3 \quad\; 0 \quad -8 \quad -11 \quad\;\; 1} \;\; \leftarrow \text{dividend} \\
\underline{-6 \quad -12 \quad -8 \quad\;\; 6} \\
3 \quad\; 6 \quad\;\; 4 \quad -3 \;\boxed{-5} \;\; \leftarrow \text{remainder} \\
\underbrace{} \\
\text{quotient}
\end{array}
$$

For reasons that will soon be apparent, we shall now rewrite this shorthand version in a slightly different manner. We replace -2 by 2 and change all the signs in the *second* row (and leave everything else alone):

$$
\begin{array}{r}
\text{divisor} \rightarrow 2\,\overline{)3 \quad 0 \quad -8 \quad -11 \quad\;\; 1} \;\; \leftarrow \text{dividend} \\
\underline{6 \quad 12 \quad\;\; 8 \quad -6} \\
3 \quad 6 \quad\;\; 4 \quad -3 \;\boxed{-5} \;\; \leftarrow \text{remainder} \\
\underbrace{} \\
\text{quotient}
\end{array}
$$

Providing that we remember the sign change on the 2, this three-line array of numbers still preserves all the essential information (divisor, dividend, quotient, and remainder). Note that the three rows are related to each other as follows:

(i) The second row can be obtained by multiplying each entry in the last row (except the remainder -5) by 2. For instance, $2 \cdot 3 = 6$, $2 \cdot 6 = 12$, and so on, as shown by the arrows below:

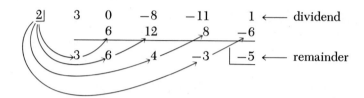

(ii) The last row can be obtained by *adding* the corresponding entries in the first and second rows. For instance, the 4 in the last row is the sum of the two numbers directly above it, $-8 + 12$.

The three-line array of numbers just obtained is a shorthand summary of the division of $3x^4 - 8x^2 - 11x + 1$ by $x - 2$. **Synthetic division** is just a method of producing this summary directly, without having to go through the entire long division process first. It is based on properties (i) and (ii) above.

Here is a step-by-step explanation of the division of $3x^4 - 8x^2 - 11x + 1$ by $x - 2$ by means of synthetic division:

Step 1. In the first row list the constant term of the divisor (namely, 2) and the coefficients of the dividend in order of decreasing powers of x (insert 0 coefficients for missing powers of x).

$$\underline{2|} \quad 3 \quad 0 \quad\quad -8 \quad\quad -11 \quad\quad 1$$

Step 2. Bring down the first dividend coefficient (namely, 3) to the third row.

$$\underline{2|} \quad 3 \quad 0 \quad\quad -8 \quad\quad -11 \quad\quad 1$$
$$\quad\quad 3$$

Step 3. Multiply $2 \cdot 3$ and insert the answer 6 in the second row, in the position shown here.

$$\underline{2|} \quad 3 \quad 0 \quad\quad -8 \quad\quad -11 \quad\quad 1$$
$$\quad\quad\quad 6$$
$$\quad\quad 3$$

Step 4. Add $0 + 6$ and write the answer 6 in the third row.

$$\underline{2|} \quad\quad 0 \quad\quad -8 \quad\quad -11 \quad\quad 1$$
$$\quad\quad\quad 6$$
$$\quad\quad 3 \quad 6$$

Step 5. Multiply $2 \cdot 6$ and insert the answer 12 in the second row.

$$\underline{2|} \quad 3 \quad 0 \quad\quad -8 \quad\quad -11 \quad\quad 1$$
$$\quad\quad\quad 6 \quad\quad 12$$
$$\quad\quad 3 \quad 6$$

Step 6. Add $-8 + 12$ and write the answer 4 in the third row.

$$
\begin{array}{r|rrrrr}
2 & 3 & 0 & -8 & -11 & 1 \\
  &   & 6 & 12 &   &   \\
\hline
  & 3 & 6 & 4 &   &   \\
\end{array}
$$

Step 7. Multiply $2 \cdot 4$ and insert the answer 8 in the second row.

$$
\begin{array}{r|rrrrr}
2 & 3 & 0 & -8 & -11 & 1 \\
  &   & 6 & 12 & 8   &   \\
\hline
  & 3 & 6 & 4 &   &   \\
\end{array}
$$

Step 8. Add $-11 + 8$ and write the answer -3 in the third row.

$$
\begin{array}{r|rrrrr}
2 & 3 & 0 & -8 & -11 & 1 \\
  &   & 6 & 12 & 8   &   \\
\hline
  & 3 & 6 & 4 & -3 &   \\
\end{array}
$$

Step 9. Multiply $2 \cdot (-3)$ and insert the answer -6 in the second row.

$$
\begin{array}{r|rrrrr}
2 & 3 & 0 & -8 & -11 & 1 \\
  &   & 6 & 12 & 8   & -6 \\
\hline
  & 3 & 6 & 4 & -3 &   \\
\end{array}
$$

Step 10. Add $1 + (-6)$ and write the answer -5 in the third row.

$$
\begin{array}{r|rrrrr}
2 & 3 & 0 & -8 & -11 & 1 \\
  &   & 6 & 12 & 8   & -6 \\
\hline
  & 3 & 6 & 4 & -3 & \underline{-5} \\
\end{array}
$$

We have arrived at the same three-line summary that we obtained earlier via long division. The divisor and dividend are listed in the first row. The quotient and remainder can be read directly from the third row:

The last number in the third row is the remainder.
The other numbers in the third row are coefficients of the quotient (arranged in order of decreasing powers of x).

Since we are dividing the *fourth-degree* polynomial $3x^4 - 8x^2 - 11x + 1$ by the *first*-degree polynomial $x - 2$, the quotient must be the polynomial of degree *three* with coefficients 3, 6, 4, -3, namely, $3x^3 + 6x^2 + 4x - 3$. The remainder is -5.

Warning Synthetic division can be used *only* when the divisor is of the form $x - c$. The constant c can be either positive or negative. In the example above, the divisor was $x - 2$, which is of the form $x - c$ with $c = 2$. On the other hand, $x + 5$ can be written as $x - (-5)$, which is of the form $x - c$ with $c = -5$. So synthetic division can be used with the divisor $x + 5$. But synthetic division *cannot* be used with divisors such as x^2 or $x^3 + 5$ or $6x - 7$ since these cannot be put in the form $x - c$.

EXAMPLE The first step in dividing $x^5 + 5x^4 + 6x^3 - x^2 + 4x + 29$ by $x + 3$ is to write the divisor in the form $x - c$: $x + 3 = x - (-3)$. The first row of the synthetic division consists of -3 and the coefficients of the dividend:

$$
\begin{array}{r|rrrrrr}
-3 & 1 & 5 & 6 & -1 & 4 & 29 \\
\end{array}
$$

We now proceed as in the preceding example and obtain:

$$
\begin{array}{r|rrrrrr}
-3 & 1 & 5 & 6 & -1 & 4 & 29 \\
   &   & -3 & -6 & 0 & 3 & -21 \\
\hline
   & 1 & 2 & 0 & -1 & 7 & \underline{8} \\
\end{array}
$$

Since we are dividing a fifth-degree polynomial by a first-degree polynomial, the quotient is a fourth-degree polynomial. The last row above shows that the quotient is $1x^4 + 2x^3 + 0x^2 - 1x + 7$, that is, $x^4 + 2x^3 - x + 7$ and that the remainder is 8.

EXAMPLE Show that $x - 7$ is a factor of $f(x) = 8x^5 - 52x^4 + 2x^3 - 198x^2 - 86x + 14$ and find the other factor. We know that $x - 7$ will be a factor exactly when division by $x - 7$ leaves remainder 0. The other factor will be the quotient of this division. Using synthetic division, we have:

$$
\begin{array}{r|rrrrrr}
7 & 8 & -52 & 2 & -198 & -86 & 14 \\
  &   & 56 & 28 & 210 & 84 & -14 \\
\hline
  & 8 & 4 & 30 & 12 & -2 & \underline{0} \\
\end{array}
$$

The last row shows that the remainder is 0 and the quotient is $8x^4 + 4x^3 + 30x^2 + 12x - 2$. Therefore $f(x)$ factors as:

$$8x^5 - 52x^4 + 2x^3 - 198x^2 - 86x + 14 = (x - 7)(8x^4 + 4x^3 + 30x^2 + 12x - 2)$$

EXERCISES

A.1. Use synthetic division to find the quotient and remainder.
(a) $(3x^4 - 8x^3 + 9x + 5) \div (x - 2)$
(b) $(4x^3 - 3x^2 + x + 7) \div (x - 2)$
(c) $(2x^4 + 5x^3 - 2x - 8) \div (x + 3)$
(d) $(3x^3 - 2x^2 - 8) \div (x + 5)$
(e) $(5x^4 - 3x^2 - 4x + 6) \div (x - 7)$
(f) $(3x^4 - 2x^3 + 7x - 4) \div (x - 3)$
(g) $(x^4 - 6x^3 + 4x^2 + 2x - 7) \div (x - 2)$
(h) $(x^6 - x^5 + x^4 - x^3 + x^2 - x + 1) \div (x + 3)$

B.1. Use synthetic division to find the quotient and remainder. In each divisor $x - c$, the number c is not an integer, but the same technique will work.
(a) $(3x^4 - 2x^2 + 2) \div (x - \frac{1}{4})$
(b) $(2x^4 - 3x^2 + 1) \div (x - \frac{1}{2})$
(c) $(2x^4 - 5x^3 - x^2 + 3x + 2) \div (x + \frac{1}{2})$
(d) $(10x^5 - 3x^4 + 14x^3 + 13x^2 - \frac{4}{3}x + \frac{7}{3}) \div (x + \frac{1}{5})$
(e) $(x^4 + (5 - \sqrt{3})x^3 - (6 + 5\sqrt{3})x^2 + (1 + 6\sqrt{3})x + (1 - \sqrt{3})) \div (x - \sqrt{3})$

B.2.   Use synthetic division to show that $f(x)$ is a factor of $g(x)$ and find the other factor.
    (a) $f(x) = x + 4$ and $g(x) = 3x^3 + 9x^2 - 11x + 4$
    (b) $f(x) = x - 5$ and $g(x) = x^5 - 8x^4 + 17x^2 + 293x - 15$
    (c) $f(x) = x - \frac{1}{2}$ and $g(x) = 2x^5 - 7x^4 + 15x^3 - 6x^2 - 10x + 5$
    (d) $f(x) = x + \frac{1}{3}$ and $g(x) = 3x^6 + x^5 - 6x^4 + 7x^3 + 3x^2 - 15x - 5$

B.3.   Use a calculator and synthetic division to find the quotient and remainder.
    (a) $(x^3 - 5.27x^2 + 10.708x - 10.23) \div (x - 3.12)$
    (b) $(2.79x^4 + 4.8325x^3 - 6.73865x^2 + .9255x - 8.125) \div (x - 1.35)$

6. FACTORING

When multiplying two algebraic expressions we begin with two expressions and find their product. Factoring is the reverse process: We begin with a *product* and find the expressions (factors) that multiply together to produce this particular product. Factoring is useful in simplifying various algebraic expressions, in solving certain equations, and in other areas.

One nice thing about factoring is that you can always check your answers. Just multiply the factors you have found to see if you get the expression you began with. Actually finding the factors to check, however, may be more difficult. There are no hard and fast rules for factoring and a fair amount of trial and error is often involved. But you can greatly increase your proficiency at factoring by learning to recognize those multiplication patterns that appear frequently. The most important patterns are listed in the boxes below, followed by several examples. You should verify that each of the given patterns is correct by multiplying out the two factors on the right-hand side of the equal sign. We begin with some patterns that were discussed in the last section.

DIFFERENCE OF SQUARES

$$u^2 - v^2 = (u + v)(u - v)$$

PERFECT SQUARES

$$u^2 + 2uv + v^2 = (u + v)^2$$
$$u^2 - 2uv + v^2 = (u - v)^2$$

EXAMPLE   The expression $4x^2 - 36x + 81$ can be written as $(2x)^2 - 36x + 9^2$. Since the first and last terms are squares, a perfect square pattern is a good bet for factoring this expression:

$$4x^2 - 36x + 81 = (2x)^2 - 36x + 9^2 = (2x)^2 - 2(2x)9 + 9^2 = (2x - 9)^2$$

EXAMPLE   Since $x^2 - 9y^2$ can be written as $x^2 - (3y)^2$, it is a difference of squares and can be factored by using the first pattern in the preceding box:

$$x^2 - 9y^2 = x^2 - (3y)^2 = (x + 3y)(x - 3y)$$

EXAMPLE $y^2 - 7$ can also be written as a difference of squares and factored:

$$y^2 - 7 = y^2 - (\sqrt{7})^2 = (y + \sqrt{7})(y - \sqrt{7})$$

In all examples we shall begin with expressions that have integer coefficients. We shall usually look only for factors that also have integer coefficients, because finding factors with noninteger coefficients may be quite difficult. But whenever it is *easy* to find factors with real number coefficients that are not integers, as in the last example, you should do so.

This pattern (in which c and d are constants) may be helpful for factoring some quadratic polynomials:

$$\boxed{x^2 + (c + d)x + cd = (x + c)(x + d)}$$

You should notice two key facts about the left-hand side of this pattern: The constant term is the *product cd* and the coefficient of x is the *sum $c + d$*.

EXAMPLE   Since the first term of $x^2 + 9x + 18$ is a square and the last term is not the square of an integer, we try to factor it as $(x + c)(x + d)$. We must find integers c and d whose *product* is the constant term 18 and whose *sum* is 9, the coefficient of x. By taking pairs of integers whose product is 18, we find some possibilities for c and d:

c	1	-1	2	-2	3	-3
d	18	-18	9	-9	6	-6
$c + d$	19	-19	11	-11	9	-9

The only pair whose sum is 9 is $c = 3$ and $d = 6$. So $x^2 + 9x + 18$ factors as $(x + 3)(x + 6)$. You can check the accuracy of this factorization by multiplying:

$$(x + 3)(x + 6) = x^2 + 3x + 6x + 3 \cdot 6 = x^2 + 9x + 18$$

EXAMPLE   One way to factor $x^2 + 6xy - 40y^2$ is to rewrite it as $x^2 + (6y)x - 40y^2$ and to consider it as a polynomial in x whose coefficients involve the number y. To factor it as $(x + c)(x + d)$, we must find quantities c and d whose product is $-40y^2$ and whose sum is $6y$, the coefficient of x. Here are some possible pairs whose product is $-40y^2$:

$$-40 \text{ and } y^2 \qquad 20y \text{ and } -2y \qquad -8y \text{ and } 5y \qquad 8y \text{ and } -5y$$

But none of these pairs has $6y$ as the sum. So we look further. Eventually, we find that $10y$ and $-4y$ have the product $-40y^2$ and the sum $6y$. Therefore the factors are $(x + 10y)$ and $(x + (-4y)) = (x - 4y)$. We check this factorization by multiplication:

$$(x + 10y)(x - 4y) = x^2 + 10xy - 4xy + 10y(-4y) = x^2 + 6xy - 40y^2$$

Here is a similar but slightly more complicated pattern:

$$\boxed{abx^2 + (ad + bc)x + cd = (ax + c)(bx + d)}$$

The key facts about the left-hand side of this pattern are that: The constant term is the product cd and the coefficient of x^2 is the product ab; the coefficient of x is the number $ad + bc$.

EXAMPLE To factor $6x^2 + 11x + 4$ as $(ax + c)(bx + d)$, we must find numbers a and b whose product is 6, the coefficient of x^2, and numbers c and d whose product is the constant term 4. Some possibilities are:

$ab = 6$

a	1	-1	2	-2	3	-3	6	-6
b	6	-6	3	-3	2	-2	1	-1

$cd = 4$

c	1	-1	2	-2	4	-4
d	4	-4	2	-2	1	-1

Notice that for *each* choice of a and b there are *six* possibilities for c and d. We must find the choice that produces a coefficient of 11 for x. Trial and error and a good deal of checking via multiplication finally shows that $(2x + 1)(3x + 4) = 6x^2 + 11x + 4$.

EXAMPLE The first step in factoring $24y^5 - 14y^4 - 5y^3$ is to factor out the lowest power of y that appears: $24y^5 - 14y^4 - 5y^3 = y^3(24y^2 - 14y - 5)$. To factor $24y^2 - 14y - 5$, we consider pairs of integers a and b whose product is 24, the coefficient of y^2, and pairs of integers c and d whose product is the constant term -5. Once again, there are many possibilities. Trial and error finally shows that $a = 6$, $b = 4$, and $c = -5$, $d = 1$ do the trick:

$$(6y - 5)(4y + 1) = 24y^2 - 14y - 5$$

Therefore the original expression factors as:

$$24y^5 - 14y^4 - 5y^3 = y^3(24y^2 - 14y - 5) = y^3(6y - 5)(4y + 1)$$

$$\boxed{\begin{array}{c} \textbf{DIFFERENCE OF CUBES} \\[4pt] u^3 - v^3 = (u - v)(u^2 + uv + v^2) \\[8pt] \textbf{SUM OF CUBES} \\[4pt] u^3 + v^3 = (u + v)(u^2 - uv + v^2) \end{array}}$$

EXAMPLE $x^3 + 125 = x^3 + 5^3 = (x + 5)(x^2 - 5x + 5^2)$
$$= (x + 5)(x^2 - 5x + 25).$$

EXAMPLE $y^3 - 7 = y^3 - (\sqrt[3]{7})^3 = (y - \sqrt[3]{7})(y^2 + \sqrt[3]{7}y + (\sqrt[3]{7})^2).$

EXAMPLE $x^3 + 8y^3 = x^3 + (2y)^3 = (x + 2y)(x^2 - x(2y) + (2y)^2)$
$$= (x + 2y)(x^2 - 2xy + 4y^2).$$

$$\boxed{\begin{array}{c} \textbf{PERFECT CUBES} \\[4pt] (c - d)^3 = c^3 - 3c^2d + 3cd^2 - d^3 \\[4pt] (c + d)^3 = c^3 + 3c^2d + 3cd^2 + d^3 \end{array}}$$

EXAMPLE $x^3 - 12x^2 + 48x - 64 = x^3 - 12x^2 + 48x - 4^3$
$$= x^3 - 3x^2 \cdot 4 + 3x \cdot 4^2 - 4^3 = (x - 4)^3.$$

Factoring expressions involving exponents larger than 3 is usually quite difficult. But sometimes it can be done.

EXAMPLE $x^6 - y^6 = (x^3)^2 - (y^3)^2 = (x^3 + y^3)(x^3 - y^3)$
$$= (x + y)(x^2 - xy + y^2)(x - y)(x^2 + xy + y^2).$$

EXAMPLE $x^8 - 1 = (x^4)^2 - 1 = (x^4 + 1)(x^4 - 1)$
$$= (x^4 + 1)(x^2 + 1)(x^2 - 1)$$
$$= (x^4 + 1)(x^2 + 1)(x + 1)(x - 1).$$

Certain expressions can be factored by using an appropriate substitution.

EXAMPLE   To factor $x^4 - 2x^2 - 3$, let $u = x^2$. Then $x^4 - 2x^2 - 3$
$$= (x^2)^2 - 2x^2 - 3 = u^2 - 2u - 3 = (u - 3)(u + 1) = (x^2 - 3)(x^2 + 1)$$
$$= (x + \sqrt{3})(x - \sqrt{3})(x^2 + 1).$$

EXAMPLE   To factor $x^6 + 2x^3 + 1$, let $u = x^3$. Then $x^6 + 2x^3 + 1$
$$= (x^3)^2 + 2x^3 + 1 = u^2 + 2u + 1 = (u + 1)^2 = (x^3 + 1)^2$$
$$= ((x + 1)(x^2 - x + 1))^2 = (x + 1)^2(x^2 - x + 1)^2.$$

Occasionally, an expression can be regrouped and the distributive law used to factor out a common factor.

EXAMPLE $3x^3 + 3x^2 + x + 1 = 3x^2(x + 1) + (x + 1) = (3x^2 + 1)(x + 1)$.

EXAMPLE $x^3 + 5x^2 - 3x - 15 = x^2(x + 5) - 3(x + 5)$
$$= (x^2 - 3)(x + 5)$$
$$= (x + \sqrt{3})(x - \sqrt{3})(x + 5).$$

COMPLETING THE SQUARE

We now introduce a technique related to factoring that will prove useful in several situations. Recall that a polynomial that can be written in the form $(x + c)^2$ for some constant c is called a **perfect square.** For example, the polynomial $x^2 + 6x$ is *not* a perfect square, but by adding 9, we obtain a perfect square:

$$x^2 + 6x + 9 = x^2 + 6x + 3^2 = (x + 3)^2$$

Notice that the number 9 is just the square of 3 and 3 is *one-half the coefficient of x* in the original polynomial $x^2 + 6x$. This process of adding a constant to a polynomial of the form $x^2 + bx$ in order to make it a perfect square is called **completing the square.**

Given any polynomial $x^2 + bx$, with b a fixed real number, what number should we add in order to obtain a perfect square? The preceding example suggests the answer. Take *one-half the coefficient of x*, namely, $b/2$, and *square it:* $(b/2)^2$. Add this number to the original polynomial $x^2 + bx$ and the result is a perfect square:

$$x^2 + bx + \left(\frac{b}{2}\right)^2 = x^2 + 2\left(\frac{b}{2}\right)x + \left(\frac{b}{2}\right)^2 = \left(x + \frac{b}{2}\right)^2$$

In other words:

To complete the square in the polynomial $x^2 + bx$, *add the square of one-half the coefficient of* x, *namely,* $\left(\dfrac{b}{2}\right)^2$.

EXAMPLE   The polynomial $x^2 - 8x$ is of the form $x^2 + bx$ with $b = -8$. To complete the square in $x^2 - 8x$, we take one-half the coefficient of x, namely, $\frac{1}{2}(-8) = -4$ and square it: 16. Adding this number to $x^2 - 8x$ produces a perfect square:

$$x^2 - 8x + 16 = x^2 - 8x + (-4)^2 = (x - 4)^2$$

EXAMPLE   To complete the square in $y^2 + 9y$, we take one-half the coefficient of y, namely, $\frac{9}{2}$, and add the square of this number, namely, $\frac{81}{4}$:

$$y^2 + 9y + \tfrac{81}{4} = y^2 + 9y + (\tfrac{9}{2})^2 = y^2 + 2(\tfrac{9}{2})y + (\tfrac{9}{2})^2 = (y + \tfrac{9}{2})^2$$

Warning   The technique just described is only valid for quadratic polynomials with leading coefficient 1. It will not work for a polynomial such as $3x^2 - 15x$, which has the leading coefficient 3. However, in these cases we can first factor out the leading coefficient: $3x^2 - 15x = 3(x^2 - 5x)$, and then complete the square in $x^2 - 5x$ by adding $(-5/2)^2$:

$$3\left(x^2 - 5x + \left(\frac{-5}{2}\right)^2\right) = 3\left(x - \frac{5}{2}\right)^2$$

EXERCISES

A.1.   Factor these expressions:
- (a) $x^2 - 4$
- (b) $x^2 + 6x + 9$
- (c) $9y^2 - 25$
- (d) $y^2 - 4y + 4$
- (e) $81x^2 + 36x + 4$
- (f) $4x^2 - 12x + 9$
- (g) $5 - x^2$
- (h) $1 - 36u^2$
- (i) $49 + 28z + 4z^2$
- (j) $25u^2 - 20uv + 4v^2$
- (k) $x^4 - y^4$
- (l) $x^2 - \frac{1}{9}$

A.2.   Factor the following expressions:
- (a) $x^2 + x - 6$
- (b) $y^2 + 11y + 30$
- (c) $z^2 + 4z + 3$
- (d) $x^2 - 8x + 15$
- (e) $y^2 + 5y - 36$
- (f) $z^2 - 9z + 14$
- (g) $x^2 - 6x + 9$
- (h) $4y^2 - 81$
- (i) $x^2 + 7x + 10$
- (j) $w^2 - 6w - 16$
- (k) $x^2 + 11x + 18$
- (l) $x^2 + 3xy - 28y^2$

A.3.   Factor the following expressions:
- (a) $3x^2 + 4x + 1$
- (b) $4y^2 + 4y + 1$
- (c) $2z^2 + 11z + 12$
- (d) $10x^2 - 17x + 3$
- (e) $9x^2 - 72x$
- (f) $4x^2 - 4x - 3$
- (g) $10x^2 - 8x - 2$
- (h) $7z^2 + 23z + 6$
- (i) $8u^2 + 6u - 9$
- (j) $2y^2 - 4y + 2$
- (k) $4x^2 + 20xy + 25y^2$
- (l) $63u^2 - 46uv + 8v^2$

A.4.   Factor the following expressions:
- (a) $x^3 - 125$
- (b) $y^3 + 64$
- (c) $x^3 + 6x^2 + 12x + 8$
- (d) $y^3 - 3y^2 + 3y - 1$
- (e) $8 + x^3$
- (f) $z^3 - 9z^2 + 27z - 27$
- (g) $-x^3 + 15x^2 - 75x + 125$
- (h) $27 - t^3$
- (i) $x^3 + 1$
- (j) $x^3 - 1$
- (k) $8x^3 - y^3$
- (l) $(x - 1)^3 + 1$

A.5.   Factor the following expressions:
- (a) $x^6 - 64$
- (b) $x^5 - 8x^2$
- (c) $y^4 + 7y^2 + 10$
- (d) $z^4 - 5z^2 - 6$
- (e) $81 - y^4$
- (f) $x^6 + 16x^3 + 64$
- (g) $z^6 - 1$
- (h) $y^6 + 26y^3 - 27$
- (i) $x^4 + 2x^2y - 3y^2$
- (j) $x^8 - 17x^4 + 16$

A.6.   Factor the following expressions by regrouping and using the distributive law:
- (a) $x^2 - yz + xz - xy$
- (b) $x^6 - 2x^4 - 8x^2 + 16$
- (c) $a^3 - 2b^2 + 2a^2b - ab$
- (d) $u^2v - 2w^2 - 2uvw + uw$
- (e) $x^3 + 4x^2 - 8x - 32$
- (f) $z^8 - 5z^7 + 2z - 10$

A.7. Complete the square:

(a) $x^2 + 4x$ (e) $x^2 + 12x$ (h) $3y^2 - 30y$
(b) $y^2 - 6y$ (f) $y^2 - 11y$ (i) $2z^2 + 14z$
(c) $z^2 + 3z$ (g) $2x^2 + 4x$ (j) $3x^2 + 5x$
(d) $x^2 - x$

B.1. Factor the following expressions by regrouping and using the distributive law:

(a) $2x^2 + 5xy - 3y^2 + 6x - 3y$ (c) $x^3 + x - 3y - 27y^3$
(b) $x^2 - 9xy + 14y^2 + 3xy^2 - 6y^3$ (d) $8u^3 + 10u + v^3 + 5v$

B.2. Factor the following expressions. For example,

$$x^2 - \frac{x}{4} - \frac{3}{8} = \left(x + \frac{1}{2}\right)\left(x - \frac{3}{4}\right).$$

(a) $x^2 - \frac{1}{64}$ (d) $x^2 + x - \frac{3}{4}$
(b) $x^3 - \frac{1}{8}$ (e) $z^2 + 3z + \frac{35}{16}$
(c) $y^2 - \frac{2y}{3} - \frac{5}{36}$ (f) $9t^2 - 3t - 2$

C.1. Show that there do *not* exist any real numbers c and d such that $x^2 + 1 = (x + c)(x + d)$.

7. FRACTIONS

When we divide one number by another, the quotient is usually written as a fraction. For example, if 7 is divided by $\pi + 3$, the quotient is $\dfrac{7}{\pi + 3}$. The same is true for algebraic expressions. For instance, if $x^2 + 2$ is divided by $4x - 5$, the quotient is $\dfrac{x^2 + 2}{4x - 5}$. In this section the basic properties of fractions are reviewed.

As you know, the same number can be expressed as a fraction in many different ways. For instance, $\frac{1}{2} = \frac{2}{4} = \frac{5}{10}$. This is just an example of the basic rule for equality of fractions:

$$\boxed{\text{For every nonzero number k,} \qquad \frac{a}{b} = \frac{ka}{kb} \quad (b \neq 0)}$$

Informally, this property is usually expressed by saying that we can cancel the factor k from the top and bottom of the fraction.

EXAMPLE $\dfrac{27}{15} = \dfrac{3 \cdot 9}{3 \cdot 5} = \dfrac{9}{5}.$

EXAMPLE $\dfrac{x^4 - 1}{x^2 + 1} = \dfrac{(x^2 + 1)(x^2 - 1)}{(x^2 + 1)1} = \dfrac{x^2 - 1}{1} = x^2 - 1.$

Warning   Cancellation is only valid for multiplicative factors. Don't try any *non-sense* operations, such as $\dfrac{3+5}{3+1} = \dfrac{5}{1} = 5$ or $\dfrac{x+2}{x+7} = \dfrac{2}{7}$.

A fraction is said to be in *lowest terms* if its numerator (top) and denominator (bottom) have no common factors. Cancellation is used to express a particular fraction in lowest terms.

EXAMPLE $\frac{8}{14}$ is *not* in lowest terms since 2 is a factor of both 8 and 14. In order to express $\frac{8}{14}$ in lowest terms, we cancel the common factor 2: $\dfrac{8}{14} = \dfrac{2 \cdot 4}{2 \cdot 7} = \dfrac{4}{7}$. The fraction $\frac{4}{7}$ *is* in lowest terms since 4 and 7 have no common factors (except, of course, the trivial factor 1).

EXAMPLE   In order to express $\dfrac{x^2 + x - 6}{x^2 - 3x + 2}$ in lowest terms we first factor both top and bottom to see if there is a common factor that can be canceled:

$$\frac{x^2 + x - 6}{x^2 - 3x + 2} = \frac{(x - 2)(x + 3)}{(x - 2)(x - 1)} = \frac{x + 3}{x - 1}$$

The fraction $\dfrac{x + 3}{x - 1}$ is in lowest terms.

ADDITION AND SUBTRACTION OF FRACTIONS

Adding (or subtracting) two fractions that have the same denominator is easy—using the distributive law as follows:

$$\frac{a}{b} + \frac{c}{b} = a\left(\frac{1}{b}\right) + c\left(\frac{1}{b}\right) = (a + c)\left(\frac{1}{b}\right) = \frac{a + c}{b} \qquad (b \neq 0)$$

Subtraction is done similarly. In summary:

$$\boxed{\ \frac{a}{b} + \frac{c}{b} = \frac{a + c}{b} \qquad and \qquad \frac{a}{b} - \frac{c}{b} = \frac{a - c}{b} \quad (b \neq 0)\ }$$

EXAMPLES $\dfrac{7}{3} + \dfrac{13}{3} = \dfrac{7 + 13}{3} = \dfrac{20}{3}$ and $\dfrac{4}{5} - \dfrac{7}{5} = \dfrac{4 - 7}{5} = \dfrac{-3}{5}$.

EXAMPLE $\dfrac{7x^2 + 2}{x^2 + 3} - \dfrac{4x^2 + 2x - 5}{x^2 + 3} = \dfrac{(7x^2 + 2) - (4x^2 + 2x - 5)}{x^2 + 3}$

$$= \frac{7x^2 + 2 - 4x^2 - 2x + 5}{x^2 + 3} = \frac{3x^2 - 2x + 7}{x^2 + 3}.$$

In order to add or subtract two fractions with different denominators, we must first find a *common denominator;* that is, we must express both fractions with the same number on the bottom.

EXAMPLE In order to add $\frac{1}{2}$ and $\frac{2}{3}$, we first write $\frac{1}{2} = \frac{3}{6}$ and $\frac{2}{3} = \frac{4}{6}$. Then

$$\frac{1}{2} + \frac{2}{3} = \frac{3}{6} + \frac{4}{6} = \frac{3+4}{6} = \frac{7}{6}$$

One way to find a common denominator for a/b and c/d (with $b \neq 0$, $d \neq 0$) is to use the product of the two denominators bd. Note that

$$\frac{a}{b} = \frac{ad}{bd} \qquad \text{and} \qquad \frac{c}{d} = \frac{bc}{bd}$$

Consequently,

$$\frac{a}{b} + \frac{c}{d} = \frac{ad}{bd} + \frac{bc}{bd} = \frac{ad + bc}{bd} \qquad (b \neq 0, d \neq 0)$$

$$\frac{a}{b} - \frac{c}{d} = \frac{ad}{bd} - \frac{bc}{bd} = \frac{ad - bc}{bd} \qquad (b \neq 0, d \neq 0)$$

The denominator bd can always be used to add or subtract a/b and c/d as in the previous box. But bd may not be the smallest (or least) common denominator for these two fractions. So the answers shown in the box may not be in lowest terms.

EXAMPLE In order to find $\frac{6}{5} + \frac{4}{7}$, we use $7 \cdot 5 = 35$ as the denominator:

$$\frac{6}{5} + \frac{4}{7} = \frac{6 \cdot 7}{5 \cdot 7} + \frac{5 \cdot 4}{5 \cdot 7} = \frac{42}{35} + \frac{20}{35} = \frac{42 + 20}{35} = \frac{62}{35}.$$

EXAMPLE
$$\frac{2x + 1}{3x} - \frac{x^2 - 2}{x - 1} = \frac{(2x + 1)(x - 1)}{3x(x - 1)} - \frac{3x(x^2 - 2)}{3x(x - 1)}$$

$$= \frac{(2x + 1)(x - 1) - 3x(x^2 - 2)}{3x(x - 1)}$$

$$= \frac{2x^2 - x - 1 - 3x^3 + 6x}{3x^2 - 3x} = \frac{-3x^3 + 2x^2 + 5x - 1}{3x^2 - 3x}.$$

EXAMPLE In order to find $\dfrac{1}{z} + \dfrac{3z}{z + 1} - \dfrac{z^2}{(z + 1)^2}$, we could use the product $z(z + 1)(z + 1)^2$ as the denominator. But it will be more efficient to use just $z(z + 1)^2$, because all three fractions can be expressed with this denominator:

$$\frac{1}{z} = \frac{(z + 1)^2}{z(z + 1)^2} \qquad \frac{3z}{z + 1} = \frac{3z \cdot z(z + 1)}{(z + 1)z(z + 1)} = \frac{3z^2(z + 1)}{z(z + 1)^2}$$

$$\frac{z^2}{(z + 1)^2} = \frac{z^2 \cdot z}{(z + 1)^2 z} = \frac{z^3}{z(z + 1)^2}$$

Therefore

$$\frac{1}{z} + \frac{3z}{z+1} - \frac{z^2}{(z+1)^2} = \frac{(z+1)^2}{z(z+1)^2} + \frac{3z^2(z+1)}{z(z+1)^2} - \frac{z^3}{z(z+1)^2}$$

$$= \frac{(z+1)^2 + 3z^2(z+1) - z^3}{z(z+1)^2}$$

$$= \frac{z^2 + 2z + 1 + 3z^3 + 3z^2 - z^3}{z(z+1)^2}$$

$$= \frac{2z^3 + 4z^2 + 2z + 1}{z(z+1)^2} = \frac{2z^3 + 4z^2 + 2z + 1}{z^3 + 2z^2 + z}.$$

MULTIPLICATION OF FRACTIONS

Multiplication of fractions is easier than addition because you do not have to find common denominators. Just multiply top by top and bottom by bottom:

$$\boxed{\frac{a}{b} \cdot \frac{c}{d} = \frac{ac}{bd} \qquad (b \neq 0, d \neq 0)}$$

EXAMPLES $\dfrac{3}{4} \cdot \dfrac{7}{5} = \dfrac{3 \cdot 7}{4 \cdot 5} = \dfrac{21}{20}$; $\dfrac{2}{3} \cdot \dfrac{5}{6} = \dfrac{2 \cdot 5}{3 \cdot 6} = \dfrac{10}{18} = \dfrac{5}{9}$.

EXAMPLE $\dfrac{x^2 - 1}{x^2 + 2} \cdot \dfrac{3x - 4}{x + 1} = \dfrac{(x^2 - 1)(3x - 4)}{(x^2 + 2)(x + 1)}$. In order to reduce this answer to lowest terms we factor and cancel:

$$\frac{(x^2 - 1)(3x - 4)}{(x^2 + 2)(x + 1)} = \frac{(x - 1)(x + 1)(3x - 4)}{(x^2 + 2)(x + 1)} = \frac{(x - 1)(3x - 4)}{x^2 + 2} = \frac{3x^2 - 7x + 4}{x^2 + 2}$$

DIVISION OF FRACTIONS

The basic rule for simplifying a complicated fraction, such as $\dfrac{a/b}{c/d}$ (with $b \neq 0$, $c \neq 0$, and $d \neq 0$), is *invert the denominator and multiply by the numerator.* The two simplest cases are:

$$\boxed{\frac{a}{c/d} = \frac{a}{1} \cdot \frac{d}{c} = \frac{ad}{c} \qquad and \qquad \frac{a/b}{c} = \frac{a}{b} \cdot \frac{1}{c} = \frac{a}{bc} \qquad (b \neq 0, c \neq 0, d \neq 0)}$$

EXAMPLES $\dfrac{7}{\frac{3}{4}} = \dfrac{7}{1} \cdot \dfrac{4}{3} = \dfrac{28}{3}$ and $\dfrac{\frac{5}{6}}{4} = \dfrac{5}{6} \cdot \dfrac{1}{4} = \dfrac{5}{24}$.

EXAMPLE $\dfrac{\dfrac{x+2}{x^2+1}}{x-3} = \dfrac{x+2}{1} \cdot \dfrac{x-3}{x^2+1} = \dfrac{(x+2)(x-3)}{x^2+1} = \dfrac{x^2-x-6}{x^2+1}.$

EXAMPLE $\dfrac{\dfrac{y^2}{y+2}}{y^3+y} = \dfrac{y^2}{y+2} \cdot \dfrac{1}{y^3+y} = \dfrac{y^2}{(y+2)(y^3+y)} = \dfrac{y^2}{(y+2)y(y^2+1)}$

$$= \dfrac{y}{(y+2)(y^2+1)} = \dfrac{y}{y^3+2y^2+y+2}.$$

The same rule (invert and multiply) applies to more complicated fractions:

$$\boxed{\dfrac{a/b}{c/d} = \dfrac{a}{b} \cdot \dfrac{d}{c} = \dfrac{ad}{bc} \qquad (b \neq 0, c \neq 0, d \neq 0)}$$

EXAMPLES $\dfrac{\frac{3}{4}}{\frac{2}{3}} = \dfrac{3}{4} \cdot \dfrac{3}{2} = \dfrac{9}{8}$ and $\dfrac{\frac{7}{2}}{\frac{15}{8}} = \dfrac{7}{2} \cdot \dfrac{8}{15} = \dfrac{56}{30} = \dfrac{28}{15}.$

EXAMPLE $\dfrac{\dfrac{16y^2z}{8yz^2}}{\dfrac{yz}{6y^3z^3}} = \dfrac{16y^2z}{8yz^2} \cdot \dfrac{6y^3z^3}{yz} = \dfrac{16 \cdot 6 \cdot y^5z^4}{8y^2z^3} = 2 \cdot 6 \cdot y^{5-2}z^{4-3} = 12y^3z.$

It is often necessary to simplify complicated algebraic expressions that involve all four operations on fractions (addition, subtraction, multiplication, and division).

EXAMPLE   In order to simplify

$$\dfrac{\dfrac{3}{x^2-4} + \dfrac{1}{x+2}}{5 - \dfrac{6}{x-2}}$$

we first use the fact that $x^2 - 4 = (x+2)(x-2)$ to find a common denominator on the top and then continue:

$$\dfrac{\dfrac{3}{x^2-4} + \dfrac{1}{x+2}}{5 - \dfrac{6}{x-2}} = \dfrac{\dfrac{3}{x^2-4} + \dfrac{x-2}{x^2-4}}{\dfrac{5(x-2)}{x-2} - \dfrac{6}{x-2}} = \dfrac{\dfrac{3+x-2}{x^2-4}}{\dfrac{5(x-2)-6}{x-2}}$$

$$= \dfrac{\dfrac{1+x}{x^2-4}}{\dfrac{5x-16}{x-2}} = \dfrac{1+x}{x^2-4} \cdot \dfrac{x-2}{5x-16} = \dfrac{(1+x)(x-2)}{(x+2)(x-2)(5x-16)}$$

$$= \dfrac{1+x}{(x+2)(5x-16)} = \dfrac{x+1}{5x^2-6x-32}$$

RATIONALIZING THE DENOMINATOR

It is sometimes convenient to write fractions in a form that has no radicals in the denominator. Consider, for example, the fraction $1/\sqrt{2}$. Using the fact that $\sqrt{2}/\sqrt{2} = 1$, we have:

$$\frac{1}{\sqrt{2}} = \frac{1}{\sqrt{2}} \cdot \frac{\sqrt{2}}{\sqrt{2}} = \frac{\sqrt{2}}{2}$$

One advantage of the form $\sqrt{2}/2$ over $1/\sqrt{2}$ becomes apparent when you need a decimal approximation for $\sqrt{2}$, say, $\sqrt{2} \approx 1.414$. In order to find the decimal approximation of $1/\sqrt{2}$, we must compute $1/1.414$, which requires some nontrivial long division. But if we use $\sqrt{2}/2$, it is easy to see that $\sqrt{2}/2 \approx 1.414/2 = .707$.

Here are some more examples of this process, which is usually called **rationalizing the denominator.** The basic idea is to multiply both numerator and denominator by the "radical quantity" appearing in the denominator:

EXAMPLE $\dfrac{1}{\sqrt{3}} = \dfrac{1}{\sqrt{3}} \cdot \dfrac{\sqrt{3}}{\sqrt{3}} = \dfrac{\sqrt{3}}{3}.$

EXAMPLE $\sqrt{\dfrac{5}{2x+1}} = \dfrac{\sqrt{5}}{\sqrt{2x+1}} = \dfrac{\sqrt{5}}{\sqrt{2x+1}} \cdot \dfrac{\sqrt{2x+1}}{\sqrt{2x+1}} = \dfrac{\sqrt{10x+5}}{2x+1}.$

Sometimes a slightly different procedure is needed to rationalize the denominator.

EXAMPLE   In order to rationalize the denominator of $\dfrac{1}{3+\sqrt{2}}$ we must multiply both the top and bottom by something that will eliminate the radical in the denominator. Observe that $(3+\sqrt{2})(3-\sqrt{2}) = 3^2 - (\sqrt{2})^2 = 9 - 2 = 7$. Therefore

$$\frac{1}{3+\sqrt{2}} = \left(\frac{1}{3+\sqrt{2}}\right)\left(\frac{3-\sqrt{2}}{3-\sqrt{2}}\right) = \frac{3-\sqrt{2}}{(3+\sqrt{2})(3-\sqrt{2})} = \frac{3-\sqrt{2}}{7}$$

EXAMPLE   To rationalize the denominator of $\dfrac{7}{\sqrt{5}-\sqrt{3}}$, we note that $(\sqrt{5}-\sqrt{3})(\sqrt{5}+\sqrt{3}) = (\sqrt{5})^2 - (\sqrt{3})^2 = 5 - 3 = 2$. Thus

$$\frac{7}{\sqrt{5}-\sqrt{3}} = \left(\frac{7}{\sqrt{5}-\sqrt{3}}\right)\left(\frac{\sqrt{5}+\sqrt{3}}{\sqrt{5}+\sqrt{3}}\right) = \frac{7(\sqrt{5}+\sqrt{3})}{(\sqrt{5}-\sqrt{3})(\sqrt{5}+\sqrt{3})} = \frac{7(\sqrt{5}+\sqrt{3})}{2}$$

EXERCISES

A.1.   Express these fractions in lowest terms:

(a) $\dfrac{63}{49}$
(b) $\dfrac{121}{33}$
(c) $\dfrac{13 \cdot 27 \cdot 22 \cdot 10}{6 \cdot 4 \cdot 11 \cdot 12}$
(d) $\dfrac{x^2 - 4}{x + 2}$

(e) $\dfrac{x^2 - x - 2}{x^2 + 2x + 1}$

(f) $\dfrac{z + 1}{z^3 + 1}$

(g) $\dfrac{a^2 - b^2}{a^3 - b^3}$

(h) $\dfrac{x^4 - 3x^2}{x^3}$

(i) $\dfrac{(x + c)(x^2 - cx + c^2)}{x^4 + c^3x}$

A.2. Perform the indicated addition or subtraction:

(a) $\dfrac{3}{7} + \dfrac{2}{5}$

(b) $\dfrac{7}{8} - \dfrac{5}{6}$

(c) $\left(\dfrac{19}{7} + \dfrac{1}{2}\right) - \dfrac{1}{3}$

(d) $\dfrac{1}{a} - \dfrac{2a}{b}$

(e) $\dfrac{c}{d} + \dfrac{3c}{e}$

(f) $\dfrac{r}{s} + \dfrac{s}{t} + \dfrac{t}{r}$

(g) $\dfrac{b}{c} - \dfrac{c}{b}$

(h) $\dfrac{a}{b} + \dfrac{2a}{b^2} + \dfrac{3a}{b^3}$

A.3. Perform the indicated addition or subtraction:

(a) $\dfrac{1}{x + 1} - \dfrac{1}{x}$

(b) $\dfrac{1}{2x + 1} + \dfrac{1}{2x - 1}$

(c) $\dfrac{1}{x + 4} + \dfrac{2}{(x + 4)^2} - \dfrac{3}{x^2 + 8x + 16}$

(d) $\dfrac{1}{x} + \dfrac{1}{xy} + \dfrac{1}{xy^2}$

(e) $\dfrac{1}{x} - \dfrac{1}{3x - 4}$

(f) $\dfrac{3}{x - 1} + \dfrac{4}{x + 1}$

(g) $\dfrac{1}{x + y} + \dfrac{x + y}{x^3 + y^3}$

(h) $\dfrac{6}{5(x - 1)(x - 2)^2} + \dfrac{x}{3(x - 1)^2(x - 2)}$

(i) $\dfrac{1}{4x(x + 1)(x + 2)^3} - \dfrac{6x + 2}{4(x + 1)^3}$

(j) $\dfrac{x + y}{(x^2 - xy)(x - y)^2} - \dfrac{2}{(x^2 - y^2)^2}$

A.4. Multiply and express in lowest terms:

(a) $\dfrac{3}{4} \cdot \dfrac{12}{5} \cdot \dfrac{10}{9}$

(b) $\dfrac{10}{45} \cdot \dfrac{6}{14} \cdot \dfrac{1}{2}$

(c) $\dfrac{3a^2c}{4ac} \cdot \dfrac{8ac^3}{9a^2c^4}$

(d) $\dfrac{6x^2y}{2x} \cdot \dfrac{y}{21xy}$

(e) $\dfrac{7x}{11y} \cdot \dfrac{66y^2}{14x^3}$

(f) $\dfrac{ab}{c^2} \cdot \dfrac{cd}{a^2b} \cdot \dfrac{ad}{bc^2}$

A.5. Multiply and express in lowest terms:

(a) $\dfrac{3x + 9}{2x} \cdot \dfrac{8x^2}{(x^2 - 9)}$

(b) $\dfrac{4x + 16}{3x + 15} \cdot \dfrac{2x + 10}{x + 4}$

(c) $\dfrac{5y - 25}{3} \cdot \dfrac{y^2}{y^2 - 25}$

(d) $\dfrac{6x - 12}{6x} \cdot \dfrac{8x^2}{x - 2}$

(e) $\dfrac{u}{u - 1} \cdot \dfrac{u^2 - 1}{u^2}$

(f) $\dfrac{t^2 - t - 6}{t^2 - 6t + 9} \cdot \dfrac{t^2 + 4t - 5}{t^2 - 25}$

(g) $\dfrac{2u^2 + uv - v^2}{4u^2 - 4uv + v^2} \cdot \dfrac{8u^2 + 6uv - 9v^2}{4u^2 - 9v^2}$

(h) $\dfrac{2x^2 - 3xy - 2y^2}{6x^2 - 5xy - 4y^2} \cdot \dfrac{6x^2 + 6xy}{x^2 - xy - 2yz}$

A.6. Compute the quotient and express in lowest terms:

(a) $\dfrac{\dfrac{5}{12}}{\dfrac{4}{14}}$

(b) $\dfrac{\dfrac{100}{52}}{\dfrac{27}{26}}$

(c) $\dfrac{\dfrac{uv}{v^2w}}{\dfrac{vw}{u^2v}}$

(d) $\dfrac{\dfrac{3x^2y}{(xy)^2}}{\dfrac{3xyz}{x^2y}}$

(e) $\dfrac{\dfrac{x+3}{x+4}}{\dfrac{2x}{x+4}}$

(f) $\dfrac{\dfrac{(x+2)^2}{(x-2)^2}}{\dfrac{x^2+2x}{x^2-4}}$

(g) $\dfrac{\dfrac{x+y}{x+2y}}{\left(\dfrac{x+y}{xy}\right)^2}$

(h) $\dfrac{\dfrac{u^3+v^3}{u^2-v^2}}{\dfrac{u^2-uv+v^2}{u+v}}$

(i) $\dfrac{\dfrac{(c+d)^2}{c^2-d^2}}{cd}$

A.7. Rationalize each denominator:

(a) $\dfrac{2}{\sqrt{5}}$

(b) $\sqrt{\dfrac{16}{5}}$

(c) $\sqrt{\dfrac{7}{10}}$

(d) $\sqrt{\dfrac{9x^4}{23}}$

(e) $\dfrac{1}{\sqrt{x}}$

(f) $\dfrac{\sqrt{6}}{\sqrt{6}+\sqrt{2}}$

(g) $\dfrac{\sqrt{r}+\sqrt{s}}{\sqrt{r}-\sqrt{s}}$

(h) $\dfrac{1}{\sqrt{a}-2\sqrt{b}}$

(i) $\dfrac{u^2-v^2}{\sqrt{u+v}-\sqrt{u-v}}$

B.1. **Errors to Avoid** Find a numerical example to show that the given statement is *false*. Then find the mistake in the statement and correct it. (See Exercise B.6 on page 41.)

(a) $\dfrac{1}{a}+\dfrac{1}{b}=\dfrac{1}{a+b}$

(b) $\dfrac{x^2}{x^2+x^6}=1+x^3$

(c) $\left(\dfrac{1}{\sqrt{a}+\sqrt{b}}\right)^2=\dfrac{1}{a+b}$

(d) $\dfrac{r+s}{r+t}=1+\dfrac{s}{t}$

(e) $\dfrac{U}{V}+\dfrac{V}{U}=1$

(f) $\dfrac{\dfrac{1}{x}}{\dfrac{1}{y}}=\dfrac{1}{xy}$

(g) $(\sqrt{x}+\sqrt{y})\dfrac{1}{\sqrt{x}+\sqrt{y}}=x+y$

Equations and Inequalities

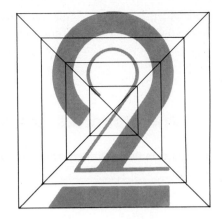

This chapter deals with equations, such as

$$3x + 2 = 17 \qquad x^2 + 8x + 3 = 0 \qquad \sqrt{2x - 3} - \sqrt{x + 7} = 2$$

and inequalities, such as

$$x^2 + 3 < 5 \qquad 4x + 3 > 9 \qquad 2x^3 - 15x < x^2 \qquad |2x^2 + 3x - 1| \geq 3$$

A **solution** of such an equation or inequality is a number that, when substituted for x,[°]
produces a true statement. For example, 5 is a solution of $3x + 2 = 17$ since $3 \cdot 5 + 2 = 17$ is a true statement. But 4 is *not* a solution of the inequality $x^2 + 3 < 5$ since it is *not true* that $4^2 + 3 < 5$. When a number *is* a solution of an equation (or inequality), we say that the number **satisfies the equation** (or inequality).

In order to deal effectively with many practical problems and other mathematical situations, you often must solve a particular equation or inequality (that is, find all its solutions). The solution of almost every equation[†] involves:

BASIC PRINCIPLES FOR SOLVING EQUATIONS

Performing any one of the following operations on an equation produces an equation with the same solutions as the original equation:

1. *Add or subtract the same quantity from both sides of the equation.*

2. *Multiply or divide both sides of the equation by the same nonzero quantity.*

° The letter x is called a variable or unknown. Any letter may be used as a variable, so we shall also deal with equations and inequalities involving letters other than x.
† Similar principles for solving inequalities are discussed in Section 5.

Two equations with the same solutions are said to be **equivalent.** The usual strategy is to use the Basic Principles repeatedly to transform a given equation into an equivalent equation whose solutions are easy to find. The examples below will clarify this procedure.

1. FIRST-DEGREE EQUATIONS

This section deals with equations and applications involving first-degree polynomials, such as

$$3x - 6 = 7x + 4 \qquad \frac{5}{x + 8} = \frac{3}{x - 2} \qquad \left| \frac{5x - 4}{3} \right| = 2$$

Here are some step-by-step examples of the solution of such equations. The reason for each step is listed at the right. In most cases the reason is just one of the Basic Principles listed above.

EXAMPLE   Here is one way the Basic Principles can be used to transform the equation $3x - 6 = 7x + 4$ into an equivalent equation whose solution is obvious:

$$3x - 6 = 7x + 4$$
$$3x = 7x + 10 \qquad \text{(add 6 to both sides)}$$
$$-4x = 10 \qquad \text{(subtract } 7x \text{ from both sides)}$$
$$x = \frac{10}{-4} = -\frac{5}{2} \qquad \text{(divide both sides by } -4\text{)}$$

Clearly, $-\frac{5}{2}$ is the only solution of this last equation. Since the last equation has the same solutions as the original one, $-\frac{5}{2}$ is the only solution of $3x - 6 = 7x + 4$.

   Warning   To guard against mistakes, check your answers by substituting each solution you obtain into the original equation to make sure it really *is* a solution. All the answers in the examples have been checked, but the details are omitted to save space.

EXAMPLE   The first step in solving $\dfrac{t + 7}{2} = \dfrac{5t - 4}{7} + t$ is to eliminate the fractions by multiplying both sides by a common denominator, say, 14:

$$14 \left(\frac{t + 7}{2} \right) = 14 \left(\frac{5t - 4}{7} + t \right)$$
$$14 \left(\frac{t + 7}{2} \right) = 14 \left(\frac{5t - 4}{7} \right) + 14t \qquad \text{(begin multiplying out right side)}$$
$$7(t + 7) = 2(5t - 4) + 14t \qquad \text{(simplify)}$$
$$7t + 49 = 10t - 8 + 14t \qquad \text{(multiply out both sides)}$$
$$7t + 49 = 24t - 8 \qquad \text{(simplify)}$$
$$7t = 24t - 57 \qquad \text{(subtract 49 from both sides)}$$

$$-17t = -57 \qquad \text{(subtract 24}t \text{ from both sides)}$$

$$t = \frac{-57}{-17} = \frac{57}{17} \qquad \text{(divide both sides by } -17)$$

The only solution of this last equation, and hence the original one, is $\frac{57}{17}$.

EXAMPLE The equation $\dfrac{5}{x+8} = \dfrac{3}{x-2}$ makes sense only when the denominators $x + 8$ and $x - 2$ are nonzero. This will be the case provided that $x \neq -8$ and $x \neq 2$. So the statement of this equation implicitly involves an *extra condition: $x \neq -8$ and $x \neq 2$*. Any solution of the equation must be consistent with this condition. To solve the equation, we first eliminate the fractions by multiplying both sides by the common denominator $(x + 8)(x - 2)$. The condition that $x \neq -8$ and $x \neq 2$ guarantees that the quantity $(x + 8)(x - 2)$ is nonzero. So we obtain this equivalent equation:

$$\frac{5}{x+8}(x+8)(x-2) = \frac{3}{x-2}(x+8)(x-2)$$

$$5(x - 2) = 3(x + 8) \qquad \text{(simplify both sides)}$$

$$5x - 10 = 3x + 24 \qquad \text{(multiply out both sides)}$$

$$5x = 3x + 34 \qquad \text{(add 10 to both sides)}$$

$$2x = 34 \qquad \text{(subtract } 3x \text{ from both sides)}$$

$$x = 17 \qquad \text{(divide both sides by 2)}$$

Since 17 is the solution of this last equation and satisfies the extra condition that $x \neq -8$ and $x \neq 2$, it is the solution of the original equation.

EXAMPLE The equation $\dfrac{x-3}{x-7} = \dfrac{3x-17}{x-7}$ is meaningful only when the denominator $x - 7$ is nonzero, that is, when $x \neq 7$. *If* this condition holds, then we can multiply both sides of the equation by the nonzero quantity $x - 7$ and obtain:

$$\frac{x-3}{x-7}(x-7) = \frac{3x-17}{x-7}(x-7)$$

$$x - 3 = 3x - 17 \qquad \text{(simplify both sides)}$$

$$x = 3x - 14 \qquad \text{(add 3 to both sides)}$$

$$-2x = -14 \qquad \text{(subtract } 3x \text{ from both sides)}$$

$$x = 7 \qquad \text{(divide both sides by } -2)$$

But *no* number can be a solution of $x = 7$ and also satisfy the condition $x \neq 7$, which is necessary for the original equation to make sense. Therefore the original equation has *no solutions*.

ABSOLUTE VALUE EQUATIONS

A geometric method of solving simple equations, such as $|x + 3| = 5$, was presented in Section 4 of Chapter 1. For slightly more complicated absolute value equations the following algebraic method of solution is usually the easiest.

EXAMPLE The key to solving $\left|\dfrac{5x-4}{3}\right| = 2$ is a basic fact discussed on page 29: There are exactly two real numbers with absolute value 2, namely, 2 and -2. So if $\left|\dfrac{5x-4}{3}\right| = 2$, then $\dfrac{5x-4}{3}$ must be either 2 or -2. Each of these possibilities leads to a solution of the original equation:

$$\text{if } \frac{5x-4}{3} = 2, \quad \text{then} \qquad \text{if } \frac{5x-4}{3} = -2, \quad \text{then}$$

$$5x - 4 = 6 \qquad\qquad 5x - 4 = -6$$

$$5x = 10 \qquad\qquad 5x = -2$$

$$x = 2 \qquad\qquad x = -\tfrac{2}{5}$$

You should verify that both 2 and $-\tfrac{2}{5}$ are solutions of the original equation.

FORMULAS

We sometimes deal with formulas and equations involving several variables, such as

$$A = \pi r^2 \qquad S = 2\pi(r^2 + rh) \qquad aw - b = cdw \qquad ax + by = 8z + 5$$

A typical problem in such situations is to express one of the variables in terms of the others. What this amounts to in practice is solving an equation for one variable while treating the others as constants.

EXAMPLE To solve the equation $aw - b = cdw$ for w, we treat w as the unknown and the other letters as constants. Then we proceed as before to collect all terms involving w on one side of the equation:

$$aw - b = cdw$$
$$aw = cdw + b \qquad \text{(add } b \text{ to both sides)}$$
$$aw - cdw = b \qquad \text{(subtract } cdw \text{ from both sides)}$$
$$(a - cd)w = b \qquad \text{(factor } w \text{ out of left-hand side)}$$

If the quantity $(a - cd)$ is nonzero, we can divide both sides of the equation by it and obtain this solution:

$$w = \frac{b}{a - cd} \qquad \text{(provided } a - cd \neq 0)$$

EXAMPLE The surface area S of a cylindrical tin can is given by the formula $S = 2\pi(r^2 + rh)$, where h is the height and r is the radius of the circular top of the can. In order to find a formula for the height in terms of the surface area and the radius, we must solve the equation $2\pi(r^2 + rh) = S$ for h:

$$2\pi(r^2 + rh) = S$$
$$2\pi r^2 + 2\pi rh = S \qquad \text{(multiply out left-hand side)}$$
$$2\pi rh = S - 2\pi r^2 \qquad \text{(subtract } 2\pi r^2 \text{ from both sides)}$$

Since the radius r of the top of the can is a positive number, we can divide both sides of this last equation by the nonzero number $2\pi r$ and obtain the solution:

$$h = \frac{S - 2\pi r^2}{2\pi r}$$

APPLICATIONS

Many practical problems can be answered by solving certain equations. Typically, you are given several quantities, some of which are not presently known, together with various relationships among these quantities. In order to find the unknown quantities, you should follow these guidelines:

GENERAL GUIDELINES FOR SOLVING "WORD PROBLEMS"

1. *Denote one of the unknown quantities by a letter, say, x.*
2. *If there are other unknown quantities, use the given information to express each of them in terms of x.*
3. *Use the given relationships among the various known and unknown quantities to set up an equation in x.*
4. *Solve the equation.*

EXAMPLE   A tea merchant wants to mix some fancy Darjeeling tea that sells for \$8.25 per pound with some common black tea that sells for \$4.50 per pound. How much of each kind of tea should she use in order to make 100 pounds of a mixture that will sell for \$6.00 per pound?

SOLUTION   Let x denote the number of pounds of Darjeeling tea in 100 pounds of the mixture. Then the remainder of the 100 pounds, namely, $(100 - x)$ pounds, will be the common tea. The price (in dollars) of x pounds of Darjeeling is the product

$$(\text{Price per pound})(\text{Number of pounds}) = 8.25x.$$

Similarly, the price of $(100 - x)$ pounds of common tea at \$4.50 per pound is $4.50(100 - x)$ dollars. The price of 100 pounds of mixture at \$6.00 per pound is $6(100) = 600$ dollars. We can now set up an equation by using this fact:

$$\begin{pmatrix} \text{Price of } x \text{ pounds} \\ \text{of Darjeeling} \end{pmatrix} + \begin{pmatrix} \text{Price of } (100 - x) \\ \text{pounds of common} \end{pmatrix} = \begin{pmatrix} \text{Price of 100 pounds} \\ \text{of mixture} \end{pmatrix}$$

$$8.25x + 4.50(100 - x) = 6(100)$$

$$8.25x + 450 - 4.50x = 600$$

$$8.25x - 4.50x = 600 - 450$$

$$3.75x = 150$$

$$x = \frac{150}{3.75} = 40$$

So she should mix 40 pounds of Darjeeling and $(100 - 40) = 60$ pounds of common tea to obtain a mixture that will sell for \$6.00 per pound.

To deal with problems involving interest, you should recall the meaning of certain terms. For example, 8 percent means .08 and 8 percent of 227 means .08 times 227 (that is, $.08(227) = 18.16$). To answer the question: 128.25 is 9 percent of what number, let x denote the unknown number and observe that:

$$9 \text{ percent of } x = 128.25 \qquad \text{or equivalently,} \qquad .09x = 128.25$$

so that $x = \dfrac{128.25}{.09} = 1425.$

EXAMPLE   A certain high-risk stock has been increasing in value at a rate of 12 percent a year while insured savings certificates at a local bank pay only 6 percent a year. If you have 9000 dollars, how much should you invest in the stock and how much in savings certificates in order to obtain a return of 8 percent per year on your investment?

SOLUTION   Let x be the amount invested in the stock. Then the rest of the 9000 dollars, namely, $(9000 - x)$ dollars, will be put in savings certificates. We want the total return on the 9000 dollars to be 8 percent. So we have:

$$\begin{pmatrix}\text{Return on } x \text{ dollars} \\ \text{of stock at 12\%} \end{pmatrix} + \begin{pmatrix}\text{Return on } (9000 - x) \\ \text{dollars of savings at 6\%}\end{pmatrix} = (8\% \text{ of 9000 dollars})$$

$$(12\% \text{ of } x \text{ dollars}) + (6\% \text{ of } (9000 - x) \text{ dollars}) = (8\% \text{ of 9000 dollars})$$

$$.12x + .06(9000 - x) = .08(9000)$$

$$.12x + .06(9000) - .06x = .08(9000)$$

$$.12x + 540 - .06x = 720$$

$$.12x - .06x = 720 - 540$$

$$.06x = 180$$

$$x = \frac{180}{.06} = 3000$$

So 3000 dollars should be invested in the stock and $(9000 - 3000) = 6000$ dollars put in savings certificates in order to obtain an 8 percent return.

EXAMPLE   Tom can paint a certain fence in 6 hours. Huck can paint the same fence in 4 hours. If they work together, how long will it take to paint the fence?

SOLUTION   Since Tom can paint the entire fence in 6 hours, he can paint $\frac{1}{6}$ of it in 1 hour. Similarly, Huck can paint $\frac{1}{4}$ of the fence in 1 hour. Let t denote the number of hours it takes to paint the fence when they work together. Then together they can paint $1/t$ of the fence in 1 hour. Therefore we have:

$$\begin{pmatrix} \text{Part of fence} \\ \text{painted by Tom} \\ \text{in 1 hour} \end{pmatrix} + \begin{pmatrix} \text{Part of fence} \\ \text{painted by Huck} \\ \text{in 1 hour} \end{pmatrix} = \begin{pmatrix} \text{Part of fence} \\ \text{painted by both} \\ \text{in 1 hour} \end{pmatrix}$$

$$\frac{1}{6} + \frac{1}{4} = \frac{1}{t}$$

We can solve this equation by multiplying both sides by a common denominator for the three fractions, such as $12t$:[*]

$$12t\left(\frac{1}{6} + \frac{1}{4}\right) = 12t\left(\frac{1}{t}\right)$$

$$2t + 3t = 12$$

$$5t = 12$$

$$t = \frac{12}{5} = 2\frac{2}{5} \text{ hours}$$

EXERCISES

A.1. Solve these equations:

(a) $3x + 2 = 26$

(b) $\dfrac{y}{5} - 3 = 14$

(c) $3z + 2 = 9z + 7$

(d) $-7(t + 2) = 3(4t + 1)$

(e) $\dfrac{3y}{4} - 6 = y + 2$

(f) $\dfrac{4y}{5} + \dfrac{5y}{4} = 1$

(g) $2x - \dfrac{x - 5}{4} = \dfrac{3x - 1}{2} + 1$

(h) $2\left(\dfrac{x}{3} + 1\right) + 5\left(\dfrac{4x}{3} - 2\right) = 2$

(i) $3\left(\dfrac{x}{2} + 2x\right) = 11 - 4\left(\dfrac{2x}{3} + 1\right)$

A.2. Solve these equations:

(a) $\dfrac{3x + 2}{x - 6} = 4$

(b) $\dfrac{3x + 2}{x - 6} = \dfrac{2}{x - 6} + 2$

(c) $\dfrac{2x - 1}{2x + 1} = \dfrac{1}{4}$

(d) $\dfrac{4}{3y + 1} = \dfrac{1}{y}$

(e) $\dfrac{-5}{t} = \dfrac{7}{t + 1}$

(f) $\dfrac{2}{x + 4} = \dfrac{5}{x - 1}$

(g) $\dfrac{2x - 7}{x + 4} = \dfrac{5}{x + 4} - 2$

(h) $\dfrac{z + 4}{z + 5} = \dfrac{-1}{z + 5}$

(i) $1 + \dfrac{1}{x} = \dfrac{2 + x}{x} + 1$

[*] The context of the problem shows that t is positive, so we are multiplying by a nonzero quantity.

A.3. Use a calculator to solve these equations and *check your answers:*
   (a) $2.37x + 3.1288 = 6.93x - 2.48$
   (b) $18.923y - 15.4228 = 10.003y + 18.161$
   (c) $6.31(x - 3.53) = 5.42(x + 1.07) - 21.1584$

A.4. Solve each equation for the indicated letter. State any conditions necessary for your answer to be valid.

   (a) $A = \dfrac{h}{2}(b + c)$ for b (f) $a(y - 7) + 2a\left(\dfrac{y}{2} + a\right) = 16$ for y

   (b) $V = \pi b^2 c$ for c (g) $ax + (4a - b)(x + 3b) = 2x - a$ for x

   (c) $V = \dfrac{\pi d^2 h}{4}$ for h (h) $at^2 - (3b + t)t - 4a + 7 = 0$ for a

   (d) $\dfrac{1}{r} = \dfrac{1}{s} + \dfrac{1}{t}$ for r (i) $(a + c)(a - b)(b + z) = 14$ for z

   (e) $S = \dfrac{b}{1 - v}$ for v (j) $S = \dfrac{H}{a(v - w)}$ for w

B.1. Solve these equations. [*Hint:* First multiply out any products that occur.]
   (a) $(x + 2)^2 = (x + 3)^2$
   (b) $x^2 + 3x - 7 = (x + 4)(x - 4)$
   (c) $(x + 1)^2 + 2(x - 3) = (x - 2)(x + 4)$

   (d) $\dfrac{x + 1}{x} + \dfrac{2 - x}{x - 1} = \dfrac{3x + 5}{x^2 - x}$

   (e) $\dfrac{3}{x + 1} + \dfrac{2}{x - 1} = \dfrac{2x + 11}{x^2 - 1}$

   (f) $(y - 1)^3 = (y + 1)^3 - 3y(1 + 2y)$

B.2. (a)   Find a number c such that 4 is a solution of $3(x + 2) + c = 12 + 7c$.
   (b)   Find a number d such that $-\frac{3}{2}$ is a solution of $4x + 4d = -d(1 + 2x)$.

B.3. A student has exam scores of 88, 62, and 79. What score does he need on the fourth exam in order to have an average of 80?

B.4. A student scored 63 and 81 on two midterm exams. Each midterm exam accounts for 30 percent of the course grade and the final exam accounts for 40 percent of the grade. What score must she get on the final exam in order to have a grade of 76?

B.5. In six years George's age will be 21 years less than three times his sister's age. Seven years ago George was four times as old as his sister. How old is George now? [*Hint:* Let x be George's age now. Then $x - 7$ was George's age seven years ago and $x + 6$ will be his age six years from now. Verify that seven years ago his sister's age was $\dfrac{x - 7}{4}$. What will the sister's age be six years from now?]

B.6. If Lionel lost 20 pounds, then he would weigh seven times as much as his pet boa constrictor. Together they weigh 200 pounds. How much does each weigh?

B.7. My father was half again as old as my uncle when my father was the age my uncle is now. My father is now 40. How old is my uncle?

B.8. If Tom can do a certain job in 9 hours and Anne can do the same job in 6 hours, how long will it take to do the job if they both work together?

B.9. Susan can paint the living room in 2 hours. Bert can paint it in 3 hours and Ernie can paint it in 4 hours. If all three work together, how long will it take?

B.10. An expert can do a certain job in 10 hours, whereas an amateur takes 16 hours to do the same job. If two experts and four amateurs work together on the job, how long will it take?

B.11. A chemist has 12 ounces of a solution that is 30 percent acid. She has another solution that is 80 percent acid. How much of the 80 percent acid solution must be added to the 30 percent solution in order to obtain a solution that is 50 percent acid? [*Hint:* Let x be the amount of 80 percent solution to be added. Then $x + 12$ is the total number of ounces in the new solution. It should contain $.5(x + 12)$ ounces of acid (why?). How much acid is in x ounces of the 80 percent solution, and how much in 12 ounces of the 30 percent solution?]

B.12. A radiator contains 12 quarts of fluid, 30 percent of which is antifreeze. How much fluid should be drained from the radiator and replaced by pure (100 percent) antifreeze in order that resulting mixture will be 50 percent anti-freeze? [*Hint:* Let x denote the quarts of fluid to be drained; then x is also the amount of antifreeze to be added. When x quarts of fluid are drained, $.3x$ quarts of antifreeze are lost (why?).]

B.13. How much pure water should be added to 75 ounces of a 30 percent salt solution in order to obtain a 12 percent salt solution?

B.14. A merchant has five pounds of mixed nuts on hand; they cost $30. He wants to add peanuts that cost $1.50 per pound and cashews that cost $4.50 per pound to obtain 50 pounds of a mixture that costs $2.90 per pound. How many pounds of peanuts and how many of cashews should he add?

B.15. An item on sale costs $13.41. All merchandise was marked down 25 percent for the sale. What was the original price of the item?

B.16. A worker gets an 8 percent pay raise and now makes $1593 per month. What was the worker's old salary?

B.17. If you borrow $500 from a credit union at 12 percent annual interest and $250 from a bank at 18 percent annual interest, what is the effective annual interest rate on the total amount borrowed?

B.18. You have already invested $550 in a stock with an annual return of 11 percent. How much of an additional $1100 should be invested at 12 percent and how much at 6 percent in order that the total return on the entire $1650 is 9 percent?

B.19.   If 9 is added to a certain number, the result is one less than three times the number. What is the number?

B.20.   What number, when added to 30, is eleven times the number?

B.21.   When 40 is added to a certain number, the result is 8 less than three times the number. What is the number?

B.22.   Find four consecutive integers whose sum is 106. [Example: 12, 13, 14, 15 are four consecutive integers whose sum is 54. Note that $13 = 12 + 1$; $14 = 12 + 2$; etc.]

B.23.   Find four consecutive *even* integers whose sum is 268. [Example: 8, 10, 12, 14 are four consecutive even integers whose sum is 44.]

B.24.   Is it possible to find four consecutive even integers whose sum is 90?

B.25.   A car passes a certain point at 1 P.M. and continues along at a constant speed of 64 kilometers per hour. A second car passes the point at 2 P.M. and goes on at a constant speed of 88 kilometers per hour, following the same route as the first car. At what time will the second car catch up with the first one? [*Hint:* Remember that

$$\text{Distance traveled} = (\text{rate of speed})(\text{time})$$

Let t denote the number of hours *after* 2 P.M. How far has each car traveled from the starting point after t hours? When the second car catches up, the two cars will be the same distance from the starting point.]

B.26.   An airplane flew with the wind for 2.5 hours and returned the same distance against the wind in 3.5 hours. If the cruising speed of the plane was a constant 360 miles per hour, how fast was the wind blowing? [*Hint:* If the wind speed is r miles per hour, then the plane travels at $(360 + r)$ miles per hour with the wind and at $(360 - r)$ miles per hour against the wind.]

B.27.   A boat traveled upstream from point A to point B in 3 hours and 20 minutes. It then traveled downstream from B to A in 2 hours. Assuming that the boat traveled at a constant speed and that the speed of the current was 3 miles per hour, what was the boat's speed? How far is it from A to B?

B.28.   A motorist drives from city C to city D at an average speed of 33 miles per hour. The motorist returns to city C by the same route at an average speed of 41.25 miles per hour. If the return trip took 40 minutes less time than the outgoing trip, how far is it from city C to city D?

DO IT YOURSELF!

DIRECT VARIATION

Recall that for an object moving at a constant speed

$$\text{Distance traveled} = \text{speed} \times \text{time}$$

For instance, a plane that flies at 400 miles for 3 hours will travel $400 \times 3 = 1200$

miles. More generally, the distance d traveled by the plane in t hours is given by the formula

$$d = 400t$$

This equation states that d is a constant multiple of t (with the constant being 400). This is one example of the following definition:

Let u *and* v *be two quantities. The statement*

v *varies directly as* u

means that v *is always a constant multiple of* u. *In other words, there is a constant* k *such that*

$$v = ku$$

The constant k *is called the* ***constant of variation.***

In the preceding airplane example we had the equation $d = 400t$. In that case the constant k is 400, and we say that d varies directly at t or, in words, distance varies directly as time.

EXAMPLE   The equation $y = 7x$ says that y varies directly as x, with the constant of variation being 7.

In many situations involving direct variation the constant k of variation is not given. In such cases you can usually use other known information to find k.

EXAMPLE   When you swim under water, the pressure in your ears varies directly with the depth at which you swim. At a depth of 20 feet the pressure is 8.6 pounds per square inch. What will the pressure be at 65 feet?

SOLUTION   Let p denote the pressure (in pounds per square inch) and let d denote the depth. Since pressure varies directly as depth, we know that p is a constant multiple of d, that is,

$$p = dk$$

for some constant k. First we use the given information to find k. We know that when the depth is 20 then the pressure is 8.6. So we substitute $d = 20$ and $p = 8.6$ into the equation and obtain:

$$8.6 = k(20)$$

Dividing both sides by 20 shows that $k = \dfrac{8.6}{20} = .43$. Therefore the equation relating pressure and depth is

$$p = .43d$$

In order to find the pressure at 65 feet, we substitute $d = 65$ in this equation and obtain $p = (.43)(65) = 27.95$ pounds per square inch.

Direct variation can be viewed from another useful perspective. In the airplane example we had the equation $d = 400t$, which states that d varies directly as t. Dividing both sides of this equation by t shows that

$$\frac{d}{t} = 400$$

Thus the *quotient* of these two quantities that vary directly is always constant. We sometimes say that the quantities d and t are **proportional.** The constant quotient 400 is precisely the constant of variation.

Conversely, suppose we know that the quantities v and u are proportional. That is, their quotient is always constant, say $v/u = 5$. By multiplying both sides of this last equation by u we obtain $v = 5u$. Thus, v varies directly as u, with constant of variation 5. These examples illustrate the truth of the following alternate description of direct variation:

> v *varies directly as* u *exactly when* v *and* u *are proportional* (*that is, when their quotient is constant*).

It often happens that you need the answer to a direct variation question but don't have to know the constant of variation explicitly. In these cases it is usually best to attack the problem in terms of proportionality.

EXAMPLE   At a certain theater popcorn sales vary directly with the length of the movie. During a 90-minute movie 320 boxes of popcorn are sold. How many boxes will be sold during a 144-minute movie?

SOLUTION   Let n denote the length of the movie (in minutes) and b the number of boxes of popcorn that are sold. We want to find the value of b when $n = 144$. We can summarize the given information in this table:

b	?	320
n	144	90

Because b varies directly as n, we know that the quotient b/n always has the same constant value. Thus the quotient when $n = 144$ must be equal to the quotient when $n = 90$, so that

$$\frac{b}{144} = \frac{320}{90}$$

We need only solve this first-degree equation to find b. Multiplying both sides by 144 we have

$$144\left(\frac{b}{144}\right) = 144\left(\frac{320}{90}\right)$$

$$b = \frac{144 \cdot 320}{90} = 512$$

ALTERNATE SOLUTION We can also find the desired value of b by first finding the constant of variation. We know that $\dfrac{b}{n} = k$ for some constant k. When $n = 90$, then $b = 320$, so that $k = \dfrac{b}{n} = \dfrac{320}{90} = 3\dfrac{5}{9}$. Therefore

$$\frac{b}{n} = 3\frac{5}{9}$$

$$b = \left(3\frac{5}{9}\right)n$$

To find the value of b when $n = 144$, just substitute $n = 144$ in this last equation:

$$b = \left(3\frac{5}{9}\right)(144) = \left(\frac{32}{9}\right)(144) = \frac{4608}{9} = 512$$

You should know one more basic fact about direct variation. Suppose, for example, that $y = 5x$. Then y varies directly as x, with constant of variation 5. Dividing both sides of the equation $y = 5x$ by 5 produces this equation:

$$x = \frac{1}{5}y$$

This equation says that x varies directly as y, with constant of variation $\frac{1}{5}$. The same phenomenon occurs in general:

---

v *varies directly as* u *exactly when* u *varies directly as* v.

If k *is the constant of variation in one case, then* $\dfrac{1}{k}$ *is the constant of variation in the other.*

INVERSE VARIATION

The basic idea in *direct* variation is that the two quantities grow or shrink together. For instance, when $v = 3u$, then as u gets large so does v. Similarly, if u is very small, for example $u = \dfrac{1}{270}$, then $v = 3\left(\dfrac{1}{270}\right) = \dfrac{1}{90}$ so that v is also small. But two quantities aren't always related in this way. Many times they behave in this fashion: As one quantity grows, the other shrinks, and vice versa.

EXAMPLE Consider the equation

$$v = \frac{5}{u}$$

When u is very large, say $u = 500$, then v is very small, namely $v = \frac{5}{500} = \frac{1}{100}$. On the other hand, when u is small, say $u = \frac{1}{30}$, then v is large, namely $v = \frac{5}{\left(\frac{1}{30}\right)} = 5 \cdot 30 = 150$.

Another way to view the equation $v = \frac{5}{u}$ is to multiply both sides by u so that $uv = 5$.

In other words, the *product* of u and v is constant. This is an example of the following concept:

Let u *and* v *be two quantities. The statement*

v varies inversely as u

and the statement

v is inversely proportional to u

mean exactly the same thing, namely: There is some constant k *such that*

$$v = \frac{k}{u} \ \textit{or, equivalently, } uv = k$$

The constant k *is called the constant of variation.*

EXAMPLE According to one of Parkinson's Laws, the amount of time a department spends discussing an item in its budget is inversely proportional to the amount of money involved. The Math Department spent 40 minutes discussing the purchase of a new ditto machine for $450. How much time will they spend discussing a $100 appropriation for the departmental picnic?

SOLUTION Let t denote time spent (in minutes) discussing a given item and d the dollars to be spent on that item. Then t is inversely proportional to d so that

$$t = \frac{k}{d}$$

for some constant k. We know that $t = 40$ when $d = 450$. Substituting these numbers in the preceding equation shows that

$$40 = \frac{k}{450}$$

Multiplying both sides of this last equation by 450 shows that $k = 40 \cdot 450 = 18,000$. Therefore t and d are related by the equation

$$t = \frac{18000}{d}$$

Substituting $d = 100$ in this equation shows that the time spent discussing the picnic is

$$t = \frac{18000}{100} = 180 \text{ minutes } (= 3 \text{ hours!})$$

ALTERNATE SOLUTION We know that the product dt is always constant. So the product when $d = 100$ must be equal to the product when $d = 450$. Since we know the value of t when $d = 450$, we have:

$$\text{product } dt \text{ when } d \text{ is } 100 = \text{product } dt \text{ when } d \text{ is } 450$$
$$100t = 450 \cdot 40$$
$$100t = 18000$$
$$t = 180$$

OTHER KINDS OF VARIATION

Direct variation is just a name for the relationship expressed by equations such as

$$y = 4x \qquad v = \tfrac{7}{3}u \qquad d = 400t$$

Now we want to give a name to the relationship expressed in equations such as these:

$$y = 5x^2 \qquad v = 7u^5 \qquad w = \tfrac{4}{5}t^3$$

In each of these equations one quantity is a constant multiple of a *power* of the other quantity. There is a difference between these equations and the preceding ones. To say, for example, that y is a constant multiple of x^2 is *not* the same as saying that y is a constant multiple of x. We shall use the following terminology to describe this new situation.

Let u *and* v *be two quantities. Let* n *be a positive integer. The statement*

v *varies directly as the* **n**-*th power of* **u**

means that v *is a constant multiple of* u^n. *In other words, there is a constant* k *such that*

$$v = ku^n$$

EXAMPLE The equation $y = 7x^4$ says that y varies directly as the fourth power of x. The formula for the area A of a circle of radius r is $A = \pi r^2$. Since π is a constant, this formula says that A varies directly as the square of r.

The word "proportional" is also used in this context. For instance, the statement "v is proportional to the 5th power of u" means "v varies directly as the 5th power of u," that is, $v = ku^5$ for some constant k.

An analogous situation occurs with inverse variation.

> Let u *and* v *be two quantities. Let* n *be a positive integer. The statement*
>
> **v *varies inversely as the* n-*th power of* u**
>
> *means that there is a constant* k *such that*
>
> $$v = \frac{k}{u^n}$$

EXAMPLE   The equation $y = \dfrac{10}{x^3}$ says that y varies inversely as the cube of x. We also say that y is inversely proportional to the cube of x.

EXAMPLE   The study of physics shows that the intensity of illumination I from a source of light varies inversely as the square of the distance d from the source. In other words, there is a constant k such that

$$I = \frac{k}{d^2}$$

JOINT VARIATION

The terminology of variation can be adapted to situations involving more than two quantities, as illustrated in the following examples.

EXAMPLE   The equation $z = 10xy$ says that z is a constant multiple of the product xy. We say that z **varies jointly as x and y.**

EXAMPLE   The equation $W = 4xy^3z^2$ says that W varies jointly as x and the cube of y and the square of z.

EXAMPLE   The equation $K = \dfrac{4t^2}{d^4}$ says that K varies directly as the square of t and inversely as the fourth power of d.

EXAMPLE   The maximum load L that can be supported by a horizontal beam varies directly as the width w and square of the height h of a cross section and inversely as the length d of the beam. Translating this statement into an equation (with k denoting the constant of variation), we have

$$L = \frac{kwh^2}{d}$$

EXAMPLE   The stopping distance S of a car varies directly with the *sum* of the *reaction distance r* (the distance traveled between the time you realize you need to stop and the time you hit the brake pedal) and the *braking distance b* (the distance traveled from the time you hit the brake pedal until you stop). That is, for some constant k,

$$S = k(r + b)$$

EXAMPLE The volume V of a compressed gas varies directly as the temperature T and inversely as the pressure p. At a temperature of $300°$ the volume of a certain gas is 60 cubic feet and the pressure is 40 pounds per square inch. If the container is enlarged so that the gas has a volume of 200 cubic feet, then what is the pressure when the temperature is $325°$?

SOLUTION Since V varies directly as T and inversely as p, we know that for some constant k,

$$V = \frac{kT}{p} \qquad \text{or, alternatively,} \qquad \frac{Tk}{p} = V$$

We are given that $V = 60$ when $T = 300$ and $p = 40$. Substituting these values in the formula and solving for k we have

$$\frac{Tk}{p} = V$$

$$\frac{300k}{40} = 60$$

$$300k = 60 \cdot 40 \qquad \text{(multiply both sides by 40)}$$

$$k = \frac{60 \cdot 40}{300} = 8 \qquad \text{(divide both sides by 300)}$$

Therefore the formula relating volume, temperature and pressure is

$$V = \frac{8T}{p}$$

In order to find p when $T = 325$ and $V = 200$, we substitute these values in the formula and solve for p:

$$V = \frac{8T}{p}$$

$$200 = \frac{8 \cdot 325}{p}$$

$$200p = 8 \cdot 325 = 2600 \qquad \text{(multiply both sides by } p\text{)}$$

$$p = \frac{2600}{200} = 13 \qquad \text{(divide both sides by 200)}$$

Therefore the pressure is 13 pounds per square inch.

EXERCISES

A.1. Assume that v varies directly as u. Find the constant of variation in each case.
   (a) $v = 8$ when $u = 2$ (c) $v = 1$ when $u = 2$
   (b) $v = -8$ when $u = 4$ (d) $v = .4$ when $u = .8$

A.2. Assume that v varies inversely as u. Find the constant of variation in each case.

(a) $v = 8$ when $u = 2$ (c) $v = .12$ when $u = .1$

(b) $v = 30$ when $u = 10$ (d) $v = \frac{1}{4}$ when $u = \frac{1}{3}$

A.3. Express each of these statements as an equation, using k for the constant of variation.

(a) a varies inversely as b (d) z varies jointly as b and c

(b) r is proportional to t (e) z varies jointly as x, y and w

(c) p is inversely proportional to T (f) R is proportional to d and inversely proportional to y

A.4. Express each of these statements as an equation, using k for the constant of variation.

(a)   The weight w of an object varies inversely as the square of the distance d from the object to the center of the earth.

(b)   The amount of interest I varies jointly as the principal P and the time t.

(c)   The distance d one can see to the horizon varies directly as the square root of the height h above sea level.

(d)   The period p of a pendulum varies directly as the square root of the length t of the pendulum and inversely as the square root of the acceleration a due to gravity.

(e)   The pressure p exerted on the floor by a person's shoe heel is directly proportional to the weight w of the person and inversely proportional to the square of the width r of the heel.

B.1. Assume that r varies directly as t.

(a)   If $r = 6$ when $t = 3$, find r when $t = 2$.

(b)   If $r = 8$ when $t = 4$, find r when $t = 6$.

(c)   If $r = 4$ when $t = 2$, find t when $r = 2$.

(d)   If $r = 24$ when $t = 6$, find t when $r = 8$.

B.2. Assume that b varies inversely as x.

(a)   If $b = 9$ when $x = 3$, find b when $x = 12$.

(b)   If $b = 20$ when $x = 4$, find b when $x = 2$.

(c)   If $b = 10$ when $x = 4$, find x when $b = 12$.

(d)   If $b = 10$ when $x = 6$, find x when $b = \frac{1}{2}$.

B.3. Express each of these statements as an equation and find the constant of variation.

(a) t varies jointly as r and s; $t = 24$ when $r = 2$ and $s = 3$.

(b) T varies jointly as x and y; $T = 1$ when $x = 4$ and $y = .5$.

(c) B varies inversely as u and v; $B = 4$ when $u = 1$ and $v = 3$.

(d) D varies inversely as x and y; $D = \frac{2}{3}$ when $x = \frac{1}{4}$ and $y = 9$.

(e) w varies jointly as x and y^2; $w = 96$ when $x = 3$ and $y = 4$.

(f) z varies jointly as x^2, y^3 and t; $z = 96$ when $x = .5$, $y = 2$ and $t = 16$.

B.4. Express each of these statements as an equation and find the constant of variation.

(a) v varies directly as the cube of T and $v = 16$ when $T = 4$.

   (b) D varies inversely as the cube of r and $D = 8$ when $r = 4$.
   (c) p varies directly as the square of z and inversely as r; $p = 32/5$ when
         $z = 4$ and $r = 10$.
   (d) r varies directly as the square of m and inversely as s; $r = 12$ when $m = 6$
         and $s = 4$.
   (e) T varies jointly as p and the cube of v and inversely as the square of u;
         $T = 24$ when $p = 3$, $v = 2$, and $u = 4$.
   (f) D varies jointly as the square of r and the square of s and inversely as the
         cube of t; $D = 18$ when $r = 4$, $s = 3$ and $t = 2$.

B.5.   Suppose w is directly proportional to the sum of u and the square of v. If
      $w = 200$ when $u = 1$ and $v = 7$, then find u when $w = 300$ and $v = 5$.

B.6.   Suppose z varies jointly as x and y.
   (a)   If $z = 30$ when $x = 5$ and $y = 2$, then find x when $z = 45$ and $y = 3$.
   (b)   If $z = .1$ when $x = .5$ and $y = .02$, then find z when $x = .05$ and $y = .4$.

B.7.   Suppose r varies inversely as s and t.
   (a)   If $r = 12$ when $s = 3$ and $t = 1$, then find r when $s = 6$ and $t = 2$.
   (b)   If $r = 50$ when $s = .2$ and $t = .5$, then find s when $r = 2$ and $t = 5$.

B.8.   Suppose u varies jointly as r and s and inversely as t. If $u = 1.5$ when $r = 2$,
      $s = 3$ and $t = 4$, then find r when $u = 27$, $s = 9$, and $t = 5$.

B.9.   Suppose D varies jointly as b and c, and inversely as the square of d. If $D = 2.4$
      when $b = 16$, $c = 3$ and $d = 5$, then find c when $D = 5$, $b = 6$ and $d = 10$.

B.10.   In the State of Confusion your income tax varies directly as your income. If the
      tax is \$200 on an income of \$16,000, find the tax on an income of \$7,000.

B.11.   By experiment you discover that the amount of water that comes from your
      garden hose varies directly with the water pressure. A pressure of 10 pounds
      per square inch is needed to produce a flow of 3 gallons per minute.
   (a)   What pressure is needed to produce a flow of 4.2 gallons per minute?
   (b)   If the pressure is 5 pounds per square inch, what is the flow rate?

B.12.   At a fixed temperature the pressure of an enclosed gas is inversely proportional
      to its volume. The pressure is 50 kilograms per square centimeter when the
      volume is 200 cubic centimeters. If the gas is compressed to 125 cubic cm,
      what is the pressure?

B.13.   The electrical resistance in a piece of wire of a given length and material varies
      inversely as the square of the diameter of the wire. If a wire of diameter .01 cm
      has a resistance of .4 ohm, what is the resistance of a wire of the same length
      and material, but with diameter .025 cm?

B.14.   The weight of a cylindrical can of glop varies jointly as the height and the
      square of the base radius. The weight is 250 ounces when the height is 20
      inches and the base radius is 5 inches. What is the height when the weight is
      960 ounces and the base radius is 8 inches?

B.15.   The force needed to keep a car from skidding on a circular curve varies inversely as the radius of the curve and jointly as the weight of the car and the square of the speed. It takes 1500 kilograms of force to keep a 1000-kilogram car from skidding on a curve of radius 200 meters at a speed of 50 kilometers per hour. What force is needed to keep the same car from skidding on a curve of radius 320 meters at 100 kilometers per hour?

B.16. The period of a pendulum is the time it takes for the pendulum to make one complete swing and return to its starting point. The period varies directly with the *square root* of the length of the pendulum. A pendulum 3 meters long has a period of 4 seconds. If a grandfather clock has a 1.92-meter pendulum, what is its period?

C.1. **(a)** Suppose v varies directly as u and u is doubled. What is the effect on v?

  (b) Suppose v varies inversely as the square of u and u is multiplied by 4. What is the effect on v?

  (c) Suppose n is a positive number and that v varies inversely as the square of u. If u is multiplied by n, what is the effect on v?

2. QUADRATIC EQUATIONS

A **quadratic** (or second-degree) equation is one that can be written in the form

$$ax^2 + bx + c = 0 \qquad \text{for some constants } a, b, \text{ and } c \text{ with } a \neq 0$$

For example, each of these is a quadratic equation:

$$3x^2 - x - 10 = 0 \qquad \text{(here } a = 3, \ b = -1, \text{ and } c = -10)$$
$$x^2 = 5x - 6 \qquad \text{(equivalent to } x^2 - 5x + 6 = 0)$$

The various methods of solving quadratic equations are presented in this section. We begin with one of the most common ones—factoring.

EXAMPLE In order to solve the equation $x^2 - 5x + 6 = 0$, we first factor the left-hand side:

$$x^2 - 5x + 6 = 0$$
$$(x - 3)(x - 2) = 0$$

Remember that the only time a product of real numbers is zero occurs when one of the factors is zero. Consequently, the last equation is equivalent to:

$$x - 3 = 0 \qquad \text{or} \qquad x - 2 = 0$$

But $x - 3 = 0$ means $x = 3$ and $x - 2 = 0$ means $x = 2$. Therefore the solutions of $x^2 - 5x + 6 = 0$ are the numbers 2 and 3, since either of these numbers satisfies the equation.

EXAMPLE Solve the equation $3x^2 - x - 10 = 0$. Once again, the left-hand side can be factored:

$$3x^2 - x - 10 = 0$$
$$(3x + 5)(x - 2) = 0$$

This last equation is equivalent to

$$3x + 5 = 0 \qquad \text{or} \qquad x - 2 = 0$$
$$3x = -5 \qquad\qquad\qquad x = 2$$
$$x = -\tfrac{5}{3}$$

Therefore the solutions are $-\tfrac{5}{3}$ and 2.

COMPLETING THE SQUARE

An equation such as $x^2 = 36$ is easy to solve. Any solution of this equation is a number whose square is 36. But there are exactly *two* such numbers, $\sqrt{36} = 6$ and $-\sqrt{36} = -6$. Here is a slight variation on the same idea.

EXAMPLE In order to solve $(x + 5)^2 = 11$, we note that $(x + 5)$ must be a number whose square is 11. Since the *only* numbers whose squares are 11 are $\sqrt{11}$ and $-\sqrt{11}$, we have:

$$x + 5 = \sqrt{11} \qquad \text{or} \qquad x + 5 = -\sqrt{11}$$

so that

$$x = \sqrt{11} - 5 \qquad \text{or} \qquad x = -\sqrt{11} - 5$$

Therefore $(x + 5)^2 = 11$ has two solutions: $\sqrt{11} - 5$ and $-\sqrt{11} - 5$.

The preceding example shows that a quadratic equation can be solved if one side can be written as a perfect square. We can always arrange for this to be the case by using the technique of completing the square that was introduced on page 51.

EXAMPLE In order to solve $x^2 + 6x + 1 = 0$, we first rewrite it as

$$x^2 + 6x = -1$$

The idea now is to add a suitable number to both sides of the equation so that the left side will factor as a perfect square $(x + ?)^2$. But we know how to find the number needed to complete the square in the expression $x^2 + 6x$: *Take half the coefficient of x,* namely, $\tfrac{6}{2} = 3$, *and square it,* thus obtaining $3^2 = 9$. Adding 9 to both sides of the equation above and factoring the left-hand side yields:

$$x^2 + 6x + 9 = -1 + 9$$
$$(x + 3)^2 = 8$$

Thus $x + 3$ must be a number whose square is 8. The only two numbers whose square is 8 are $\sqrt{8}$ and $-\sqrt{8}$. Therefore

$$x + 3 = \sqrt{8} \qquad \text{or} \qquad x + 3 = -\sqrt{8}$$
$$x = \sqrt{8} - 3 \qquad\qquad\qquad x = -\sqrt{8} - 3$$

Consequently, the solutions are $\sqrt{8} - 3$ and $-\sqrt{8} - 3$ or, in more compact notation, $\pm\sqrt{8} - 3$.

EXAMPLE   In order to solve $3x^2 + 11x + 5 = 0$ by completing the square, we must have 1 as the coefficient of x^2. So we divide both sides of the equation by 3 and *then* proceed as before:

$$x^2 + \frac{11}{3}x + \frac{5}{3} = 0$$

$$x^2 + \frac{11}{3}x = \frac{-5}{3} \qquad \left(\text{subtract } \frac{5}{3} \text{ from both sides}\right)$$

$$x^2 + \frac{11}{3}x + \left(\frac{11}{6}\right)^2 = \left(\frac{11}{6}\right)^2 - \frac{5}{3} \qquad \Bigg(\text{add the square of half the coefficient}$$
$$\text{of } x, \text{ namely, } \left(\frac{1}{2} \cdot \frac{11}{3}\right)^2 = \left(\frac{11}{6}\right)^2, \text{ to}$$
$$\textit{both } \text{sides}\Bigg)$$

$$\left(x + \frac{11}{6}\right)^2 = \left(\frac{11}{6}\right)^2 - \frac{5}{3} \qquad \text{(factor left-hand side as a perfect square)}$$

$$\left(x + \frac{11}{6}\right)^2 = \frac{121}{36} - \frac{5}{3} = \frac{61}{36} \qquad \text{(put right-hand side over a common denominator)}$$

Thus the *square* of $x + \frac{11}{6}$ is $\frac{61}{36}$, so we must have:

$$x + \frac{11}{6} = \sqrt{\frac{61}{36}} \qquad \text{or} \qquad x + \frac{11}{6} = -\sqrt{\frac{61}{36}}$$

or in more compact notation:

$$x + \frac{11}{6} = \pm\sqrt{\frac{61}{36}} = \pm\frac{\sqrt{61}}{6}$$

Subtracting $\frac{11}{6}$ from both sides yields

$$x = \frac{-11}{6} \pm \frac{\sqrt{61}}{6} = \frac{-11 \pm \sqrt{61}}{6}$$

Therefore the solutions are $\dfrac{-11 + \sqrt{61}}{6}$ and $\dfrac{-11 - \sqrt{61}}{6}$.

THE QUADRATIC FORMULA

The technique just described can be used to find a formula for the solution of *any* quadratic equation. Here is a step-by-step solution of the general equation $ax^2 + bx + c = 0$. The reason for each step is given at the right. Although it may look complicated, the procedure is *exactly* the same as that used in the preceding example, where we had $a = 3$, $b = 11$, and $c = 5$. If you have trouble following this argument, just compare it step for step with the preceding example.

$$ax^2 + bx + c = 0$$

$$x^2 + \frac{b}{a}x + \frac{c}{a} = 0 \qquad \text{(divide both sides by } a\text{)}$$

$$x^2 + \frac{b}{a}x = -\frac{c}{a} \qquad \left(\text{subtract } \frac{c}{a} \text{ from both sides}\right)$$

Now we want to complete the square in the expression $x^2 + \dfrac{b}{a}x$. To do this, we *take one-half the coefficient of* x, *namely,* $\dfrac{1}{2} \cdot \dfrac{b}{a}$, *and square it:* $\left(\dfrac{1}{2} \cdot \dfrac{b}{a}\right)^2 = \left(\dfrac{b}{2a}\right)^2$. Adding this quantity to both sides of the last equation yields:

$$x^2 + \frac{b}{a}x + \left(\frac{b}{2a}\right)^2 = \left(\frac{b}{2a}\right)^2 - \frac{c}{a}$$

$$\left(x + \frac{b}{2a}\right)^2 = \left(\frac{b}{2a}\right)^2 - \frac{c}{a} \qquad \text{(factor left-hand side as a perfect square)}$$

$$\left(x + \frac{b}{2a}\right)^2 = \frac{b^2}{4a^2} - \frac{c}{a} = \frac{b^2 - 4ac}{4a^2} \qquad \text{(put right-hand side over common denominator)}$$

Thus the *square* of $x + \dfrac{b}{2a}$ is $\dfrac{b^2 - 4ac}{4a^2}$, so that;

$$x + \frac{b}{2a} = \sqrt{\frac{b^2 - 4ac}{4a^2}} \qquad \text{or} \qquad x + \frac{b}{2a} = -\sqrt{\frac{b^2 - 4ac}{4a^2}}$$

or in more compact notation:

$$x + \frac{b}{2a} = \pm\sqrt{\frac{b^2 - 4ac}{4a^2}} = \pm\frac{\sqrt{b^2 - 4ac}}{2a}$$

Subtracting $b/2a$ from both sides yields:

$$x = -\frac{b}{2a} \pm \frac{\sqrt{b^2 - 4ac}}{2a} = \frac{-b \pm \sqrt{b^2 - 4ac}}{2a}$$

We have proved

THE QUADRATIC FORMULA

The solutions of the quadratic equation $ax^2 + bx + c = 0$ *are the numbers*

$$x = \frac{-b \pm \sqrt{b^2 - 4ac}}{2a}$$

You should memorize the quadratic formula and be able to use it easily.

EXAMPLE   In order to solve $x^2 + 8x + 3 = 0$, apply the quadratic formula with $a = 1$, $b = 8$, and $c = 3$:

$$x = \frac{-b \pm \sqrt{b^2 - 4ac}}{2a} = \frac{-8 \pm \sqrt{8^2 - 4 \cdot 1 \cdot 3}}{2 \cdot 1} = \frac{-8 \pm \sqrt{64 - 12}}{2} = \frac{-8 \pm \sqrt{52}}{2}$$

$$= \frac{-8 \pm \sqrt{4 \cdot 13}}{2} = \frac{-8 \pm \sqrt{4}\sqrt{13}}{2} = \frac{-8 \pm 2\sqrt{13}}{2} = -4 \pm \sqrt{13}$$

Therefore there are exactly two real number solutions: $-4 + \sqrt{13}$ and $-4 - \sqrt{13}$.

EXAMPLE   In order to solve $\frac{1}{3}x^2 - 2x + 3 = 0$, apply the quadratic formula with $a = \frac{1}{3}$, $b = -2$, and $c = 3$:

$$x = \frac{-b \pm \sqrt{b^2 - 4ac}}{2a} = \frac{-(-2) \pm \sqrt{(-2)^2 - 4(\frac{1}{3})3}}{2\frac{1}{3}} = \frac{2 \pm \sqrt{4 - 4}}{\frac{2}{3}}$$

$$= \frac{3}{2}(2 \pm \sqrt{0}) = 3$$

Thus 3 is the one and only solution of the equation.

EXAMPLE   To solve $2x^2 + x + 3 = 0$, apply the quadratic formula with $a = 2$, $b = 1$, and $c = 3$:

$$x = \frac{-b \pm \sqrt{b^2 - 4ac}}{2a} = \frac{-1 \pm \sqrt{1 - 4 \cdot 2 \cdot 3}}{2 \cdot 2} = \frac{-1 \pm \sqrt{1 - 24}}{4}$$

But $\sqrt{b^2 - 4ac} = \sqrt{1 - 24} = \sqrt{-23}$ is *not* a real number. There are *no solutions* in the real number system.

The term $b^2 - 4ac$ in the quadratic formula is called the **discriminant.** As the three preceding examples illustrate, the discriminant determines the *number* of real solutions° of the equation $ax^2 + bx + c = 0$:

Discriminant $b^2 - 4ac$	Number of Real Solutions° of $ax^2 + bx + c = 0$	Example
> 0	Two distinct real solutions	$x^2 + 8x + 3 = 0$
$= 0$	One real solution	$\frac{1}{3}x^2 - 2x + 3 = 0$
< 0	No real solutions	$2x^2 + x + 3 = 0$

FORMULAS AND APPLICATIONS

The preceding techniques for solving quadratic equations work equally well for quadratic equations or formulas involving several variables.

° The term "real solution" means a solution that is a real number.

EXAMPLE To express the radius r of the top of a cylindrical can in terms of the surface area S and the height h of the can, we must solve the surface area formula $S = 2\pi(r^2 + rh)$ for r. We have:

$$2\pi(r^2 + rh) = S$$

$$2\pi r^2 + (2\pi h)r - S = 0$$

This is a quadratic equation *in* r. We can apply the quadratic formula, substituting r for x and $a = 2\pi$, $b = 2\pi h$, and $c = -S$:

$$r = \frac{-b \pm \sqrt{b^2 - 4ac}}{2a} = \frac{-2\pi h \pm \sqrt{(2\pi h)^2 - 4(2\pi)(-S)}}{2(2\pi)} = \frac{-2\pi h \pm \sqrt{4\pi^2 h^2 + 8\pi S}}{4\pi}$$

$$= \frac{-2\pi h \pm \sqrt{4(\pi^2 h^2 + 2\pi S)}}{4\pi} = \frac{-2\pi h \pm 2\sqrt{\pi^2 h^2 + 2\pi S}}{4\pi} = \frac{-\pi h \pm \sqrt{\pi^2 h^2 + 2\pi S}}{2\pi}$$

Because the radius cannot be negative, the only solution that makes sense in this problem is

$$r = \frac{-\pi h + \sqrt{\pi^2 h^2 + 2\pi S}}{2\pi}$$

The equation in the previous example had two solutions, but only one was meaningful in the given context. This situation often occurs in applications.

EXAMPLE An investor buys some stock for 2400 dollars. If each share had cost 4 dollars less, the investor could have bought 30 more shares for the same 2400 dollars. How many shares did the investor actually buy? What was the price per share?

Solution: Let x be the number of shares purchased. The basic relationship here is:

$$\text{Total investment} = (\text{Price per share})(\text{Number of shares})$$

$$2400 = (\text{Price per share})x.$$

Thus the price per share is $\dfrac{2400}{x}$ dollars. If the price per share had been 4 dollars less, namely, $\left(\dfrac{2400}{x} - 4\right)$ dollars, the investor would have bought $(x + 30)$ shares. In this case we would have:

$$\text{Total investment} = (\text{Price per share})(\text{Number of shares})$$

$$2400 = \left(\frac{2400}{x} - 4\right)(x + 30)$$

We can now multiply out the right-hand side and solve this equation for x:

$$2400 = \frac{2400}{x} \cdot x - 4x + 30 \cdot \frac{2400}{x} - 4 \cdot 30$$

$$2400 = 2400 - 4x + \frac{72,000}{x} - 120$$

$$0 = -4x + \frac{72,000}{x} - 120$$

Multiplying both sides by x (which must be nonzero in this case) yields:

$$0 = -4x^2 + 72{,}000 - 120x$$

$$4x^2 + 120x - 72{,}000 = 0$$

Now divide both sides by 4 and factor:

$$x^2 + 30x - 18{,}000 = 0$$

$$(x + 150)(x - 120) = 0$$

$$x + 150 = 0 \qquad \text{or} \qquad x - 120 = 0$$

$$x = -150 \qquad\qquad x = 120$$

Only the positive solution makes sense here (you don't buy a negative number of shares). Therefore the investor bought 120 shares at a price of $\frac{2400}{120} = 20$ dollars per share.

EXERCISES

A.1. Solve these equations by factoring:

(a) $x^2 - x - 12 = 0$

(b) $15x^2 + 7x - 2 = 0$

(c) $x^2 + 9x + 14 = 0$

(d) $4t^2 + 9t + 2 = 0$

(e) $2y^2 + 5y = 3$

(f) $3u^2 = 4 - u$

(g) $5x^2 + 5 = -26x$

(h) $3y^2 = 10y + 8$

A.2. Solve these equations:

(a) $x^2 = 64$

(b) $x^2 + 7 = 32$

(c) $z^2 = 56$

(d) $(x - 7)^2 = 16$

(e) $(y + 2)^2 = 5$

(f) $x^2 + 2x + 1 = 9$

(g) $y^2 - 6y + 9 = 0$

(h) $9x^2 + 12x + 4 = 14$

A.3. Solve these equations by completing the square:

(a) $x^2 - 2x - 15 = 0$

(b) $x^2 - x - 1 = 0$

(c) $x^2 - 4x = 32$

(d) $2y^2 + y = 15$

(e) $3t^2 = 1 - 2t$

(f) $3u^2 + 3 = 8u$

A.4. Use the quadratic formula to solve these equations:

(a) $x^2 + 8x + 15 = 0$

(b) $4x^2 - 8x + 1 = 0$

(c) $2t^2 + 4t + 1 = 0$

(d) $3t^2 + 4t + 2 = 0$

(e) $5u^2 + 8u = -2$

(f) $\dfrac{2u^2}{3} + \dfrac{2}{3} = u$

(g) $4x^2 = 3x + 5$

(h) $\dfrac{3x^2}{4} + \dfrac{x}{4} + \dfrac{1}{2} = 1$

A.5. Find the *number* of real solutions of each equation by computing the discriminant:

(a) $x^2 + 4x + 1 = 0$

(d) $9t^2 + 15 = 30t$

(b) $4x^2 - 4x - 3 = 0$ **(e)** $25t^2 + 49 = 70t$

(c) $9x^2 = 12x + 1$ **(f)** $49t^2 + 5 = 42t$

A.6. Solve these equations using any method:

(a) $3t^2 - 11t - 20 = 0$ (d) $2x^2 = 7x + 15$

(b) $t^2 + 4t + 13 = 0$ (e) $25y^2 = 20y + 1$

(c) $4x(x + 1) = 1$ (f) $5x^2 + 2x = -2$

A.7. Use a calculator and the quadratic formula to find (approximate) solutions of these equations. Do your answers check? Why?

(a) $4.42x^2 - 10.14x + 3.79 = 0$

(b) $8.06x^2 + 25.8726x - 25.047256 = 0$

(c) $3x^2 - 82.74x + 570.4923 = 0$

(d) $7.63x^2 + 2.79x = 5.32$

B.1. Solve these equations. [*Hint:* In (a) the only numbers with absolute value 4 are 4 and -4; see the first-degree example on page 64.]

(a) $|x^2 + 4x - 1| = 4$ (c) $|x^2 + 3x + 2| = 5$

(b) $|x^2 - 5x + 1| = 3$ (d) $|x^2 + 7x - 2| = 3$

B.2. Find a number k such that the given equation has exactly one real number solution:

(a) $x^2 + kx + 25 = 0$ (d) $kx^2 + 24x + 16 = 0$

(b) $x^2 - kx + 49 = 0$ (e) $9x^2 + k = 30x$

(c) $kx^2 + 8x + 1 = 0$ (f) $4u^2 + ku + 9 = 0$

B.3. Find a number k such that 4 and 1 are the solutions of $x^2 - 5x + k = 0$.

B.4. Find a quadratic equation that has the given numbers as its only solutions:

(a) $1, -2$ (b) $0, 7$ (c) $\frac{3}{5}$ (d) $\sqrt{3}$ (e) $-\pi, 2\pi$ (f) $2, -2\sqrt{2}$

B.5. Solve each equation for the indicated letter. State any conditions that are necessary for your answer to be valid.

(a) $E = mc^2$ for c

(b) $V = 4\pi r^2$ for r

(c) $A = \pi rh + \pi r^2$ for r

(d) $d = -16t^2 + vt$ for t

(e) $3x^2 + xy - 4y^2 = 9$ for x

(f) $3x^2 + xy - 4y^2 = 9$ for y

(g) $kx^2 + 2x = 3kx + 6$ for x

(h) $2x^2 - 2ax + 4 = (a + b)^2 + 2bx$ for x

B.6. Suppose a, b, and c are fixed real numbers such that $b^2 - 4ac \geq 0$. Let r and s be the solutions of $ax^2 + bx + c = 0$.

(a) Use the quadratic formula to show that $r + s = -b/a$ and $rs = c/a$.

(b) Use part (a) to verify that $ax^2 + bx + c = a(x - r)(x - s)$.

(c) Use part (b) to factor these polynomials: $x^2 - 2x - 1$ and $5x^2 + 8x + 2$.

B.7. Find two consecutive integers whose product is 272. [*Hint:* If x is an integer, then $x + 1$ is the next consecutive integer.]

B.8. Find two consecutive integers, the sum of whose squares is 313.

B.9.   The diameter of a circle is 16 inches. By what amount must the radius be decreased in order to decrease the area of the circle by 48π square inches?

B.10.   A group of people agree to share equally in the $162 cost of printing some campaign literature for their candidate. Later 18 more people join the group and this reduces each person's share by $12. How much did it cost each group member before?

B.11.   A rectangular theater seats 1620 people. If each row had six more seats in it, the number of rows would be reduced by nine. How many seats would *then* be in each row?

B.12.   A 13-foot long ladder leans on a wall. The bottom of the ladder is 5 feet from the wall. If the bottom is pulled out 3 feet farther from the wall, how far does the top of the ladder move down the wall? [*Hint:* The ladder, ground, and wall form a right triangle. Draw pictures of this triangle before and after the ladder is moved. Use the Pythagorean Theorem to set up an equation.]

B.13.   A 15-foot long pole leans against a wall. The bottom is 9 feet from the wall. How much farther should the bottom be pulled away from the wall so that the top moves the same amount down the wall? [See the Hint for Exercise B.12.]

B.14.   When an object is dropped or thrown downward (and air resistance is neglected), then after t seconds the object will have fallen s feet, where $s = 16t^2 + v_0 t$, where v_0 is the initial velocity of the object.
   (a)   Suppose an object is dropped from the top of a 640-foot high building. How long does it take to reach the ground? [*Hint:* At the instant it is dropped the object's speed (the initial velocity) is 0 feet per second.]
   (b)   If the object is thrown downward and leaves the top of the building at a rate of 52 feet per second, how long does it take to reach the ground?

B.15.   A woman and her son working together can paint a garage in 4 hours and 48 minutes. The woman working alone can paint it in 4 hours less than the son would take to do it alone. How long would it take the son to paint the garage alone?

B.16.   Two ships leave the same point at the same time, one going due north and the other due east. The northbound ship travels 5 knots (= nautical miles per hour) faster than the eastbound one. After 6 hours the ships are 150 nautical miles apart. Find the speed of each ship.

B.17.   A right triangle has hypotenuse of length 12.054 meters. The sum of the lengths of the other two sides is 16.96 meters. How long is each side? [Use of a calculator is encouraged.]

3. HIGHER DEGREE POLYNOMIAL EQUATIONS

In this section we explore techniques that can be used to solve certain polynomial equations of degree 3 or more. If such an equation is in "quadratic form" it can be solved by the methods used in the last section.

EXAMPLE   To solve $2x^4 - 5x^2 - 3 = 0$, we first make a substitution in such a way that the equation becomes quadratic. Let $u = x^2$; then we have:

$$2x^4 - 5x^2 - 3 = 0$$
$$2(x^2)^2 - 5x^2 - 3 = 0$$
$$2u^2 - 5u - 3 = 0$$

But now we have a quadratic equation *in* u, it can be solved by factoring:

$$2u^2 - 5u - 3 = 0$$
$$(2u + 1)(u - 3) = 0$$

$$2u + 1 = 0 \qquad \text{or} \qquad u - 3 = 0$$
$$2u = -1 \qquad\qquad\qquad u = 3$$
$$u = -\tfrac{1}{2}$$

Since $u = x^2$ we see that

$$x^2 = -\tfrac{1}{2} \qquad \text{or} \qquad x^2 = 3$$

Now $x^2 = -\tfrac{1}{2}$ has no real number solutions because the square of every real number is nonnegative. But $x^2 = 3$ has $\sqrt{3}$ and $-\sqrt{3}$ as solutions. So $\sqrt{3}$ and $-\sqrt{3}$ are the only real number solutions of the original fourth-degree equation.

EXAMPLE   To solve $x^4 - 4x^2 + 1 = 0$, we let $u = x^2$ so that the equation becomes $u^2 - 4u + 1 = 0$. This quadratic equation in u can be solved via the quadratic formula:

$$u = \frac{-b \pm \sqrt{b^2 - 4ac}}{2a} = \frac{-(-4) \pm \sqrt{(-4)^2 - 4 \cdot 1 \cdot 1}}{2 \cdot 1} = \frac{4 \pm \sqrt{12}}{2} = \frac{4 \pm \sqrt{4 \cdot 3}}{2}$$
$$= \frac{4 \pm 2\sqrt{3}}{2} = 2 \pm \sqrt{3}$$

Since $u = x^2$, we have the equivalent statement:

$$x^2 = 2 + \sqrt{3} \qquad \text{or} \qquad x^2 = 2 - \sqrt{3}$$
$$x = \pm\sqrt{2 + \sqrt{3}} \qquad \text{or} \qquad x = \pm\sqrt{2 - \sqrt{3}}$$

Taking square roots in this last step is valid since both $2 + \sqrt{3}$ and $2 - \sqrt{3}$ are positive real numbers. Therefore the original equation has four solutions.

Occasionally, a higher degree polynomial equation can be solved by factoring.

EXAMPLE   Factoring the left-hand side of $x^7 - 7x^5 - 18x^3 = 0$ yields:

$$x^3(x^4 - 7x^2 - 18) = 0$$
$$x^3(x^2 - 9)(x^2 + 2) = 0$$
$$x^3(x + 3)(x - 3)(x^2 + 2) = 0$$

Since a product is zero only when at least one of the factors is zero, this last equation is equivalent to:

$$x^3 = 0 \quad \text{or} \quad x + 3 = 0 \quad \text{or} \quad x - 3 = 0 \quad \text{or} \quad x^2 + 2 = 0$$

$$x = 0 \quad \text{or} \quad x = -3 \quad \text{or} \quad x = 3 \quad \text{or} \quad x^2 = -2$$

Since $x^2 = -2$ has no real number solutions, the only real number solutions of the original equation are 0, 3, and -3.

The easiest equations to solve are those that are presented in factored form. You can simply read the solutions directly from the equation.

EXAMPLE   The solutions of $3(x - 2)^3(x + \frac{5}{2})^2(x - \sqrt{6}) = 0$ are 2, $-\frac{5}{2}$, and $\sqrt{6}$. This claim can be proved by first writing the equation as

$$3(x - 2)(x - 2)(x - 2)(x + \tfrac{5}{2})(x + \tfrac{5}{2})(x - \sqrt{6}) = 0$$

Since a product is zero only when at least one of the factors is zero, this equation is equivalent to:

$$x - 2 = 0 \quad \text{or} \quad x + \tfrac{5}{2} = 0 \quad \text{or} \quad x - \sqrt{6} = 0$$

$$x = 2 \quad \text{or} \quad x = -\tfrac{5}{2} \quad \text{or} \quad x = \sqrt{6}$$

Thus the only solutions are 2, $-\frac{5}{2}$, and $\sqrt{6}$ as claimed.

THE FACTOR THEOREM

In the last example, $(x - 2)$ was a factor of the polynomial and 2 was a solution of the equation. Similarly, $-\frac{5}{2}$ was a solution and $(x - (-\frac{5}{2})) = (x + \frac{5}{2})$ was a factor. This relationship between factors of the form $x - c$ and solutions holds true for any polynomial equation:

THE FACTOR THEOREM

The number c is a solution of the polynomial equation $f(x) = 0$ *exactly when* $(x - c)$ *is a factor of the polynomial* $f(x)$.°

If you know at least one solution of a polynomial equation the Factor Theorem can sometimes be used to obtain a factorization of the polynomial and hence the other solutions of the equation.

EXAMPLE   Given that 2 is a solution, find all solutions of the equation

$$x^3 - 4x^2 + 2x + 4 = 0.$$

SOLUTION   By the Factor Theorem, $(x - 2)$ must be a factor of $x^3 - 4x^2 + 2x + 4$. Using synthetic or long division, we find that the other factor is $x^2 - 2x - 2$ (verify!). We use this factorization to solve the equation:

° The Factor Theorem will be proved in Section 1 of Chapter 5.

$$x^3 - 4x^2 + 2x + 4 = 0$$

$$(x - 2)(x^2 - 2x - 2) = 0$$

$$x - 2 = 0 \quad \text{or} \quad x^2 - 2x - 2 = 0$$

We can use the quadratic formula on $x^2 - 2x - 2 = 0$ and conclude that

$$x = 2 \text{ or } x = \frac{-(-2) \pm \sqrt{(-2)^2 - 4 \cdot 1(-2)}}{2} = \frac{2 \pm \sqrt{12}}{2} = \frac{2 \pm 2\sqrt{3}}{2} = 1 \pm \sqrt{3}$$

Therefore the solutions of $x^3 - 4x^2 + 2x + 4 = 0$ are 2, $1 + \sqrt{3}$, and $1 - \sqrt{3}$.

RATIONAL NUMBER SOLUTIONS

The effective use of the Factor Theorem in the preceding example depended on knowing one solution of the equation to begin with. The following result can sometimes be used to find that first solution.

RATIONAL SOLUTIONS TEST[*]

Consider the polynomial equation

$$a_n x^n + a_{n-1} x^{n-1} + \cdots + a_1 x + a_0 = 0$$

where the coefficients a_n, $a_{n-1}, \ldots,$ a_0 *are integers. If a rational number* $\dfrac{r}{s}$ *(expressed in lowest terms) is a solution of this equation, then* r *is a factor of the constant term* a_0 *and* s *is a factor of the leading coefficient* a_n.

The proof of the Rational Solutions Test depends on some elementary number theory. Since the proof sheds little light on how the result is actually *used*, it will be omitted.

EXAMPLE   The equation $2x^4 + x^3 - 21x^2 - 14x + 12 = 0$ may or may not have any solutions that are rational numbers. But *if* some rational number r/s is a solution, then, according to the Rational Solutions Test, the number s must be a factor of the leading coefficient 2. Since the only integer factors of 2 are 1, -1, 2, and -2, s must be one of these numbers. Similarly, the number r must be a factor of the constant term 12. Therefore r must be one of 1, -1, 2, -2, 3, -3, 4, -4, 6, -6, 12, or -12. Consequently, the only possibilities for the quotient r/s (in lowest terms) are:

$$1, \ -1, \ 2, \ -2, \ 3, \ -3, \ 4, \ -4, \ 6, \ -6, \ 12, \ -12, \ \tfrac{1}{2}, \ -\tfrac{1}{2}, \ \tfrac{3}{2}, \ -\tfrac{3}{2}$$

Now all 16 of these numbers certainly won't be solutions. But *if* there is any rational number solution, it *must* be one of these 16 numbers. By substituting each of these numbers in the equation, we can find out which, if any, actually *are* solutions. Al-

---

[*] The Rational Solutions Test is sometimes called the Rational Root Test.

though this is a tedious procedure, it can be done. If you do it, you will find that both -3 and $\frac{1}{2}$ are solutions and that none of the other numbers on the list are solutions. So the *only* rational number solutions are -3 and $\frac{1}{2}$.

We have just seen that the only rational number solutions of $2x^4 + x^3 - 21x^2 - 14x + 12 = 0$ are -3 and $\frac{1}{2}$. Any other solutions of the equation must be irrational numbers. We now use the Factor Theorem to find them. Since -3 and $\frac{1}{2}$ are solutions we know by the Factor Theorem that $x - (-3) = x + 3$ and $x - \frac{1}{2}$ are factors of the polynomial $f(x) = 2x^4 + x^3 - 21x^2 - 14x + 12$. Therefore $f(x) = q(x)(x + 3)(x - \frac{1}{2})$ for some polynomial $q(x)$. We can find $q(x)$ by dividing $f(x)$ by $(x + 3)(x - \frac{1}{2}) = x^2 + \frac{5}{2}x - \frac{3}{2}$:

$$
\begin{array}{r}
2x^2 - 4x - 8 \\
\hline
x^2 + \tfrac{5}{2}x - \tfrac{3}{2}\,{\overline{\smash{\big)}\,2x^4 + x^3 - 21x^2 - 14x + 12}} \\
2x^4 + 5x^3 - 3x^2 \\
\hline
-4x^3 - 18x^2 - 14x + 12 \\
-4x^3 - 10x^2 + 6x \\
\hline
-8x^2 - 20x + 12 \\
-8x^2 - 20x + 12 \\
\hline
0
\end{array}
$$

We now use this information to factor the original equation and to find all its solutions:

$$2x^4 + x^3 - 21x^2 - 14x + 12 = 0$$
$$\left(x^2 + \tfrac{5}{2}x - \tfrac{3}{2}\right)(2x^2 - 4x - 8) = 0$$
$$(x + 3)\left(x - \tfrac{1}{2}\right)2(x^2 - 2x - 4) = 0$$

This last equation is equivalent to

$$x + 3 = 0 \quad \text{or} \quad x - \tfrac{1}{2} = 0 \quad \text{or} \quad x^2 - 2x - 4 = 0$$

Using the quadratic formula on the last equation on the right, we see that

$$x = -3 \quad \text{or} \quad x = \frac{1}{2} \quad \text{or} \quad x = \frac{2 \pm \sqrt{4 - 4(-4)}}{2} = \frac{2 \pm \sqrt{20}}{2}$$

$$= \frac{2 \pm 2\sqrt{5}}{2} = 1 \pm \sqrt{5}$$

So the equation $2x^4 + x^3 - 21x^2 - 14x + 12 = 0$ has two rational number solutions, -3 and $\frac{1}{2}$, and two irrational number solutions, $1 + \sqrt{5}$ and $1 - \sqrt{5}$.

EXAMPLE   To find the rational number solutions of $x^5 + 4x^4 + x^3 - x^2 = 0$ (or of any polynomial equation with constant term 0), begin by factoring out the highest possible power of x from *all* terms:

$$x^2(x^3 + 4x^2 + x - 1) = 0$$

Obviously, $x = 0$ is a rational number solution. The other solutions are the solutions of

$$x^3 + 4x^2 + x - 1 = 0$$

Now *if* this equation has a rational number solution r/s, then by the Rational Solutions Test

r is a factor of the constant term -1 and

s is a factor of the leading coefficient 1

Therefore the only possibilities for both r and s are 1 and -1. Hence the only possibilities for r/s are 1 and -1 as well. But you can easily verify that neither 1 nor -1 is a solution of $x^3 + 4x^2 + x - 1 = 0$. So this equation has no rational number solutions. Consequently, 0 is the only rational number solution of the original equation. If that equation has any other real number solutions, they must be irrational numbers.

EXERCISES

A.1. Solve these equations:

(a) $x^4 - 7x^2 + 10 = 0$

(b) $2y^4 - 9y^2 + 4 = 0$

(c) $6z^4 = z^2 + 2$

(d) $-10x^4 - 3x^2 + 1 = 0$

(e) $y^4 + 7 = 6y^2$

(f) $z^4 - 8z^2 = -9$

(g) $x^4 = 2x^2 + 1$

(h) $x^4 = 1 - 2x^2$

A.2. Solve these equations:

(a) $x^{127}(x - 4)^{15} = 0$

(b) $(4t - 1)^3(t + 7)^2 = 0$

(c) $(x + 100)^7(x + 7)^{100}(x - 2)^7(x - 7)^2 = 0$

(d) $(t + 5)(5t - 5)(t - 5)^5(t + 10)^5 = 0$

A.3. Use the Factor Theorem to determine whether the first polynomial is a factor of the second:

(a) $x - 1;$ $x^5 + 1$

(b) $x - \frac{1}{2};$ $2x^4 + x^3 + x - \frac{3}{4}$

(c) $x + 2;$ $x^3 - 3x^2 - 4x + 12$

(d) $x + 1;$ $x^3 - 4x^2 + 3x + 8$

(e) $x + 2;$ $x^3 + x^2 - 4x + 4$

(f) $x - 1;$ $14x^{99} - 65x^{56} + 51$

A.4. Find all the rational number solutions of these equations:

(a) $x^3 + 3x^2 - x - 3 = 0$

(b) $x^3 - x^2 - 3x + 3 = 0$

(c) $x^3 + 5x^2 - x - 5 = 0$

(d) $3x^3 + 8x^2 - x - 20 = 0$

(e) $2x^3 + 5x^2 = 11x - 4$

(f) $2x^3 = 3x^2 + 7x + 6$

A.5. Find all the rational number solutions of these equations:

(a) $\frac{1}{12}x^3 - \frac{1}{12}x^2 - \frac{2}{3}x + 1 = 0$ [*Hint:* First multiply both sides by 12.]

(b) $\frac{2}{3}x^4 + \frac{1}{2}x^3 - \frac{5}{4}x^2 - x - \frac{1}{6} = 0$ (d) $\frac{1}{3}x^3 + \frac{1}{6} = \frac{1}{2}x^2 + \frac{1}{6}x$

(c) $\frac{1}{3}x^4 - x^3 - x^2 + \frac{13}{3}x - 2 = 0$ (e) $\frac{2}{3}x^3 + \frac{2}{3}x = \frac{1}{2}x^2 + \frac{1}{2}$

B.1. Solve these equations. [*Hint:* The factoring patterns in Section 6 of Chapter 1 may be helpful here.]

(a) $x^3 - 1 = 0$

(b) $x^3 + 8 = 0$

(c) $x^4 - 125x = 0$

(d) $x^3 + 64 = 0$

(e) $12x^5 + 2x^4 - 2x^3 = 0$

(f) $t^8 + t^4 = 2$

(g) $x^3 - 12x^2 + 48x - 64 = 0$

(h) $x^3 - 3x^2 + 3x - 1 = 0$

(i) $x^6 - 7x^3 = 8$

B.2. One solution of each equation is given. Find all the real number solutions:

(a) $x^3 + 7x = 5x^2 + 2$; $x = 2$

(b) $3x^3 = 10x^2 + 23x + 10$; $x = -1$

(c) $8x^3 + 22x^2 = 7x + 3$; $x = -3$

(d) $x^3 + 9x + 5 = 7x^2$; $x = 5$

(e) $x^4 + 6x^3 = 7x^2$; $x = 0$

(f) $2x^3 = x^2 + 3x + 1$; $x = -\frac{1}{2}$

B.3. Use the Factor Theorem to show that for every real number c, $x - c$ is *not* a factor of $x^4 + x^2 + 1$.

B.4. Let c be a real number and n a positive integer.

(a) Show that $x - c$ is a factor of $x^n - c^n$.

(b) If n is even, show that $x + c$ is a factor of $x^n - c^n$. [Remember that $x + c = x - (-c)$.]

(c) If n is odd, give an example to show that $x + c$ may not be a factor of $x^n - c^n$.

(d) If n is odd, show that $x + c$ is a factor of $x^n + c^n$.

B.5. Find a number k such that

(a) $x + 2$ is a factor of $x^3 + 3x^2 + kx - 2$

(b) $x - 3$ is a factor of $x^4 - 5x^3 + kx^2 + 18k + 18$

(c) $x - 1$ is a factor of $k^2x^4 - 2kx^2 + 1$

(d) $x + 2$ is a factor of $x^3 - kx^2 + 3x + 7k$

B.6. Find all the real number solutions of these equations. [*Hint:* First find all the rational number solutions.]

(a) $2x^3 - 5x^2 + x + 2 = 0$

(b) $t^4 - t^3 + 2t^2 - 4t - 8 = 0$

(c) $6x^3 - 11x^2 + 6x = 1$

(d) $z^3 + z^2 + 2z + 2 = 0$

(e) $x^4 = x^3 + x^2 + x + 2$

(f) $3x^5 + 2x^4 - 7x^3 = -2x^2$

(g) $3y^3 + 3y = 2y^2 + 2$

(h) $x^5 + x = x^3$

C.1. Prove that $\sqrt{2}$ is not a rational number. [*Hint:* Use the Rational Solutions Test on $x^2 - 2 = 0$.]

DO IT YOURSELF!

APPROXIMATING SOLUTIONS

Polynomial equations of high degree can be quite difficult to solve, even *with* the help of a computer. Consequently, it is often necessary to *approximate* the solutions of a given equation to some stated degree of accuracy. The Location Theorem, stated here, is one method of doing this. The statement of this theorem uses the following notation:

If $f(x)$ denotes a polynomial and c is a real number, then the symbol $f(c)$ denotes the *number* obtained by substituting c for x in the polynomial $f(x)$. For instance, if $f(x)$ is the polynomial $x^2 - 5x + 2$, then $f(3)$ is the number $3^2 - 5 \cdot 3 + 2 = -4$ and $f(-1)$ is the number $(-1)^2 - 5(-1) + 2 = 8$.

LOCATION THEOREM

If f(x) *is a polynomial and* c *and* d *are real numbers such that the numbers* f(c) *and* f(d) *have opposite signs, then the equation* f(x) = 0 *has at least one solution between* c *and* d.

A rigorous proof of this theorem is beyond the scope of this book. The underlying reason why the theorem is true will become clear when we study the graphs of polynomial functions in Chapter 5. For now we simply illustrate the meaning and uses of the Location Theorem.

EXAMPLE Suppose $f(x)$ is the polynomial $x^3 + 2x^2 - 7x + 1$ and that $c = -2$ and $d = 1$. Then

$$f(c) = f(-2) = (-2)^3 + 2(-2)^2 - 7(-2) + 1 = 15 \qquad \text{and}$$
$$f(d) = f(1) = 1^3 + 2(1)^2 - 7(1) + 1 = -3$$

Since 15 and -3 have opposite signs, we know from the Location Theorem that the equation

$$f(x) = 0, \qquad \text{that is,} \qquad x^3 + 2x^2 - 7x + 1 = 0$$

has at least one solution between -2 and 1. The solutions of this equation are discussed further in the next example.

EXAMPLE If we apply the Rational Solutions Test to the equation $x^3 + 2x^2 - 7x + 1 = 0$, we find that the only *possible* rational number solutions (± 1) are *not* solutions. So the real number solutions, if any, must be irrational numbers. We can approximate these solutions by repeated use of the Location Theorem. We begin by evaluating the polynomial $f(x) = x^3 + 2x^2 - 7x + 1$ at various numbers:

x	-4	-3	-2	-1	0	1	2
$f(x) = x^3 + 2x^2 - 7x + 1$	-3	13	15	9	1	-3	3

In the preceding example we saw that the equation has a solution between -2 and 1. Now we can locate that solution a bit more precisely. The table shows that $f(0) = 1$ and $f(1) = -3$ have opposite signs. So the Location Theorem guarantees that there is a solution of the equation between 0 and 1. Similarly, $f(-4) = -3$ and $f(-3) = 13$ have opposite signs and hence there must be a solution between -4 and -3. Finally, since $f(1) = -3$ and $f(2) = 3$ have opposite signs, there is also a solution between 1 and 2.

To obtain a better approximation of one of these solutions, say, the one between 0 and 1, you need only evaluate the polynomial $f(x)$ at several numbers between 0 and 1. Using a calculator, we evaluate $f(x)$ at $x = .1$, $x = .2$, $x = .3$, and so on. We immediately find that

$$f(.1) = .321 \quad \text{and} \quad f(.2) = -.312$$

Since $f(.1)$ and $f(.2)$ have opposite signs, the solution actually lies between .1 and .2. For a more accurate approximation we evaluate the polynomial in increments of .01:

x	.11	.12	.13	.14	.15
$f(x) = x^3 + 2x^2 - 7x + 1$	.255531	.190528	.125997	.061944	$-.001625$

Since $f(.14)$ and $f(.15)$ have opposite signs, the solution lies betwen .14 and .15. Further calculation shows that

$$f(.1497) \approx .00027° \quad \text{and} \quad f(.1498) \approx -.00036$$

Thus the solution lies between .1497 and .1498; that is, .1497 is within .0001 units of the solution. For many purposes this is a sufficient degree of accuracy. But an even more accurate approximation of this solution could be obtained by further calculation.

EXERCISES

A.1.   Locate *one* irrational number solution of the given equation between two consecutive integers:

(a) $12x^3 - 28x^2 - 7x - 10 = 0$ (d) $x^3 + 9 = 3x^2 + 6x$

(b) $x^5 + x^2 - 7 = 0$ (e) $t^4 + 2t^3 - 10t^2 - 6t + 1 = 0$

(c) $x^3 + 4x^2 + 10x + 15 = 0$ (f) $u^4 + 8u^3 + 17u^2 + 4u = 2$

B.1.   Use a calculator to approximate at least one irrational number solution of each of the equations in Exercise A.1 to within .01 units.

4. RADICAL EQUATIONS

The information developed in earlier sections can now be used to solve equations involving radicals, such as

$$\sqrt[3]{2x^2 + 7x - 6} = \sqrt[3]{9} \qquad \sqrt{3 - x} = x - 3 \qquad \sqrt[3]{x^2} - 2\sqrt[3]{x} - 15 = 0$$

But first we must introduce one more basic principle for solving equations.

  If two numbers are equal, say, $a = b$, then it is certainly true that $a^2 = b^2$ and $a^3 = b^3$. In fact,

$$\text{if } a = b, \quad \text{then } a^r = b^r \text{ for every number } r$$

° $\approx$ means "is approximately equal to."

This statement is also valid for algebraic expressions that represent real numbers. For example,

$$\text{if } x - 2 = 3, \quad \text{then } (x - 2)^2 = 3^2$$

In particular, every solution of the equation $x - 2 = 3$ is also a solution of $(x - 2)^2 = 9$. But *be careful*. This usually works only in *one* direction. In this case it is *not* true that every solution of $(x - 2)^2 = 9$ is a solution of $x - 2 = 3$. You can easily verify that $x = -1$ is a solution of $(x - 2)^2 = 9$, but $x = -1$ is *not* a solution of $x - 2 = 3$. This example is a good illustration of the

---

POWER PRINCIPLE

Every solution of the equation A = B *is also a solution of the equation* $A^r = B^r$, *but not necessarily vice versa.*

The following examples show how the Power Principle can be used to solve various equations involving radicals.

EXAMPLE In order to solve the equation $\sqrt[3]{2x^2 + 7x - 6} = \sqrt[3]{9}$, we cube both sides and obtain:

$$(\sqrt[3]{2x^2 + 7x - 6})^3 = (\sqrt[3]{9})^3$$
$$2x^2 + 7x - 6 = 9$$

Any solution of the original equation must also be a solution of this last equation by the Power Principle. But this last equation can easily be solved:

$$
\begin{aligned}
2x^2 + 7x - 6 &= 9 \\
2x^2 + 7x - 15 &= 0 \quad &&\text{(subtract 9 from both sides)} \\
(2x - 3)(x + 5) &= 0 \quad &&\text{(factor left-hand side)} \\
2x - 3 = 0 \quad &\text{or} \quad x + 5 = 0 \\
2x = 3 \quad &\text{or} \quad x = -5 \\
x = \tfrac{3}{2} \quad &\text{or} \quad x = -5
\end{aligned}
$$

Therefore the only *possible* solutions of the original equation are $x = \tfrac{3}{2}$ and $x = -5$. By substituting these numbers in the original equation, we can determine its solutions. Since

$$\sqrt[3]{2(-5)^2 + 7(-5) - 6} = \sqrt[3]{50 - 35 - 6} = \sqrt[3]{9} \quad \text{and}$$
$$\sqrt[3]{2(\tfrac{3}{2})^2 + 7(\tfrac{3}{2}) - 6} = \sqrt[3]{2(\tfrac{9}{4}) + \tfrac{21}{2} - 6} = \sqrt[3]{\tfrac{9}{2} + \tfrac{21}{2} - \tfrac{12}{2}} = \sqrt[3]{\tfrac{18}{2}} = \sqrt[3]{9}$$

both $x = \tfrac{3}{2}$ and $x = -5$ are solutions of the equation $\sqrt[3]{2x^2 + 7x - 6} = \sqrt[3]{9}$.

EXAMPLE In order to solve

$$3 + \sqrt{3 - x} - x = 0$$

we rearrange terms and square:

$$\sqrt{3 - x} = x - 3$$
$$(\sqrt{3 - x})^2 = (x - 3)^2$$
$$3 - x = x^2 - 6x + 9$$

According to the Power Principle, the only *possible* solutions of the original equation are the solutions of this last equation. It can be solved as follows:

$$3 - x = x^2 - 6x + 9$$
$$0 = x^2 - 5x + 6$$
$$0 = (x - 3)(x - 2)$$
$$x = 3 \quad \text{or} \quad x = 2$$

Substituting these numbers in the left-hand side of the original equation $3 + \sqrt{3 - x} - x = 0$ yields:

$$3 + \sqrt{3 - 3} - 3 = 3 + \sqrt{0} - 3 = 0$$
$$3 + \sqrt{3 - 2} - 2 = 3 + \sqrt{1} - 2 = 4 - 2 = 2$$

Therefore $x = 2$ is *not* a solution of the original equation; the only solution is $x = 3$.

EXAMPLE   In order to solve the equation $\sqrt{2x - 3} - \sqrt{x + 7} = 2$, we first rearrange terms so that one side of the equation contains only a *single* radical term:

$$\sqrt{2x - 3} = \sqrt{x + 7} + 2$$

Squaring both sides and simplifying yields:

$$(\sqrt{2x - 3})^2 = (\sqrt{x + 7} + 2)^2$$
$$2x - 3 = (\sqrt{x + 7})^2 + 2 \cdot 2\sqrt{x + 7} + 2^2$$
$$2x - 3 = x + 7 + 4\sqrt{x + 7} + 4$$
$$x - 14 = 4\sqrt{x + 7}$$

In order to eliminate the radical, we square both sides again and simplify:

$$(x - 14)^2 = (4\sqrt{x + 7})^2$$
$$x^2 - 28x + 196 = 4^2 \cdot (\sqrt{x + 7})^2$$
$$x^2 - 28x + 196 = 16(x + 7)$$
$$x^2 - 28x + 196 = 16x + 112$$
$$x^2 - 44x + 84 = 0$$

According to the Power Principle, applied *twice*, the solutions of the original equation must also be solutions of this last equation. Its solutions are found as follows:

$$x^2 - 44x + 84 = 0$$
$$(x - 2)(x - 42) = 0$$
$$x - 2 = 0 \quad \text{or} \quad x - 42 = 0$$
$$x = 2 \quad \text{or} \quad x = 42$$

Substituting $x = 2$ and $x = 42$ in the left-hand side of the original equation $\sqrt{2x - 3} - \sqrt{x + 7} = 2$, we find that $x = 42$ *is* a solution, but $x = 2$ is *not*.

EXAMPLE A different technique is needed to solve $\sqrt[3]{x^2} - 2\sqrt[3]{x} - 15 = 0$. The fact that $\sqrt[3]{x^2} = (\sqrt[3]{x})^2$ suggests that we let $u = \sqrt[3]{x}$ so that the equation becomes:

$$\sqrt[3]{x^2} - 2\sqrt[3]{x} - 15 = 0$$
$$(\sqrt[3]{x})^2 - 2\sqrt[3]{x} - 15 = 0$$
$$u^2 - 2u - 15 = 0$$
$$(u - 5)(u + 3) = 0$$

$$u - 5 = 0 \quad \text{or} \quad u + 3 = 0$$
$$u = 5 \quad \text{or} \quad u = -3$$
$$\sqrt[3]{x} = 5 \quad \text{or} \quad \sqrt[3]{x} = -3$$

Since $x = (\sqrt[3]{x})^3$, the only possible solutions are $5^3 = 125$ and $(-3)^3 = -27$. Substituting $x = 125$ and $x = -27$ in the left-hand side of the original equation shows that *both* numbers are solutions. (Verify!)

EXERCISES

A.1. Use the Power Principle to solve these equations. Be sure to *check your answers* in the original equation.

(a) $\sqrt[3]{x^2 - 1} = 2$

(b) $\sqrt{4x + 9} = 5$

(c) $\sqrt[3]{4 - 11x} = 3$

(d) $\sqrt[3]{4x^2 + 1} = 5$

(e) $\sqrt{x + 7} = x - 5$

(f) $\sqrt{x + 5} = x - 1$

B.1. Solve these equations:

(a) $\sqrt[3]{(x - 3)^2} = 2$

(b) $\sqrt{(x^2 + 2x + 1)^3} = 8$

(c) $\sqrt[5]{x^2 - x + 123} = \sqrt[5]{125}$

(d) $\sqrt[4]{x^2 - 4x + 3} = \sqrt[4]{8}$

(e) $\sqrt[3]{x + 5} = \sqrt[3]{(x + 3)^2}$

(f) $\sqrt[7]{2x^2 + 17x + 17} = \sqrt[7]{(2x + 4)^2}$

B.2. Solve these equations:

(a) $\sqrt{5x + 6} = 3 + \sqrt{x + 3}$

(b) $\sqrt{3y + 1} - 1 = \sqrt{y + 4}$

(c) $\sqrt{2x - 5} = 1 + \sqrt{x - 3}$

(d) $\sqrt{x - 3} + \sqrt{x + 5} = 4$

(e) $\sqrt{3x + 5} + \sqrt{2x + 3} + 1 = 0$

(f) $\sqrt{20 - x} = \sqrt{9 - x} + 3$

(g) $\sqrt{6y + 7} - \sqrt{3y + 3} = 1$

(h) $\sqrt{t + 2} + \sqrt{3t + 4} = 2$

B.3. Assume that all letters represent positive numbers and solve each equation for the required letter:

(a) $A = \sqrt{1 + \dfrac{a^2}{b^2}}$ for b

(b) $T = 2\pi\sqrt{\dfrac{m}{g}}$ for g

(c) $K = \sqrt{1 - \dfrac{x^2}{u^2}}$ for u

(d) $R = \sqrt{d^2 + k^2}$ for d

B.4. Solve these equations by making an appropriate substitution:

(a) $2\sqrt[3]{x^2} - \sqrt[3]{x} - 6 = 0$ (d) $\sqrt[3]{x} + \sqrt[6]{x} - 2 = 0$

(b) $\sqrt[3]{x^2} - 2\sqrt[3]{x} - 8 = 0$ (e) $x - 10\sqrt{x} + 9 = 0$

(c) $\sqrt{x} - \sqrt[4]{x} - 2 = 0$ [*Hint:*
note that $(\sqrt[4]{x})^2 = \sqrt{x}$ since   (f) $2x - 9\sqrt{x} + 4 = 0$
$[(\sqrt[4]{x})^2]^2 = x.$]   (g) $(1 + \sqrt{x})^2 + (1 + \sqrt{x}) = 6$

B.5. Solve these equations. [*Hint:* In part (a), use the substitution $u = x^{-1}$, then factor and solve.]

(a) $x^{-2} - x^{-1} - 6 = 0$ (c) $x^{-1} + 2(\sqrt{x})^{-1} - 3 = 0$

(b) $2x^{-2} + x^{-1} - 1 = 0$ (d) $(\sqrt[3]{x})^{-2} - (\sqrt[3]{x})^{-1} - 6 = 0$

C.1. A stone is dropped from the top of a cliff. Five seconds later the sound of the stone hitting the ground is heard. Ignore wind resistance and assume the speed of sound is 1100 feet per second. Find the height of the cliff. [*Hint:* With no wind resistance an object falls $16t^2$ feet in t seconds. What is the *sum* of the number of seconds it takes for the stone to fall and the number of seconds it takes for the sound of its hitting to rise the same distance?]

5. LINEAR INEQUALITIES

This section deals with methods for solving linear inequalities, such as

$$\frac{3x + 5}{3} + 2x < \frac{2x - 1}{3} \qquad -5 < 7 - 2x \leq 9 \qquad |5x + 2| > 3$$

We begin with inequalities that do not involve absolute value. With one exception, noted below, the strategy for solving such inequalities is the same as that used to solve equations. It depends on:

BASIC PRINCIPLES FOR SOLVING INEQUALITIES

Performing any one of the following operations on an inequality produces an inequality with the same solutions as the original inequality:

1. *Add or subtract the same quantity from both sides of the inequality.*

2. *Multiply or divide both sides of the inequality by a* positive *quantity.*

3. *Multiply or divide both sides of the inequality by a* negative *quantity and* **reverse the direction of the inequality.**

You should note Principle 3 carefully: It is the major difference between solving inequalities and solving equations. For example, $-3 < 5$, but multiplying both sides by the negative number -2 produces the inequality $+6 > -10$ (note direction of inequality sign).

Two inequalities that have the same solutions are said to be **equivalent.** The fundamental idea here, as with equations, is to use the Basic Principles to transform a given inequality into an equivalent one, whose solutions we know how to find.

EXAMPLE Here is a step-by-step solution of the inequality $5x + 3 \leq 6 + 7x$. The reason for each step is given at the right.

$$5x + 3 \leq 6 + 7x$$

$\quad -2x + 3 \leq 6$ $\qquad$ (subtract $7x$ from both sides)

$\qquad -2x \leq 3$ $\qquad$ (subtract 3 from both sides)

$\qquad\quad x \geq -\frac{3}{2}$ $\qquad$ (divide both sides by -2 and *reverse the direction of the inequality*)

The solutions of this last inequality are obvious: every real number that is greater than or equal to $-\frac{3}{2}$ is a solution. In other words, the solutions are all numbers in the interval $[-\frac{3}{2}, \infty)$, as shown in Figure 2-1.

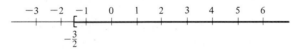

Figure 2-1

EXAMPLE The first step in solving the inequality $\dfrac{3x + 5}{2} + 2x < \dfrac{2x - 1}{3}$ is to eliminate the fractions. Since 6 is a common denominator of the two fractions, we multiply both sides of the inequality by 6 and obtain:

$$6\left(\frac{3x - 5}{2}\right) + 6 \cdot 2x < 6\left(\frac{2x + 1}{3}\right)$$

$$3(3x - 5) + 12x < 2(2x + 1)$$

Now multiply the various terms and proceed as before to collect all x terms on one side and constants on the other:

$$3(3x - 5) + 12x < 2(2x + 1)$$

$\quad 9x - 15 + 12x < 4x + 2$ $\qquad$ (multiply out both sides)

$\qquad\quad 17x - 15 < 2$ $\qquad$ (subtract $4x$ from both sides)

$\qquad\qquad 17x < 17$ $\qquad$ (add 15 to both sides)

$\qquad\qquad\quad x < 1$ $\qquad$ (divide both sides by 17)

The solutions of this last inequality, and hence the solutions of the original one, are all numbers in the interval $(-\infty, 1)$, as shown in Figure 2-2 on the next page.

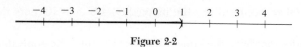

Figure 2-2

EXAMPLE A solution of the two-part inequality $-5 < 7 - 2x \le 9$ is any number that is a solution of *both* of these inequalities:

$$-5 < 7 - 2x \quad\text{and}\quad 7 - 2x \le 9$$

Each of these last inequalities can be solved by the methods just shown. For the first one, we have:

$-5 < 7 - 2x$

$-12 < -2x$ (subtract 7 from both sides)

$6 > x$, or equivalently, $x < 6$ (divide both sides by -2 and reverse the direction of the inequality)

The second inequality is solved similarly:

$7 - 2x \le 9$

$-2x \le 2$ (subtract 7 from both sides)

$x \ge -1$, or equivalently, $-1 \le x$.   (divide both sides by -2 and reverse the direction of the inequality)

The solutions of the original inequality are the numbers x that satisfy *both* $-1 \le x$ *and* $x < 6$. Therefore the solutions are precisely the numbers in the interval $[-1, 6)$, as shown in Figure 2-3.

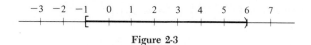

Figure 2-3

Alternate Shorthand Method You probably noticed that in the last example we followed exactly the same steps for both inequalities. Consequently, it is usually easier and faster to handle double inequalities such as this one by solving both halves at the same time:

$-5 < 7 - 2x \le 9$

$-12 < -2x \le 2$ (subtract 7 from each part)

$6 > x \ge -1$ (divide each part by -2 and reverse the (direction of the inequalities)

Reading this last inequality from right to left, we see once again that the solutions are precisely the numbers in the interval $[-1, 6)$.

LINEAR ABSOLUTE VALUE INEQUALITIES

The solution of inequalities such as

$$|3x - 7| \leq 5, \qquad |5x + 2| > 3, \qquad |4x - 1.5| < 10, \qquad |8 - \tfrac{3}{4}x| \geq \tfrac{5}{3}$$

depends on the following basic facts about absolute value (which are also true with $<$ and $>$ in place of $\leq$ and $\geq$).

Let k *be a fixed positive number. Then for any real number* r:

$$|r| \leq k \text{ exactly when } -k \leq r \leq k.$$

$$|r| \geq k \text{ exactly when } r \leq -k \text{ or } r \geq k.$$

This statement says, for example, that $|r| \leq 5$ exactly when r is a number satisfying $-5 \leq r \leq 5$, and that $|r| \geq 5$ exactly when r is a number satisfying either $r \leq -5$ or $r \geq 5$. This is easily seen to be true on the number line. Since $|r|$ is the distance from r to 0, the condition $|r| \leq 5$ means that r lies *at most* 5 units from 0, as shown in Figure 2-4.

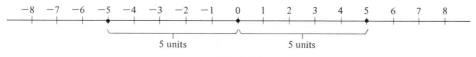

Figure 2-4

But this means that r lies between -5 and 5, that is, $-5 \leq r \leq 5$. Similarly, the condition $|r| \geq 5$ means that r lies 5 *or more* units from 0. And this occurs only when r lies on or to the left of -5 (that is, $r \leq -5$) or when r lies on or to the right of 5 (that is, $r \geq 5$). This same argument works in the general case (with k in place of 5).

EXAMPLE In order to solve $|3x - 7| \leq 5$, apply the fact in the box above with $3x - 7$ in place of r and 5 in place of k. It states that

$$|3x - 7| \leq 5 \qquad \text{exactly when} \qquad -5 \leq 3x - 7 \leq 5$$

Consequently, we need only solve the inequality on the right. This can be done by the methods discussed earlier:

$$-5 \leq 3x - 7 \leq 5$$
$$2 \leq 3x \leq 12 \qquad \text{(add 7 to each part)}$$
$$\tfrac{2}{3} \leq x \leq 4 \qquad \text{(divide each part by 3)}$$

The solutions of this last inequality, and hence of the original one, are all of the numbers in the interval $[\tfrac{2}{3}, 4]$, as shown in Figure 2-5 on the next page.

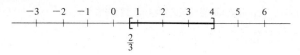

Figure 2-5

EXAMPLE   In order to solve $|5x + 2| > 3$, we apply the fact in the box above with $5x + 2$ in place of r and 3 in place of k, and $>$ in place of $\geq$:

$$|5x + 2| > 3 \quad \text{exactly when} \quad 5x + 2 < -3 \quad \text{or} \quad 5x + 2 > 3$$

Now we need only solve the two inequalities at the right:

$$
\begin{array}{ll}
5x + 2 < -3 & 5x + 2 > 3 \\
5x < -5 & 5x > 1 \\
x < -1 & x > \tfrac{1}{5}
\end{array}
$$

The solutions of the original inequality are the numbers that satisfy *either* of these last two inequalities. Thus the solutions are all numbers that are in either of the intervals $(-\infty, -1)$, or $(\tfrac{1}{5}, \infty)$, as shown in Figure 2-6.

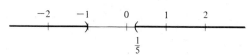

Figure 2-6

EXERCISES

A.1.   Solve these inequalities.

(a) $6x + 3 \leq x - 5$

(b) $3 + 5x \leq 2x + 7$

(c) $5 - 7x < 2x - 4$

(d) $3x + 5 > 7x - 3$

(e) $2x + 7(3x - 2) < 2(x - 1)$

(f) $x + 3(x - 5) \geq 2x + 2(x + 1) - x$

B.1.   Solve these inequalities.

(a) $\dfrac{x + 1}{2} - 3x \leq \dfrac{x + 5}{3}$

(b) $\dfrac{x - 1}{4} + 2x \geq \dfrac{2x + 1}{3} + 2$

(c) $\dfrac{2x - 5}{3} + 1 < 2 - \dfrac{x + 7}{6}$

(d) $\dfrac{3(x - 1)}{2} + 4x > \dfrac{2(x + 1)}{3} + 4$

B.2.   Solve these inequalities.

(a) $\dfrac{1}{2}x + \dfrac{3}{4} < 3 - \dfrac{1}{4}x$

(b) $\dfrac{3}{2} - \dfrac{5x}{2} \geq 2x - \dfrac{1}{4}$

(c) $2.3 - 1.1x \leq 2.9x - 1.7$

(d) $4.2x + 5.3 > 2.7x + 2.3$

B.3. Solve these inequalities.

(a) $(x - 1)(x + 2) \le (x + 5)(x - 2)$

(b) $(x - 3)^2 + 4 > (x - 1)(x + 1) + 3$

(c) $\dfrac{(x - 2)(x + 5)}{2} < (x + 1)^2 + 4 - \dfrac{x^2}{2}$

(d) $\dfrac{(x - 1)(x + 3)}{3} \ge \dfrac{(x + 1)(x - 2)}{2} + 1 - \dfrac{x^2}{6}$

B.4. Solve these inequalities.

(a) $2 < 3x - 4 < 8$

(b) $1 < 5x + 6 < 9$

(c) $-3 \le 4x + 5 \le 2$

(d) $-5 \le -3x + 1 < 10$

(e) $2x + 3 \le 5x + 6 < -3x + 7$

(f) $4x - 2 < x + 8 < 9x + 1$

B.5. Solve these inequalities.

(a) $-4 \le \dfrac{4 - 2x}{3} \le 4$

(b) $-1 \le \dfrac{2 - 3x}{2} < 1$

(c) $\dfrac{2x + 1}{3} < \dfrac{5x - 2}{2} \le \dfrac{x - 1}{6}$

(d) $1 + 2x \ge \dfrac{x - 5}{2} \ge \dfrac{3x - 1}{2} + 3$

B.6. Solve these inequalities.

(a) $|3x + 2| \le 2$

(b) $|5x - 1| < 3$

(c) $|3 - 2x| < \frac{2}{3}$

(d) $|4 - 5x| \le 4$

(e) $|2x + 3| - 2 < 0$

(f) $3 + |1 - 2x| < 7$

B.7. Solve these inequalities.

(a) $|2x + 3| > 1$

(b) $|3x - 1| \ge 2$

(c) $|5x + 2| \ge \frac{3}{4}$

(d) $|2 - 3x| > 4$

(e) $|4 - 7x| > 1$

(f) $|2x - 3| \ge \frac{1}{2}$

B.8. Solve these inequalities.

(a) $\left| \dfrac{12}{5} + 2x \right| > \dfrac{1}{4}$

(b) $\left| \dfrac{5}{6} + 3x \right| < \dfrac{7}{6}$

(c) $\left| \dfrac{3 - 4x}{2} \right| > 5$

(d) $\left| \dfrac{2 - 5x}{3} \right| \ge 2$

(e) $\left| \dfrac{2 - 3x}{4} \right| \le \dfrac{3}{2}$

(f) $\left| \dfrac{5 - 2x}{3} \right| < \dfrac{3}{4}$

B.9. Use a calculator to solve these inequalities.

(a) $7.35x - 6.42 > 5.37 - 12.24x$

(b) $8.21 - 6.75x \le 3.59x + 2.74$

(c) $8.53 (2.11x + 5.32) < 2.65 (3.21 - 6.42x)$

(d) $(2.57 - 3.26x) 6.25 \ge 1.73 (2.71x + 4.32)$

B.10. Solve these inequalities and explain your answers.

(a) $|2x + 1| \ge -1$

(b) $|3x + 2| < 0$

(c) $|5x - 1| < 0$

(d) $|7x + 3| \ge 0$

(e) $|x - 3| \le -2$

C.1. Let a and b be fixed real numbers with $a < b$. Show that the solutions of

$$\left| x - \frac{a + b}{2} \right| < \frac{b - a}{2}$$

are all x with $a < x < b$.

C.2.   Let E be a fixed real number. Show that every solution of $|x - 3| < E/5$ is also a solution of $|(5x - 4) - 11| < E$.

6. POLYNOMIAL AND RATIONAL INEQUALITIES

In this section we discuss the solutions of inequalities involving polynomial and rational expressions, such as

$$2x^3 - 15x < x^2 \qquad \frac{x + 3}{x - 1} \geq -2 \qquad \left| \frac{3x + 2}{x - 2} \right| \leq 5 \qquad |x^2 - x - 4| > 2$$

The strategy for solving inequalities that do not involve absolute values is exactly the same as that used to solve linear inequalities, such as $7 - 2x \leq 3$. So you should begin by reviewing the Basic Principles for Solving Inequalities listed on page 100. You should also review interval notation in Section 3 of Chapter 1 since it will be used frequently here.

EXAMPLE   To solve $x^2 - x - 6 \geq 0$, we first factor the left-hand side and obtain this equivalent inequality:

$$(x + 2)(x - 3) \geq 0$$

A number x is a solution of this inequality precisely when the product $(x + 2)(x - 3)$ is nonnegative. To determine when this is the case, we only need to know when each factor is zero, positive, or negative. Now

$$x + 2 = 0 \qquad \text{exactly when} \qquad x = -2 \qquad \text{and}$$
$$x - 3 = 0 \qquad \text{exactly when} \qquad x = 3$$

The numbers -2 and 3 divide the number line into three intervals, as shown here:

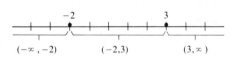

Now $(x + 2) < 0$ exactly when $x < -2$, that is, when x is in any interval to the *left* of -2. Also $(x + 2) > 0$ exactly when $x > -2$, that is, when x is in any interval to the *right* of -2. Similarly, $(x - 3)$ is negative when x is to the *left* of 3 and positive when x is to the *right* of 3, as summarized in Figure 2-7.

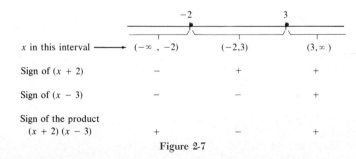

x in this interval ⟶	$(-\infty, -2)$	$(-2, 3)$	$(3, \infty)$
Sign of $(x + 2)$	$-$	$+$	$+$
Sign of $(x - 3)$	$-$	$-$	$+$
Sign of the product $(x + 2)(x - 3)$	$+$	$-$	$+$

Figure 2-7

From the last line of the chart in Figure 2-7, we see that

$(x + 2)(x - 3) > 0$ for every number x in the intervals $(-\infty, -2)$ and $(3, \infty)$

Combining this information with the fact that $(x + 2)(x - 3) = 0$ for $x = -2$ and $x = 3$ we see that

$(x + 2)(x - 3) \geq 0$ for every number x in the intervals $(-\infty, -2]$ and $[3, \infty)$.

In other words, the solutions of $(x + 2)(x - 3) \geq 0$ are all numbers x such that

$$x \leq -2 \quad \text{or} \quad x \geq 3$$

EXAMPLE   The first step in solving the inequality $2x^3 - 15x < x^2$ is to collect all the terms on the same side of the inequality sign and to simplify and factor the resulting expression:

$$2x^3 - 15x < x^2$$
$$2x^3 - x^2 - 15x < 0 \quad \text{(subtract } x^2 \text{ from both sides)}$$
$$(2x^2 - x - 15)x < 0 \quad \text{(factor } x \text{ out of left-hand side)}$$
$$(2x + 5)(x - 3)x < 0 \quad \text{(factor left-hand side further)}$$
$$2(x + \tfrac{5}{2})(x - 3)x < 0 \quad \text{(factor 2 out of } 2x + 5)$$
$$(x + \tfrac{5}{2})(x - 3)x < 0 \quad \text{(divide both sides by 2)}$$

From the steps used to obtain this last inequality, we know that it is equivalent to the original one. A solution of this last inequality is any number x that makes the product $(x + \tfrac{5}{2})(x - 3)x$ negative. As in the preceding example, the critical numbers for determining the sign of this product are the numbers for which

$$x + \tfrac{5}{2} = 0 \quad \text{or} \quad x - 3 = 0 \quad \text{or} \quad x = 0$$

namely, $-\tfrac{5}{2}$, 3, and 0. These numbers divide the number line into four intervals, as shown in Figure 2-8. The factor $(x + \tfrac{5}{2})$ is positive when $x > -\tfrac{5}{2}$ (that is, when x lies to the right of $-\tfrac{5}{2}$) and negative when $x < -\tfrac{5}{2}$ (that is, when x lies to the left of $-\tfrac{5}{2}$). The signs of the other factors on each interval can be determined similarly, as summarized in Figure 2-8.

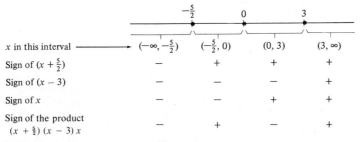

x in this interval	$(-\infty, -\tfrac{5}{2})$	$(-\tfrac{5}{2}, 0)$	$(0, 3)$	$(3, \infty)$
Sign of $(x + \tfrac{5}{2})$	$-$	$+$	$+$	$+$
Sign of $(x - 3)$	$-$	$-$	$-$	$+$
Sign of x	$-$	$-$	$+$	$+$
Sign of the product $(x + \tfrac{5}{2})(x - 3)x$	$-$	$+$	$-$	$+$

Figure 2-8

The last line of the chart in Figure 2-8 gives us all the information we need:

$(x + \tfrac{5}{2})(x - 3)x < 0$ for every number x in the intervals $(-\infty, -\tfrac{5}{2})$ and $(0, 3)$

In other words, the solutions of the inequality $(x + \frac{5}{2})(x - 3)x < 0$, and hence of the original inequality $2x^3 - 15x < x^2$, are all numbers x such that

$$x < -\tfrac{5}{2} \quad \text{or} \quad 0 < x < 3$$

EXAMPLE   In order to solve $\dfrac{x + 3}{x - 1} \geq -2$, we begin by collecting all terms on one side, writing this side as a rational expression, factoring, and simplifying:

$$\frac{x + 3}{x - 1} \geq -2$$

$$\frac{x + 3}{x - 1} + 2 \geq 0 \quad \text{(add 2 to both sides)}$$

$$\frac{x + 3}{x - 1} + \frac{2(x - 1)}{x - 1} \geq 0 \quad \text{(put left-hand side over common denominator)}$$

$$\frac{x + 3 + 2x - 2}{x - 1} \geq 0 \quad \text{(multiply out left-hand side)}$$

$$\frac{3x + 1}{x - 1} \geq 0 \quad \text{(simplify)}$$

$$\frac{3(x + \frac{1}{3})}{x - 1} \geq 0 \quad \text{(factor 3 out of } 3x + 1\text{)}$$

$$\frac{x + \frac{1}{3}}{x - 1} \geq 0 \quad \text{(divide both sides by 3)}$$

The original inequality is equivalent to this last inequality. A solution of this last one is any number x that makes the quotient a nonnegative real number. To determine the sign of the quotient, we need only check the signs of the factors $(x + \frac{1}{3})$ and $(x - 1)$. Just as before, the critical numbers for doing this are the numbers for which

$$x + \tfrac{1}{3} = 0 \quad \text{or} \quad x - 1 = 0$$

namely, $-\frac{1}{3}$ and 1. They divide the number line into three intervals, as shown in Figure 2-9. We can check the signs of $(x + \frac{1}{3})$ and $(x - 1)$ on each of these intervals, as before (see Figure 2-9).

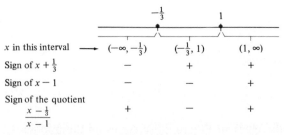

Figure 2-9

The last line of the chart in Figure 2-9 shows that

$$\frac{x + \frac{1}{3}}{x - 1} > 0 \quad \text{for every number } x \text{ such that } x < -\frac{1}{3} \text{ or } x > 1$$

The quotient $\dfrac{x + \frac{1}{3}}{x - 1}$ is 0 only when the numerator is 0 and the denominator is nonzero.°

This occurs when $x = -\frac{1}{3}$. Consequently, the solutions of $\dfrac{x + \frac{1}{3}}{x - 1} \geq 0$, and hence of the original inequality, are all numbers x such that:

$$x \leq -\frac{1}{3} \quad \text{or} \quad x > 1$$

that is, all numbers in the intervals $(-\infty, -\frac{1}{3}]$ and $(1, \infty)$.

EXAMPLE† To solve the quadratic inequality $x^2 - 6x + 1 < 0$, we must first factor the left-hand side. To do this, we first find the solutions of the equation $x^2 - 6x + 1 = 0$ via the quadratic formula:

$$x = \frac{-(-6) \pm \sqrt{(-6)^2 - 4 \cdot 1 \cdot 1}}{2 \cdot 1} = \frac{6 \pm \sqrt{32}}{2} = \frac{6 \pm \sqrt{16 \cdot 2}}{2} = \frac{6 \pm 4\sqrt{2}}{2}$$
$$= 3 \pm 2\sqrt{2}$$

Since $(3 + 2\sqrt{2})$ is a solution, the Factor Theorem assures us that $(x - (3 + 2\sqrt{2}))$ is a *factor* of $x^2 - 6x + 1$. Similarly, the solution $(3 - 2\sqrt{2})$ leads to the factor $(x - (3 - 2\sqrt{2}))$. By multiplying out the right-hand side of the following equation, you can verify that $x^2 - 6x + 1$ factors as:

$$x^2 - 6x + 1 = [x - (3 + 2\sqrt{2})][x - (3 - 2\sqrt{2})].$$

So the original inequality is equivalent to

$$[x - (3 + 2\sqrt{2})][x - (3 - 2\sqrt{2})] < 0$$

This inequality can be solved as in the earlier examples by checking the signs of the factors on the three intervals determined by the numbers $3 + 2\sqrt{2}$ and $3 - 2\sqrt{2}$ (see Figure 2-10).

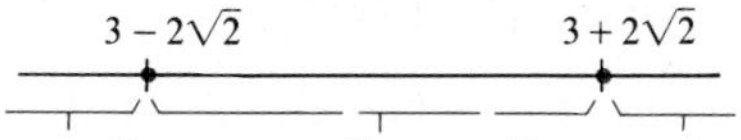

	$3 - 2\sqrt{2}$		$3 + 2\sqrt{2}$
x in this interval ⟶	$(-\infty, 3 - 2\sqrt{2})$	$(3 - 2\sqrt{2}, 3 + 2\sqrt{2})$	$(3 + 2\sqrt{2}, \infty)$
Sign of $(x - (3 + 2\sqrt{2}))$	$-$	$-$	$+$
Sign of $(x - (3 - 2\sqrt{2}))$	$-$	$+$	$+$
Sign of the product $(x - (3 + 2\sqrt{2}))(x - (3 - 2\sqrt{2}))$	$+$	$-$	$+$

Figure 2-10

° Note that when the denominator is 0 (that is, when $x = 1$), the quotient is *not defined*.

† This example is optional. You may wish to omit it if you haven't studied the Factor Theorem in Section 3.

The last line of the chart in Figure 2-10 shows that the solutions of the inequality are all numbers x such that $(3 - 2\sqrt{2}) < x < (3 + 2\sqrt{2})$.

ABSOLUTE VALUE INEQUALITIES

A great many inequalities involving absolute values, such as

$$\left|\frac{x + 3}{x - 1}\right| < 2 \qquad \left|\frac{3x + 2}{x - 2}\right| \leq 2 \qquad |2x^2 + 3x - 1| > 3 \qquad |x^2 - 5| < 4$$

can be solved by using the methods presented earlier in this section, together with certain fundamental facts about absolute value. These are the same facts that were used in section 5 to solve linear inequalities, such as $|2x - 3| < 7$. For convenience, we repeat those facts here (they are also true with $<$ and $>$ in place of $\leq$ and $\geq$):

Let k *be a fixed positive number. Then for any real number* r:

$|r| \leq k$ *exactly when* $-k \leq r \leq k$ *and*

$|r| \geq k$ *exactly when* $r \geq k$ *or* $r \leq -k$

EXAMPLE In order to solve $\left|\dfrac{x + 3}{x - 1}\right| < 2$, we observe that for any real number x (except $x = 1$), $\dfrac{x + 3}{x - 1}$ is also a real number. Using $\dfrac{x + 3}{x - 1}$ in place of r and 2 in place of k in the preceding box, we see that

$$\left|\frac{x + 3}{x - 1}\right| < 2 \qquad \text{exactly when} \qquad -2 < \frac{x + 3}{x - 1} < 2$$

As usual, $-2 < \dfrac{x + 3}{x - 1} < 2$ is shorthand for the statement

$$\frac{x + 3}{x - 1} > -2 \qquad \text{and} \qquad \frac{x + 3}{x - 1} < 2$$

Consequently, we need only find all the numbers that are solutions of *both* these inequalities. The first one was solved on page 108, where we found that its solutions are all numbers in the intervals $(-\infty, -\frac{1}{3})$ and $(1, \infty)$. The second inequality can also be solved by reducing it to an equivalent one and checking signs:

$$\frac{x + 3}{x - 1} < 2$$

$$\frac{x + 3}{x - 1} - 2 < 0 \qquad \text{(subtract 2 from both sides)}$$

$$\frac{x + 3 - 2(x - 1)}{x - 1} < 0 \qquad \text{(put left-hand side over common denominator)}$$

$$\frac{-x + 5}{x - 1} < 0 \qquad \text{(simplify)}$$

$$\frac{(-1)(x - 5)}{x - 1} < 0 \qquad \text{(factor } -1 \text{ out of } -x + 5)$$

$$\frac{x - 5}{x - 1} > 0 \qquad \text{(divide both sides by } -1 \text{ and reverse direction of inequality)}$$

To determine the values of x for which the quotient $\dfrac{x - 5}{x - 1}$ is positive, we check the signs of the factors $x - 5$ and $x - 1$ in the usual way (see Figure 2-11).

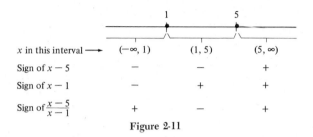

x in this interval $\longrightarrow$	$(-\infty, 1)$	$(1, 5)$	$(5, \infty)$
Sign of $x - 5$	$-$	$-$	$+$
Sign of $x - 1$	$-$	$+$	$+$
Sign of $\frac{x - 5}{x - 1}$	$+$	$-$	$+$

Figure 2-11

Therefore the solutions of $\dfrac{x - 5}{x - 1} > 0$, and hence of the original inequality $\dfrac{x + 3}{x - 1} < 2$, are all numbers in the intervals $(-\infty, 1)$ and $(5, \infty)$.

It will be helpful to sketch graphically the solutions of these two inequalities as shown in Figure 2-12.

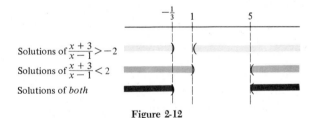

Solutions of $\dfrac{x + 3}{x - 1} > -2$

Solutions of $\dfrac{x + 3}{x - 1} < 2$

Solutions of *both*

Figure 2-12

The solutions of the original inequality are the numbers that are solutions of both the inequalities above. As Figure 2-12 shows, x is a solution of *both* inequalities precisely when

$$x < -\tfrac{1}{3} \qquad \text{or} \qquad x > 5$$

Therefore the solutions of the original inequality $\left|\dfrac{x + 3}{x - 1}\right| < 2$ are all numbers in the intervals $(-\infty, -\tfrac{1}{3})$ and $(5, \infty)$.

EXAMPLE To solve $|x^2 - x - 4| > 2$, we put $x^2 - x - 4$ in place of r and 2 in place of k in the box on page 110 and see that

$$|x^2 - x - 4| > 2 \quad \text{exactly when} \quad x^2 - x - 4 < -2 \quad \text{or} \quad x^2 - x - 4 > 2$$
$$|x^2 - x - 4| > 2 \quad \text{exactly when} \quad x^2 - x - 2 < 0 \quad \text{or} \quad x^2 - x - 6 > 0$$

Thus the solutions of $|x^2 - x - 4| > 2$ are all numbers that are solutions of *either one* of the last two inequalities on the right above. In the example on page 106 we saw that the solutions of $x^2 - x - 6 > 0$ are all numbers in the intervals $(-\infty, -2)$ and $(3, \infty)$. The solutions of the other inequality may be obtained by factoring and proceeding as before:

$$x^2 - x - 2 < 0$$
$$(x + 1)(x - 2) < 0$$

You should verify that the solutions of this last inequality are all numbers in the interval $(-1, 2)$. Sketching all these solutions on the same number line, we have Figure 2-13.

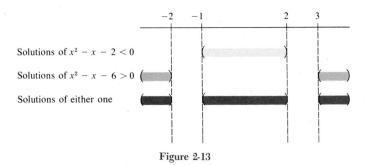

Figure 2-13

Therefore the solutions $|x^2 - x - 4| > 2$ are all numbers in the intervals $(-\infty, -2)$, $(-1, 2)$ and $(3, \infty)$.

EXERCISES

A.1. Solve these polynomial inequalities:
  (a) $x^2 + x - 2 > 0$
  (b) $2x^2 - 5x - 3 < 0$
  (c) $x^3 - x \geq 0$
  (d) $x^2 \leq 9$
  (e) $x^2 > 7$
  (f) $x^3 + 2x^2 > -x$
  (g) $x^2(x - 4) \leq 5x$
  (h) $4x^2 + 10x > -4x^2 - 10x + 12$

B.1. Solve these inequalities:

  (a) $\dfrac{x - 2}{x - 1} < 1$

  (b) $\dfrac{1}{x} < 3$

  (c) $\dfrac{-1}{x + 1} > 2$

  (d) $\dfrac{-x + 5}{2x + 3} \geq 2$

  (e) $\dfrac{x - 3}{x + 3} \leq 5$

  (f) $\dfrac{2x + 1}{x - 4} > 3$

B.2. Solve these inequalities:

(a) $(x - 1)(x - 2)(x + 3) \geq 0$

(d) $\dfrac{x^2 - 9}{x^2 + 3x - 10} > 0$

(b) $(x^2 - 1)(x^2 - 4) < 0$

(e) $\dfrac{x^2 + 6x + 9}{(x - 1)(x - 2)(x + 5)} \leq 0$

(c) $\dfrac{(x + 3)(x + 2)}{x(x - 1)} \geq 0$

(f) $(x - 2)^2(x^2 - 1)(x - 3) > 0$

B.3. Solve these inequalities. [*Hint:* Begin by collecting all nonzero terms on one side; find a common denominator and express this side as a single fraction. Then proceed as in Exercise B.2.]

(a) $\dfrac{2}{x + 3} \geq \dfrac{1}{x - 1}$

(c) $\dfrac{1}{x - 1} < \dfrac{1}{x}$

(b) $\dfrac{1}{x + 1} > \dfrac{2}{x}$

(d) $\dfrac{1}{x - 1} < \dfrac{-1}{x + 2}$

B.4. Solve these inequalities:

(a) $\dfrac{9}{x + 3} > \dfrac{4}{x + 2} + 1$

(c) $\dfrac{1}{2x - 2} + \dfrac{9}{2x - 6} \geq \dfrac{4}{x - 2}$

(b) $1 + \dfrac{1}{x - 2} \geq \dfrac{1}{x + 2}$

B.5. Solve these inequalities. [*Hint:* See the optional example on page 109.]
(a) $x^2 - 2x - 1 \leq 0$
(b) $x^2 + 2x > 2$

(c) $2x^2 \geq 2x + 1$
(d) $x^2 < 3x + 1$

B.6. Solve these inequalities:

(a) $\left| \dfrac{x - 1}{x + 2} \right| \leq 3$

(d) $\left| \dfrac{x + 1}{x + 2} \right| \geq 2$

(b) $\left| \dfrac{x + 1}{3x + 5} \right| < 2$

(e) $\left| \dfrac{1 - 4x}{2 + 3x} \right| < 1$

(c) $\left| \dfrac{2x - 1}{x + 5} \right| > 1$

(f) $\left| \dfrac{3x + 1}{1 - 2x} \right| \geq 2$

B.7. Solve these quadratic inequalities:
(a) $|x^2 - 2| < 1$
(b) $|x^2 - 4| \leq 3$
(c) $|x^2 - 4| < 5$

(d) $|x^2 - 5| > 4$
(e) $|x^2 - 2| > 4$
(f) $\left| \dfrac{1}{x^2 - 1} \right| \leq 2$

B.8. Solve these inequalities.
(a) $|x^2 + x - 1| \geq 1$
(b) $|x^2 + x - 4| \leq 2$
(c) $|3x^2 - 8x + 2| < 2$

(d) $|x^2 + 3x - 4| < 6$
(e) $|x^2 - 5x - 5| > 9$
(f) $|x^2 - 4x - 4| \geq 8$

B.9. Solve these inequalities. [*Hint:* The basic procedure is the same as in the last two examples in the text. But to complete the solutions you may have to use the technique described in the optional example on page 109.]

(a) $|3x^2 + 13x - 3| \geq 7$ (c) $|2x^2 + 5x - 1| < 2$

(b) $|x^2 + 4x - 2| \leq 3$ (d) $|3x^2 - 7x - 14| > 6$

B.10. (a) Solve the inequalities $x^2 < x$ and $x^2 > x$.

(b) Use the results of part (a) to show that for any nonzero real number c with $|c| < 1$, it is always true that $c^2 < |c|$.

(c) Use the results of part (a) to show that for any nonzero real number c with $|c| > 1$, it is always true that $c^2 > c$.

B.11. It costs a certain company $(25x + 20{,}000)$ dollars to manufacture x widgets. The income from the sale of x widgets is $(475x - x^2)$ dollars. What is the smallest number and the largest number of widgets on which the company can make a profit? [*Hint:* Profit = income − cost. The profit should be a positive number.]

B.12. The length of a rectangle is 5 inches more than its width. What possible widths can the rectangle have if its area is at least 66 square inches?

B.13. One gallon of paint will cover 400 square feet. What are the possible dimensions of a triangular area such that:

The base of the triangle is 20 feet longer than the height; *and* it takes at least one and one-half gallons, but not more than two gallons, of paint to cover the area?

Basic Analytic Geometry

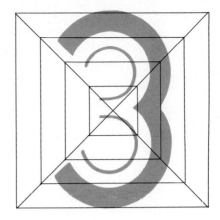

One of the great discoveries of seventeenth century mathematics was that the techniques of algebra could be applied to geometry. The resulting subject was called **analytic geometry.** The insights it provided into the interplay between algebra and geometry not only led to advances in both those areas, but also opened the way for the invention of calculus. This chapter does not attempt to cover all of analytic geometry. But it does provide the basic knowledge needed in calculus and other parts of college mathematics.

1. GRAPHS AND THE COORDINATE PLANE

In Chapter 1, we associated numbers with the points on the line. Now we are going to associate pairs of real numbers with the points in the plane. This will allow us to interpret many algebraic ideas geometrically, so that our geometric intuition can aid us. At the same time we can use algebraic methods to help solve geometric problems.

Let's use this page to represent a plane. Draw a horizontal and a vertical line. The point where they intersect is called the **origin.** Taking the origin as zero, make the horizontal line into a number line with positive numbers to the right and negative numbers to the left. Make the vertical line into a number line with positive numbers going up and negative numbers going down (Figure 3-1 on the next page).

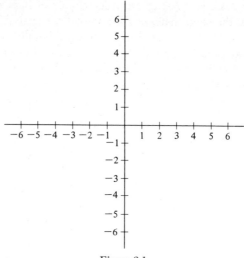

Figure 3-1

We call the horizontal line the **horizontal axis** and the vertical line the **vertical axis.** Together these two axes are called the **coordinate axes.** A plane equipped with coordinate axes is called a **coordinate plane.**

We often label the axes by letters of the alphabet. It is traditional to label the horizontal axis by x and the vertical axis by y. Then the horizontal axis is called the **x-axis,** the vertical axis the **y-axis,** and the coordinate plane the **xy-plane.** However, there is nothing sacred about the letters x and y. Whenever convenient we shall use other letters.

THE COORDINATES OF A POINT

Let P be any point in the plane. Draw two straight lines through P, one vertical, the other horizontal. These lines intersect the horizontal axis and the vertical axis at some numbers c and d, as illustrated in Figure 3-2 for two typical situations.

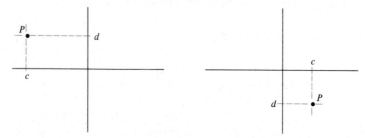

Figure 3-2

The point P is now associated with an ordered pair of numbers (c, d).° We say (ungrammatically) that the **coordinates** of P are the ordered pair (c, d), or more briefly, that P has coordinates (c, d). This means that c is the number directly above or below P on the horizontal axis, and d is the number directly to the left or right of P on the vertical axis. The number c is called the **first coordinate** of P and d is called the **second coordinate** of P. If the horizontal and vertical axes are labeled by letters—say, x and y—and the point P has coordinates (c, d), then we say that P has **x-coordinate** c and **y-coordinate** d.

EXAMPLE Convince yourself that the points in Figure 3-3 are labeled with the correct coordinates.

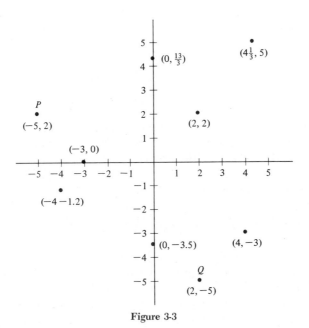

Figure 3-3

It is important to realize what the word "ordered" means in the term "ordered pair." In Figure 3-3, the point P with coordinates $(-5, 2)$ is quite different from the point Q with coordinates $(2, -5)$. The same numbers -5 and 2 occur both times, but in *different order*. The first coordinate of P is -5, but the first coordinate of Q is 2. Likewise, the second coordinates of P and of Q differ.

We have begun with a point P and labeled it by an ordered pair of numbers, the coordinates of P. Conversely, given an ordered pair of numbers (r, s), it is easy to find the point with coordinates (r, s). Because of this correspondence between points and

---

° The notation (c, d) is also used for an open interval on the number line (see p. 24). This won't cause any difficulty since the context will always make it clear whether (c, d) denotes an interval or the coordinates of a point.

ordered pairs, we often "identify" a point with its coordinates. For example, we usually say "the point $(3.9, -5)$" instead of "the point with coordinates $(3.9, -5)$."

QUADRANTS

The coordinate axes divide the plane into four regions which are numbered counter-clockwise starting from the upper right, as shown in Figure 3-4.

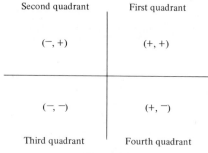

Figure 3-4

We can easily tell which quadrant a point is in by noticing which of its coordinates are positive and which are negative. Points in the first quadrant have both coordinates positive, points in the second quadrant have negative first coordinates and positive second coordinates, and so on, as shown in Figure 3-4. Note that points on the axes do not lie in any of the quadrants.

STANDARD NOTATION FOR COORDINATES

Let P and Q be two points in the plane. We could use letters such as (c, d) for the coordinates of P and (r, s) for those of Q as we did above. But whenever two points, P and Q, are to be discussed simultaneously, it is more convenient to denote the coordinates of P by (x_1, y_1) and those of Q by (x_2, y_2). The symbol "x_1" (read "x-one") is a single symbol denoting the first coordinate of the first point, just as the letter c did above. Similarly, y_1 is a single symbol, as are x_2 and y_2.

The chief advantage of using (x_1, y_1) and (x_2, y_2) is that it makes it easy to keep everything straight; for instance,

All first coordinates are x's: x_1, x_2.
All second coordinates are y's: y_1, y_2.
The coordinates of the first point have subscript 1: (x_1, y_1).
The coordinates of the second point have subscript 2: (x_2, y_2).

GRAPHS

In its most general usage the word "graph" means any set of points in the plane. The graphs that are of the most interest and usefulness are those that provide a geometric visualization of various algebraic or verbal statements. One way such graphs arise is in connection with equations and inequalities.

Throughout the rest of this chapter, the words "equation" and "inequality" always mean an equation or inequality in *two* variables. Consequently, we shall interpret equations such as $x = 7$ or $6y + 3 = 0$ as equations in two variables, one of which has coefficient zero: $x + 0y = 7$ or $0x + 6y + 3 = 0$; and similarly for inequalities.

A **solution of an equation or inequality** in two variables x and y, such as

$$7y = 4x - 2 \quad \text{or} \quad (x - 2)^2 + (y + 1)^2 = 16 \quad \text{or} \quad \frac{x^2}{9} + \frac{y^2}{4} \le 1$$

is a pair of numbers such that the substitution of the first number for x and the second for y in the equation yields a true statement. In this case, we say that the given pair of numbers **satisfies the equation.**

EXAMPLE   The pair $(2, \frac{6}{7})$ is a solution of $7y = 4x - 2$ since substituting $x = 2$ and $y = \frac{6}{7}$ yields the true statement $7\left(\dfrac{6}{7}\right) = 4 \cdot 2 - 2$. But $(3, 4)$ is *not* a solution since the substitutions $x = 3$ and $y = 4$ produce a *false* statement $7 \cdot 4 = 4 \cdot 3 - 2$.

The **graph of an equation or inequality** in two variables is the set of points in the plane whose coordinates are solutions of the given equation or inequality. Thus the graph is a *geometric picture of the solutions.*

EXAMPLE   The point $(4, 2)$ is on the graph of the equation $7y = 4x - 2$ since $7(2) = 4(4) - 2$. The point $(-3, -2)$ is also on the graph since $7(-2) = 4(-3) - 2$. Later in this section we shall see that the entire graph consists of the points on the straight line joining $(4, 2)$ and $(-3, -2)$, as shown in Figure 3-5. In Section 4 we shall see that the graph of the inequality $(x - 2)^2 + (y + 1)^2 \le 16$ consists of the points on the circular disc shown in Figure 3-5.

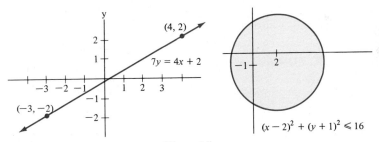

Figure 3-5

INTERCEPTS

The points (if any) where a graph crosses the x- or y-axis often play an important role. If the graph crosses the x-axis at the point $(a, 0)$, then the number a is called an **x-intercept** of the graph. Similarly if the graph crosses the y-axis at the point $(0, b)$, then the number b is called a **y-intercept** of the graph. For example, see Figure 3-6 on the next page.

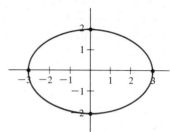

x-intercept −2
y-intercept 1

x-intercepts 3 and −3
y-intercepts 2 and −2

Figure 3-6

The intercepts of the graph of an equation can be determined *algebraically*, without drawing the graph. For instance, the y-intercepts are the numbers b such that $(0, b)$ satisfies the given equation. They may be found by setting $x = 0$ in the equation and solving for y. The x-intercepts may be determined in a similar fashion by setting $y = 0$ and solving for x.

EXAMPLE To find the y-intercepts of the equation $3x - 5y - 12 = 0$, we set $x = 0$ and solve for y:

$$3 \cdot 0 - 5y - 12 = 0$$
$$-5y = 12$$
$$y = -\tfrac{12}{5}$$

Therefore the only y-intercept is $-\tfrac{12}{5}$ and the graph crosses the y-axis at $(0, -\tfrac{12}{5})$. To find the x-intercepts, we set $y = 0$ and solve for x:

$$3x - 5 \cdot 0 = 12$$
$$x = 4$$

Consequently, the only x-intercept is 4 and the graph crosses the x-axis at $(4, 0)$.

THE DISTANCE FORMULA

A natural question to ask about two points in the plane is, "How far apart are they?" Here is a simple formula for answering this question:

THE DISTANCE FORMULA

The distance between the point (x_1, y_1) *and the point* (x_2, y_2) *is the number*

$$\sqrt{(x_1 - x_2)^2 + (y_1 - y_2)^2}$$

Before we prove that the distance formula is correct, let's see how it works in some examples.

EXAMPLE Find the distance from $(-8, -5)$ to $(1, -2)$. Let $(-8, -5)$ play the role of (x_1, y_1) and $(1, -2)$ that of (x_2, y_2) in the distance formula. Then the distance between them is

$$\sqrt{(x_1 - x_2)^2 + (y_1 - y_2)^2} = \sqrt{(-8 - 1)^2 + (-5 - (-2))^2}$$
$$= \sqrt{(-9)^2 + (-5 + 2)^2} = \sqrt{81 + (-3)^2}$$
$$= \sqrt{81 + 9} = \sqrt{90} = \sqrt{9}\sqrt{10} = 3\sqrt{10}$$

The order in which the two points are listed doesn't make any difference. If we use $(1, -2)$ for (x_1, y_1) and $(-8, -5)$ for (x_2, y_2), we obtain the same answer:

$$\sqrt{(x_1 - x_2)^2 + (y_1 - y_2)^2} = \sqrt{(1 - (-8))^2 + (-2 - (-5))^2}$$
$$= \sqrt{9^2 + 3^2} = \sqrt{81 + 9} = \sqrt{90} = 3\sqrt{10}$$

EXAMPLE Let a and b be fixed real numbers. What is the distance from the point (a, b) to the point $(2a, -b)$? Don't let the letters confuse you. We can apply the distance formula just as before. In this case (a, b) is the first point [corresponding to (x_1, y_1) in the distance formula] and $(2a, -b)$ is the second point [corresponding to (x_2, y_2) in the formula]. Consequently, in the distance formula we substitute a for x_1, b for y_1, $2a$ for x_2, and $-b$ for y_2:

$$\sqrt{(x_1 - x_2)^2 + (y_1 - y_2)^2} = \sqrt{(a - 2a)^2 + (b - (-b))^2}$$
$$= \sqrt{(-a)^2 + (b + b)^2} = \sqrt{a^2 + (2b)^2} = \sqrt{a^2 + 4b^2}$$

Since $a^2 + 4b^2 \geq 0$, no matter what a and b are, the distance $\sqrt{a^2 + 4b^2}$ is a well-defined real number.

DERIVATION OF THE DISTANCE FORMULA

Let P with coordinates (x_1, y_1) and Q with coordinates (x_2, y_2) be two points in the plane that do not lie on the same vertical or on the same horizontal line. We want to find the distance from P to Q. We shall illustrate the argument with pictures of one possible case, but the validity of the argument does *not* depend on the pictures.

First, draw a *vertical* line through P and a *horizontal* line through Q. Denote the point where these two lines intersect by R, as shown in Figure 3-7.

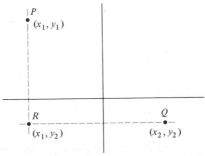

Figure 3-7

Since R is on the same vertical line as P, it has the same first coordinate as P, namely, x_1. Since R is on the same horizontal line as Q, it has the same second coordinate as Q, namely, y_2.

We now find the length of the line segments from P to R and Q to R. The line segment RQ is parallel to the horizontal axis, as shown in Figure 3-8.

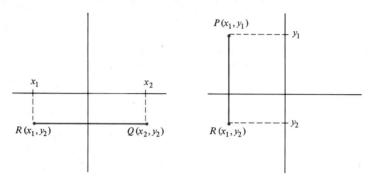

Figure 3-8

Consequently, the length of RQ is the same as the distance from x_1 to x_2 on the axis, namely, $|x_1 - x_2|$. Similarly, the segment PR is parallel to the vertical axis (see Figure 3-8). Thus its length is the distance from y_1 to y_2 on the axis, namely, $|y_1 - y_2|$.

We now know the lengths of two sides of the right triangle PRQ (Figure 3-9).

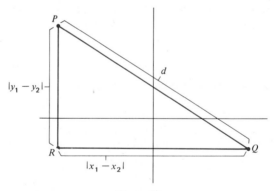

Figure 3-9

The length d of the third side of the triangle is precisely the distance from P to Q. According to the Pythagorean Theorem,[°]

$$d^2 = |x_1 - x_2|^2 + |y_1 - y_2|^2$$

Since $|c|^2 = c^2$ for any real number c (see page 27), this equation becomes

$$d^2 = (x_1 - x_2)^2 + (y_1 - y_2)^2$$

Thus d is a number whose square is the number $(x_1 - x_2)^2 + (y_1 - y_2)^2$. Since d is a length, we know that $d \geq 0$. Therefore we must have

$$d = \sqrt{(x_1 - x_2)^2 + (y_1 - y_2)^2}$$

[°] If you don't remember this, see the Geometry Review on page 444.

Thus we have proved the distance formula for any two points that don't lie on the same vertical or horizontal line.

Suppose now that (x_1, y_1) and (x_2, y_2) *do* lie on the same vertical line. Then they must have the same first coordinate; that is, $x_1 = x_2$, as shown in Figure 3-10.

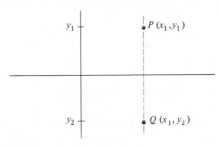

Figure 3-10

The distance from P to Q is the same as the distance from y_1 to y_2 on the number line, namely, $|y_1 - y_2|$. Since $|y_1 - y_2| \geq 0$ and since $|c|^2 = c^2$ for any number c, we have:

$$|y_1 - y_2| = \sqrt{|y_1 - y_2|^2} = \sqrt{(y_1 - y_2)^2} = \sqrt{0 + (y_1 - y_2)^2}$$

Since $x_1 = x_2$ here, $x_1 - x_2 = 0$, so that

$$|y_1 - y_2| = \sqrt{0 + (y_1 - y_2)^2} = \sqrt{(x_1 - x_2)^2 + (y_1 - y_2)^2}$$

Therefore the distance formula is correct in this case too. A similar argument takes care of the case when (x_1, y_1) and (x_2, y_2) lie on the same horizontal line; that is, when $y_1 = y_2$.

EXERCISES

A.1. Find the coordinates of each of the points in Figure 3-11.

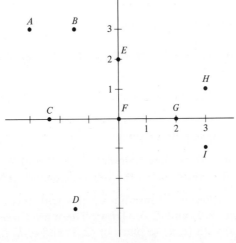

Figure 3-11

A.2. We often call the process of drawing coordinate axes and locating a point on the plane **plotting a point.** Plot the points $(0, 0)$, $(-3, 2.1)$, $(2.1, -3)$, $(-\frac{4}{3}, 1)$, $(5, \pi)$, $(2, \sqrt{2})$, $(-3, \pi)$, $(4, 6)$, $(-\sqrt{3}, \sqrt{3})$, $(\sqrt{3}, -\sqrt{3})$, $(\frac{5}{2}, \frac{17}{3})$.

✗ **A.3.** Various geometric arguments, using similar triangles, show that the **midpoint** of the line segment joining points (x_1, y_1) and (x_2, y_2) is the point with the coordinates

$$\left(\frac{x_1 + x_2}{2}, \frac{y_1 + y_2}{2}\right)$$

do not plot.

An easy way to remember this is that the first coordinate of the midpoint is the average of the two first coordinates x_1 and x_2; and similarly for the second coordinate. Plot each of the following pairs of points on a coordinate plane. Find the midpoint of the line segment joining them and plot it.

(a) $(1, 2)$, $(-4, 6)$ (c) $(-2, 3)$, $(7, 9)$ (e) $(\frac{5}{2}, 1)$, $(4, -\frac{4}{3})$
(b) $(0, 1)$, $(5, -2)$ (d) $(0, 0)$, $(-6, -3)$ (f) $(-3, \sqrt{2})$, $(-8, -2)$

✶ **A.4.** Is the given point on the graph of the given equation? Why or why not?
(a) $(1, -2)$; $3x - y - 5 = 0$
(b) $(2, -1)$; $x^2 + y^2 - 6x + 8y = -15$
(c) $(6, 2)$; $3y + x = 12$
(d) $(1, -2)$; $3y + x = 12$
(e) $(3, 4)$; $(x - 2)^2 + (y + 5)^2 = 4$

(f) $(1, -1)$; $\dfrac{x^2}{2} + \dfrac{y^2}{3} = 1$

✶ **A.5.** Find the x-intercepts and the y-intercepts of the graph of the given equation:
(a) $y = 7x - 5$ (d) $3x^2 = 12 - 2y^2$
(b) $2x - 3y = 6$ (e) $(x - 7)^2 + y^2 = 64$
(c) $9x^2 + y^2 = 9$ (f) $(x - 5)^2 + (y + 6)^2 = 50$

✶ **A.6.** Find the distance between each pair of points:
(a) $(-3, 5)$, $(2, -7)$ (c) $(\frac{1}{2}, 3)$, $(\frac{9}{2}, 6)$ (e) (a, b), (b, a)
(b) $(1, -5)$, $(2, -1)$ (d) $(\sqrt{2}, 1)$, $(\sqrt{3}, 2)$ (f) (s, t), $(0, 0)$

B.1. (a) Plot the following points on one coordinate plane: $(-4, 5)$, $(-4, 1)$, $(-4, -7.7)$, $(-4, 0)$, $(-4, -\frac{9}{2})$, $(-4, \frac{8}{13})$.
(b) Describe the geometric figure formed by the set of all points whose first coordinate is -4.

B.2. Fill in the blanks: If the first and second coordinates of a point P are equal, then either P is $(0, 0)$ or P is in the

_____ quadrant, or the _____ quadrant.

✶ **B.3.** One diagonal of a square has endpoints $(-3, 1)$ and $(2, -4)$. What are the coordinates of the endpoints of the other diagonal? [*Hint:* Draw a sketch].

✶ **B.4.** (a) Find the vertices of all possible squares with this property: Two of the vertices are $(2, 1)$ and $(2, 5)$. [*Hint:* There are three such squares.]
(b) Do part (a) with (c, d) in place of $(2, 1)$ and (c, k) in place of $(2, 5)$.

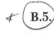 **B.5.** What are the coordinates of the point that lies on the line from $(-8, -3)$ to $(6, 9)$, one-fourth of the way from $(-8, -3)$? [*Hint:* Exercise A.3 may be helpful.]

B.6. Use algebraic or geometric reasoning to sketch the graph of the given equation or inequality. For example, the graph of the equation $y = 5$ consists of all points (x, y) with $y = 5$. But the points with second coordinate 5 form a horizontal straight line 5 units above the x-axis (Why?). Now the graph is easily sketched.

(a) $x = 3$ (d) $xy = 0$ (When is a product zero?)
(b) $y = -7$ (e) $xy > 0$ (When is a product positive?)
(c) $x = y$ (f) $xy < 0$

B.7. Sketch the graph of the given statement [that is, plot all points (x, y) for which the given statement is true]. For example, the statement $|x| \leq 1$ is true for every point (x, y) whose first coordinate satisfies $|x| \leq 1$; that is, whose first coordinate satisfies $-1 \leq x \leq 1$. Thus the graph is the shaded area in Figure 3-12.

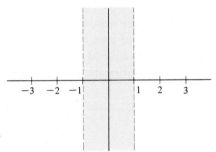

Figure 3-12

(a) $|x| \leq 1$ and $|y| \leq 1$ (d) $|x| \geq 1$
(b) x and y are positive   (e) $|x| \geq 1$ and $|y| \leq 1$
(c) $1 \leq x \leq 3$ and $|y| \leq 2$ (f) $|x| \geq 2$ and $|y| \geq 1$

 B.8. Show that each triple of points given below forms a right triangle. In each case give the length of the hypotenuse and sketch the triangle. [*Hint:* You may assume that a triangle with sides of length a, b, and c is a right triangle with hypotenuse c, *provided* $c^2 = a^2 + b^2$]

(a) $(0, 0), (1, 1), (2, -2)$ (c) $(3, -2), (0, 4), (-2, 3)$

(b) $\left(\dfrac{\sqrt{2}}{2}, 0\right), \left(\dfrac{\sqrt{2}}{2}, \dfrac{\sqrt{2}}{2}\right), (0, 0)$

 B.9. What is the perimeter of the triangle with vertices $(1, 1), (5, 4),$ and $(-2, 5)$?

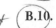 **B.10.** (a) Find all points P on the x-axis that are 5 units from the point $(3, 4)$. [*Hint:* P must have coordinates $(x, 0)$ for some number x and the distance from P to $(3, 4)$ is 5.]

(b) Find all points on the y-axis that are 8 units from $(-2, 4)$. [*Hint:* Reduce the equation you set up to the form $(y - 4)^2 = $ constant; then solve as in the second example on page 81.]

    (c) Find all points with first coordinate 3 that are 6 units from $(-2, -5)$.

    (d) Find all points with second coordinate -1 that are 4 units from $(2, 3)$.

B.11. Let S be the triangle with vertices $(\frac{1}{2}, 4)$, $(-3, \frac{1}{2})$, and $(1, -\frac{1}{2})$ and T the triangle with vertices $(4, 5)$, $(3, 1)$, and $(7, 2)$. Are S and T congruent? [*Remember:* Two triangles are congruent if the corresponding sides have the same length.]

C.1. Suppose every point on the coordinate plane gets moved 5 units straight up.

    (a) To what points do each of these points go: $(0, -5)$, $(2, 2)$, $(5, 0)$, $(5, 5)$, $(4, 1)$?

    (b) Which points go to each of the points in part (a)?

    (c) To what point does (a, b) go?

    (d) To what point does $(a, b - 5)$ go?

    (e) What point goes to $(-4a, b)$?

    (f) What points go to themselves?

2. SLOPES OF LINES

Throughout this section and the next, the word "line" is understood to mean "straight line." The question of how steeply a line rises is easy to understand *geometrically*. In Figure 3-13 line L does not rise at all. Line M rises, but not very steeply, and line N rises quite steeply. (It may help to think of lines as roads on which you are walking.)

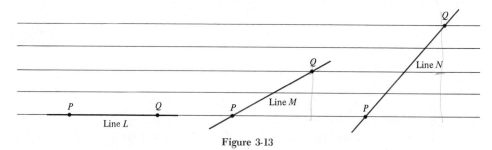

Figure 3-13

We would like to find a *numerical* way to describe the steepness of these lines. Since line L doesn't rise at all, it is reasonable to use the number 0 to describe its steepness. Line M rises 2 units as you go from P to Q. But the steeper line N rises 4 units as you go from P to Q. So steepness seems to be related to the *vertical rise* of the line.

    On the other hand, consider the three lines in Figure 3-14.

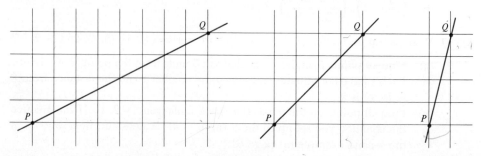

Figure 3-14

All of them have a vertical rise of 4 units as you go from P to Q. But the lines obviously don't have the same steepness. The difference is this: on the left-hand line, as you go from P to Q, you run 8 units horizontally while you rise 4 units vertically. But on the middle line you run only 4 units horizontally while rising 4 units vertically. And on the right-hand line you run just 1 unit horizontally while rising 4 units vertically.

The preceding examples suggest that the steepness of a straight line between points P and Q on the line is determined by *comparing* two factors:

The **vertical rise** from P to Q.
The **horizontal run** from P to Q.

The three lines above show how these two factors should be compared. In the left-hand line (the least steep) the rise (4 units) is only *half* the run (8 units). In the steeper middle line, the rise (4 units) is the *same* as the run (4 units). In the right-hand line (the steepest one) the rise (4 units) is *four times* larger than the run (1 unit). We can express these facts in terms of fractions by looking at the fraction $\dfrac{\text{rise}}{\text{run}}$, as illustrated in Figure 3-15.

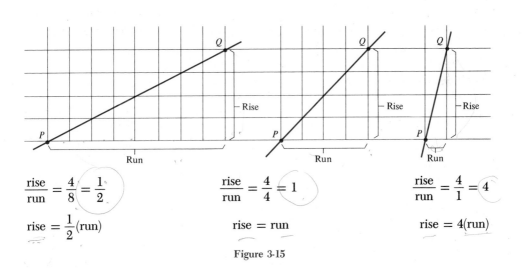

$$\frac{\text{rise}}{\text{run}} = \frac{4}{8} = \frac{1}{2}$$

$$\text{rise} = \frac{1}{2}(\text{run})$$

$$\frac{\text{rise}}{\text{run}} = \frac{4}{4} = 1$$

$$\text{rise} = \text{run}$$

$$\frac{\text{rise}}{\text{run}} = \frac{4}{1} = 4$$

$$\text{rise} = 4(\text{run})$$

Figure 3-15

The numbers $\frac{1}{2}$, 1, and 4 are increasing just as the steepness of the corresponding lines increases. Thus the fraction $\dfrac{\text{rise}}{\text{run}}$ seems to provide a numerical means of describing the steepness of a line. But there are still some unanswered questions:

Question (i)   Is there some easy way to compute $\dfrac{\text{rise}}{\text{run}}$ without using a ruler or graph paper?

Question (ii)   If we choose two points on the line other than P and Q to compute $\dfrac{\text{rise}}{\text{run}}$, will we get the same answer?

Answer to Question (i)   Suppose P and Q are points on the line L. If P has coordinates (x_1, y_1) and Q has coordinates (x_2, y_2), then Figure 3-16

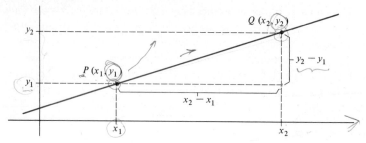

Figure 3-16

shows clearly that the vertical rise as you move from P to Q is the number $y_2 - y_1$ and the horizontal run is the number $x_2 - x_1$. Therefore

$$\frac{\text{rise}}{\text{run}} = \frac{y_2 - y_1}{x_2 - x_1}$$

Answer to Question (ii)   Now suppose R with coordinates (x_3, y_3) and S with coordinates (x_4, y_4) are also points on L. Then there are two possible ways to compute $\dfrac{\text{rise}}{\text{run}}$, using P and Q or R and S, as shown in Figure 3-17.

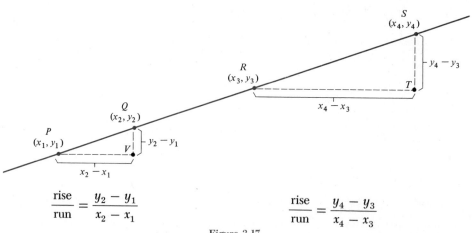

$$\frac{\text{rise}}{\text{run}} = \frac{y_2 - y_1}{x_2 - x_1} \qquad\qquad \frac{\text{rise}}{\text{run}} = \frac{y_4 - y_3}{x_4 - x_3}$$

Figure 3-17

We *claim* that the end result in each case is the same, namely,

> *For any distinct points* (x_1, y_1), (x_2, y_2), (x_3, y_3), (x_4, y_4) *on* L,
>
> $$\frac{y_2 - y_1}{x_2 - x_1} = \frac{y_4 - y_3}{x_4 - x_3}$$

In other words, the answer to Question (ii) is yes: we can use *any two points* on L to compute $\dfrac{\text{rise}}{\text{run}}$ and we'll get the *same answer* every time.

Here is a short proof of the claim made in the box above. Consider the triangles PQV and RST (as in Figure 3-17). Since angle V and angle T are both right angles, they are equal. Basic facts about parallel lines show that

$$\text{angle } P = \text{angle } R \qquad \text{angle } Q = \text{angle } S$$

Therefore triangles PQV and RST are similar.° Consequently, the ratios of the corresponding sides of the triangles are equal. In particular,

$$\frac{\text{length } QV}{\text{length } PV} = \frac{\text{length } ST}{\text{length } RT}$$

But we can express these lengths in terms of the coordinates of the points, as shown in Figure 3-17:

$$\frac{y_2 - y_1}{x_2 - x_1} = \frac{\text{length } QV}{\text{length } PV} = \frac{\text{length } ST}{\text{length } RT} = \frac{y_4 - y_3}{x_4 - x_3}$$

This proves the claim made in the preceding box.

We can now make an important definition:

Let L *be a nonvertical straight line. The* **slope of** L *is the number*

$$\frac{y_2 - y_1}{x_2 - x_1}$$

where (x_1, y_1) *and* (x_2, y_2) *are any two distinct points on* L. *In short,*

$$slope = \frac{rise}{run}.$$

As the preceding discussion suggests,

The slope of a line is a number which measures the steepness of the line.

The slope is independent of the points on the line used to compute it [see the answer to Question (ii) above]. Finally, since

$$\frac{y_1 - y_2}{x_1 - x_2} = \frac{(-1)(y_2 - y_1)}{(-1)(x_2 - x_1)} = \frac{y_2 - y_1}{x_2 - x_1}$$

it doesn't matter in what order we use the points: we can take (x_2, y_2) as the first point and (x_1, y_1) as the second, or the other way around.

° The basic facts about similar triangles are discussed in the Geometry Review on page 447.

EXAMPLE The lines L_1, L_2, L_3, L_4, and L_5 shown in Figure 3-18 are determined by these points:

L_1: $(-2, -1)$ and $(-1, 6)$ L_2: $(-2, -1)$ and $(1, 8)$ L_3: $(-2, -1)$ and $(2, 3)$
L_4: $(-2, -1)$ and $(1, 0)$ L_5: $(-2, -1)$ and $(5, -1)$

We can compute the slopes of these lines as shown in Figure 3-18.

slope $L_1 = \dfrac{6-(-1)}{-1-(-2)} = \dfrac{7}{1} = 7$

slope $L_2 = \dfrac{8-(-1)}{1-(-2)} = \dfrac{9}{3} = 3$

slope $L_3 = \dfrac{3-(-1)}{2-(-2)} = \dfrac{4}{4} = 1$

slope $L_4 = \dfrac{0-(-1)}{1-(-2)} = \dfrac{1}{3}$

slope $L_5 = \dfrac{-1-(-1)}{5-(-2)} = \dfrac{0}{7} = 0$

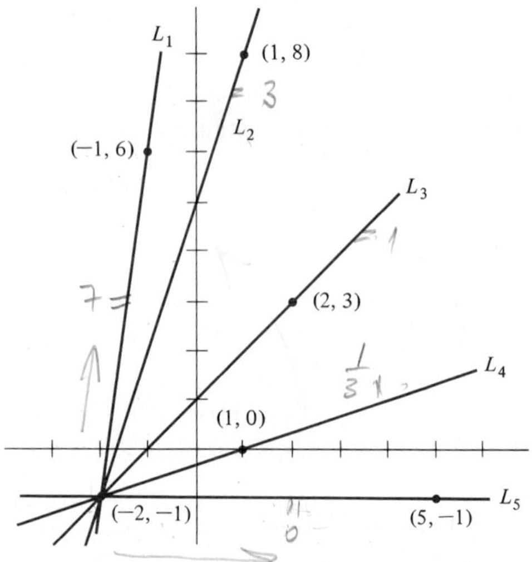

Figure 3-18

Observe how the slopes correspond to the steepness of the lines: horizontal lines have slope 0 and *the larger the slope, the more steeply the line rises* from left to right.

As you may have noticed, we have not yet considered any lines which *fall* from left to right, such as those shown in Figure 3-19.

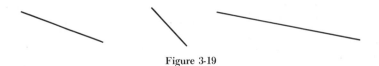

Figure 3-19

But the slope, as defined above, can be computed for *any* line. So let's see what the slopes of falling lines look like.

EXAMPLE The lines L_6, L_7, L_8, and L_9 shown on the next page are determined by these points:

L_6: $(-3, 2)$ and $(4, 1)$ L_7: $(-3, 2)$ and $(2, -4)$
L_8: $(-3, 2)$ and $(0, -6)$ L_9: $(-3, 2)$ and $(-2, -3)$

We can compute the slopes of these lines as shown in Figure 3-20.

$$\text{slope } L_6 = \frac{1-2}{4-(-3)} = \frac{-1}{7}$$

$$\text{slope } L_7 = \frac{-4-2}{2-(-3)} = \frac{-6}{5} = -1\frac{1}{5}$$

$$\text{slope } L_8 = \frac{-6-2}{0-(-3)} = \frac{-8}{3} = -2\frac{2}{3}$$

$$\text{slope } L_9 = \frac{-3-2}{-2-(-3)} = \frac{-5}{1} = -5$$

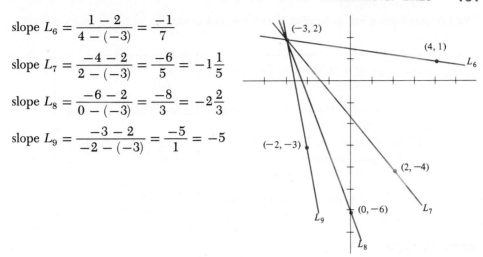

Figure 3-20

Each of these lines moves *downward* from left to right and each slope is a *negative* number. In this case too, the slopes correspond to the steepness with which the lines fall: *the larger the slope in absolute value,* * *the more steeply the line falls* from left to right.

Thus our definition of slope is a good numerical measurement of how steeply *any* nonvertical line rises or falls. Note that the slope formula doesn't work for vertical lines. The reason is that any two points on the same vertical line have the same first coordinate, say $x = c$ (see Figure 3-21).

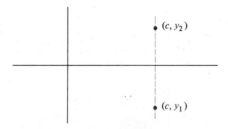

Figure 3-21

If we try to apply the slope formula, we get $\dfrac{y_2 - y_1}{c - c} = \dfrac{y_2 - y_1}{0}$. But this is *not* a real number. Therefore,

Slope is not defined for vertical lines.

---

* Remember that as negative numbers get farther and farther from 0 (such as $-\frac{1}{7}$, $-\frac{6}{5}$, $-\frac{8}{3}$, -5, -10, -50, -1000), their absolute values get *larger*. Thus a negative number of large absolute value is a number, such as -1000, which is far from 0. Such numbers are sometimes inaccurately but succinctly called "large negative numbers." Lines whose slopes are "large negative numbers" fall very steeply from left to right.

We can summarize the preceding discussion as follows:

> *The slope of a nonvertical line is a number* m
> *which measures how steeply the line rises or falls:*
>
> *If* m *is positive, the line rises to the right; the larger* |m| *is, the more*
>   *steeply the line rises.*
> *If* m *is negative, the line falls to the right; the larger* |m| *is, the more*
>   *steeply the line falls.*
> *If* m = 0, *the line is horizontal.*
>
> *Slope is not defined for vertical lines.*

APPLICATIONS

Here are some examples that show how the slope of a line can be used to find out other information about the line.

EXAMPLE   If L is a line with slope $\frac{1}{3}$ and $(2, -4)$ is a point on L, find three more points on L.

SOLUTION   To say that the slope of L is $\frac{\text{rise}}{\text{run}} = \frac{1}{3}$ means that if you start at a point on L, run 3 units to the *right*, then *rise* 1 unit, you will end up at another point on L. For instance, see Figure 3-22.

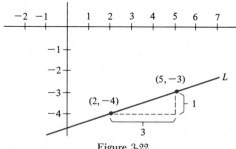

Figure 3-22

Therefore, $(5, -3)$ is a point on L. But $\frac{\text{rise}}{\text{run}} = \frac{1}{3} = \frac{2}{6}$, so we can also say that if you start at a point on L, run 6 units to the *right*, then *rise* 2 units, you will end up at a point on L. If you do this, beginning at $(5, -3)$, you end up at the point $(11, -1)$ on L, as in Figure 3-23. Finally, it is also true that $\frac{\text{rise}}{\text{run}} = \frac{1}{3} = \frac{-1}{-3}$. This means that if you start at a point on L, say, $(11, -1)$, and run 3 units to the *left* (negative horizontal direction), then *fall* 1 unit (negative vertical direction), you will end up at a point on L; namely, $(8, -2)$, as shown in Figure 3-23.

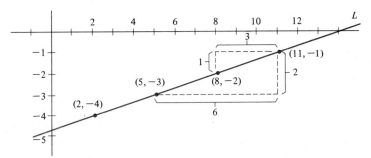

Figure 3-23

The reason the techniques in the preceding example work is that the slope is a *ratio*. Each of the fractions $\frac{1}{3}, \frac{2}{6}, \frac{-1}{-3}$, and so on, expresses the same basic fact: the rise is one-third of the run.

EXAMPLE If L is the line with slope -3, passing through the point $(1, 2)$, find the point P where L intersects the vertical line through $(5, 0)$. Since L has negative slope, it falls to the right and we can sketch a *rough* picture of the situation (Figure 3-24).

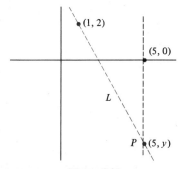

Figure 3-24

Since P lies on the same vertical line as $(5, 0)$, P has coordinates $(5, y)$ for some number y. We must find the number y. To do this we shall find an equation involving only y and various constants, as follows. Use the points $(1, 2)$ and $(5, y)$ to compute the slope of L:

$$\text{slope of } L = \frac{y - 2}{5 - 1} = \frac{y - 2}{4}$$

But L has slope -3. Therefore we have an equation that can be solved for y:

$$\frac{y - 2}{4} = \text{slope} = -3$$

$$4\left(\frac{y-2}{4}\right) = 4(-3)$$

$$y - 2 = -12$$

$$y = -10$$

Thus the point P is the point $(5, -10)$.

PARALLEL LINES

The slope of a line measures how steeply it rises or falls. Since parallel lines rise or fall *equally steeply,* it seems plausible that:

> *Two nonvertical straight lines are parallel exactly when they have the same slope.*

Here is a partial proof of this statement. Suppose L and M are parallel lines, with M lying b vertical units above L, as shown in Figure 3-25. Let (x_1, y_1) and (x_2, y_2) be two points on L.

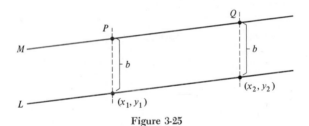

Figure 3-25

Then the slope of L is $(y_2 - y_1)/(x_2 - x_1)$. Consider the point P on M which lies directly above (x_1, y_1). Since it lies on the same vertical line as (x_1, y_1), the first coordinate of P must be x_1. Since the vertical distance from L to M is b, the second coordinate of P must be $y_1 + b$. Thus P is the point $(x_1, y_1 + b)$. A similar argument shows that the point Q which lies on M directly above (x_2, y_2) has coordinates $(x_2, y_2 + b)$. We can now use P and Q to compute the slope of M:

$$\text{slope } M = \frac{(y_2 + b) - (y_1 + b)}{x_2 - x_1} = \frac{y_2 + b - y_1 - b}{x_2 - x_1} = \frac{y_2 - y_1}{x_2 - x_1} = \text{slope } L$$

Therefore parallel lines have the same slope. The rest of the proof (namely, that two lines with the same slope are parallel) is considered in Exercise C.3 in Section 3.

EXAMPLE Let L be the line through $(0, 2)$ and $(1, 5)$. Let M be the line through $(2, 1)$ and $(3, 4)$. Then

$$\text{slope } L = \frac{5-2}{1-0} = \frac{3}{1} = 3 \quad \text{and} \quad \text{slope } M = \frac{4-1}{3-2} = \frac{3}{1} = 3$$

Therefore L and M are parallel. You can check this visually by drawing the lines on the coordinate plane.

PERPENDICULAR LINES

Two lines that meet at a right angle (90-deg angle) are said to be perpendicular. As you might suspect, there is a close relationship between the slopes of two perpendicular lines.

> *Let* L *be a line with slope* k *and* M *a line with slope* m. *Then* L *and* M *are perpendicular exactly when* km = −1.

We shall illustrate this fact with an example. If you're interested in a proof of it, see Exercise C.4 in Section 3.

EXAMPLE   Let L be the line through $(0, 2)$ and $(1, 5)$. Let M be the line through $(-6, -1)$ and $(3, -4)$. Then

$$\text{slope } L = \frac{5-2}{1-0} = 3 \quad \text{and} \quad \text{slope } M = \frac{-4-(-1)}{3-(-6)} = \frac{-3}{9} = -\frac{1}{3}$$

Since $3(-\frac{1}{3}) = -1$, the lines L and M are perpendicular. You can check this visually by drawing the lines on the coordinate plane.

EXERCISES

A.1. Find the slope of the line through the two given points.
  (a) $(1, 2), (3, 7)$ **(d)** $(-7, -7), (-5, -5)$ **(g)** $(3, \sqrt{2}), (-4, -\sqrt{5})$
  (b) $(-1, -2), (2, -1)$ **(e)** $(3, -2), (-4, 6)$ **(h)** $(\sqrt{2}, -1), (2, -9)$
  (c) $(\frac{1}{4}, 0), (\frac{3}{4}, 2)$ **(f)** $(\frac{1}{3}, 0), (0, \frac{1}{3})$ **(i)** $(\pi, 1), (-1, \pi)$

A.2. On one graph, sketch five lines satisfying these conditions: (i) one line has slope 0, two lines have positive slope, and two lines have negative slope; (ii) all five lines meet at a single point.

A.3. **(a)** On one graph sketch five lines, not all meeting at a single point, whose slopes are five different positive numbers. Do this in such a way that the left-hand line has the largest slope, the second line from the left the next largest slope, and so on.
  (b) Do part (a) with nine lines, four of which have positive slope, one of which has slope 0, and four of which have negative slope.

A.4. In each case determine whether the line through P and Q is parallel or perpendicular to the line through R and S, or neither. Then draw the two lines.

    (a) $P = (1, 0)$ $Q = (2, -3)$ $R = (-1, -6)$ $S = (2, -15)$
    (b) $P = (1, -4)$ $Q = (2, -3)$ $R = (-1, 3)$ $S = (2, 0)$
    (c) $P = (2, 5)$ $Q = (-1, -1)$ $R = (4, 2)$ $S = (6, 1)$
    (d) $P = (0, \frac{3}{2})$ $Q = (1, 1)$ $R = (2, 7)$ $S = (3, 9)$
    (e) $P = (-3, \frac{1}{3})$ $Q = (1, -1)$ $R = (2, 0)$ $S = (4, -\frac{2}{3})$
    (f) $P = (3, 3)$ $Q = (-3, -1)$ $R = (2, -2)$ $S = (4, -5)$

B.1. Find five points on the given line, in addition to the given points.
    (a)   line with slope $\frac{3}{2}$ through $(3, 4)$
    (b)   line with slope 5 through $(1, -2)$ (Remember $5 = \frac{5}{1}$)
    (c)   line with slope $-\frac{7}{4}$ through $(0, -2)$

B.2. Graph the following lines:
    (a)   through $(1, 2)$ with slope 1 (d)   through $(-2, 3)$ with no slope
    (b)   through $(-3, 4)$ with slope -1 (e)   through $(0, 0)$ with slope 3
    (c)   through $(6, 1)$ with slope 0 (f)   through $(0, 1)$ with slope 3

B.3. The door of a campus building is 5 ft above ground level. To allow wheelchair access the steps in front of the door are to be replaced by a straight ramp with constant slope $\frac{1}{12}$, as shown in Figure 3-26. How long must the ramp be?

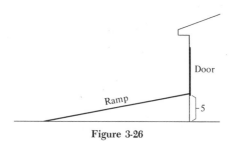

Door

Ramp

5

Figure 3-26

B.4. Use slopes to show that the points $(-4, 6)$, $(-1, 12)$, and $(-7, 0)$ all lie on the same straight line.

B.5. (a)   Use slopes to show that the points $(-5, -2)$, $(-3, 1)$, $(3, 0)$, and $(5, 3)$ are the vertices of a parallelogram.
    (b)   Are the points $(-10, 9)$, $(-\frac{16}{3}, \frac{13}{3})$, $(-3, -2)$, and $(4, -9)$ the vertices of a parallelogram?

B.6. Use slopes to determine if the three given points are the vertices of a right triangle.
    (a) $(9, 6)$, $(-1, 2)$, $(1, -3)$ (b) $(1, 6)$, $(-5, -8)$, $(5, -4)$

B.7. Let L be the line through $(-4, 5)$ which is perpendicular to the line through $(1, 3)$ and $(-4, 2)$. Find three points on L.

B.8. Find a number t such that the line passing through the two given points has slope -2.

(a) $(0, t), (9, 4)$ (c) $(-2, t), (-1, -7)$ (e) $\left(\dfrac{t}{3}, -2\right), \left(4, \dfrac{t}{4}\right)$

(b) $(1, t), (-3, 5)$ (d) $(t, t), (5, 9)$ (f) $(t + 1, 5), (6, -3t + 7)$

C.1. (a) Let L be a nonvertical straight line through the origin. L intersects the vertical line through $(1, 0)$ at a point P. Show that the second coordinate of P is the slope of L.

(b) Use part (a) to sketch quickly eleven lines through the origin having these slopes: 6, 4, 3, 2, 1, 0, -1, -2, -3, -5, -7.

(c) Let b be a real number and L a nonvertical line through $(0, b)$. Let P be the point where L intersects the vertical line through $(1, 0)$. Show that the second coordinate of P is (slope of L) $+ b$.

C.2. For which line segment in Figure 3-27 is the slope the
(a) largest?
(b) smallest?
(c) largest in absolute value?
(d) closest to zero?

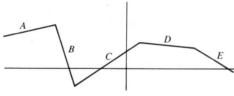

Figure 3-27

3. EQUATIONS OF LINES

We now begin a systematic program of relating simple algebraic equations and inequalities with familiar geometric shapes. In this section we shall use our knowledge of slopes to show that every straight line is the graph of a first-degree equation and vice versa. Second-degree equations will be considered in the next section.

The simplest case is that of vertical lines, that is, lines parallel to the y-axis. Suppose a vertical line L has x-intercept c. This means that L crosses the x-axis at the point $(c, 0)$, as shown in Figure 3-28.

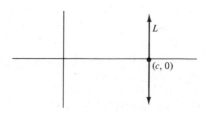

Figure 3-28

Then *every* point on L has the *same* x-coordinate—namely, c—and every point with x-coordinate c lies on L. Therefore

---

The vertical line through $(c, 0)$ *is the graph of the equation* $x = c$.

We often say **"the equation of the line"** instead of "the equation whose graph is the line."

EXAMPLE The vertical line L through $(14, 79)$ is the same as the vertical line through $(14, 0)$. Therefore the equation of L is $x = 14$.

NONVERTICAL LINES

If (x_1, y_1) is a point and m is a real number, it is geometrically clear that there is exactly one line through (x_1, y_1) with slope m. Here is an algebraic description of this line.

POINT-SLOPE FORM OF THE EQUATION OF A LINE

The line L *with slope* m *through the point* (x_1, y_1) *is the graph of the equation*

$$y - y_1 = m(x - x_1)$$

In order to *prove* that the line L coincides with the graph of $y - y_1 = m(x - x_1)$ we must show *two* things: (1) every point on L satisfies the equation *and* (2) every point that satisfies the equation is actually on L. First, suppose (c, d) is any point on L other than (x_1, y_1). Using these two points to compute the slope of L yields

$$\frac{d - y_1}{c - x_1} = \text{slope } L = m, \quad \text{or equivalently,} \quad d - y_1 = m(c - x_1)$$

Therefore (c, d) satisfies the equation $y - y_1 = m(x - x_1)$. Since (x_1, y_1) obviously satisfies this equation, we have proved part 1.

Now for part 2: we know (x_1, y_1) is on L. If (r, s) is any point other than (x_1, y_1) which satisfies the equation, then

$$s - y_1 = m(r - x_1), \quad \text{or equivalently,} \quad \frac{s - y_1}{r - x_1} = m$$

The last equation says that the line M joining (r, s) and (x_1, y_1) has slope m, the same slope as the line L. In Section 2 we saw that two *distinct* lines with the same slope are parallel. Since (x_1, y_1) lies on both L and M, the only possibility here is that L and M are actually the *same* line. Thus (r, s) does lie on L and the proof is complete.

What we have just proved is that if you know *one point* and the *slope* of a line, then you know the equation of the line.

EXAMPLE   The line L with slope 5 through the point $(3, -4)$ is the graph of the equation $y - y_1 = m(x - x_1)$, with $m = 5$ and $(x_1, y_1) = (3, -4)$; that is,

$$y - (-4) = 5(x - 3)$$
$$y + 4 = 5x - 15$$
$$y = 5x - 19$$

Observe that the slope of the line L is 5 and the y-intercept of L (obtained by setting $x = 0$ in the equation) is precisely the number -19.

The equation of a line can also be found when you know only *two points* on the line.

EXAMPLE   Let M be the line through $(1, 2)$ and $(-5, 6)$. Then the slope of M is $\dfrac{6 - 2}{-5 - 1} = \dfrac{4}{-6} = -\dfrac{2}{3}$. By using $m = -\dfrac{2}{3}$ and $(x_1, y_1) = (1, 2)$, we see that the equation of M is

$$y - y_1 = m(x - x_1)$$
$$y - 2 = -\tfrac{2}{3}(x - 1)$$

We can simplify this equation as follows:

$$y - 2 = -\tfrac{2}{3}x + \tfrac{2}{3}$$
$$y = -\tfrac{2}{3}x + (\tfrac{2}{3} + 2) = -\tfrac{2}{3}x + \tfrac{8}{3}$$

You might be wondering what would happen if we used the point $(-5, 6)$ for (x_1, y_1) instead of $(1, 2)$:

$$y - y_1 = m(x - x_1)$$
$$y - 6 = -\tfrac{2}{3}(x - (-5))$$

Now this doesn't look much like the equation obtained above, but some routine algebra shows that it is actually an equivalent form of the same equation:

$$y - 6 = -\tfrac{2}{3}(x - (-5)) = -\tfrac{2}{3}x - \tfrac{10}{3}$$
$$y = -\tfrac{2}{3}x - \tfrac{10}{3} + 6$$
$$y = -\tfrac{2}{3}x + \tfrac{8}{3}$$

Note that the slope of the line M is $-\tfrac{2}{3}$ and the y-intercept is $\tfrac{8}{3}$ [since $(0, \tfrac{8}{3})$ satisfies the equation].

The final form of the equations in the preceding examples suggests that you can find the equation of a line, provided you know its *slope* and y-intercept:

SLOPE-INTERCEPT FORM OF THE EQUATION OF A LINE

The line with slope m *and y-intercept* b *is the graph of the equation*
$y = mx + b.$

This fact is easily proved as follows. A line with y-intercept b goes through the point $(0, b)$. But as we saw above, the line through $(0, b)$ with slope m is just the graph of the equation

$$y - b = m(x - 0) = mx$$
$$y = mx + b$$

As the earlier examples showed, the equation of any nonvertical line can be obtained in several ways. But in every case, the equation can always be written in the slope-intercept form $y = mx + b$. This is probably the most useful form of the equation of a line, since you can *immediately* read off the slope and the y-intecept of the line.

EXAMPLE In order to find the graph of the equation $2x - 3y + 14 = 6x + 5y$, we first rewrite the equation in an equivalent form:

$$2x - 3y + 14 = 6x + 5y$$
$$-3y - 5y = 6x - 2x - 14$$
$$-8y = 4x - 14$$
$$y = -\tfrac{4}{8}x - (-\tfrac{14}{8}) = -\tfrac{1}{2}x + \tfrac{7}{4}$$

Now that the equation is in the form $y = mx + b$, we can just *read off the basic facts:* the graph is a line with slope $m = -\tfrac{1}{2}$ and y-intercept $b = \tfrac{7}{4}$. The y-intercept $\tfrac{7}{4}$ tells us that the point $(0, \tfrac{7}{4})$ is on the graph. To obtain another point on the graph, we can substitute any nonzero number for x—say, $x = 2$—in the equation $y = -\tfrac{1}{2}x + \tfrac{7}{4}$ and obtain $y = -\tfrac{1}{2}(2) + \tfrac{7}{4} = \tfrac{3}{4}$. Therefore $(2, \tfrac{3}{4})$ is on the graph and the graph looks like the one in Figure 3-29.

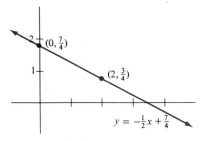

Figure 3-29

EXAMPLE The equation $y = 3$ can be written as $y = 0x + 3$. Therefore its graph is a straight line with slope 0 and y-intercept 3, that is, a horizontal line through $(0, 3)$, as shown in Figure 3-30.

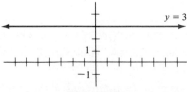

Figure 3-30

EXAMPLE Find the equation of the line L through $(2, -1)$, which is parallel to the line M whose equation is $3x - 2y + 6 = 0$. The equation $3x - 2y + 6 = 0$ may be rewritten

$$-2y = -3x - 6$$
$$y = \tfrac{3}{2}x + 3$$

The slope-intercept form of the equation of M tells us that M has slope $\tfrac{3}{2}$. Therefore the parallel line L has the *same* slope $\tfrac{3}{2}$. Using the point $(2, -1)$ on L and the slope $\tfrac{3}{2}$, we see that the equation of L is

$$y - (-1) = \tfrac{3}{2}(x - 2) = \tfrac{3}{2}x - 3$$
$$y = \tfrac{3}{2}x - 4$$

FIRST-DEGREE EQUATIONS

The preceding examples show that the equation of any straight line is a **first-degree equation,** that is, an equation which can be written in the form

$$Ax + By + C = 0,$$

where A, B, C are real numbers with at least one of A or B nonzero. For instance,

$y = 5x - 19$	can be written	$5x - y - 19 = 0$
$x = -6$	can be written	$x + 0y + 6 = 0$
$y - 2 = -3(x - 4)$	can be written	$3x + y - 14 = 0$

Conversely, consider any first-degree equation $Ax + By + C = 0$. Either $B = 0$ or $B \neq 0$. If $B = 0$, then $A \neq 0$ and the equation becomes

$$Ax + C = 0$$
$$Ax = -C$$
$$x = \frac{-C}{A}$$

Its graph is a vertical line. On the other hand, if $B \neq 0$, then the equation becomes

$$Ax + By + C = 0$$
$$By = -Ax - C$$
$$y = \frac{-A}{B}x - \frac{C}{B}$$

Its graph is a line with slope $-A/B$ and y-intercept $-C/B$. We have proved:

> *The graph of every first-degree equation* $Ax + By + C = 0$ *is a straight line and every straight line is the graph of a first-degree equation.*

For obvious reasons, first-degree equations are often called **linear equations.** We frequently refer to "the line $Ax + By + C = 0$" instead of using the proper phrase "the line that is the graph of $Ax + By + C = 0$."

LINEAR INEQUALITIES

The techniques for graphing linear equations can also be used to graph linear inequalities.

EXAMPLE   The graph of $y \le 2x + 1$ consists of all points (x, y) in the plane whose coordinates satisfy this inequality. Since all points on the line $y = 2x + 1$ obviously satisfy the inequality, this line is *part* of the graph of $y \le 2x + 1$. Any point (x, y) that is *not* on the line $y = 2x + 1$ must lie either above or below the line (see Figure 3-31).

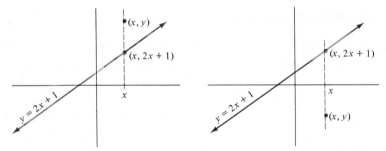

Figure 3-31

As Figure 3-31 shows, (x, y) lies directly above or directly below the point $(x, 2x + 1)$ on the line. Now the relative position of two points on the same vertical line is determined by their second coordinates. So if (x, y) lies above $(x, 2x + 1)$, we must have $y > 2x + 1$. Thus no point (x, y) above the line satisfies the inequality $y \le 2x + 1$. On the other hand, if (x, y) lies below $(x, 2x + 1)$, we must have $y < 2x + 1$, so that (x, y) *does* satisfy the inequality $y \le 2x + 1$. Therefore the graph of $y \le 2x + 1$ is the half-plane consisting of *all points on or below the line* $y = 2x + 1$, as shown in Figure 3-32.

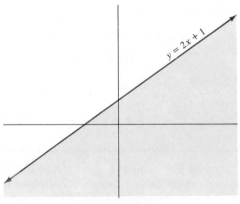

Figure 3-32

The argument in the preceding example also shows that the graph of the inequality $y \geq 2x + 1$ consists of the points *on or above* the line $y = 2x + 1$. A similar argument works for all linear inequalities:

> *The graph of* $y \leq mx + b$ *is the half-plane consisting of all points on or below the line* $y = mx + b.$
>
> *The graph of* $y \geq mx + b$ *is the half-plane consisting of all points on or above the line* $y = mx + b.$

EXERCISES

A.1. Find the equation of the line with given slope m and passing through the given point and graph the line.

   (a) $m = 1;$ $(3, 5)$ **(d)** $m = 0;$ $(-4, -5)$

   (b) $m = 2;$ $(-2, 1)$ **(e)** $m = \frac{1}{2};$ $(-3, 1)$

   (c) $m = -1;$ $(6, 2)$ **(f)** $m = -3;$ $(2, \sqrt{3})$

A.2. Find the equation of the line through the two given points.

   (a) $(0, -5)$ and $(-3, -2)$ **(e)** $(8.7, 1)$ and $(0, 0)$

   (b) $(4, 3)$ and $(2, -1)$ **(f)** $(6, 7)$ and $(6, 15)$

   (c) $(\frac{4}{3}, \frac{2}{3})$ and $(\frac{1}{3}, 3)$ **(g)** $(\sqrt{8}, \sqrt{2})$ and $(-\sqrt{2}, \sqrt{6})$

   (d) $(-10, 11)$ and $(12, 1)$ **(h)** $(\frac{1}{2}, 4)$ and $(\frac{5}{2}, \frac{6}{5})$

A.3. Find the equation of the line with given slope m and given y-intercept b; and graph the line.

   (a) $m = 1;$ $b = 2$ **(c)** $m = -4;$ $b = 2$ **(e)** $m = \frac{1}{2};$ $b = 3$

   (b) $m = 2;$ $b = 5$ **(d)** $m = -5;$ $b = -2$ **(f)** $m = \frac{4}{3};$ $b = -\frac{5}{3}$

A.4. Find the slope and y-intercept of each line whose equation is given below and graph the line. (*Hint:* put the equation in slope-intercept form.)

   (a) $2x - y + 5 = 0$ **(d)** $2(x + y + 1) = 5x - 3$

   (b) $3x + 4y = 7$ **(e)** $3(x - 2) + y = 7 - 6(y + 4)$

   (c) $7 + 2y = -8x$ **(f)** $2(y - 3) + (x - 6) = 4(x + 1) - 2$

B.1. Find an equation for the line satisfying the given conditions and graph the line.

   (a) through $(-2, 1)$ with slope 3

   (b) y-intercept -7 and slope 1

   (c) through $(2, 3)$ and parallel to $3x - 2y = 5$

   (d) through $(1, -2)$ and perpendicular to $y = 2x - 3$

   (e) x-intercept 5 and y-intercept -5

   (f) through $(-5, 2)$ and parallel to the line through $(1, 2)$ and $(4, 3)$

   (g) through $(-1, 3)$ and perpendicular to the line through $(0, 1)$ and $(2, 3)$

   (h) through $(-5, 6)$ and perpendicular to the x-axis

   (i) through $(-5, 2)$ and parallel to the x-axis

   (j) y-intercept 3 and perpendicular to $2x - y + 6 = 0$

(k) y-intercept 0 and parallel to $x - 3y + 7 = 0$

(l)   parallel to $3x - 3y + 5 = 7$, with the same y-intercept as $2x - 5y + 7 = 4$

B.2.   Determine whether the following pairs of lines are parallel, perpendicular, or neither. (*Hint:* put the equations in slope-intercept form and use well-known facts about slopes.)

(a) $2x + y - 2 = 0$ and $4x + 2y + 18 = 0$

(b) $3x + y - 3 = 0$ and $6x + 2y + 17 = 0$

(c) $x + 2y - 3 = 0$ and $2x - y + 3 = 0$

(d) $x - 3y + 7 = 0$ and $y - 3x + 3 = 0$

(e) $x + y - 3 = 0$ and $y - x + 2 = 0$

(f) $y - ax + 5 = 0$ and $ay + x - 7 = 0$ (where a is a constant)

B.3.   **(a)**   Find a real number k such that $(3, -2)$ is on the line $kx - 2y + 7 = 0$.

(b)   Find a real number k such that the line $3x - ky + 2 = 0$ has y-intercept -3.

B.4.   Let A, B, C, D be nonzero real numbers. Show that the lines $Ax + By + C = 0$ and $Ax + By + D = 0$ are parallel.

B.5.   Suppose A and B are real numbers, at least one of which is nonzero. Prove that the graph of $Ax + By = 0$ is a straight line through the origin.

B.6.   Let L be a line which is neither vertical nor horizontal and which does *not* pass through the origin. Show that L is the graph of $\dfrac{x}{a} + \dfrac{y}{b} = 1$, where a is the x-intercept and b the y-intercept of L.

B.7.   Graph the equation $|x| + |y| = 1$. [*Hint:* just look at one quadrant at a time. For instance, all points (x, y) in the second quadrant have $x < 0$ and $y > 0$, so that $|x| = -x$ and $|y| = y$. Thus in the second quadrant the graph of $|x| + |y| = 1$ is the same as the graph of $-x + y = 1$. Deal with the other quadrants similarly.]

B.8.   Graph these inequalities.

(a) $y \leq -3x + 2$

(b) $y \geq x + 4$

(c) $y < 2x - 1$
(*Hint:* follow the same procedure above; but the line $y = 2x - 1$ is *not* part of the graph.)

(d) $y > 3x + 1$

(e) $y > -3x + 1$

(f) $4x + 2y - 1 \leq 0$
(*Hint:* first solve for y.)

(g) $-3x + 4y + 8 > 0$

(h) $-5x + 3y - 6 < 0$

B.9.   Graph these systems of inequalities (that is, plot the points that are on the graphs of *all* the inequalities in the given system).

(a) $y \leq x + 1$
$y \leq -2x + 3$

(b) $y \leq 2x - 1$
$y \geq -x$

(c) $3x - 2y - 2 \leq 0$
$y \leq 1$

(d) $y \geq x + 1$ **(e)** $2x - y \leq -1$

$\quad\quad y \leq -2x + 1$ $4x + y \leq 3$

$\quad\quad x \geq -2$ $x + y \geq -1$

C.1. Let (x_1, y_1), (x_2, y_2), (x_3, y_3) be any three points on the line $y = mx + b$, where $x_1 < x_2 < x_3$. Show that the distance from (x_1, y_1) to (x_3, y_3) is the sum of the distance from (x_1, y_1) to (x_2, y_2) and the distance from (x_2, y_2) to (x_3, y_3). (*Hint:* $y_1 = mx_1 + b$.)

C.2. A road is being built along the floor of a valley. At the end of the valley it must pass over the hill, as shown in Figure 3-33.

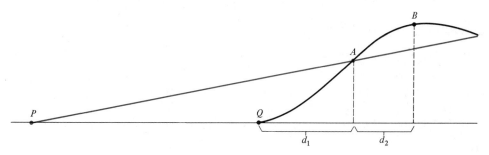

Figure 3-33

Because of soil conditions and other factors, the road is to lie along a straight line of slope $\frac{1}{25}$ which passes through point A (as indicated by the colored line above). The top of the hill will be cut away, and the bottom of the hill will be filled in to road level. The point A lies 400 ft above the floor of the valley. The peak of the hill (point B) lies 500 ft above the valley floor. The horizontal distance d_1 is 600 ft; distance d_2 is 300 ft.

(a) Find the point where the road should meet the valley floor by determining the distance from P to Q. (*Hint:* sketch the picture on a coordinate system, with the valley floor as the x-axis and the vertical line through A as the y-axis.)

(b) Find out how much of the hilltop must be cut off by determining the vertical distance from point B to the road.

C.3. This exercise completes the proof of the statement in the box on page 134. Show that two nonvertical lines with the same slope are parallel. (*Hint:* write the equations of the lines in slope-intercept form and show that the vertical distance between the two lines is the same for any value of x.)

C.4. This exercise provides a proof of the statement in the box on page 135. Let L be a line with slope k and M a line with slope m and assume *both* L and M pass through the origin.

(a) Show that L passes through $(1, k)$ and M passes through $(1, m)$.

(b) Compute the length of each side of the triangle with vertices $(0, 0)$, $(1, k)$ and $(1, m)$.

(c) Suppose L and M are perpendicular. Then the triangle of part (b) has a right angle at $(0, 0)$. Use part (b) and the Pythagorean Theorem to find an equation involving k, m, and various constants. Simplify this equation to show that $km = -1$.

(d) Suppose instead that $km = -1$ and prove that L and M are perpendicular. [*Hint:* you may assume that a triangle whose sides a, b, c satisfy $a^2 + b^2 = c^2$ is a right triangle with hypotenuse c. Use this fact and $km = -1$ to "reverse" the argument in part (c).]

(e) Finally, assume L and M are any two nonvertical lines (which don't necessarily go through the origin), with slope $L = k$ and slope $M = m$. Use the preceding material to prove that L is perpendicular to M exactly when $km = -1$. (*Hint:* every line is parallel to a line through the origin and parallel lines have the same slope.)

4. CONIC SECTIONS

In this section we discuss algebraic descriptions (in terms of second-degree equations) of several frequently seen geometric curves: circles, ellipses, and hyperbolas. These curves, together with parabolas (which will be discussed in Chapter 4), are called **conic sections.**

Warning All the graphs in this section are obtained with a minimal amount of plotting of points. Usually geometric or algebraic information is used to produce the entire graph very quickly. In one sense, this illustrates the power of analytic geometry. In another sense, however, it is quite misleading. The techniques presented here work very well for uncomplicated second-degree equations. But determining the graph of an arbitrary equation almost always involves plotting points, as well as some educated guesswork, as we shall see in Chapter 4.

CIRCLES

If P is a point in the plane and r is a positive real number, then the **circle with center P and radius r** is the set of all points in the plane whose distance from P is precisely r units, as shown below. Suppose the point P has coordinates (a, b). Then the point (x, y) is on the circle with center P and radius r exactly when the distance from (x, y) to (a, b) is r, as shown in Figure 3-34.

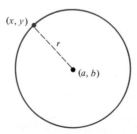

Figure 3-34

Using the distance formula on the points (x, y) and (a, b), we can rewrite this statement as

$$\sqrt{(x - a)^2 + (y - b)^2} = r$$

Squaring both sides of this equation yields

$$(x - a)^2 + (y - b)^2 = r^2$$

Therefore we have proved that

The circle with center (a, b) *and radius* r *is the graph of the equation*

$$(x - a)^2 + (y - b)^2 = r^2$$

We sometimes say that $(x - a)^2 + (y - b)^2 = r^2$ is the **equation of the circle** with center (a, b) and radius r. If the center of the circle is at the origin (so that $a = 0$ and $b = 0$ in the discussion above), then the equation of the circle takes a simple form:

The circle with center $(0, 0)$ *and radius* r *is the graph of the equation*
$$x^2 + y^2 = r^2$$

EXAMPLE The circle with radius 1 and center $(0, 0)$ is the graph of the equation $x^2 + y^2 = 1$, as shown in Figure 3-35. This circle is usually called the **unit circle.**

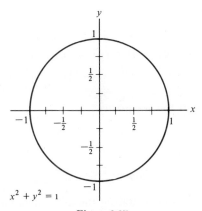

$x^2 + y^2 = 1$

Figure 3-35

EXAMPLE The circle with center $(-3, 2)$ and radius 2 is the graph of the equation

$$(x - (-3))^2 + (y - 2)^2 = 2^2$$

which can also be written as

$$(x + 3)^2 + (y - 2)^2 = 4$$

The graph is shown in Figure 3-36.

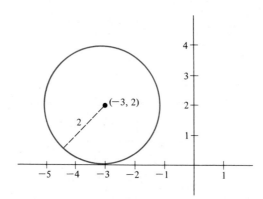

Figure 3-36

EXAMPLE   What is the equation whose graph is the circle with center $(2, -1)$ which passes through the origin? In order to write the equation of this circle, we must first find its radius. The radius is the distance from any point on the circle to the center, $(2, -1)$. Since $(0, 0)$ is on the circle, the radius is the distance from $(0, 0)$ to $(2, -1)$, namely,

$$\sqrt{(0 - 2)^2 + (0 - (-1))^2} = \sqrt{4 + 1} = \sqrt{5}$$

Finally, the equation of the circle with radius $\sqrt{5}$ and center $(2, -1)$ is

$$(x - 2)^2 + [y - (-1)]^2 = (\sqrt{5})^2$$

which can be written as:

$$(x - 2)^2 + (y + 1)^2 = 5$$
$$(x^2 - 4x + 4) + (y^2 + 2y + 1) = 5$$
$$x^2 + y^2 - 4x + 2y = 0$$

EXAMPLE   If (x, y) satisfies the inequality

$$(x - 1)^2 + y^2 \geq 4$$

then (x, y) necessarily satisfies

$$\sqrt{(x - 1)^2 + (y - 0)^2} \geq 2$$

But this is just an algebraic way of stating the geometric fact that

The distance from (x, y) to $(1, 0)$ is greater than or equal to 2.

Therefore the points (x, y) which satisfy $(x - 1)^2 + y^2 \geq 4$ lie *outside or on* the circle with center $(1, 0)$ and radius 2. In other words, the graph of the inequality $(x - 1)^2 + y^2 \geq 4$ is the shaded area in Figure 3-37.

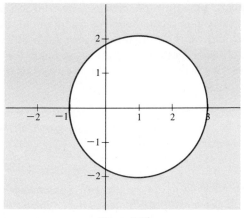

Figure 3-37

Similarly, the points (x, y) that satisfy the inequality

$$(x - 1)^2 + y^2 < 4$$

also satisfy

$$\sqrt{(x - 1)^2 + (y - 0)^2} < 2$$

This last inequality states that the distance from (x, y) to $(1, 0)$ is less than 2, so that (x, y) lies *inside* the circle with center $(1, 0)$ and radius 2. Therefore the graph of $(x - 1)^2 + y^2 < 4$ is the white circular disc in Figure 3-37.

ELLIPSES

Let P and Q be two points in the plane and r a positive real number. The set of all points X such that

$$(\text{distance from } P \text{ to } X) + (\text{distance from } Q \text{ to } X) = r$$

is called an **ellipse.** Points P and Q are called the **foci** of the ellipse ("foci" is the plural of "focus"). The midpoint of the line segment from P to Q is called the **center** of the ellipse. The number r is called the **distance sum.**

One way to see what an ellipse looks like is to take a string of length r and pin its ends on the points P and Q. Then put your pencil against the string so that the string is taut (as indicated by the dotted line in Figure 3-38). If you move the pencil point X, keeping the string taut, you will trace out an ellipse, as shown in Figure 3-38.

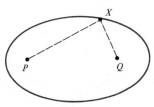

Figure 3-38

Ellipses arise frequently in nature and science. The orbit of a planet around the sun is an ellipse with the sun as one focus. Satellites travel in elliptical orbits around the earth. Elliptical gears and cams are used in various kinds of machinery.

Ellipses can be described as graphs of equations, in much the same way we did for circles above. However, we shall present only the case of ellipses whose center is at the origin.

Let a *and* b *be positive real numbers. The graph of the equation*

$$\frac{x^2}{a^2} + \frac{y^2}{b^2} = 1$$

is an ellipse centered at the origin with x-intercepts $\pm$a *and y-intercepts* $\pm$b. *Every ellipse centered at the origin, with foci on one of the coordinate axes, is the graph of an equation of this form.*

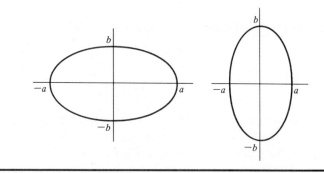

The proof of this claim is basically an exercise in the use of the distance formula. Those interested should consult Exercise C.3.

EXAMPLE   In order to graph the equation $\dfrac{x^2}{9} + \dfrac{y^2}{4} = 1$, we first rewrite the equation as $\dfrac{x^2}{3^2} + \dfrac{y^2}{2^2} = 1$. Now the equation has the form $\dfrac{x^2}{a^2} + \dfrac{y^2}{b^2} = 1$ with $a = 3$ and $b = 2$. Therefore the graph is an ellipse with x-intercepts ±3 and y-intercepts ±2, as shown in Figure 3-39.

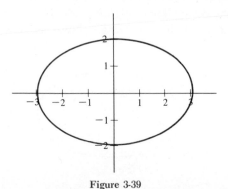

Figure 3-39

$y = -(b/a)x = -(3/2)x$. We first draw the asymptotes and plot the points $(-2, 0)$ and $(2, 0)$. Then the graph of the hyperbola can be sketched easily, as shown in Figure 3-42.

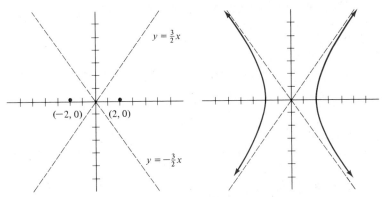

Figure 3-42

Let a and b be positive real numbers. The graph of the equation

$$\frac{y^2}{b^2} - \frac{x^2}{a^2} = 1$$

is a hyperbola with y-intercepts $\pm b$ and asymptotes the lines $y = \dfrac{b}{a}x$ and $y = -\dfrac{b}{a}x$,

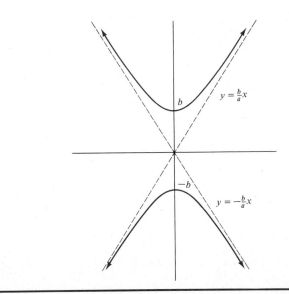

EXAMPLE   To find the graph of the equation $75x^2 - 4y^2 + 100 = 0$, we first rewrite the equation

$$75x^2 - 4y^2 + 100 = 0$$

$$75x^2 - 4y^2 = -100$$

$$\frac{75x^2}{-100} - \frac{4y^2}{-100} = \frac{-100}{-100}$$

$$-\frac{3}{4}x^2 + \frac{y^2}{25} = 1$$

$$\frac{y^2}{25} - \frac{x^2}{(4/3)} = 1$$

$$\frac{y^2}{5^2} - \frac{x^2}{(2/\sqrt{3})^2} = 1$$

The equation now has the form $\dfrac{y^2}{b^2} - \dfrac{x^2}{a^2} = 1$ with $b = 5$ and $a = \dfrac{2}{\sqrt{3}}$. Therefore the graph is a hyperbola with y-intercepts ± 5 and asymptotes the lines

$$y = \frac{b}{a}x = \frac{5}{2/\sqrt{3}}x = \frac{5\sqrt{3}}{2}x \quad \text{and} \quad y = -\frac{b}{a}x = \frac{-5}{2/\sqrt{3}}x = \frac{-5\sqrt{3}}{2}x$$

as shown in Figure 3-43.

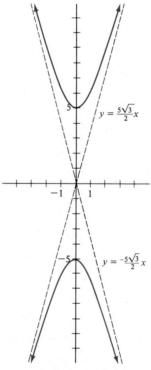

Figure 3-43

Note The two hyperbola equations presented above are easy to confuse with one another. Here is a "memory hook" for distinguishing the graphs of the equations

$$\frac{x^2}{a^2} - \frac{y^2}{b^2} = 1 \quad \text{and} \quad \frac{y^2}{b^2} - \frac{x^2}{a^2} = 1$$

In the first equation, the coefficient of x^2 (namely, $1/a^2$) is *positive* and the coefficient of y^2 (namely, $-1/b^2$) is *negative:* the hyperbola crosses the x-axis but *not* the y-axis. In the second equation, the coefficient of y^2 is positive and that of x^2 negative: the hyperbola crosses the y-axis but not the x-axis.

SECOND-DEGREE EQUATIONS

A **second-degree equation** in x and y is any equation of the form

$$Ax^2 + By^2 + Cxy + Dx + Ey + F = 0$$

where A, B, C, D, E, F are fixed real numbers and at least one of A, B, or C is nonzero.

EXAMPLE The circle with center $(1, 2)$ and radius 5 is the graph of the equation $(x - 1)^2 + (y - 2)^2 = 5^2$. This equation can easily be seen to be a second-degree equation.

$$(x - 1)^2 + (y - 2)^2 = 5^2$$
$$(x^2 - 2x + 1) + (y^2 - 4y + 4) = 25$$
$$x^2 + y^2 - 2x - 4y - 20 = 0$$

This last version of the equation is of the form $Ax^2 + By^2 + Cxy + Dx + Ey + F = 0$ with $A = 1$, $B = 1$, $C = 0$, $D = -2$, $E = -4$, and $F = -20$.

Although we have not discussed all the possibilities, it is in fact true that

> *Every conic section is the graph of a second-degree equation.*

The converse of this statement (namely, the graph of every second-degree equation is a conic section) is *essentially* true, provided you allow for a few so-called degenerate cases. These exceptions and the graphs of various second-degree equations are considered in the DO IT YOURSELF! segment at the end of this section.

EXERCISES

A.1. Find the equation of the circle with the given center and given radius r.

(a) $(-3, 4)$; $r = 2$

(b) $(-2, -1)$; $r = 3$

(c) $(0, 0)$; $r = \sqrt{2}$

(d) $(5, -2)$; $r = 1$

(e) $(4, 7)$; $r = \frac{1}{2}$

(f) $(\frac{1}{2}, \frac{5}{2})$; $r = \frac{7}{3}$

(g) $(3, \frac{8}{3})$; $r = \sqrt{3}$

(h) $(100, \sqrt{50})$; $r = \dfrac{4\sqrt{2}}{3}$

A.2. Sketch the graph of each equation:

(a) $(x - 2)^2 + (y - 4)^2 = 1$

(f) $\dfrac{x^2}{25} + \dfrac{y^2}{4} = 1$

(b) $(x + 1)^2 + (y - 3)^2 = 9$

(g) $\dfrac{x^2}{6} + \dfrac{y^2}{16} = 1$

(c) $(x - 5)^2 + (y + 2)^2 = 5$

(h) $\dfrac{x^2}{10} - 1 = \dfrac{y^2}{36}$

(d) $(x + 6)^2 + y^2 = 4$

(i) $\dfrac{y^2}{49} + \dfrac{x^2}{81} = 1$

(e) $x^2 + y^2 = 16$

A.3. Find an equation whose graph is an ellipse with the given intercepts.
(a) x-intercepts ± 7 and y-intercepts ± 2
(b) x-intercepts ± 1 and y-intercepts ± 8
(c) x-intercepts ± 9 and y-intercepts ± 10.

A.4. The area of the ellipse $\dfrac{x^2}{a^2} + \dfrac{y^2}{b^2} = 1$ is πab. Find the area of these ellipses:

(a) $\dfrac{x^2}{16} + \dfrac{y^2}{4} = 1$ (c) $3x^2 + 4y^2 = 12$ (e) $6x^2 + 2y^2 = 14$

(b) $\dfrac{x^2}{9} + \dfrac{y^2}{5} = 1$ (d) $7x^2 + 5y^2 = 35$ (f) $5x^2 + y^2 = 5$

A.5. Find an equation whose graph is a hyperbola
(a) with asymptotes $y = \frac{3}{2}x$ and $y = -\frac{3}{2}x$ and x-intercepts ± 2
(b) with asymptotes $y = \frac{3}{4}x$ and $y = -\frac{3}{4}x$ and x-intercepts ± 4.

B.1. Find the equation of each of the circles described below.
(a) center $(2, 2)$; passes through the origin
(b) center $(-1, -3)$; passes through $(-4, -2)$
(c) center $(1, 2)$; x-intercepts -1 and 3
(d) center $(3, 1)$; diameter 2
(e) center $(4, 3)$; area 81π (*Hint:* the area of a circle of radius r is πr^2)
(f) center $(0, 0)$; circumference 2π (*Hint:* the circumference of a circle of radius r is $2\pi r$)
(g) center $(-5, 4)$; tangent (touching at one point) to the x-axis
(h) center $(2, -6)$; tangent to the y-axis.

B.2. Without drawing any graphs, determine whether the given point lies inside, outside, or on the given circle.
(a) $(1.5, -1.5)$; circle of radius 4.5 centered at the origin
(b) $(2, 1)$; circle with center $(-1, 4)$ and radius 4
(c) $(-2, 0)$; circle with center $(-1, -2)$ and radius 2.1
(d) $(-2, 3)$; circle with center $(3, 4)$ and radius 5
(e) $(\sqrt{3}, \sqrt{3})$; circle with center $(2, -5)$ and radius $\sqrt{43}$.

B.3. Sketch the graph of these inequalities (see the example on pp. 148–149).

(a) $x^2 + y^2 \leq 1$

(b) $x^2 + y^2 \geq 1$

(c) $x^2 + y^2 > 4$

(d) $(x + 3)^2 + (y - 5)^2 \leq 9$

(e) $(x - 2)^2 + y^2 \leq 4$

(f) $(x - 1)^2 + (y + 2)^2 < 5$

B.4. Graph these systems of inequalities (that is, plot the points that satisfy *all* the inequalities in the given system).

(a) $x^2 + y^2 \leq 25$
$y \leq 2x$

(b) $(x - 4)^2 + (y - 1)^2 \leq 36$
$y > 3x - 1$

(c) $x^2 + y^2 \leq 16$
$x - 2y + 4 \geq 0$
$3x + 4y + 12 \geq 0$

(d) $x^2 + y^2 \geq 9$
$x + 1 \geq 0$
$x + y - 7 \leq 0$

(e) $x^2 + y^2 \leq 16$
$x^2 + y^2 \geq 9$

(f) $x^2 + y^2 \geq 1$
$x^2 + y^2 \leq 4$

(g) $(x + 3)^2 + (y - 1)^2 \geq 1$
$(x + 3)^2 + (y - 1)^2 \leq 9$

(h) $(x - 2)^2 + (y + 2)^2 \leq 36$
$(x - 2)^2 + (y + 2)^2 \geq 16$

B.5. For each real number k, the graph of $(x - k)^2 + y^2 = k^2$ is a circle. Describe all possible such circles.

B.6. Sketch the graph of each equation. If the graph is a hyperbola, also sketch the asymptotes.

(a) $4x^2 - y^2 = 16$

(b) $4x^2 + 3y^2 = 12$

(c) $\dfrac{x^2}{6} - \dfrac{y^2}{16} = 1$

(d) $3y^2 - 5x^2 = 15$

(e) $\dfrac{x^2}{4} + \dfrac{y^2}{9} = 2$

(f) $4x^2 + 4y^2 = 1$

(g) $x^2 + 4y^2 = 1$

(h) $x^2 - 4y^2 = 1$

(i) $3x^2 + 2y^2 = 6$

(j) $2x^2 - y^2 = 4$

(k) $18y^2 - 8x^2 - 2 = 0$

(l) $x^2 - 2y^2 = -1$

(m) $(y - 3)^2 - 10 = -x^2 + 2x - 1$

(n) $(x + y)(x - y) + x^2 = 4$

(o) $(2x - y)(x + 4y) - 7xy = 8$

(p) $15y^2 + 12x^2 - 30 = 0$

B.7. If $a > b > 0$, then the number $e = (\sqrt{a^2 - b^2})/a$ is called the **eccentricity** of the ellipse $\dfrac{x^2}{a^2} + \dfrac{y^2}{b^2} = 1$.

(a) Show that $0 < e < 1$.

(b) Determine the eccentricity of each of the following ellipses:

$$\frac{x^2}{100} + \frac{y^2}{99} = 1, \qquad \frac{x^2}{25} + \frac{y^2}{18} = 1, \qquad \frac{x^2}{16} + \frac{y^2}{2} = 1$$

(c)   Describe the general shape of an ellipse when the eccentricity is very close to 1; when the eccentricity is very close to 0. [*Hint:* part (b) may be helpful.]

B.8.   Find a number k such that $(-2, 1)$ lies on the graph of $3x^2 + ky^2 = 4$. Then graph the equation.

C.1.   The punchbowl and a table holding the punch cups are placed 50 ft apart at a yard party. A portable fence is then set up so that any guest inside the fence can walk straight to the table, then to the punchbowl, and then return to his or her starting point without traveling more than 150 ft. Describe the longest possible such fence.

C.2.   An arched footbridge over a 100-ft wide river is shaped like half an ellipse. The maximum height of the bridge over the river is 20 ft. Find the height of the bridge over a point in the river, exactly 25 ft from the center of the river.

C.3.   Here is a partial proof that the graph of $\dfrac{x^2}{a^2} + \dfrac{y^2}{b^2} = 1$ is an ellipse. Assume first that $a > b$ and let $c = \sqrt{a^2 - b^2}$. Let E be the ellipse with foci $(-c, 0)$ and $(c, 0)$ and distance sum $2a$. E consists of all points (x, y) such that

(distance from $(-c, 0)$ to (x, y)) + (distance from (x, y) to $(c, 0)$) = $2a$

(a)   Use the distance formula to show that every point on E satisfies the equation
$$\sqrt{(x + c)^2 + y^2} = 2a - \sqrt{(x - c)^2 + y^2}$$

(b)   Square both sides of the equation in part (a) and show that the resulting equation simplifies to
$$\sqrt{(x - c)^2 + y^2} = a - \frac{c}{a}x$$

(c)   Square both sides of the equation in (b) and show that the resulting equation simplifies to
$$\frac{a^2 - c^2}{a^2}x^2 + y^2 = a^2 - c^2$$

(d)   Use the fact that $c = \sqrt{a^2 - b^2}$ to show that the equation in part (c) is equivalent to
$$\frac{x^2}{a^2} + \frac{y^2}{b^2} = 1$$

(e)   Use parts (a)–(d) to verify that every point on the ellipse E is on the graph of the equation $\dfrac{x^2}{a^2} + \dfrac{y^2}{b^2} = 1$. The rest of the proof (namely, that every point on the graph is on the ellipse) is a bit tricky and is omitted here.

(f)   If $b > a$, let $c = \sqrt{b^2 - a^2}$ and show that every point on the ellipse with foci $(0, -c)$ and $(0, c)$ and distance sum $2b$ is on the graph of $\dfrac{x^2}{a^2} + \dfrac{y^2}{b^2} = 1$. (*Hint:* adapt parts (a)–(e) in the obvious fashion.)

DO IT YOURSELF!

GRAPHS OF SECOND-DEGREE EQUATIONS

The following examples show how the technique of completing the square° can be used to find the graph of any second-degree equation of the form $Ax^2 + By^2 + Dx + Ey + F = 0$, where *both* A and B are nonzero. The graph is usually a conic section, but there are exceptions, as noted below.

CIRCLES

EXAMPLE   To find the graph of the equation $x^2 + y^2 - 3x + 12y + 28 = 0$, we begin by rearranging the terms:

$$(x^2 - 3x) + (y^2 + 12y) = -28$$

Now we complete the square in the expression $x^2 - 3x$ by adding the square of half the coefficient of x, namely, $[\frac{1}{2}(-3)]^2 = \frac{9}{4}$, so that $(x^2 - 3x + \frac{9}{4}) = (x - \frac{3}{2})^2$. In order to leave the equation unchanged we add $\frac{9}{4}$ to *both* sides:

$$(x^2 - 3x + \tfrac{9}{4}) + (y^2 + 12y) = -28 + \tfrac{9}{4}$$
$$(x - \tfrac{3}{2})^2 + (y^2 + 12y) = -28 + \tfrac{9}{4}$$

In order to complete the square in $y^2 + 12y$ we must add $(\frac{1}{2} \cdot 12)^2 = 36$. Since we want to leave the equation unchanged, we add 36 to both sides:

$$(x - \tfrac{3}{2})^2 + (y^2 + 12y + 36) = -28 + \tfrac{9}{4} + 36$$
$$(x - \tfrac{3}{2})^2 + (y + 6)^2 = 8 + \tfrac{9}{4} = \tfrac{41}{4}$$
$$(x - \tfrac{3}{2})^2 + (y + 6)^2 = (\sqrt{\tfrac{41}{4}})^2$$

Therefore the graph is a circle with center $(\frac{3}{2}, -6)$ and radius $\sqrt{\dfrac{41}{4}} = \dfrac{\sqrt{41}}{2}$.

EXAMPLE   To find the graph of $3x^2 + 3y^2 - 12x - 30y + 60 = 0$, we write the equation as

$$(3x^2 - 12x) + (3y^2 - 30y) = -60$$

Dividing both sides by 3 yields

$$(x^2 - 4x) + (y^2 - 10y) = -20$$

In order to complete the square in $x^2 - 4x$ we must add 4. In order to complete the square in $y^2 - 10y$ we must add 25:

$$(x^2 - 4x + 4) + (y^2 - 10y + 25) = -20 + 4 + 25$$
$$(x - 2)^2 + (y - 5)^2 = 9 = 3^2$$

Therefore the graph is the circle with center $(2, 5)$ and radius 3.

° This technique is explained on page 51.

EXAMPLE   The equation $(x - 1)^2 + (y + 4)^2 = -9$ has no solutions and *no graph*. For every real number x, the number $(x - 1)^2$ is ≥ 0. Similarly, $(y + 4)^2 \geq 0$ for *every* y. Thus $(x - 1)^2 + (y + 4)^2 \geq 0$ always, and hence $(x - 1)^2 + (y + 4)^2 = -9$ has no solutions.

EXAMPLE   The only solution of $x^2 + y^2 = 0$ is $(0, 0)$, so the graph consists of the *single point* $(0, 0)$. You can consider the graph to be a "degenerate" circle with center $(0, 0)$ and radius 0.

In the preceding examples x^2 and y^2 always had the same coefficient. (That is, $A = B$ in $Ax^2 + By^2 + Dx + Ey + F = 0$.) These examples illustrate the fact that

> *The graph of* $Ax^2 + Ay^2 + Dx + Ey + F = 0$ *is either a circle or a single point, or there is no graph.*

ELLIPSES AND HYPERBOLAS

The next two examples are included for the sake of completeness, even though they require a bit more information about the graphs of ellipses and hyperbolas than was presented earlier in the text.

EXAMPLE   To graph the equation $4x^2 + 9y^2 - 32x - 90y + 253 = 0$, we first write the equation as

$$(4x^2 - 32x) + (9y^2 - 90y) = -253$$
$$4(x^2 - 8x) + 9(y^2 - 10y) = -253$$

Now complete the square in $x^2 - 8x$ and $y^2 - 10y$:

$$4(x^2 - 3x + 16) + 9(y^2 - 10y + 25) = -253 + ? + ?$$

Be careful here: on the left side we haven't just added 16 and 25. When the left side is multiplied out we have actually added in $4 \cdot 16 = 64$ and $9 \cdot 25 = 225$. Therefore to leave the original equation unchanged, we must add these numbers on the right:

$$4(x^2 - 8x + 16) + 9(y^2 - 10y + 25) = -253 + 64 + 225$$
$$4(x - 4)^2 + 9(y - 5)^2 = 36$$
$$\frac{4(x - 4)^2}{36} + \frac{9(y - 5)^2}{36} = \frac{36}{36}$$
$$\frac{(x - 4)^2}{9} + \frac{(y - 5)^2}{4} = 1$$

The only difference between this equation and the equations of ellipses seen above is that x has been replaced by $(x-4)$ and y by $(y-5)$. In order to see how this change affects the graph, it may be helpful to recall the similar situation with circles:

the circle $x^2 + y^2 = 1$ has center $(0, 0)$, but

the circle $(x - 4)^2 + (y - 5)^2 = 1$ has center $(4, 5)$.

The same phenomenon occurs here, so that the graph of the equation

$$\frac{(x - 4)^2}{3^2} + \frac{(y - 5)^2}{2^2} = 1$$

is an ellipse with center $(4, 5)$, as shown in Figure 3-44. The numbers 3 and 2 in the denominators of the equation tell us that the ellipse extends 3 units to the right and to the left of the center $(4, 5)$ and that it extends 2 units above and below the center.

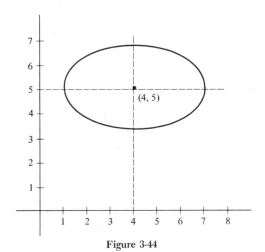

Figure 3-44

EXAMPLE The equation $2x^2 - y^2 + 4x + 6y - 11 = 0$ can be written

$$2(x^2 + 2x) - (y^2 - 6y) = 11$$

Completing the square in $x^2 - 2x$ and $y^2 - 6y$ (and adding the same amount to the right side of the equation) yields:

$$2(x^2 + 2x + 1) - (y^2 - 6y + 9) = 11 + 2 + (-9)$$
$$2(x + 1)^2 - (y - 3)^2 = 4$$
$$\frac{(x + 1)^2}{2} - \frac{(y - 3)^2}{4} = 1$$
$$\frac{(x - (-1))^2}{2} - \frac{(y - 3)^2}{4} = 1$$

The last equation shows that the graph is a hyperbola with center $(-1, 3)$, as shown in Figure 3-45 on the next page.

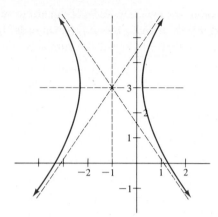

Figure 3-45

EXAMPLE Consider the equation $x^2 - y^2 = 0$. We can factor the left side and obtain $(x + y)(x - y) = 0$. Since a product is zero only when one of the factors is zero, the equation $(x + y)(x - y) = 0$ is equivalent to

$$x + y = 0 \qquad \text{or} \qquad x - y = 0$$

Thus the graph consists of all (x, y) that are solutions of *either* of the linear equations $x + y = 0$ or $x - y = 0$. Therefore the graph consists of two straight lines, as shown in Figure 3-46.

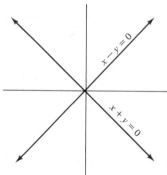

Figure 3-46

The examples above all dealt with the equations $Ax^2 + By^2 + Cxy + Dx + Ey + F = 0$ in which $C = 0$. If the coefficient of xy is nonzero, then the graph is usually a conic which is rotated from its standard position. Trigonometry is often needed to deal effectively with rotation of axes and the graphs of such equations.

EXERCISES

A.1. Find the center and radius of each of the circles whose equations are:
    (a) $x^2 + y^2 + 8x - 6y - 15 = 0$ (e) $x^2 + y^2 + 25x + 10y + 12 = 0$
    (b) $15x^2 + 15y^2 = 10$ (f) $3x^2 + 3y^2 + 12 - 18y + 12 = 0$
    (c) $x^2 + y^2 + 6x - 4y - 15 = 0$ (g) $2x^2 + 2y^2 + x - y - 3 = 0$
    (d) $x^2 + y^2 + 10x - 75 = 0$ (h) $5x^2 + 5y^2 + 30y = 0$

B.1. **(a)** Find the equation, center, and radius of the circle that passes through $(1, 0)$, $(-1, 0)$, and $(0, 2)$. [*Hint:* the equation must be of the form $x^2 + y^2 + Dx + Ey + F = 0$. Since $(1, 0)$ satisfies the equation, we must have $1 + 0 + D + E \cdot 0 + F = 0$, or equivalently, $D + F = -1$. Similarly, since $(-1, 0)$ and $(0, 2)$ are also solutions, we have $-D + F = -1$ and $2E + F = -4$. Solve these three equations for D, E, and F. Then use the usual completing-the-square technique to find the center and radius.]

(b) Do the same for the circle that passes through $(0, 0)$, $(1, 0)$, and $(2, 1)$.

(c) Do the same for the circle that passes through $(0, 5)$, $(2, 5)$, and $(2, -1)$.

(d) Do the same for the circle that passes through $(-1, -2)$, $(1, -1)$, and $(0, 0)$.

B.2. Graph these equations. [*Hint:* first complete the square in x and y (if necessary), then follow the pattern illustrated in the last three examples above.]

(a) $\dfrac{(x - 1)^2}{4} + \dfrac{(y - 5)^2}{9} = 1$

(d) $4x^2 - y^2 + 8x - 4y - 4 = 0$

(b) $x^2 - 16y^2 = 0$

(e) $9x^2 + 4y^2 + 54x - 8y + 49 = 0$

(c) $\dfrac{(y + 3)^2}{25} - \dfrac{(x + 1)^2}{16} = 1$

(f) $9x^2 - 4y^2 + 54x + 8y + 45 = 0$

5. GRAPH READING

In Sections 3 and 4 we showed how to translate certain algebraic statements (first- and second-degree equations and inequalities) into equivalent graphical pictures. In this section we shall move in the other direction and translate graphical information into equivalent verbal or algebraic statements. There are no hard and fast rules for handling all such "graph reading" situations, so we shall present several varied examples.

EXAMPLE The graph in Figure 3-47 shows the distance traveled by a car during an hour's time.

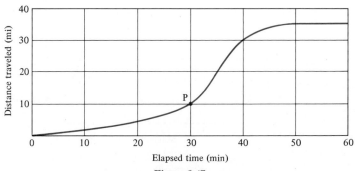

Figure 3-47

For example, the point $(30, 10)$ is on the graph. This indicates that after 30 minutes (min), the car has traveled 10 miles (mi). The question,

How many miles does the car travel in the first 40 min?

can be answered by examining the point on the graph with first coordinate 40 (representing the elapsed time of 40 min). This point is (40, 30). Therefore the car traveled 30 mi in the first 40 min. The question,

How long does it take the car to travel the first 5 mi?

requires some careful measurement to answer. If you examine the point on the graph with *second* coordinate 5 (representing 5 mi traveled) you will see that it is (approximately) the point (20,5). Therefore it took 20 min to travel the first 5 mi. The graph also provides the answer to this question:

Does the car ever stop during the hour? If so, for how long?

Observe that the point (50, 35) is on the graph, meaning that after 50 min the car has traveled 35 mi. But the graph is *horizontal* to the right of this point, so that every point on the graph to the right of (50, 35) has the same second coordinate, 35. This means that at every time from 50 min to 60 min, the total distance traveled remained 35 mi. In other words, the car did not move during the 10-min period from 50 to 60 min. Finally,

During what 10-min period was the car traveling at the fastest speed?

In the 10-min period from 30 to 40 min the graph rises more steeply than in any other 10-min period. This means that a greater distance was traveled during this 10-min period than during any other one (why?). But a greater distance can be traveled in the same length of time only by going at a faster rate. Therefore the speed was fastest from 30 to 40 min. In fact, it was too fast for safety: the graph shows that the car has traveled 10 mi after 30 min and 30 mi after 40 min. Thus it traveled 20 mi during that 10 min period. But 20 mi per 10 min is equivalent to 120 miles per hour.

EXAMPLE The weather bureau has a device which records the temperature over the 24 hr of a given day in the form of a graph (Figure 3-48). Time is measured in hours after midnight along the horizontal axis.

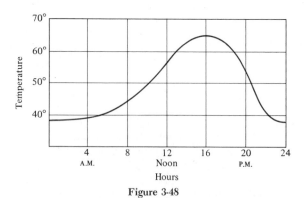

Figure 3-48

This graph can be used to answer several questions, including:

At what times during the day was the temperature 40° or more?

Any time at which the temperature is 40° or more is represented on the graph by a point whose *second* coordinate is ≥ 40. Thus the time period when the temperature was 40° or more is the period during which the graph lies on or above the horizontal line through 40°. An examination of the graph shows that it lies on or above this line (approximately) from 5:24 A.M. ($= 5\frac{2}{5}$ hr after midnight) to 10:00 P.M. ($= 22$ hr after midnight).°

> *During what period did the temperature rise most slowly?*

We can't answer this question exactly, but we can give a reasonable estimate. The graph is almost horizontal from midnight to 4:00 A.M., but rises very slightly during this time interval. This means that at 4:00 A.M. the temperature was only a tiny bit higher than at midnight. No other portion of the graph is both rising and so close to horizontal. So this is the period during which the temperature rose most slowly.

EXAMPLE   At a city reservoir water is let in at one end and out at the other. At each of these two gates there is a meter measuring the *rate* at which the water is flowing in or out (in gallons per hr). The two graphs in Figure 3-49 record the incoming and outgoing rate of flow at any time from noon to 5:00 P.M.

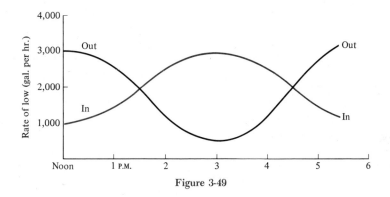

Figure 3-49

First question:

> *If you watch the reservoir from noon to 1:00 P.M.,*
> *what change do you see in the water level?*

Note that the water level will rise if more water is coming in than going out and it will fall if more water is going out than in. Figure 2-13 shows that between noon and 1:00 the outflow graph lies above the inflow graph. This means that at any time from noon to 1:00, water was flowing out at a greater rate than it was flowing in. Therefore the water level in the reservoir was *falling* during this hour.

> *At what time between 2:00 and 4:00 P.M. is the water level*
> *in the reservoir rising at the fastest rate?*

° The measurements here and below were made on the original hand-drawn graphs. Consequently they may occasionally differ slightly from measurements made on the printed graph that appears here.

At any given time the difference between the inflow rate and the outflow rate is the rate at which the amount of water in the reservoir is increasing. When this difference is greatest, the water level will be rising at the fastest rate. Between 2:00 and 4:00 P.M. the inflow graph is always above the outflow graph, so the water level is rising. The vertical distance between the two graphs is greatest at approximately 3:00 P.M. This means that at 3:00 P.M. the rate at which the water in the reservoir is increasing, and hence the rate at which the water level is rising, is greatest.

EXERCISES

C.1. A certain mathematics class recently turned in a six-problem homework assignment. Each problem was graded either right or wrong (no partial credit!), so the number of correct problems a student did was one of these numbers: 0, 1, 2, 3, 4, 5, or 6. The graph in Figure 3-50 shows how many students got 0, 1, 2, 3, 4, 5, or 6 correct problems. For example, the point $(1, 4)$ indicates that 4 students got only 1 problem correct.

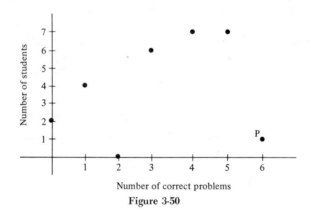

Figure 3-50

(a) How many people got exactly four correct problems?
(b) Find a number x so that exactly two students have x correct problems.
(c) How many students got less than three problems correct?
(d) If exactly one student got t correct answers, then what is t?
(e) How many students got more than four problems correct?
(f) How many students handed in this assignment?

C.2. The Pink Chopper Company produces motorbikes especially designed to please those people between 18 and 21 years old. In order to estimate the demand for motorbikes in the years to come, the company uses the graph in Figure 3-51. It shows the expected population of the 18–21 age group in future years.

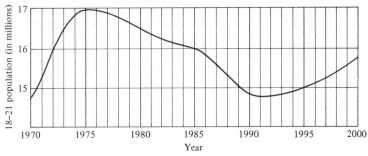

Figure 3-51

(a) How many 18–21 year olds are there in 1980?

(b) How many 18–21 year olds will there be in 1984? in 1988? in 1992?

(c) Find a year in which the population of 18–21 year olds is 16 million.

(d) Find all years in which the population of 18–21 year olds is *less* than 15 million.

(e) If from one year to the next, the number of 18–21 year olds increases, the demand for motorbikes will probably also increase and the Pink Chopper Company will have to make plans ahead of time to increase production. Similarly, if from one year to the next the number of 18–21 year olds decreases, the Pink Chopper Company must make plans to decrease production. With this in mind, indicate in the following table whether production has to be increased or decreased in the next year.

Year	Increased	Decreased
1982		
1988		
1990		
1995		

(f) It takes three years to ge a new plant ready for production of motorbikes. In which years would it be a definite mistake to start construction of a new plant? Explain.

C.3. The graphs in Figure 3-52 on the next page show the price per share of four stocks during the period from March 1 to June 1.

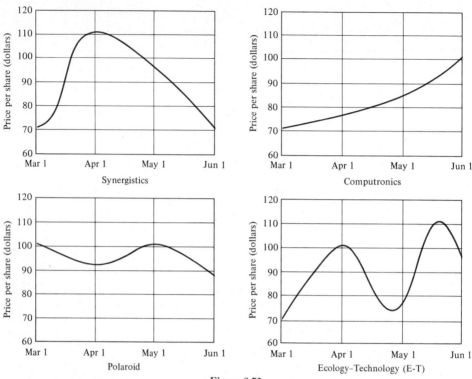

Figure 3-52

In the questions below, when we speak of "holding" a given stock over some time period we mean to buy the stock at the beginning of the period and sell it at the end.

(a) For maximum profit, would Computronics or E-T have been a better holding over the period March 1 to June 1?

(b) The increase in the price per share for Computronics from March 1 to June 1 is the same as the increase in price per share of E-T from March 1 to April 1. Is there any basis for arguing that holding Computronics for the three months is better or worse than holding E-T for one? Explain.

(c) Synergistics did not do well over the three-month period while Computronics did very well. On the other hand, is there some 10-day period when a holding of Synergistics would have brought more profit than any 10-day period of Computronics? Explain.

(d) The graphs are not sufficiently detailed to calculate profits or losses for holding periods of three days in length. However, is there something about the shapes of these graphs to justify holding one stock for three days rather than another stock? Explain.

C.4. The graph in Figure 3-53 gives the cost of producing a certain number of items. The items bear serial numbers in the order they are produced, the first one bearing the number 1. At 0 the curve shows $1000, meaning that the fixed costs for rent, equipment, and so on, are $1000 even if no items are produced.

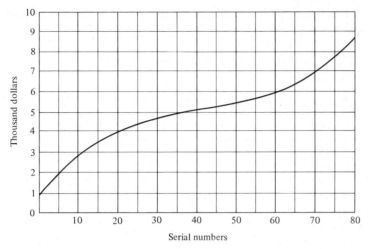

Figure 3-53

(a) How many items can you produce if you want to spend $5000?
(b) What is the cost of producing the items numbered 35 through 80?
(c) What is the average cost per item of the first 25 items? the first 45 items?
(d) What is the average cost of items 25 through 45?
(e) Which consecutively numbered 20 items cost the most to produce? Which cost the least? How can you decide this question with your ruler?
(f) Suppose you want to stop production when the average cost per item is least. At which serial number would you have to stop?

C.5. Two cars start a trip at the same time, but from opposite ends of a 40-mi-long road. The distance traveled after time t is graphed for each car in Figure 3-54.

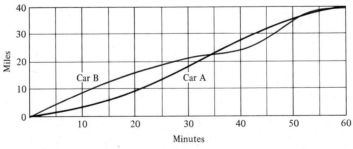

Figure 3-54

(a) How far did car A travel in the first 25 min?
(b) How long did it take car A to travel the first 25 mi?
(c) How far did car B travel between 15 and 30 min after start?

(d)   Over which 10-min interval did car A cover the most distance? and car B?

(e)   What was the average speed (in miles per minute) for car A over the entire trip? for car B?

(f)   What was the average speed for car A over the time interval from 10 to 35 min after start? And for car B?

(g)   Over which 10-min interval did car A have the greatest average speed? And car B? How can you decide this question quickly with a ruler?

(h)   How far had car A traveled in the first 10 min? And car B? How far were they apart after the first 10 min of travel? How far apart were they after the first 15 min?

C.6.   A gauge is attached to the city water reservoir which measures the depth of the water. City water officials can then figure out how much water is in the reservoir. Water is being pumped both in and out of the reservoir so that the water level may rise if the water is being pumped in faster than it is being pumped out, or the water level may fall if the water is being pumped out faster than it is being pumped in. The graph in Figure 3-55 shows the recorded depths over a 12-hr period.

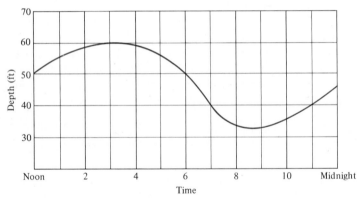

Figure 3-55

(a)   Give the change in the depth for the following time periods:

(i)   noon to 3:00. [Solution: the depth at noon is 50 feet (ft) and the depth at 3:00 is 60 ft. The *change* in the depth would be (60 ft − 50 ft) or 10 ft.]

(ii)   noon to 2:00.   (iii)   noon to 6:00.   (iv)   7:00 to midnight.

(b)   Name the 1-hr period (that is, from 1:00 to 2:00, or 4:00 to 5:00, and so forth) in which the amount of change was the greatest. Name the 1-hr period in which the amount of change was the least.

(c)   The actual change in depth between noon and 3:00 was 10 ft. The actual change in depth between 7:30 and midnight was also 10 ft. Is it possible to compare the *rates* of change over these two time periods? In which of these two time periods would you say that the rate of change was the greatest, or in other words, over which time period did the water level rise the fastest? Explain.

(**d**) The actual change in depth between noon and 2:00 was 8 ft, and the change between 10:00 and 11:00 was 4 ft. Can you compare the rates of change in these two time periods? Does one rate of change seem bigger than the other, or are they about the same? Explain.

(**e**) The change in depth was 26 ft between 3:00 and 8:00. Can you find some 1-hr period between 3:00 and 8:00 where the *rate* of change over the 1-hr period is the same as the *rate* of change between 3:00 and 8:00? If so, which period? Can you find a 1-hr period where the rate of change over that hour is less than the rate of change from 3:00 to 8:00? If so, which period?

Functions

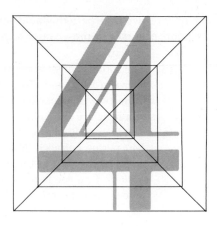

You have probably seen the term "function" before. Nevertheless, you may feel that you don't really understand just *what* a function is or *why* functions are important. Both the what and the why of functions are explained in detail in this chapter.

1. FUNCTIONS

There are many situations in which two numerical quantities depend on each other, or vary with each other, or determine each other. The following three examples of such situations will be used continually throughout this chapter and will be referred to by the numbers used here.

EXAMPLE 1 In a certain state, the amount of state income tax you pay depends on your income.° The income determines the tax. Here the two numerical quantities are:

(i)   the income; and
(ii) the amount of tax.

The way the income determines the tax is laid down by law.

° For simplicity we assume that this particular state bases its income tax on your entire income, regardless of number of dependents, source of income, federal taxes, or other factors.

EXAMPLE 2   Weather stations have a device which records the temperature over the 24 hours of a day in the form of a graph (Figure 4-1).

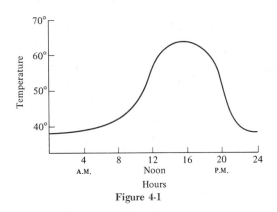

Figure 4-1

Here the two numerical quantities are

   (i)   the hours of the day, that is, the time elapsed since midnight; and
   (ii)   the temperature.

The way time and temperature are related to each other is indicated by the height of the graph over the horizontal axis. The height of the graph at 12 noon is the temperature at noon. The temperature at 6:06 P.M. (that is, 18.1 hr after midnight) is the height of the graph at 18.1, and so on.

EXAMPLE 3   You drop a rock straight down and want to know how far the rock will have fallen after 1 second, 2 seconds, 3 seconds, and so on. Here the two numerical quantities are

   (i)   the time elapsed after you drop the rock; and
   (ii)   the distance the rock has traveled.

The way in which the distance traveled depends on the time elapsed is given by a formula discovered by physicists: after t sec, the rock has traveled $16t^2$ ft.

   The three preceding examples deal with things very much *different* from each other:

Income and income tax.
Times of the day and temperature.
How far a rock has traveled after so many seconds.

However, the examples also have important *common* features. The first is that

   In each example, we have two sets of numbers.

This is indicated in the following chart:

	Set 1	Set 2
Example 1	All possible incomes	All possible amounts of tax
Example 2	The various times of the day	The various possible temperatures
Example 3	The seconds elapsed after dropping the rock	The distances the rock has traveled

The second common feature of our three examples is that

In each example, there is a very definite way in which an element of set 1 determines an element of set 2, or, alternatively, in which an element of set 2 is associated with an element of set 1.

For instance,

The income determines the income tax by law (Example 1).

The device measures and registers the temperature at any given time of the day (Example 2).

The formula of the physicists predicts how far the rock has traveled in any span of time (Example 3).

Let us call any such situation with these two features a **functional situation.** By the word "functional" we want to express such ideas as:

The tax is a *function* of, or *depends* on, the income (Example 1).

The location of the needle recording the temperature *varies* according to the time (Example 2).

The distance traveled is *determined* by the time elapsed (Example 3).

Instead of studying each functional situation *separately,* the mathematician focuses on the *common* features of the various functional situations. His or her goal is to design tools to handle *all* functional situations simultaneously. For this, the mathematician must strip the different functional situations of their connections with time, tax, temperature, and so on, and deal only with what is common to all functional situations.

For the mathematician,

A *function* consists of three items:

(*i*)   a set of numbers, called the **domain.**
(*ii*) another set of numbers, called the **range.**
(*iii*) a **rule** that assigns to each number in the domain one and only
        one *number in the range.*

The domain corresponds to Set 1 and the range to Set 2 in the three examples above.

EXAMPLE 1   The *domain* is the set of all possible incomes. The *range* is the set of all possible tax amounts. The *rule* is the law that decrees the amount of tax to be paid on each income.

EXAMPLE 2   The *domain* is the set of various times during the day (measured in hours after midnight), that is, all real numbers from 0 to 24. The *range* is the set of possible temperatures. The *rule* is the graphical temperature record, which shows the temperature at any given time during the day.

EXAMPLE 3   The *domain* consists of the possible numbers of seconds elapsed after dropping the rock, that is, the set of all nonnegative real numbers.° The *range* is the set of possible distances traveled by the rock, that is, the set of all nonnegative real numbers.° The *rule* is the physical law discovered by the physicists:

$$\text{distance} = 16t^2 \text{ ft, where } t = \text{time elapsed in seconds}$$

You should be sure you understand the meaning of the phrase *"one and only one"* in the description of the rule of a function [item (iii) in the box above]:

EXAMPLE 1   For a particular income—say, $7500—there is *exactly* one tax amount. Indeed, a tax law that said something like "the tax on $7500 is $155 or $187 or $210" would be ludicrous. For each income (number in the domain), there is *one and only one* tax amount (number in the range).

EXAMPLE 2   At a specific time during the day—say, 12:00 noon, the temperature is exactly 56°. It is impossible to have two different temperatures at the same time. In other words, for each time (number in the domain), there is *one and only one* temperature (number in the range).

Notice, however, that it is quite possible to have the *same temperature* at two *different times.* For instance, the graph on page 173 shows that the temperature is 56° at

---

° We assume here, for convenience, that the rock can drop infinitely far. In actual practice, there would be some maximum distance and hence some maximum time.

12:00 noon and at 7:30 P.M. (= 19.5 hours after midnight). In this case, two different numbers in the domain (times) are associated with the same number in the range (temperature).

Example 3 and some further aspects of this topic are discussed in Exercises B.2–B.4. For now we can summarize the discussion as follows:

> *The rule of a function assigns to each number in the domain* one and only one *number in the range. But the rule may possibly assign to two (or more)* different *numbers in the domain the* same *number in the range.*

Functions in the abstract sense just discussed (domain, range, rule) are at the core of all functional situations. Thus the *motivation* for studying functions is the fact that particular concrete functional situations (such as those in Examples 1–3) regularly occur in the real world. But the *manner* in which functions are actually studied by mathematicians is something else again.

The mathematician usually restricts his or her view to the abstract concept of a function. The typical mathematics text rarely discusses just how or why a particular function might be connected with (or arise from) some concrete functional situation. It deals almost exclusively with properties of functions that are common to all functional situations.

In this book we shall try to remind you regularly of the origin of functions in real-life situations. But you will also have to get accustomed to dealing with functions as entities in themselves, independent of possible interpretations in concrete situations.

EXAMPLE   The rule of the **identity function** assigns to each real number the number itself. Thus 4 is assigned to 4, -7 to -7, $\pi + 3$ to $\pi + 3$,   and so on. The domain of the identity function is the set of all real numbers; the range is the same set.

EXAMPLE   The domain of the **absolute value function** is the set of all real numbers. Its rule assigns to each real number x the number $|x|$. For instance,

$$|-6| = 6 \text{ is assigned to } -6.$$
$$|\pi - 3| = \pi - 3 \text{ is assigned to } \pi - 3.$$

Since $|x| \geq 0$ for every number x, the range is the set of all nonnegative real numbers, that is, the interval $[0, \infty)$.

EXAMPLE   The function whose rule assigns to every real number the number 6 is called a **constant function**. Its domain is the set of all real numbers; its range consists of the single number 6. More generally, if c is a fixed real number, then there is a constant function whose rule assigns to each real number the number c.

EXAMPLE   For each real number s let $[s]$ denote the *integer* which is closest to s on the *left* side of s on the number line. If s is itself an integer, we define $[s] = s$. Some examples are given in Figure 4-2.

$$[-4.7] = -5 \qquad [-3] = -3 \qquad [-1.5] = -2 \qquad [0] = 0 \qquad [\tfrac{5}{3}] = 1 \qquad [\pi] = 3$$

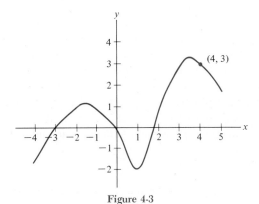

Figure 4-2

The function whose domain is the set of all real numbers and whose rule is:

assign to the real number x the integer $[x]$

is called the **greatest integer function.** The range of the greatest integer function is the set of all integers.

EXAMPLE   The graph in Figure 4-3

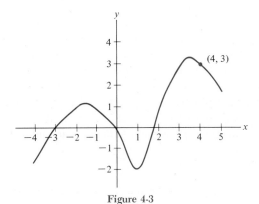

Figure 4-3

defines a function whose domain is the interval $[-4, 5]$ and whose rule is:

Assign to a number x the number y such that (x, y) lies on the graph.

For instance, the rule assigns to 4 the number 3 since $(4, 3)$ is on the graph. Since all the second coordinates of points on the graph lie between -2 and 3.3, the range of this function is the interval $[-2, 3.3]$.

   Warning Not every graph defines a function in this way. See Exercises B.6 and B.7.

   Remark The definition of "function" given in this section assumes that the elements of both the domain and the range are real numbers. Consequently, such a function is sometimes called a **real-valued function of a real variable.** The vast majority of the functions you will encounter in this book and in calculus are of this type. However, the term "function" can be defined in a more general way by allowing the domain or range (or both) to consist of elements other than real numbers.

EXERCISES

A.1. **(a)** The notation $[r]$ used here is explained in the Example of the greatest integer function on page 177. In each of the following statements, give examples of two pairs of numbers for which the statement is true and two pairs for which it is false:

    (i) $[u + v] = [u]$;   (ii) $[r] + [s] < [r + s]$;   (iii) $[st] > [s][t]$.

  (b) Evaluate $[-\frac{4}{3}]$, $[-\frac{10}{3}]$, $[-16\frac{1}{2}]$, $[.75]$, $[6.75]$, $[-9]$, $[\frac{2}{3}]$.

B.1. Each of the following functional situations involves at least one function. Verbally describe the domain, range, and rule of each such function, providing there is sufficient information to do so. For example,

> *Situation:* Harry Hamburger owns a professional baseball team. He decides that the only factor to be considered in determining a player's salary for this year is his batting average last season. *Function:* Salaries are a function of batting averages. *Domain:* All possible batting averages. *Range:* All possible salaries. *Rule:* There isn't enough information given to determine the rule.

  (a) The area of a circle depends on its radius.
  (b) If you drive your car at a constant rate of 55 mph, then your distance from the starting point varies with the time elapsed.
  (c) When more is spent on advertising at Grump's Department Store, sales increase. If less is spent on advertising, sales drop.
  (d) A widget manufacturer has a contract to produce widgets at a price of $1 each. His profit per widget is determined by the cost of manufacturing the widget. (Note that if it costs more than one dollar to make a widget, he loses money; interpret such a loss as "negative profit.") Find an algebraic formula for the rule of this function.

B.2. In Example 1 of the text, suppose that the state income tax law reads as follows:

Annual Income	Amount of Tax
Less than $2000	0
$2000–$6000	2% of income over $2000
More than $6000	$80 plus 5% of income over $6000

  (a) Find the number in the range (tax amount) that is assigned to each of the following numbers in the domain (incomes):

    $500, $1509, $3754, $6783, $12,500, $55,342

  (b) Find four different numbers in the domain of this function that are associated with the same number in the range.

(c) Explain why your answer in part (b) does *not* contradict item (iii) in the definition of a function (in the box on page 175).

(d) Is it possible to do part (b) if all four numbers in the domain are required to be greater than 2000? Why or why not?

B.3. The amount of postage required to mail a first-class letter is determined by its weight. In this situation, is weight a function of postage? or vice-versa? or both?

B.4. Some (but not all) functions have the following property: any two different numbers in the domain are always assigned to different numbers in the range. Such functions are said to be **one-to-one** or **injective.**

(a) Show that the function in Example 3 of the text *is* one-to-one; that is, two different numbers in the domain (times) are always assigned to two different numbers in the range (distances). (This may be intuitively clear to you, but give a mathematical argument, using the formula of the physicists.)

(b) Give examples of two functions which are *not* one-to-one. [Hint: see Exercise B.2.(b) for one.]

(c) Give another example of a function which *is* one-to-one.

B.5. Could the following statement ever be the rule of a function?

Assign to a number x in the domain the number in the range whose square is x.

Why or why not? If there is a function with this rule, what is its domain and range?

B.6. Each of the graphs in Figure 4-4 defines a function as in the Example on page 177. In each case,

(i) State the domain and range of the function.

(ii) By measuring as carefully as you can, state what numbers in the range the function assigns to each of the following numbers in the domain: -2, -1, 0, $\frac{1}{2}$, $\frac{3}{2}$.

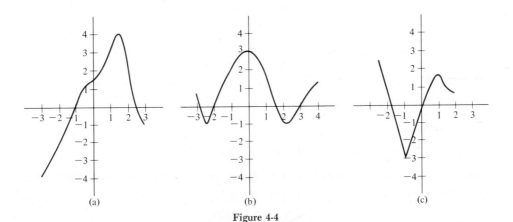

(a)   (b)   (c)

Figure 4-4

B.7.   Explain why *none* of the graphs in Figure 4-5 defines a function according to the procedure in Exercise B.6. What goes wrong?

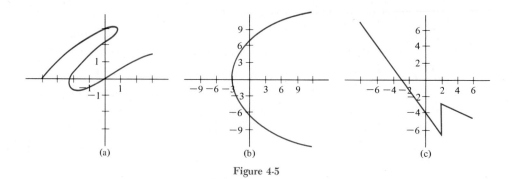

(a)   (b)   (c)

Figure 4-5

2. FUNCTIONAL NOTATION

Like most mathematical symbolism, functional notation has its origins in real-life situations. It was developed in such functional situations in order to facilitate discussion and analysis of various problems. Examples 1–3 of Section 1 provide good illustrations of the need for and development of functional notation. So we begin with them.

EXAMPLE 1—INCOME TAX   In a certain state, the income tax is determined by the following law.

If the Annual Income Is	Then the Amount of Income Tax Is
Less than $2000	0
$2000–$6000	2% of income over $2000
More than $6000	$80 plus 5% of income over $6000

Let's write i for the income (in dollars). The tax due on income i will be written $T(i)$, which is read "T of i." The T indicates "tax" and the i in parentheses indicates that the tax depends on, or varies with, the income i. In this way, the long sentence,

The income tax on an income of $5512 is $70.24,

is abbreviated as

$$T(5512) = 70.24$$

which is read "T of 5512 equals 70.24." Similarly, if your income is $12,500, then according to the table above the income tax is $405. So we write

$$T(12,500) = 405$$

which is *read* "*T* of 12,500 equals 405" and *means*

The income tax on an income of $12,500 is $405.

Note 1 There is nothing that forces us to choose the letters *i* and *T* as abbreviations. We might just as well have chosen α for income and *s* for tax and written $s(\alpha)$:

Any choice of letters or symbols will do, provided we make clear what is meant by the letters or symbols chosen.

Note 2 The symbol $T(i)$ is to be treated as *one* thing. The parentheses are *not* the parentheses of elementary algebra, as in the equation

$$3(a + b) = 3a + 3b.$$

The parentheses in $T(i)$ express the fact that the amount *T* of tax is forced upon us by the income *i*. For example,

$$T(236.14 + 8750)$$

stands for the amount of tax due on an income of $236.14 + $8750 = $8986.14.

EXAMPLE 2—TEMPERATURE Write *t* for the time elapsed (in hours since midnight) and tem for temperature. Then tem(*t*) represents the temperature at time *t*. The sentence,

At 11:30 A.M. the temperature was 52°,

is now written

$$\text{tem}(11.5) = 52$$

which is read

tem of 11.5 equals 52

Since time in this example is measured in hours after midnight, 3:15 P.M. is written as 15.25 hr after midnight. Thus the sentence,

At 3:15 P.M. the temperature was 63°,

is the same as the sentence,

At 15.25 hr after midnight the temperature was 63°,

which is abbreviated

$$\text{tem}(15.25) = 63.$$

EXAMPLE 3—FALLING ROCK Let *t* denote the time (in seconds) after the rock is released. As we saw in Section 1, the physicists have found a formula to compute the distance (in feet) the rock has traveled after *t* sec, namely, $16t^2$. Let $d(t)$ denote the distance (in feet) the rock has traveled after *t* sec [so that $d(t) = 16t^2$]. In functional notation the sentence,

After 1 sec the rock has traveled 16 ft,

is written

$$d(1) = 16$$

Similarly, $d(4) = 256$ means that "after 4 sec the rock has traveled 256 ft." The sentence, "After 5 sec the rock has traveled 400 ft," is written $d(5) = 400$.

Note 1   The formula for computing the distance traveled $d(t)$ after t sec is

$$d(t) = 16t^2$$

Suppose we had chosen different letters, say, the Greek letter θ for time and F for distance. Then the *same* formula reads:

$$F(\theta) = 16\theta^2$$

The letters here are not important. What matters is the information they convey. Both formulas, $d(t) = 16t^2$ and $F(\theta) = 16\theta^2$, describe exactly the same function, namely, the function that assigns to any number the number obtained by squaring the original number and then multiplying this result by 16.

Note 2   Once again, the parentheses in the symbol "$d(t)$" do *not* indicate multiplication. For instance,

$$d(1 + 4) \neq d(1) + d(4)$$

For $d(1)$ is the "distance traveled after 1 sec," namely, 16 ft; $d(4)$ is the "distance traveled after 4 sec," namely, 256 ft. Thus

$$d(1) + d(4) = 16 + 256 = 272$$

But $d(1 + 4)$ is the "distance traveled after $1 + 4 = 5$ sec," namely, 400 ft. Thus

$$d(1 + 4) = 400, \qquad \text{but} \qquad d(1) + d(4) = 272$$

MORE FUNCTIONAL NOTATION

In Examples 1–3 above, functional notation was used to abbreviate certain sentences in the English language. We now want to adapt this convenient shorthand notation to the usual mathematical setting, where the particulars of time, temperature, distance, and so on, are eliminated. In this abstract situation we don't deal with sentences such as, "At 11:30 the temperature was 52°," but there *are* sentences which can be conveniently abbreviated by a similar sort of functional notation.

Let the letter x represent a number in the domain of a function and y a number in the range. Denote the function by the letter f. In functional notation, the sentence,

> The rule of the function f assigns to the number
> x in the domain the number y in the range,

is written

$$f(x) = y \qquad \text{[or equivalently, } y = f(x)\text{]}$$

which is read

$$f \text{ of } x \text{ equals } y \qquad \text{[or equivalently, } y \text{ equals } f \text{ of } x\text{]}$$

EXAMPLE $f(5) = 7$ (read "f of 5 equals 7") means "the rule of the function f assigns to the number 5 in the domain the number 7 in the range."

Sometimes just the symbol $f(x)$ (read "f of x") is used alone. Consistent with the usage above,

> f(x) *denotes the number in the range which is assigned to the* *number* x *in the domain by the rule of the function* f.

EXAMPLE $f(-6)$ denotes the number in the range which is assigned to the number -6 in the domain by the rule of the function f.

The meaning of the symbols $f(x)$ and $y = f(x)$ as just explained differs slightly from the way functional notation was used in Examples 1–3 above. But the basic idea is the same:

> *Functional notation is just a convenient shorthand for phrases and* *sentences in the English language.*

Once they have made a careful definition, most mathematicians tend to become quite casual about their language. Instead of the precise sentence,

> The rule of the function f assigns to the number
> x in the domain the number y in the range,

or its symbolic abbreviation $y = f(x)$, you are quite likely to hear one or more of the following statements. Each of them is intended to mean *exactly the same thing* as the precise sentence above:

> The **value of the function** f at x is y.
> The **value** of f at x is y.
> The function f **maps** x to y.
> y is the **image** of x under (the function) f

Similarly, the number $f(x)$ in the range which is assigned to the number x in the domain by the rule of the function f is sometimes called

"the **value** (of the function) f at x," or
"the **image** of x (under the function f)."

There is nothing sacred about the letters x, y, and f. Just as in Examples 1–3 above, *we are free to choose any letters we want,* so long as we clearly explain their meanings. You can frequently reconstruct from the circumstances which letters have been used for domain, range, and rule. In particular, there are several **universally used conventions for interpreting certain algebraic expressions as functions,** as illustrated in the following examples.

EXAMPLE   An algebraic formula, such as

$$f(x) = \sqrt{x + 1}$$

is understood to denote a function f, as follows. The letter x denotes an element of the domain. The *rule* of the function f is understood to assign to the number x in the domain, the number $\sqrt{x + 1}$ in the range. For instance,

$$f(2) = \sqrt{2 + 1} = \sqrt{3} \text{ is the number assigned to } 2$$
$$f(-1) = \sqrt{-1 + 1} = 0 \text{ is the number assigned to } -1$$
$$f(\pi + 3) = \sqrt{(\pi + 3) + 1} = \sqrt{\pi + 4} \text{ is the number assigned to } \pi + 3$$

The *domain* of the function f is determined by this convention:

> *Unless specific information to the contrary is given, the domain of a function* f *is taken to be the set consisting of every real number for which the rule of* f *produces a well-defined real number.*

In this case, $\sqrt{x + 1}$ is a well-defined real number only when

$$x + 1 \geq 0 \qquad \text{or equivalently} \qquad x \geq -1$$

Consequently, the domain of this function is the set of all real numbers that are ≥ -1, that is, the interval $[-1, \infty)$. The *range* of this function is some set of real numbers. For most purposes in this course and in calculus, it is not necessary to specify the range more precisely. Consequently, we shall often omit any mention of the range. Determining the domain, however, is often essential.

EXAMPLE   The expression

$$h(u) = \frac{u^2 + 3}{u^2 - 9u + 20}$$

is understood to define a function (denoted h) whose rule is: assign to a number u in the domain the number $\dfrac{u^2 + 3}{u^2 - 9u + 20}$ in the range. For example,

$$h(-2) = \frac{(-2)^2 + 3}{(-2)^2 - 9(-2) + 20} = \frac{4 + 3}{4 + 18 + 20} = \frac{7}{42} = \frac{1}{6}$$

Since no contrary information is given, the domain consists of all real numbers for which $\dfrac{u^2 + 3}{u^2 - 9u + 20}$ is a well-defined real number. The only time when $\dfrac{u^2 + 3}{u^2 - 9u + 20}$ is *not* a real number occurs when the denominator $u^2 - 9u + 20$ is zero. Note that $u^2 - 9u + 20 = (u - 4)(u - 5)$. Clearly, this expression is 0 precisely when $u = 4$ or $u = 5$ and is nonzero for all other values of u. Therefore, the domain of the function h is the set of all real numbers, *except* 4 and 5.

EXAMPLE   An expression such as

$$y = t^3 + 6t^2 - 5, \qquad t \geq 0$$

is understood to define a function whose rule is: assign to a number t in the domain the number $t^3 + 6t^2 - 5$ in the range. In this case, we are given the additional information that $t \geq 0$. So the domain of the function is taken to be the set of all real numbers t such that $t^3 + 6t^2 - 5$ is a real number *and* $t \geq 0$. Since $t^3 + 6t^2 - 5$ is a real number whenever t is, the domain consists of all nonnegative real numbers, that is, the interval $[0, \infty)$. Restrictions on the domain, such as $t \geq 0$ here, sometimes occur with functions that arise in practical problems. For instance, negative values of t might not be meaningful in a physical situation where t represents total distance traveled, even though the mathematical rule of the function makes sense for such values.

EXAMPLE   The equation in the preceding example defined a function since for each number t there was one and only one number y that made the equation true. But this isn't always the case. The equation $y^2 = 4t^2$ does *not* define a function as it stands. For instance, if $t = 3$, then $4t^2 = 36$. There are two possible values of y that satisfy $y^2 = 36$, namely, $y = 6$ and $y = -6$. Thus it is not true that each number t in the domain is assigned to *one and only one* number in the range. Therefore, this equation is *not* the rule of a function. On the other hand, the statement $y^2 = 4t^2$ is true exactly when $y = \sqrt{4t^2}$ *or* $y = -\sqrt{4t^2}$. The equation $y = \sqrt{4t^2}$ *does* define a function whose domain is the set of all real numbers and whose rule is: assign to the number t the number $\sqrt{4t^2}$. This function assigns to the number 3 the number $\sqrt{4 \cdot 3^2} = 6$. The equation $y = -\sqrt{4t^2}$ also defines a function whose domain is all real numbers, but it is a *different* function since it has a different rule: assign to each number t the number $-\sqrt{4t^2}$. This function assigns to the number 3 the number -6.

EXAMPLE   The statement

$$f(x) = \begin{cases} 2x + 3 & \text{if } x < 4 \\ x^2 - 1 & \text{if } 4 \leq x \leq 10 \end{cases}$$

defines a function f as follows. The rule of the function assigns to every number x that is *less than* 4 the number $2x + 3$. For instance,

$$f(-50) = 2(-50) + 3 = -97 \qquad \text{and} \qquad f(\tfrac{7}{4}) = 2(\tfrac{7}{4}) + 3 = \tfrac{13}{2}$$

The rule of the function f assigns to every number in the interval $[4, 10]$ the number $x^2 - 1$. For example,

$$f(\tfrac{9}{2}) = (\tfrac{9}{2})^2 - 1 = \tfrac{77}{4} \qquad \text{and} \qquad f(8) = 8^2 - 1 = 63$$

Since the rule of the function is defined only for numbers that are less than or equal to 10, the domain is the interval $(-\infty, 10]$.

Don't let the preceding examples mislead you into thinking that the rule of *every* function is given by an algebraic formula or by several algebraic formulas. For instance, in Example 2 above, where temperature is a function of time, the rule is given by the graph on page 173. It is very unlikely that there is *any* simple algebraic formula to describe this rule.

USING FUNCTIONAL NOTATION

Let f be the function whose rule is

$$f(x) = \sqrt{x^2 + 1}$$

The rule of f can be written in words as:

Assign to a given number the number obtained by squaring the given number, adding 1 to the result, and then taking the square root of this sum.

Keeping this fact in mind will help you to understand such symbols as:

$$f(a), \quad f(a + b), \quad f\left(\frac{1}{a}\right), \quad f(\sqrt{c}), \quad f(c^4)$$

Each of them denotes

The number obtained by applying the rule of the function f to the number in parentheses, namely: square it, add 1, then take the square root of the sum.

Thus

$$f(a) = \sqrt{a^2 + 1}$$
$$f(a + b) = \sqrt{(a + b)^2 + 1} = \sqrt{a^2 + 2ab + b^2 + 1}$$
$$f\left(\frac{1}{a}\right) = \sqrt{\left(\frac{1}{a}\right)^2 + 1} = \sqrt{\frac{1}{a^2} + 1} = \sqrt{\frac{1 + a^2}{a^2}}$$
$$f(\sqrt{c}) = \sqrt{(\sqrt{c})^2 + 1} = \sqrt{c + 1}$$
$$f(c^4) = \sqrt{(c^4)^2 + 1} = \sqrt{c^8 + 1}$$

The very same principle applies to expressions such as

$$f(x - 1), \quad f(x + h), \quad f(x^3), \quad f\left(\frac{1}{x}\right), \quad f(-x)$$

To compute these numbers, proceed as above and *apply the rule of the function to the number in parentheses*. In this case, the rule is $f(x) = \sqrt{x^2 + 1}$; that is, "square it, add 1, take the square root of the sum." Consequently,

$$f(x - 1) = \sqrt{(x - 1)^2 + 1} = \sqrt{x^2 - 2x + 1 + 1} = \sqrt{x^2 - 2x + 2}$$
$$f(x + h) = \sqrt{(x + h)^2 + 1} = \sqrt{x^2 + 2xh + h^2 + 1}$$
$$f(x^3) = \sqrt{(x^3)^2 + 1} = \sqrt{x^6 + 1}$$
$$f\left(\frac{1}{x}\right) = \sqrt{\left(\frac{1}{x}\right)^2 + 1} = \sqrt{\frac{1}{x^2} + 1} = \sqrt{\frac{1 + x^2}{x^2}}$$
$$f(-x) = \sqrt{(-x)^2 + 1} = \sqrt{x^2 + 1}$$

EXAMPLE   Suppose $g(x) = \dfrac{|x + 5|}{x^3}$. Then:

$$g(t) = \frac{|t + 5|}{t^3} \qquad\qquad g(x + h) = \frac{|(x + h) + 5|}{(x + h)^3}$$

$$g(x + 4) = \frac{|(x + 4) + 5|}{(x + 4)^3} \qquad\qquad g(-x) = \frac{|-x + 5|}{(-x)^3}$$

$$g(x + \Delta x) = \frac{|(x + \Delta x) + 5|}{(x + \Delta x)^3} \qquad\qquad g\left(\frac{1}{x}\right) = \frac{|(1/x) + 5|}{(1/x)^3}$$

COMMON MISTAKES WITH FUNCTIONAL NOTATION

Consider the function f whose domain and range are the set of all real numbers and whose rule is: assign to the number x the number x^3. According to the conventions introduced earlier, all this information is contained in the notation

$$f(x) = x^3 \qquad \text{or} \qquad y = x^3$$

Note that each of the symbols

$$f(x), \qquad x^3, \qquad \text{and} \qquad y$$

represents a *number,* namely the number assigned to the number x by the rule of the function. Consequently, all of the following statements are *logically incorrect* even though their intended meaning may seem clear:

> "the function $f(x)$"
> "the function x^3"
> "the function y"

For a *function* is *not* a number; it consists of two sets (domain and range) and a rule that assigns to each number in the domain one and only one number in the range.

Nevertheless, the use of such inaccuracies as "the function $f(x)$" or "the function x^3" or "the function $y = f(x)$" is so widespread that you may as well get accustomed to it. So long as you know that these phrases *are* inaccurate and know the precise statements they represent, you won't have any difficulty.

Similarly, mathematicians often say things like "the function assigns $\sqrt{x + 3}$ to x," meaning that the *rule* of the function assigns $\sqrt{x + 3}$ to x. Once again, there is no problem in understanding what is intended.

Unfortunately, there are more serious mistakes in the use of functional notation. These are not just inaccuracies of language in situations where the intended meaning is clear, but out-and-out *falsehoods.* Usually they result from an attempt to treat functional notation as if it were ordinary algebraic notation, instead of a very specialized *shorthand language.* Here are examples of the most common errors.

Note There may be some functions for which one or more of the statements below are true. But all of these statements are *false* for most functions.

> **MISTAKES:** $f(a + b) = f(a) + f(b)$
> $f(a - b) = f(a) - f(b)$

EXAMPLE If $f(x) = x^2$, then $f(3 + 2) = (3 + 2)^2 = 25$, but $f(3) + f(2) = 3^2 + 2^2 = 9 + 4 = 13$.   Hence $f(3 + 2) \neq f(3) + f(2)$.   Furthermore, $f(3 - 2) = (3 - 2)^2 = 1$, but $f(3) - f(2) = 3^2 - 2^2 = 9 - 4 = 5$, Hence $f(3 - 2) \neq f(3) - f(2)$.

$$\boxed{\textbf{MISTAKE:}\quad f(ab) = f(a)f(b)}$$

EXAMPLE   If $f(x) = x + 7$,   then $f(3 \cdot 4) = (3 \cdot 4) + 7 = 12 + 7 = 19$,   but $f(3)f(4) = (3 + 7)(4 + 7) = 10 \cdot 11 = 110$. Hence $f(3 \cdot 4) \neq f(3)f(4)$.

$$\boxed{\begin{array}{l}\textbf{MISTAKES:}\quad f(ab) = af(b)\\ \phantom{\textbf{MISTAKES:}\quad} f(ab) = bf(a)\end{array}}$$

EXAMPLE   If $f(x) = x^2 + 1$, then $f(2 \cdot 3) = (2 \cdot 3)^2 + 1 = 36 + 1 = 37$, but $2f(3) = 2(3^2 + 1) = 2(10) = 20$ and $3f(2) = 3(2^2 + 1) = 3(5) = 15$.   Hence $f(2 \cdot 3) \neq 2f(3) \neq 3f(2)$.

EXERCISES

A.1. Let f be the function defined by the expression $f(x) = \sqrt{x + 3} - x + 1$. Evaluate:

(a) $f(0)$ (c) $f(\tfrac{5}{2})$ (e) $f(\sqrt{2})$ (g) $f(-2)$
(b) $f(1)$ (d) $f(\pi)$ (f) $f(\sqrt{2} - 1)$ (h) $f(-\tfrac{3}{2})$

A.2. Let h be the function defined by $h(x) = x^2 + \dfrac{1}{x} + 2$. Evaluate:

(a) $h(3)$ (c) $h(\tfrac{3}{2})$ (e) $h(a + k)$ (g) $h(2 - x)$
(b) $h(-4)$ (d) $h(\pi + 1)$ (f) $h(-x)$ (h) $h(x - 3)$

A.3. Let g be the function defined by $g(t) = t^2 - 1$. Evaluate:
(a) $g(3)$ (d) $g(x)$ (g) $g(-t)$

(b) $g(-2)$ (e) $g(s + 1)$ (h) $g(t + h)$

(c) $g(0)$ (f) $g(1 - r)$ (i) $g\left(\dfrac{1}{t}\right)$

A.4. Let f be the function defined by $f(x) = |2 - x| + \sqrt{x - 2} + x^2$. Evaluate:
(a) $f(2)$ (d) $f(5) + f(11)$ (g) $f(-x)$
(b) $f(11)$ (e) $f(5 - 2)$ (h) $f(5 - x)$
(c) $f(5 + 11)$ (f) $f(5) - f(2)$ (i) $f(5) - f(x)$

A.5. For each of the following functions, compute $f(2)$; $f(\tfrac{16}{3})$; $f(2) - f(\tfrac{16}{3})$; $f(r)$;

$f(r) - f(x)$; and $\dfrac{f(r) - f(x)}{r - x}$ (assume $r \neq x$ and simplify your answer to the last

one). For example, if $f(x) = x^2$, then

$$f(2) = 4, \quad f\left(\frac{16}{3}\right) = \frac{16^2}{3^2} = \frac{256}{9}, \quad f(2) - f\left(\frac{16}{3}\right) = 4 - \frac{256}{9} = -\frac{220}{9},$$

$$f(r) = r^2, \quad f(r) - f(x) = r^2 - x^2,$$

$$\frac{f(r) - f(x)}{r - x} = \frac{r^2 - x^2}{r - x} = \frac{(r + x)(r - x)}{r - x} = r + x \quad (r \neq x)$$

(a) $f(x) = x$ (d) $f(x) = -10x + 12$ (g) $f(x) = x - x^2$

(b) $f(x) = -10x$ (e) $f(x) = 3x + 7$ (h) $f(x) = \sqrt{x}$

(c) $f(x) = 12$ (f) $f(x) = x^3$ (i) $f(x) = \dfrac{1}{x}$

A.6. Each of the graphs in Figure 4-6 defines a function f with domain $[-3, 4]$. In each case, find $f(-3), f(-\frac{3}{2}), f(0), f(1), f(\frac{5}{2}), f(4)$. Careful approximate answers are acceptable.

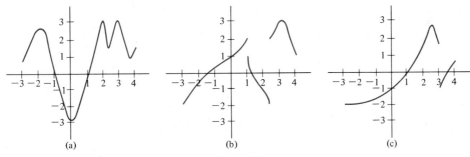

Figure 4-6

A.7. For each of the functions in Exercise A.6., find $f(-3) + f(-\frac{3}{2})$; $f(0) - f(2)$; $f(\frac{5}{2}) - f(3)$; $f(4) + 3f(-2)$.

A.8. In Washington state the sales tax $T(p)$ on an item of price p (*dollars*) equals 5% of p.

(a) Which of the following formulas gives the correct sales tax in all cases?
   (i) $T(p) = p + 5$ (iv) $T(p) = p + (5/100)p = p + .05p$
   (ii) $T(p) = 1 + 5p$ (v) $T(p) = (5/100)p = .05p$
   (iii) $T(p) = p/20$

(b) Find $T(3.6)$, $T(4.8)$, $T(0.6)$, and $T(0)$.

B.1. The sales tax law of state X reads as follows: "on any item up to and including 99¢, the sales tax is 5¢. On an item of \$1.00 or more, the tax is 5¢ *plus* 3% of the amount in excess of \$1.00."

(a) Find an algebraic rule for the sales tax (in dollars) in state X on an item of price p dollars.

(b) We want to compare the 5% Washington state sales tax (as discussed in Exercise A.8. immediately above) with the tax in state X. To keep the two taxes straight, we write $T_X(p)$, which is read "T sub X of p," for the tax in state X, and continue writing $T(p)$ for the tax in Washington. Which of the following statements are true, which false?

(i) $T(2) > T_X(2)$ (iv) $T(2 \cdot 3) = T(2)T(3)$

(ii) $T_X(2 + 6) = T_X(2) + T_X(6)$ (v) $T_X(1) = T(1)$

(iii) $T_X(p) < T(p)$ for $0 \le p \le 0.99$

B.2. **(a)** Which of the following statements are true for *all* numbers x in the domain of the identity function [whose rule is $f(x) = x$]? If a statement is not true for some x in the domain, give an example to demonstrate this fact.

(i) $f(x^2) = (f(x))^2$ (iii) $f(-x) = f(x)$

(ii) $f(|x|) = |f(x)|$ (iv) $f(3x) = 3f(x)$

(b) Do part (a) for the function $f(x) = 4x$.

(c) Do part (a) for the absolute value function $f(x) = |x|$.

(d) Do part (a) for the function $f(x) = x^2$.

B.3. Determine the *domain* of each of the following functions, according to the usual conventions.

(a) $f(x) = x^2$ (g) $k(x) = |x| + \sqrt{x} - 1$

(b) $g(x) = \dfrac{1}{x^2} + 2$ (h) $h(x) = \sqrt{(x + 1)^2}$

(c) $h(t) = |t| - 1$ (i) $f(x) = x - [x]$

(d) $k(u) = \sqrt{u}$ (j) $r(t) = [t] + [-t]$

(e) $f(x) = [x]^2$ (k) $g(u) = \dfrac{|u|}{u}$

(f) $g(t) = |t - 1|$ (l) $h(x) = \begin{cases} -x & \text{if } x < 1 \\ 4x - 5 & \text{if } x \ge 1 \end{cases}$

B.4. Give an example of two different functions f and g which have all of the following properties:

$$f(-1) = 1 = g(-1) \quad \text{and} \quad f(0) = 0 = g(0) \quad \text{and} \quad f(1) = 1 = g(1).$$

B.5. **(a)** Give an example of a function h which has the property that $h(u) = h(2u)$ for every real number u.

(b) Give an example of a function f which has the property that $f(x) = 2f(x)$ for every real number x.

B.6. Determine the *domain* of each of the following functions, according to the usual conventions.

(a) $f(x) = |-x|$ (g) $h(x) = \sqrt{(1 - x)^3}$

(b) $h(x) = \dfrac{\sqrt{x - 1}}{x^2 - 1}$ (h) $y = \dfrac{1}{x} + \dfrac{1}{x - 1} + \dfrac{1}{x + 2}$

(c) $g(t) = \sqrt{t^2}$ (i) $g(u) = \dfrac{u^2 + 1}{u^2 - u - 6}$

(d) $y = x^3 + 2$ (j) $f(t) = \sqrt{4 - t^2}$

(e) $g(y) = [-y]$ (k) $y = -\sqrt{9 - (x - 9)^2}$

(f) $f(t) = \sqrt{-t}$

B.7. Let the symbol Δx represent a *nonzero* number. (That is, Δx represents a *single* number; it does *not* mean Δ times x.) For each of the following functions, compute $f(x + \Delta x)$.   *Example:* if $f(x) = x^2 + 1$, then

$$f(x + \Delta x) = (x + \Delta x)^2 + 1$$
$$= x^2 + 2x\,\Delta x + (\Delta x)^2 + 1$$

(a) $f(x) = x$	**(d)** $h(x) = x^3$	**(g)** $f(x) = x + 5$
(b) $f(x) = x^2$	**(e)** $k(x) = \dfrac{1}{x}$	**(h)** $f(x) = 7x + 2$
(c) $g(x) = 12$	**(f)** $g(x) = -10x$	**(i)** $k(x) = x^2 + 3x - 7$

B.8. For each of the functions in Exercise B.7 compute and simplify the **difference quotient**, which is the quotient $\dfrac{f(x + \Delta x) - f(x)}{\Delta x}$. The difference quotient is used extensively in calculus.   *Example:* if $f(x) = x^2 + 1$, then

$$\frac{f(x + \Delta x) - f(x)}{\Delta x} = \frac{[(x + \Delta x)^2 + 1] - (x^2 + 1)}{\Delta x}$$

$$= \frac{x^2 + 2x\,\Delta x + (\Delta x)^2 + 1 - x^2 - 1}{\Delta x} = \frac{(2x + \Delta x)\,\Delta x}{\Delta x} = 2x + \Delta x \quad (\Delta x \neq 0)$$

B.9. (a) Evaluate each of the difference quotients in Exercise B.8 when x is fixed and $\Delta x = 2$; $\Delta x = 1$; $\Delta x = .5$; $\Delta x = .1$; and $\Delta x = .01$.   *Example:* if $f(x) = x^2 + 1$, then

$$\frac{f(x + \Delta x) - f(x)}{\Delta x} = 2x + \Delta x \quad (\Delta x \neq 0)$$

Hence,

Δx	2	1	.5	.1	.01
$2x + \Delta x$	$2x + 2$	$2x + 1$	$2x + .5$	$2x + .1$	$2x + .01$

(b) When Δx is a nonzero number very close to 0, what is the difference quotient very close to? (In the example above, the difference quotient $2x + \Delta x$ is very close to $2x$ when Δx is very close to 0.)

C.1. As explained in Example 3 of the text, the distance traveled by a falling rock after t sec is $16t^2$. In functional notation, $d(t) = 16t^2$.
(a) Find $d(0)$ and $d(2)$.
(b) Find $d(1)$ and $d(3)$.
(c) Find $d(2)$ and $d(4)$.
(d) How far does the rock travel during the first 2 sec?
(e) How far does the rock travel during the second and third seconds (that is, what distance is traveled from $t = 1$ to $t = 3$)?

(f) How far does the rock travel from $t = 2$ to $t = 4$?

(g) Use functional notation to express the distance traveled by the rock from time t_1 to time t_2.

(h) Use functional notation to express the distance traveled by the rock during a 4-sec period beginning at time t.

C.2. This exercise deals with Example 2 in the text; use the graph shown in Figure 4-1 (p. 173).

(a) By measuring as carefully as you can, fill the blanks in the following statements. There may be more than one correct answer in some cases.

   (i)   The temperature at 8 A.M. was _____ degrees.

   (ii) The temperature at 8 P.M. was _____ degrees.

   (iii) The temperature at 8 A.M. was the same as the temperature at

   _____ .

   (iv) The difference between the temperatures at noon and at 6 P.M. was _____ degrees.

   (v)   The temperature at _____ was greater than the temperature at 8 P.M.

   (vi) The temperature at _____ P.M. was less than the temperature at _____ A.M.

   (vii) The temperature at 10 A.M. was _____ than the temperature at 5 P.M.

   (viii) The temperature at noon was _____ than the temperature at 8 P.M. but _____ than the temperature at 4 P.M.

(b) After filling the blanks in part (a), write each of the statements in the functional notation introduced on page 181.

DO IT YOURSELF!

BACK TO REAL LIFE

This chapter began with some real-life situations which suggested various kinds of functions and functional notation. These in turn led to the abstract concept of function in a purely mathematical setting, together with more functional notation. Now that you have some familiarity with functional notation, it's time to return to the starting point. If you want to understand mathematics fully or to apply it, you must be able to:

Recognize functional situations in real-life settings.

Determine which quantities are functions of others.

Find a mathematical description of the function involved (including, it is to be hoped, an algebraic formula for the rule of the function).

There are no hard and fast rules for doing these things. The only way to become proficient at them is to work through some examples and then do some exercises on your own.

SITUATION A 20-in. square sheet of tin is to be used to make an open-top box by cutting a small square from each corner of the sheet and bending up the sides (see Figure 4-7).

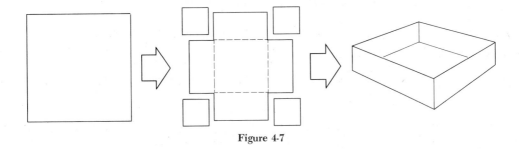

Figure 4-7

Approximately what size square should be cut out of each corner in order to obtain a box with the largest possible volume?

Analysis It is clear that the volume of the box depends on the size of the square cut from the corners. The size of the square is determined by the length of its side. Call this length x. Then the *volume is a function of the length x of the side* of the square to be cut from the corners. Since the whole sheet of tin is 20×20 in., we see that each of the dotted lines in Figure 4-8 has the length $20 - 2x$ in.

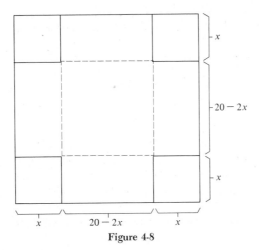

Figure 4-8

When the sides are folded up, the bottom of the box will measure $(20 - 2x)$ by $(20 - 2x)$ in. and its height will be x in. Therefore its volume will be

$$\text{height} \times \text{length} \times \text{width} = x(20 - 2x)(20 - 2x) = x(20 - 2x)^2$$

Thus the volume is a function of the length x and the *rule* of the function is:

$$V(x) = x(20 - 2x)^2$$

What is the *domain* of this function? Certainly $V(x) = x(20 - 2x)^2$ is a well-defined real number for any real number x. But in this situation the only numbers which *make sense* are those numbers x with $0 < x < 10$. For you can't cut a zero or negative amount from the corners. Nor can you cut four squares each of side length 10 in. or more from a 20×20-in. sheet (and still have something left). Consequently, we write

$$V(x) = x(20 - 2x)^2 \qquad 0 < x < 10$$

to indicate that the domain is the interval $(0, 10)$.

Here are some values of the function for different numbers:

x	1	2	3	4	5	6	9
$V(x) = x(20 - 2x)^2$	324	512	588	576	500	384	36

It appears that a box of largest possible volume will be obtained by cutting out a square of side *approximately* 3 in. This is the best we can do with purely algebraic techniques. In calculus you will learn how to find the *exact* value of x which makes the volume $V(x)$ a maximum. (It turns out to be $x = \frac{10}{3}$, which gives a box of volume $\frac{16,000}{27} = 592.59$ cu in.)

SITUATION   A manufacturer has found that she can't sell any widgets at a price of $2.00 or more. But for each 10¢ decrease in the price per widget, she can sell 1000 widgets a week (that is, she can sell 1000 at $1.90 each, 2000 at $1.80 each, and so on). It costs 50¢ to manufacture one widget. Fixed expenses (mortgage, taxes, and the like) run $2000 per week. The maximum number of widgets that can be manufactured in one week is 17,000. How is the manufacturer's weekly *profit* affected by the number of widgets she sells?

Analysis   Let x be the number of widgets sold per week. To measure the number of widgets sold *in thousands* we must divide x by 1000. For instance, 2500 is the same as $2.5 \left(= \frac{2500}{1000} \right)$ *thousands*. No widgets can be sold at a price of $2.00. For each thousand widgets to be sold, the price must be decreased by 10¢. So to sell x widgets per week the price per widget (in dollars) must be:

$$2 - (\text{number of thousands sold})(.10) = 2 - \left(\frac{x}{1000} \right)(.10) = 2 - \frac{x}{10,000}$$

For instance, if $x = 5000$, the price is $2 - \frac{5000}{10,000} = 2 - .5 = \$1.50$. Therefore the *income* from selling x widgets is

$$(\text{price per widget}) \times (\text{number sold}) = \left(2 - \frac{x}{10,000} \right) x$$

The *cost* of manufacturing x widgets per week is

$$(\text{cost per widget}) \times (\text{number sold}) + (\text{fixed expenses}) = .50x + 2000$$

The manufacturer's profit is

$$\text{income} - \text{cost} = \left(2 - \frac{x}{10,000}\right)x - (.50x + 2000)$$

$$= 2x - \frac{x^2}{10,000} - .5x - 2000$$

$$= 1.5x - \frac{x^2}{10,000} - 2000$$

Thus *profit is a function P of the number x of widgets sold:*

$$P(x) = 1.5x - \frac{x^2}{10,000} - 2000$$

Note that $P(x)$ is a well-defined real number for any real number x. But in this situation the only numbers which make sense for x are integers from 0 to 17,000. Thus the domain of P is all integers in the interval $[0, 17,000]$.

The preceding examples illustrate a common phenomenon:

> *A real-life functional situation may lead to a function whose domain does not include all real numbers, even though the rule of the function may make sense for all real numbers.*

EXERCISES

A.1. Suppose a car travels at a constant rate of 55 mph for 2 hr, and travels at 45 mph thereafter. Show that distance traveled is a function of time and find the rule of the function.

A.2. **(a)** The distance between city C and city S is 2000 mi. A plane flying directly to S passes over C at noon. If the plane travels at 475 mph, express the distance of the plane from *city* S as a function of time.
(b) Do part (a) for a plane which travels at 325 mph.

A.3. The list price of a textbook is $12. But if 10 or more copies are purchased, then the price per copy is reduced by 25¢ for every copy above 10. (That is, $11.75 per copy for 11 copies, $11.50 per copy for 12 copies, and so on.)
(a) The price per copy is a function of the number of copies purchased. Find the rule of this function.
(b) The total cost of a quantity purchase is (number of copies) × (price per copy). Show that the total cost is a function of the number of copies and find the rule of the function.

A.4. A potato chip factory has a daily overhead from salaries and building costs of $1800. The cost of ingredients and packaging to produce a pound of potato chips is 50¢. A pound of potato chips sells for $1.20. Show that the factory's daily profit is a function of the number of pounds of potato chips sold and find the rule of this function. (Assume that the factory sells all the potato chips it produces each day.)

B.1. (a) A rectangular region of 6000 sq ft is to be fenced in on three sides with fencing costing $3.75 per ft and on the fourth side with fencing costing $2.00 per ft. Express the cost of the fence as a function of the length x of the fourth side.

(b) Estimate the value of x which produces the cheapest fence.

(c) Do parts (a) and (b) assuming that the side opposite the fourth side is a river, so that no fencing is required there.

B.2. The fast food king Ray Rotgut can sell 10,000 hamburgers per day at a price of 75¢ each. Each price increase of 10¢ per hamburger results in 1000 fewer hamburgers being sold.

(a) Express the number of hamburgers sold as a function of the price per hamburger.

(b) Express the total income from hamburger sales as a function of the price per hamburger.

(c) Rotgut's fixed costs (salaries, building, equipment, and so on) are $1100 per day The ingredients for one hamburger costs 40¢. Express Rotgut's daily profit as a function of the price per hamburger.

(d) Use the function in part (c) to estimate the price Rotgut should charge per hamburger in order to maximize his daily profit.

B.3. A box with a square base measuring $t \times t$ ft is to be made of three kinds of wood. The cost of the wood for the base is 85¢ per sq ft; the wood for the sides costs 50¢ per sq ft and the wood for the top $1.15 per sq ft. The volume of the box is to be 10 cu ft.

(a) Express the total cost of the box as a function of the length t.

(b) Estimate the value of t which makes the cost as low as possible.

B.4. An open-top rectangular box is to be made from a piece of cardboard 10 in. wide and 16 in. long by cutting a square from each corner and bending up the sides. The volume of the box is a function of the length t of the side of the cut square. Find the rule of this function and *estimate* the value of t which will produce a box of maximum volume.

3. GRAPHS OF FUNCTIONS

The next step in analyzing functional situations is to draw a picture. The graph of a function is essentially just a picture of the function. We have seen such pictures before, when we considered graphs of equations in Chapter 3. The graph of an *equation*, such as $y = 7x^2$ or $y = 3x - 4$, is just the set of all points (x, y) in the coordinate plane whose coordinates, x and y, satisfy the given equation. The graph of a *function* is similar:

> *The **graph of the function** f is the graph of the equation* y = f(x).

Thus the point (x, y) is on the graph of the function f precisely when x is a number in the domain of f and y is the number $f(x)$, the value of the function at x. In other words,

> *The graph of the function* f *consists of all points* (x, f(x)), *where* x *is any number in the domain of* f.

The letters used are not important. For instance, if the function is denoted by g, then its graph is the set of all points $(t, g(t))$, where t is any number in the domain of the function.

Graphs allow us to apply various geometric insights to the study of function. Properties of a function, which may not be immediately apparent, often become obvious when you look at the graph. This interaction between geometry and algebra is crucial in the development of the mathematics needed to cope with numerous problems in the real world.

In theory, once you know the function f, you automatically know its graph: just plot each of the points $(x, f(x))$ for every number x in the domain. In practice, however, you can actually plot only finitely many points and usually must make an "educated guess" about the rest. For most of the functions in this course and in calculus, you should follow this general procedure:

How to Graph the Function *f*

1. *Choose a few numbers* x *in the domain of* f *and compute the corresponding numbers* f(x).
2. *Plot the points* (x, f(x)) *determined in step 1. In many cases, they will suggest a geometric pattern.*
3. *Apply any other algebraic or geometric information that may be available about the function* f *in order to determine the general shape of the entire graph.*
4. *Using the points plotted in step 2 and the information developed in step 3, sketch the graph. Unless the information from step 3 indicates otherwise, the graph will usually be an unbroken curve.°*

This general procedure, especially step 3, isn't very enlightening until you have seen it applied in examples. As you will see, it isn't necessary to be rigid about the order in which you do steps 1–3.

EXAMPLE Let g be the **square root function,** given by $g(x) = \sqrt{x}$. We know that $\sqrt{x}$ is defined only when $x \geq 0$ and that in such cases $\sqrt{x} \geq 0$. Therefore the only points

°The word "curve" here includes the possibility of straight line segments.

$(x, g(x)) = (x, \sqrt{x})$ on the graph are those with both coordinates ≥ 0. Thus the entire graph lies in the first quadrant. With the use of the table on page 451, or a calculator, we see that

$$g(0) = \sqrt{0} = 0, \qquad g(.25) = \sqrt{.25} = .5, \qquad g(1) = \sqrt{1} = 1,$$
$$g(2) = \sqrt{2} \approx 1.414, \qquad g(3) = \sqrt{3} \approx 1.732, \qquad g(4) = \sqrt{4} = 2,$$
$$g(6) = \sqrt{6} \approx 2.449, \qquad g(9) = \sqrt{9} = 3, \qquad g(10) = \sqrt{10} \approx 3.162$$

If we plot the corresponding points, we have Figure 4-9.

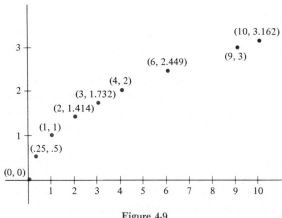

Figure 4-9

In this case there is some additional algebraic information:

$$\text{if } 0 \leq b < c, \qquad \text{then } \sqrt{b} < \sqrt{c}$$

In graphical terms this means that;

> If c lies to the *right* of b on the horizontal axis,
> then the graph at c is *higher* than the graph at b

In other words, as you move to the *right,* the graph always *rises.* Consequently, the entire graph looks like the one shown in Figure 4-10 (where the arrow indicates that the graph continues upward to the right).

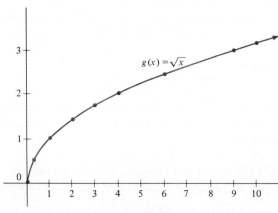

Figure 4-10

EXAMPLE The graph of $f(x) = x^2$ consists of all points (x, x^2). Since $x^2 \geq 0$ for every x, every point on the graph lies on or above the x-axis. By computing x^2 for various values of x, we are able to locate some points on the graph, as shown in Figure 4-11.

x	$f(x) = x^2$
-2.5	6.25
-2	4
-1.5	2.25
-1	1
$-.5$	.25
0	0
.5	.25
1	1
1.5	2.25
2	4
2.5	6.25

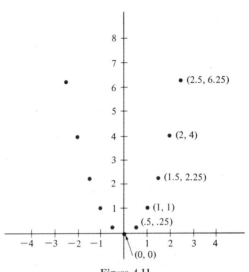

Figure 4-11

As x gets very large in absolute value, x^2 gets even larger. Consequently, the graph of $f(x) = x^2$ looks like the one shown in Figure 4-12 (where the arrows indicate that the graph continues sharply upward and outward).

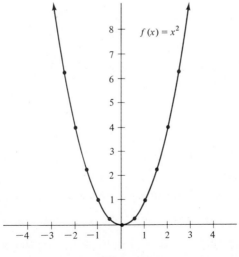

Figure 4-12

A curve shaped like the graph of $f(x) = x^2$ is called a **parabola**. Its lowest point [in this case $(0, 0)$] is called the **vertex** of the parabola. Parabolas are discussed further in Section 6.

EXAMPLE To graph the function $f(x) = \dfrac{1}{x^2 + 1}$, we first find some points on the graph by computing the value of the function at several numbers:

x	-10	-7	-3	-1	$-\frac{1}{2}$	0	$\frac{1}{3}$	1	2	3	7	10
$f(x) = \dfrac{1}{x^2 + 1}$	$\frac{1}{101}$	$\frac{1}{50}$	$\frac{1}{10}$	$\frac{1}{2}$	$\frac{4}{5}$	1	$\frac{9}{10}$	$\frac{1}{2}$	$\frac{1}{5}$	$\frac{1}{10}$	$\frac{1}{50}$	$\frac{1}{101}$

Observe that as x gets larger and larger in absolute value, $f(x) = \dfrac{1}{x^2 + 1}$ is a positive number that gets closer and closer to zero. In geometric terms this means that as you move to the far left or far right ($|x|$ large), the graph lies above the x-axis [$f(x)$ positive] but gets closer and closer to the x-axis. Furthermore, $x^2 + 1 \geq 1$ for every number x, so that $f(x) = \dfrac{1}{x^2 + 1} \leq 1$. Geometrically, this means that the graph always lies below the horizontal line $y = 1$. Using these facts and the points obtained from the table above, we see that the entire graph looks like the one shown in Figure 4-13.

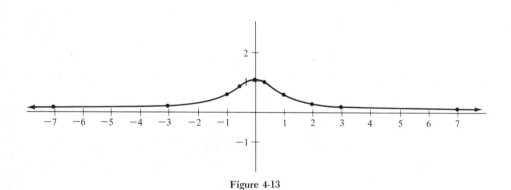

Figure 4-13

EXAMPLE No such elaborate analysis is needed to graph **linear functions** such as

$$f(x) = 3x - 4, \qquad g(t) = 7t + 2, \qquad h(x) = -6$$

For instance, the graph of $f(x) = 3x - 4$ is, by definition, the graph of the equation $y = f(x)$, that is, $y = 3x - 4$. From Section 3 of Chapter 3 we know that the graph of any linear equation, such as $y = 3x - 4$, $y = 7t + 2$, and so on, is just a straight line. Hence we need only plot two points in each case to determine the entire graph, as shown in Figure 4-14.

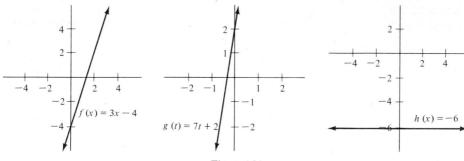

Figure 4-14

EXAMPLE   Let f be the absolute value function, given by $f(x) = |x|$. If we write down the definition of $|x|$, we see that the rule of this function is in two parts:

$$f(x) = |x| = \begin{cases} x & \text{if } x \geq 0 \\ -x & \text{if } x < 0 \end{cases}$$

Thus we first consider those points on the graph with $x \geq 0$. If $x \geq 0$, then $|x| = x$ and the equation $y = f(x)$ becomes $y = |x| = x$. But we know from Section 3 of Chapter 3 that the graph of $y = x$ (with $x \geq 0$) is just half of the straight line $y = x$, as shown in Figure 4-15.

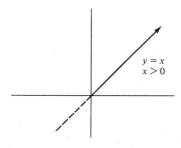

Figure 4-15

Similarly, when $x < 0$, then $|x| = -x$, and the equation $y = f(x)$ becomes $y = |x| = -x$. Once again we know that the graph of $y = -x$ (with $x < 0$) is just half of the straight line $y = -x$, as shown in Figure 4-16.

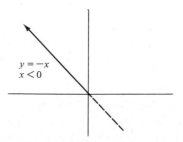

Figure 4-16

Combining this information, we see that the entire graph of $f(x) = |x|$ looks like the one in Figure 4-17.

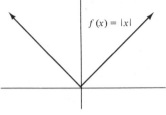

Figure 4-17

EXAMPLE Just plotting points may not be enough to find the graph of the function h given by

$$h(t) = \begin{cases} t^2 & \text{if } t < 0 \\ t & \text{if } 0 \le t < 5 \\ -2t + 11 & \text{if } t \ge 5 \end{cases}$$

If you simply compute $h(t)$ for some selected values of t, plot the corresponding points, and join them by a single curve, you'll probably get the graph wrong. To obtain the correct graph in cases such as this, you need a careful analysis of the separate parts of the graph, corresponding to the three-part rule of the function.

$t < 0$ The graph of h is the graph of the equation $y = h(t)$. When $t < 0$, this equation is $y = t^2$. From the example on page 199 we know that the graph of $y = t^2$ with $t < 0$ is the left half of the parabola $y = t^2$, as plotted in Figure 4-18.

t	-1	-2
$h(t) = t^2$	1	4

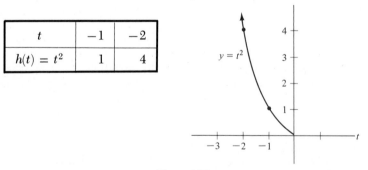

Figure 4-18

$0 \le t < 5$ For these values of t the rule of the function is $h(t) = t$. So the graph of $y = h(t)$ is just the graph of $y = t$. Since the entire graph of $y = t$ is a straight line, the graph of the function h over the interval $[0, 5)$ is just a segment of that line, as plotted in Figure 4-19.

t	0	3	4
$h(t) = t$	0	3	4

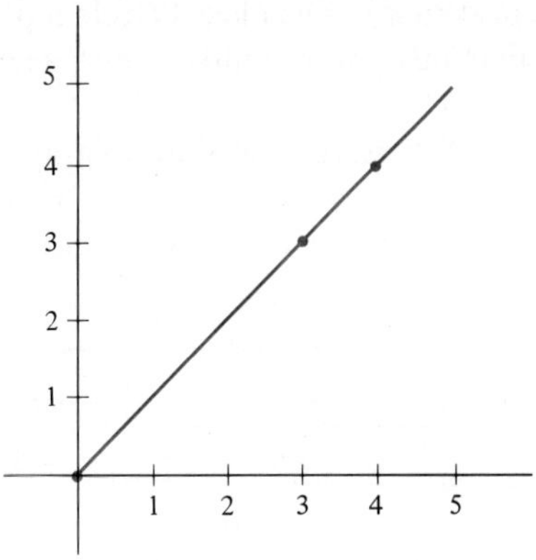

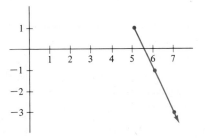

Figure 4-19

$t \geq 5$ Over the interval $[5, \infty)$, the graph of h is the graph of $y = h(t) = -2t + 11$, namely, a half line, as plotted in Figure 4-20.

t	5	6	7
$h(t) = -2t + 11$	1	-1	-3

Figure 4-20

Combining the above information yields the entire graph of the function h, as shown in Figure 4-21.

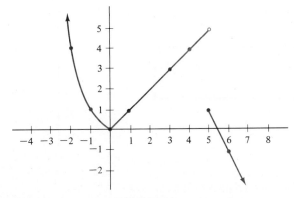

Figure 4-21

The open circle indicates that the point $(5, 5)$ is *not* on the graph of h (it is on the graph of $y = t$, of course). The closed circle indicates that the point $(5, 1)$ *is* on the graph of h. Note that this graph, unlike the others discussed so far, is *not* an *unbroken* curve.

EXAMPLE Whenever you want to graph a function whose rule involves the greatest integer function, such as $g(x) = x - [x]$, the best procedure is to consider what the function and graph look like between each two consecutive integers. For instance,

If	Then $[x] =$	So That $x - [x] =$
$-2 \leq x < -1$	-2	$x - (-2) = x + 2$
$-1 \leq x < 0$	-1	$x - (-1) = x + 1$
$0 \leq x < 1$	0	x
$1 \leq x < 2$	1	$x - 1$
$2 \leq x < 3$	2	$x - 2$

Thus the rule of the function g really consists of many parts:

$$g(x) = \begin{cases} \vdots & \\ x + 2 & \text{if } -2 \leq x < -1 \\ x + 1 & \text{if } -1 \leq x < 0 \\ x & \text{if } \;\; 0 \leq x < 1 \\ x - 1 & \text{if } \;\; 1 \leq x < 2 \\ x - 2 & \text{if } \;\; 2 \leq x < 3 \\ \vdots & \end{cases}$$

Its graph can be found by considering the function over each of the intervals . . . , $[-2, -1), [-1, 0), [0, 1), [1, 2), \ldots$, and so on. Over each such interval the graph is a segment of a straight line. For instance, when $1 \leq x < 2$, we have the graph shown in Figure 4-22.

x	1	$\frac{3}{2}$	$\frac{7}{4}$
$g(x) = x - 1$	0	$\frac{1}{2}$	$\frac{3}{4}$

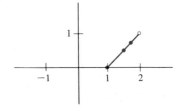

Figure 4-22

The open circle indicates that the point $(2, 1)$ is not on the graph.

A similar analysis shows that for $-2 \leq x < 3$, the graph of g looks like the one in Figure 4-23.

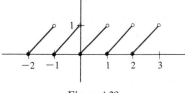

Figure 4-23

You should convince yourself that this same pattern continues both to the left and the right.

A WARNING AND A PREVIEW

The examples above are a bit misleading. It is not *always* possible to find the graph simply by plotting a few points and making a simple algebraic analysis of the function. Even when plotting points *does* suggest a general pattern, you may not be able to answer questions such as these:

(i) When the graph rises from one point to another, which way does it bend?

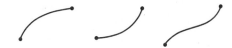

(ii) Does the graph wiggle between two points?

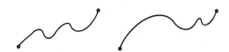

(iii) When the graph appears to change from rising to falling between points P and Q, exactly where does it change?

(iv) Is the graph a continuous, unbroken curve between two points? Or are there gaps, jumps, holes, or isolated points?

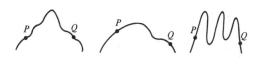

The last of these four questions is especially important. In many of the examples above, it was possible only to plot a finite number of points. Unless there was specific information to the contrary, we *assumed* that the graph between two such points was a continuous, unbroken curve. Although this assumption may seem *reasonable*, we can't be absolutely *sure* it is true without some proof. The techniques needed to provide this proof, as well as to answer all of the questions above, are developed in calculus. Until then, you should continue to make such reasonable assumptions and apply the general graphing procedure outlined above as carefully as possible.

EXERCISES

A.1. Sketch the graph of the function d in Example 3 (page 181).

A.2. Sketch the graph of $g(x) = x^3$.

A.3. Sketch the graph of $f(x) = -x^3 + 1$.

A.4. Sketch the graph of the cube root function h, given by $h(x) = \sqrt[3]{x}$. (*Hint:* the table of cube roots on p. 451 may be helpful.)

A.5. Graph each of the following functions.

(a) $f(x) = \begin{cases} x^2 & \text{if } x \geq -1 \\ 2x + 3 & \text{if } x < -1 \end{cases}$

(b) $g(x) = \begin{cases} |x| & \text{if } x < 1 \\ -3x + 4 & \text{if } x \geq 1 \end{cases}$

(c) $h(x) = \begin{cases} x - 2 & \text{if } x < 4 \\ x & \text{if } x \geq 4 \end{cases}$

(d) $f(t) = \begin{cases} t & \text{if } t < -3 \\ t^2 & \text{if } -3 \leq t \leq 3 \\ 2t & \text{if } t > 3 \end{cases}$

(e) $k(u) = \begin{cases} -2u - 2 & \text{if } u < -3 \\ u - [u] & \text{if } -3 \leq u \leq 1 \\ 2u^2 & \text{if } u > 1 \end{cases}$

(f) $f(x) = \begin{cases} x^2 & \text{if } x < -2 \\ x & \text{if } -2 \leq x < 4 \\ \sqrt{x} & \text{if } x \geq 4 \end{cases}$

B.1. The greatest integer function f, whose rule is $f(x) = [x]$, is called a **step function.** To see why, carefully sketch the graph of f. (*Hint:* what does the graph look like on the interval $[0, 1)$? on $[1, 2)$? on $[-1, 0)$? on $[-2, -1)$? and so forth.)

B.2. (a) Graph $f(x) = -[x]$ for $-3 \leq x \leq 3$.
(The hint for Exercise B.1 also applies here.)
(b) Graph $g(x) = [-x]$ for $-3 \leq x \leq 3$. (*Note:* this *not* the same as $-[x]$.)
(c) Graph $h(x) = [x] + [-x]$ for $-3 \leq x \leq 3$.

B.3. The amount of postage required for each ounce of first-class mail, or fraction thereof, is k cents. (At this writing $k = 18$.) The *number* of k-cent stamps required to mail a first-class letter is a function of the weight of the letter (in ounces). Call this function the postage stamp function.
(a) Describe the rule of the postage stamp function algebraically.
(b) Graph the postage stamp function.
(c) Graph the function f whose rule is $f(x) = p(x) - [x]$, where p is the postage stamp function.

B.4. Sketch the graph of $f(x) = 1/x$. (*Hints:* the function is not defined when $x = 0$;

what does the graph look like *near x = 0*? What does the graph look like when $|x|$ is very large?)

B.5. (a) Sketch the graph of the function given by $y = x + |x|$.
  (b) Sketch the graph of the function given by $y = x|x|$.

B.6. Sketch the graph of $f(x) = x^3 - x$. [*Hints:* determine whether $f(x)$ is always positive or always negative in each of the intervals $(-\infty, -1)$, $(-1, 0)$, $(0, 1)$, $(1, \infty)$. What happens at $x = -1$, $x = 0$, $x = 1$?]

B.7. Sketch the graphs of the following functions. (*Hint:* think circular.)
  (a) $f(x) = \sqrt{1 - x^2}$ (c) $f(x) = \sqrt{4 - (x - 1)^2} + 2$
  (b) $g(t) = -\sqrt{16 - t^2}$ (d) $g(t) = \sqrt{16 - (t + 3)^2} - 5$

B.8. In each part, graph the two given functions (one of them was graphed in the text). What is the geometric relationship between the two graphs?
  (a) $f(x) = |x|$ and $h(x) = |x| + 1$ (e) $g(x) = \sqrt{x}$ and $k(x) = -\sqrt{x}$
  (b) $f(x) = |x|$ and $k(x) = |x| - 4$ (f) $f(x) = |x|$ and $h(x) = |x - 5|$
  (c) $g(x) = \sqrt{x}$ and $r(x) = \sqrt{x} - 1$ (g) $f(x) = |x|$ and $v(x) = |x + 5|$
  (d) $g(x) = \sqrt{x}$ and $s(x) = \sqrt{x} + 2$

B.9. When you have done Exercises A.2 and A.4, answer this question: how is the graph of $g(x) = x^3$ related geometrically to the graph of $h(x) = \sqrt[3]{x}$?

B.10. Let f be a *function*. Suppose x and r are two *different* numbers in the domain of f. Then the points $(r, f(r))$ and $(x, f(x))$ are on the graph of f.
  (a) Why is it *impossible* for $(r, f(r))$ and $(x, f(x))$ to be on the same *vertical* straight line?
  (b) Draw three different graphs which are *not* the graphs of functions.

B.11. Graph each of these functions as best you can (some of them may be harder than the examples and other exercises).
  (a) $f(x) = 2x^2 - 3x + 2$ (d) $f(u) = \dfrac{1}{u^3 + 1}$

  (b) $g(x) = -3x^2 + 4x - 7$ (e) $k(x) = x^3 - 3x + 1$

  (c) $h(t) = \dfrac{t}{1 - t}$ (f) $h(x) = \dfrac{x}{x^2 + 1}$

4. MORE GRAPH READING

In order to understand the interaction of algebra and geometry in the study of functions, or to apply this knowledge to practical problems, you must be able to "translate" statements from one to another of three different "languages":

The English language.
Formula language (algebraic and functional notation).
Graphical language (graphs).

The emphasis in this section is on translating graphical information into equivalent statements in English or functional notation; in short, graph reading. We begin with a familiar example from Sections 1 and 2.

EXAMPLE 2—TEMPERATURE The recording device at the weather bureau in city F directly produces the graph of the function which relates the time of day (measured in hours after midnight) to the temperature, as shown below (Figure 4-24). Using functional notation we write tem(t) for the temperature at t hours after midnight. The graph consists of all points with coordinates (t, tem(t)). For instance, since the point (4, 39) is on the graph,° we know that the temperature at 4:00 A.M. was 39°. To determine the time period during which the temperature was below 50°, we must *first* find every point (t, tem(t)) on the graph whose second coordinate, tem(t) is < 50, that is, every point which lies *below* the horizontal line through 50, as shown in Figure 4-24.

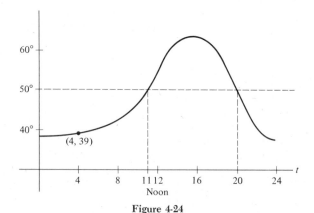

Figure 4-24

Having found all such points, we now must determine their first coordinates, for these first coordinates are precisely the times when the temperature is less than 50°. A careful examination of the graph above suggests that tem(t) < 50 whenever

$$0 \leq t \leq 11 \quad \text{or} \quad 20 \leq t \leq 24$$

In other words, the temperature was below 50° from midnight to 11:00 A.M. and again from 8:00 P.M. ($t = 20$) to midnight.

EXAMPLE 2 (PART 2) A slightly more complicated problem is to determine the time period *before* 4 P.M. during which the temperature was *at least* 60°. To do so, we translate these requirements into functional notation and graphical terms. Remember that 4:00 P.M. is 16 hours after midnight:

° Here and below our results are only as accurate as our measuring ability. But the basic idea should be clear.

Statement	Functional Notation	Graph
The time is before 4:00 P.M.	$t < 16$	$(t, \text{tem}(t))$ lies to the left of the vertical line through $t = 16$
The temperature is at least 60°	$\text{tem}(t) \geq 60$	$(t, \text{tem}(t))$ lies on or above the horizontal line through 60

Using this information and examining the graph in Figure 4-25

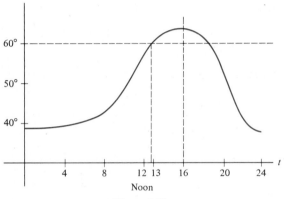

Figure 4-25

shows that the points $(t, \text{tem}(t))$ with $t < 16$ and $\text{tem}(t) \geq 60$ are those with first coordinates between 12.8 and 16. Thus the temperature was at least 60° from 12:48 P.M. ($t = 12.8$) to 4:00 P.M. ($t = 16$).

EXAMPLE 2 (PART 3) Suppose the temperature graph for a second city (city S) is superimposed on the temperature graph given above for city F, as shown in Figure 4-26.

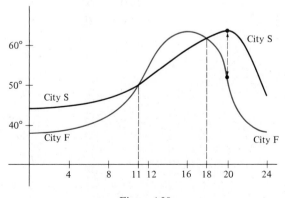

Figure 4-26

We continue to denote the temperature function for our original city (city F) by tem(t). We shall denote the temperature function for the second city (city S) by tem$_S$(t). By examining the graphs of tem(t) and tem$_S$(t) carefully, we can answer such questions as:

(i)   During what time period was it warmer in city F than in city S?
(ii) Was there any time during the day when it was at least 10 degrees warmer in city S than in city F?

Once again it is a matter of three-way translation from English language to functional notation to graphical terms:

Statement	Functional Notation	Graph
City F is warmer than city S at time t	tem(t) > tem$_S$(t)	The point $(t, \text{tem}(t))$ lies directly above $(t, \text{tem}_S(t))$
City S is at least 10 degrees warmer than city F at time t	tem$_S$(t) ≥ tem(t) + 10	The point $(t, \text{tem}_S(t)$ is at least 10 units above the point $(t, \text{tem}(t))$

Examination and careful measurement on the graph on page 209 shows that

(i)   tem(t) > tem$_S$(t) for all t in the interval (11, 18).
(ii) tem$_S$(t) ≥ tem(t) + 10 for many values of t, including $t = 20$.

In other words,

(i)   It was warmer in city F than in city S between 11:00 A.M. and 6:00 P.M. ($t = 18$).
(ii) It was at least 10 degrees warmer in city S at 8:00 P.M. ($t = 20$) and at other times.

Of course, in the usual mathematical setting for graph reading, there is no reference to times, temperatures, and so on. You are simply required to use the graphs of functions to determine information about the functions and vice-versa.

EXAMPLE   Figure 4-27 shows the graphs of functions g and h over the interval $[-5, 7]$.

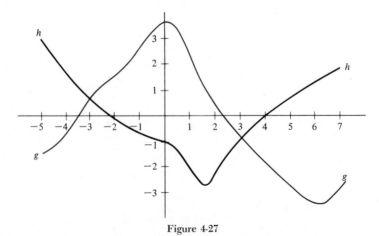

Figure 4-27

We can use these graphs to solve such problems as:

(i)   Find all numbers x in the interval $[-3, 3]$ such that $g(x) = 2$.

(ii) Find the largest interval over which the graph of g is rising, the graph of h is falling,° and $h(x) \geq g(x)$ for every number x in the interval.

In problem (i), for instance, the numbers x with x in $[-3, 3]$ and $g(x) = 2$ are the first coordinates of all points $(x, g(x))$ on the graph of g which lie on or between the vertical lines through -3 and 3, and on the horizontal line through 2, as shown in Figure 4-28.

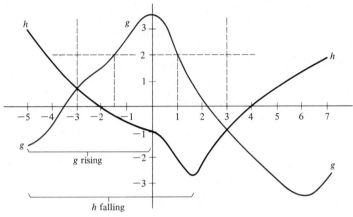

Figure 4-28

Thus the answer is $x = -1.5$ and $x = 1$.

To solve problem (ii), observe first that the graph of h is falling over the interval $[-5, 1.5]$. Over *that* interval, the graph of g is rising only when $-5 \leq x \leq 0$. Thus the only interval over which the graph of g is rising *and* the graph of h is falling is $[-5, 0]$. Clearly, $h(x) \geq g(x)$ exactly when the point $(x, h(x))$ lies on or above the point $(x, g(x))$. The only time this occurs over the interval $[-5, 0]$ is when $-5 \leq x \leq -3$, as shown above. Therefore the interval asked for in (ii) is the interval $[-5, -3]$.

EXERCISES

B.1.   Let g be the function with the graph shown in Figure 4-29.

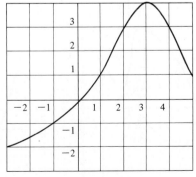

Figure 4-29

° Here and below "rising" and "falling" refer to movement from left to right.

(a) If $t = 1.5$, then $g(2t) = ?$

(b) If $t = 1.5$, then $2g(t) = ?$

(c) If $y = 2$, then $g(y + 1.5) = ?$

(d) If $y = 2$, then $g(y) + g(1.5) = ?$

(e) If $y = 2$, then $g(y) + 1.5 = ?$

(f) $g(0) = ?$

(g) If $v = 1.5$, then $g(3v - 1.5) = ?$

(h) If $s = 2$, then $g(-s) = ?$

(i) For what values of z is $g(z) = 1?$

(j) For what values of z is $g(z) = -1?$

(k) What is the largest interval over which the graph is rising?

(l) At what number t in the interval $[-1, 2]$ is $g(t)$ largest?

B.2. (a) Draw the graph of a function f, which satisfies the following four conditions: (i) domain $f = [-2, 4]$; (ii) range $f = [-5, 6]$; (iii) $f(-1) = f(2)$; (iv) $f(\tfrac{1}{2}) = 0$.

(b) Draw the graph of a function different from the one in part (a), which also satisfies all the conditions of part (a).

B.3. Figure 4-30 shows the entire graph of a function f.

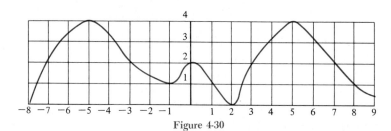

Figure 4-30

(a) What is the domain of f?

(b) What is the range of f?

(c) Find all numbers x such that $f(x) = 2$.

(d) Find all numbers x such that $f(x) > 2$.

(e) Find at least three numbers x such that $f(x) = f(-x)$.

(f) Find a number x such that $f(x + 1) = 0$.

(g) Find two numbers x such that $f(x - 2) = 4$.

(h) Find a number x such that $f(x + 1) = f(x - 2)$.

(i) Find a number x such that $f(x) + 1 = f(x - 4)$.

B.4. Figure 4-31 shows the entire graphs of functions f and g.

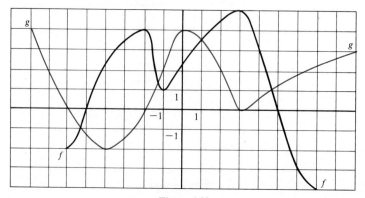

Figure 4-31

(a) What is the domain of f? the domain of g?
(b) What is the range of f? the range of g?
(c) Find all numbers x in the interval $[-3, 1]$ such that $f(x) = 2$.
(d) Find all numbers x in the interval $[-3, 3]$ such that $g(x) \geq 2$.
(e) Find the number x for which $f(x) - g(x)$ is largest.
(f) For how many values of x is it true that $f(x) = g(x)$?
(g) Find all intervals over which both functions are defined, the graph of f is falling *and* the graph of g is rising (from left to right).
(h) Find all intervals over which the graph of $g(x)$ is falling *and* $0 \leq f(x) \leq 2$.

B.5. The owners of the Rieben & Tabares Deluxe Widget Works have determined that both their weekly manufacturing expenses and their weekly sales income are functions of the number of widgets manufactured each week. Figure 4-32 shows the graphs of these two functions.

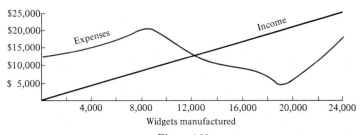

Figure 4-32

(a) Use careful measurement on the graph and the fact that profit = income − expenses to determine the weekly profit if 5000 widgets are manufactured.
(b) Do the same if 10,000, 14,000, 18,000, or 22,000 widgets are manufactured.
(c) What is the smallest number of widgets that can be manufactured each week without losing money?
(d) What is the largest number of widgets that can be manufactured without losing money?
(e) The owners build a new lounge and swimming pool for their employees. This raises their expenses by approximately $5000 per week. Draw the graph of the new "expense function."
(f) Due to competitive pressure, widget prices cannot be increased and the income function remains the same. Answer parts (a)–(d) with the new expense function in place of the old.

B.6. A weather bureau device records the graph of the temperature as a function of time as shown in Figure 4-33 on the next page.

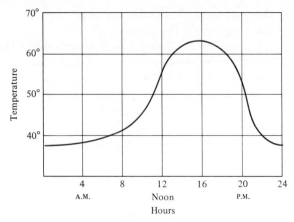

Figure 4-33

We write tem(t) for the temperature at t hours after midnight.

(a) Find tem(10). Find tem(3 + 12).
(b) Is tem(6) bigger than, equal to, or less than tem(18)?
(c) At which time is the temperature 50°?
(d) Find a 4-hr period for which tem(h) > 40 for all h in this 4-hr period.
(e) Find the difference in temperature at 10 and 16 hours. Identify this difference in the graph; that is, express difference in terms of points and their location on the graph.
(f) Is it true that tem(6) = tem(8)? Explain in terms of the graph.
(g) Is it true that tem(6 · 2) = 6 · tem(2)?
(h) The temperature graph above was recorded in city F. City B is 500 miles to the south of city F, and its temperature is 7° higher all day long. Sketch into the above drawing the temperature for city B during the same day.
(i) Find an hour h at which the temperature in city B is the same as tem(12) in city F.

5. THE SHAPE OF A GRAPH

We now consider various *geometric* properties a graph might have. Each of them is easily understood simply by looking at the *shape* of the graph. But a careful analysis is needed to understand just what these geometric properties mean in terms of the *algebraic* behavior of the function.

The ability to translate graphical properties into algebraic terms, and vice-versa, can be very helpful in graphing. For instance, by using algebra we may be able to tell *in advance* that the graph of a given function will have certain geometric features. This will not only make it easier to graph the function but will often result in a much more accurate graph as well.

SYMMETRY WITH RESPECT TO THE y-AXIS

Geometric Description Figure 4-34 shows some graphs which are **symmetric with respect to the y-axis.**

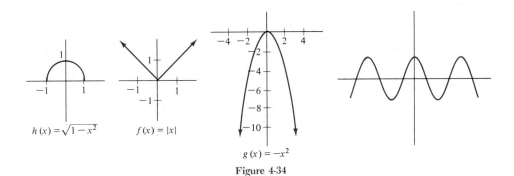

Figure 4-34

In each case the part of the graph on the right side of the y-axis is the *mirror image* of the part of the graph on the left side of the y-axis (with the y-axis being the mirror). In more technical terms, the left half of the graph can be obtained by *reflecting* the right half in the y-axis. This means that if you fold the plane along the y-axis, so that the right-hand half of the plane goes on top of the left-hand half, then the right-hand half of the graph will *fit exactly* on the left-hand half. A point on the right half of the graph will be folded onto its mirror image point on the left-hand half of the graph. For example, in each of the graphs shown in Figure 4-35, all of which are symmetric with respect to the y-axis, P is the mirror image of Q:

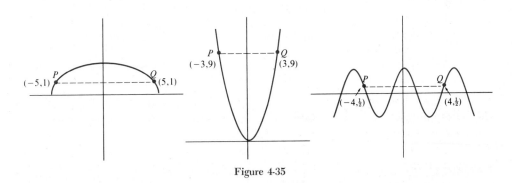

Figure 4-35

Algebraic Description Observe that each pair of mirror image points P and Q in Figure 4-35 has these two properties:

(i) P and Q are the same vertical distance from the x-axis. Hence P and Q have the same *second* coordinates.

   (ii)   *P* and *Q* are the same horizontal distance from the *y*-axis, on opposite sides of the axis. Hence the *first* coordinates of *P* and *Q* are negatives of each other.

The same facts are true for *any* pair of mirror image points *P* and *Q* on the graph of a function *f*. If *Q* has coordinates $(c, f(c))$, then the first coordinate of *P* must be $-c$, as shown in Figure 4-36.

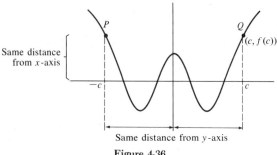

Figure 4-36

But *P* is on the graph of the function *f*, so its second coordinate is $f(-c)$. Since *P* and *Q* are the same distance from the *x*-axis (as shown in Figure 4-36), they must have the same second coordinate. This means that $f(-c)$ and $f(c)$ must be the same number. The fact that $f(-c) = f(c)$ for mirror image points provides this *algebraic* description of functions that are symmetric with respect to the *y*-axis:

The graph of a function f *is* **symmetric with respect to the y-axis** *provided*

$$f(-x) = f(x)$$

for every number x *in the domain of* f. *Such a function is said to be an* **even function.**

    When the rule of the function *f* is given by an algebraic formula involving *x*, then the condition that $f(-x) = f(x)$ means that **the formula remains the *same* when *x* is replaced by** $-x$.

EXAMPLE   The function $f(x) = \dfrac{1}{x^2 + 1}$ is an even function because for every real number *x*

$$f(-x) = \frac{1}{(-x)^2 + 1} = \frac{1}{x^2 + 1} = f(x)$$

This explains algebraically why the graph of *f* (which is sketched on page 200) is symmetric with respect to the *y*-axis.

EXAMPLE   On the other hand, the function $f(x) = 2x + 5$ is *not* an even function since

$$f(-x) = 2(-x) + 5 = -2x + 5, \qquad \text{while } f(x) = 2x + 5$$

Thus $f(-x)$ is *not equal* to $f(x)$ when $x \neq 0$. So the graph of f is *not* symmetric with respect to the y-axis. You can confirm this geometrically by sketching the graph (it's a straight line).

In order to find the *graph of an even function* f, you need only consider points $(x, f(x))$ with $x \geq 0$. Once you have this part of the graph, you can immediately obtain the other half by using symmetry with respect to the y-axis.

PERIODIC FUNCTIONS

Geometric Description   A function whose graph repeats the same pattern at regular intervals is said to be **periodic**. If the shortest length in which the graph completes a pattern is c units, then the function is said to have **period** c. For instance, see Figure 4-37.

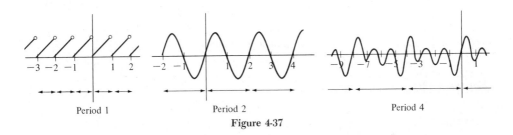

Period 1   Period 2   Period 4

Figure 4-37

The critical fact about the graph of a periodic function of period c is that you need only determine the graph over a single interval of length c. For instance, you can consider only points with $0 \leq x \leq c$. The rest of the graph will just be a repetition of this part.

Algebraic Description   Suppose P, with coordinates $(b, f(b))$, is a point on the graph of a periodic function f with period c. We can think of the basic graph pattern as starting at P and extending to the right for c units, as shown in Figure 4-38.

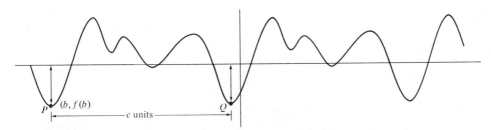

Figure 4-38

The point Q at which the pattern begins to repeat is c units to the *right* of P. Since P has first coordinate b, the point Q must have first coordinate $b + c$. But Q is on the graph of the function f, so its second coordinate must be $f(b + c)$. Since the pattern begins at P and starts to repeat at Q, these two points must lie the same distance from the x-axis, as shown in Figure 4-38. In other words, the second coordinates of P and Q are equal; that is,

$$f(b) = f(b + c)$$

This analysis applies to *any* point $(x, f(x))$ on the graph. The second coordinate of $(x, f(x))$ is the same as the second coordinate of the point c units to the right $(x + c, f(x + c))$. Consequently,

> *A function* f *is **periodic with period** c *provided* c *is the smallest positive number such that*
>
> $$f(x) = f(x + c)$$
>
> *for every number* x *in the domain of* f.

The function $g(x) = x - [x]$, whose graph is on page 205, is periodic.

INCREASING FUNCTIONS

Geometric Description A function is said to be **increasing on an interval** if the graph of the function always *rises* as you move from left to right in the interval. For example, each of the functions shown in Figure 4-39 is increasing on the stated intervals.

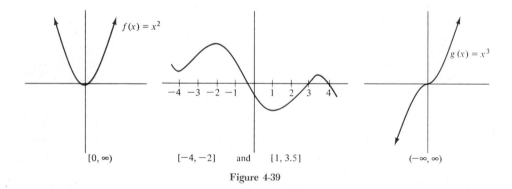

Figure 4-39

Obviously, if a function is increasing on an interval I, it is also increasing on any interval contained in I. A function, such as the function g in Figure 4-39, which is increasing on *every* interval in its domain is called an **increasing function**.

Algebraic Description Suppose the function f is increasing on an interval and that c and d are numbers in the interval with $c < d$. Since $c < d$, the point $(d, f(d))$ lies to the *right* of the point $(c, f(c))$ on the graph. Since f is increasing, its graph is rising from left to right. Therefore the right-hand point $(d, f(d))$ must be *higher* than the left-hand point $(c, f(c))$, as shown in Figure 4-40.

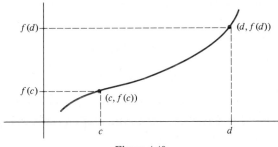

Figure 4-40

Consequently, the second coordinate of $(d, f(d))$ must be *larger* than the second coordinate of $(c, f(c))$; that is, $f(c) < f(d)$. Thus

> A function f *is **increasing on an interval** provided that for any numbers* c *and* d *in the interval,*
>
> $$\textit{whenever } \mathrm{c} < \mathrm{d}, \qquad \textit{then } \mathrm{f(c)} < \mathrm{f(d)}$$

EXAMPLE We know from the graph of the function $f(x) = x^2$ (Figure 4-39) that f is increasing on $[0, \infty)$. Since $f(c) = c^2$ and $f(d) = d^2$, the algebraic meaning of this fact is:

$$\text{whenever } 0 \le c < d, \qquad \text{then } c^2 < d^2$$

DECREASING FUNCTIONS

Geometric Description A function is said to be **decreasing on an interval** if the graph of the function always *falls* as you move from left to right in the interval. A function which is decreasing on *every* interval in its domain is called a **decreasing function.**

Algebraic Description Suppose the function f is decreasing on an interval and that c and d are numbers in the interval with $c < d$. Then the point $(d, f(d))$ lies to the *right* of the point $(c, f(c))$ on the graph. Since f is decreasing, its graph is *falling* from left to right. Therefore, the right-hand point $(d, f(d))$ must be *lower* than the left-hand point $(c, f(c))$, as shown in Figure 4-41 on the next page.

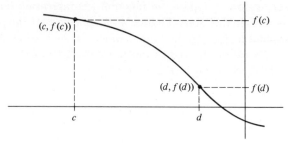

Figure 4-41

Consequently, $f(c) > f(d)$ and we have:

> *The function* f *is **decreasing on an interval** provided that for any numbers* c *and* d *in the interval,*
>
> *whenever* c < d, *then* f(c) > f(d)

SUMMARY

The following chart summarizes the preceding discussion; it also mentions "odd functions," which are explained in the DO IT YOURSELF! segment at the end of this section.

Geometric Description	Algebraic Description	Name of Property
Graph of f is *symmetric with respect to y-axis*	$f(-x) = f(x)$ for all x in domain of f	f is *even*
Graph of f repeats its pattern every c units	$f(x) = f(x + c)$ for all x in domain of f	f is *periodic with period c*
Graph of f *rises* from left to right over the interval I	Whenever $b < c$, then $f(b) < f(c)$ for all b, c in I	f is *increasing on I*
Graph of f *falls* from left to right over the interval I	Whenever $b < c$, then $f(b) > f(c)$ for all b, c in I	f is *decreasing on I*
Graph of f is *symmetric with respect to the origin*	$f(-x) = -f(x)$ for all x in the domain of f	f is *odd*

EXERCISES

A.1. Without graphing, decide which of the following functions have graphs which are symmetric to the y-axis (that is, which functions are *even*).

(a) $f(x) = |x| + 3$

(b) $g(x) = |x - 1|$

(c) $y = x^2 - |x|$

(d) $k(t) = t^4 - 6t^2 + 5$

(e) $f(u) = (u + 2)^2 + u^4 + 2$

(f) $g(x) = x^3(3x + x^5) + 6x^2 + 3$

(g) $h(x) = x^2(x^3 - 3x^5) + 5$

(h) $y = \sqrt{t^2 - 5}$

A.2. Each of the graphs in Figure 4-42 is the graph of a function. For each of these graphs answer the following questions:

(i) Is the function even?

(ii) Is the function periodic?

(iii) Is the function increasing on $[1, 5]$?

(iv) Is the function decreasing on $[-3, 2]$?

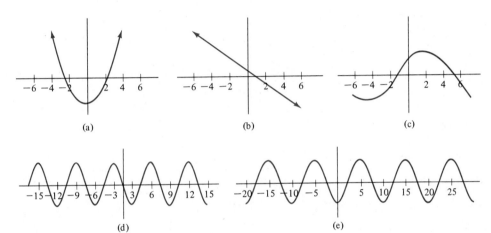

Figure 4-42

A.3. For each of the functions whose graphs appear in Figure 4-43, state the intervals on which the function is increasing and the intervals on which it is decreasing.

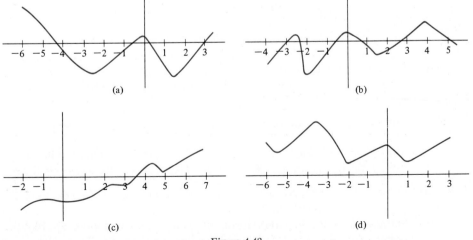

Figure 4-43

B.1.   Sketch the graph of a function f which satisfies these five conditions:

(i) $f(-1) = 2$ (iii) $f(x)$ starts decreasing when $x = 1$

(ii) $f(x) \geq 2$ when x is in   (iv) $f(3) = 3 = f(0)$

the interval $(-1, \frac{1}{2})$ (v) $f(x)$ starts increasing when $x = 5$

(*Note:* the function whose graph you sketch need not be given by an algebraic formula.)

B.2.   Examine Figure 4-44.

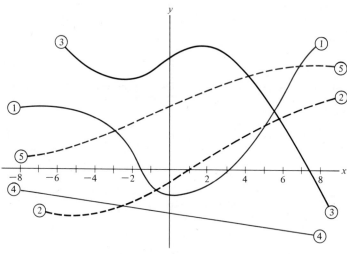

Figure 4-44

(a)   For *each* of the following *five* statements, find one (or more) functions (among the five whose graphs appear in Figure 4-44) for which the statement is true.

(i) $f(2) < f(1)$

(ii) $f(x)$ is negative and increasing from $x = 1$ to $x = 2$

(iii) $f(0) < 0$ but $f(2) > 0$

(iv) $f(x)$ is negative and decreasing from $x = -4$ to $x = -3$

(v) $f(x) > f(-x)$ for some number x with $|x| \leq 5$

(b)   For each of the following six statements, find a pair of functions (or several pairs) from among the five whose graphs appear in Figure 4-44 for which the statement is true.

(i) $f(1) - g(1) > 0$ (iv) $\dfrac{f(x)}{g(x)} < 1$ for some $x < 0$

(ii) $f(x) < g(3)$ for $0 \leq x \leq 2$ (v) $f(x) = g(x)$ for some x with $|x| \geq 2$

(iii) $f(x)g(x) < 0$ for $x > 4$ (vi) $f(x) \leq g(-x)$ for some x with $|x| < 4$

B.3. (a)   Draw some coordinate axes and plot the points $(0, 1)$, $(1, -3)$, $(-5, 2)$, $(-3, -5)$, $(2, 3)$, and $(4, 1)$.

(b)   Suppose the points in part (a) lie on the graph of an *even* function f. Plot the points $(0, f(0))$, $(-1, f(-1))$, $(5, f(5))$, $(3, f(3))$, $(-2, f(-2))$, and $(-4, f(-4))$.

B.4. Draw the graph of an *even* function which includes the points $(0, -3)$, $(-3, 0)$, $(2, 0)$, $(1, -4)$, $(2.5, -1)$, $(-4, 3)$ and $(-5, 3)$. (*Note:* there are many possible correct answers here.)

B.5. Suppose f is a periodic function with period c and that for some number x, $f(x) = k$.
   (a) Find $f(x + c)$, $f(x + 2c)$, $f(x + 3c)$, $f(x + 4c)$, $f(x + 5c)$. (*Hint:* how far apart are $x + c$ and $x + 2c$? How far apart are $x + 2c$ and $x + 3c$?)
   (b) Find $f(x - c)$, $f(x - 2c)$, $f(x - 3c)$, $f(x - 4c)$, $f(x - 5c)$. (*Hint:* how far apart are $x - c$ and x? How far apart are $x - 2c$ and $x - c$?)
   (c) Find $f(x + nc)$ for any integer n. [See part (a) when $n = 1, 2, 3, 4$, or 5 and part (b) when $n = -1, -2, -3, -4$, or -5.]

B.6. Figure 4-45 shows the graphs of some periodic functions. What is the period of each?

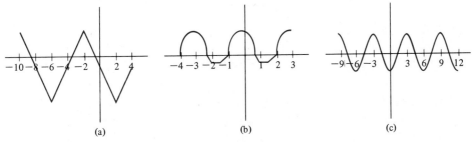

Figure 4-45

B.7. Draw the graph of an even function which is periodic of period 3. (There are many possible correct answers.)

B.8. Use algebra to show that each of the functions below is increasing on the interval $(0, 10]$. Some of them may also be increasing on other intervals. You may assume the usual facts about inequalities, including the following:

$$\text{if } 0 \le c < d, \quad \text{then } c^2 < d^2;$$
$$\text{if } c < d, \quad \text{then } c^3 < d^3;$$
$$\text{if } 0 \le c < d, \quad \text{then } \sqrt{c} < \sqrt{d}.$$

   (a) $f(x) = x^2 + 3$
   (b) $g(x) = x^3 - 10{,}000$
   (c) $h(t) = t^2 + t + 5$
   (d) $k(u) = u^3 + u^2 + 1$
   (e) $h(x) = \sqrt{x + 3}$
   (f) $g(x) = x^3 + x^2$
   (g) $k(x) = \sqrt{x^3 + 2x - 1}$
   (h) $f(x) = -\dfrac{1}{x}$

B.9. Suppose an equation in x and y has the following property: the equation remains the same when y is replaced by $-y$. For example, each of these equations has this property:

$$x = y^2, \quad |x| + |y| = 1, \quad x^2 + y^2 - 2x + 1 = 0, \quad 16x^2 + 9y^2 + 16x = 20.$$

   (a) If the point (c, d) is on the graph of the equation, what other point is *necessarily* on the graph as well?

(b)   How does the part of the graph of the equation *above* the x-axis look in comparison with the part of the graph *below* the x-axis? (*Hint:* see the analogous, but different, discussion on pp. 215–217.)

(c)   In view of your answer to part (b), what would be a good name for the property defined above?

(d)   Is the graph of such an equation *ever* the same as a graph of some function?

C.1.   (a)   Suppose x is a real number and [x] = k. Show that [x + 1] = k + 1. (Note that k and k + 1 are consecutive integers.)

(b)   Let g(x) = x − [x]. Use part (a) to give an algebraic proof that g(x) = g(x + 1) for every number x. Hence g is periodic of period (at most) 1.

(c)   Use an algebraic argument to show that the function f(x) = [x] + [−x] is periodic of period 1.

DO IT YOURSELF!

SYMMETRY WITH RESPECT TO THE ORIGIN

Geometric Description   A graph is said to be symmetric with respect to the origin if rotating the graph through an angle of 180° around the origin results in exactly the same graph. Every straight line through the origin has this property, as shown on the left-hand side of Figure 4-46.

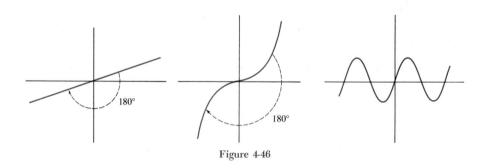

Figure 4-46

The other graphs in Figure 4-46 are also symmetric with respect to the origin, although rotating them is harder to visualize. [It may help to think of the plane as a giant turntable, revolving around the origin.]

Algebraic Description   Suppose P is a point on the graph of a function f, which is symmetric with respect to the origin. When the graph is rotated 180° around the origin, P will land on another point Q on the graph, as shown in Figure 4-47.

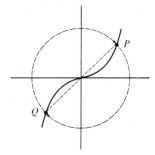

Figure 4-47

Observe that the line segment PQ is just the diameter of a circle with center at the origin. As the graph rotates $180°$, P and Q move along the circle and exchange places. We claim that:

The coordinates of Q are the *negatives* of the coordinates of P.

For instance, if P has coordinates $(4, 3)$, then Q has coordinates $(-4, -3)$. This claim should appear plausible and we shall assume its truth here. A proof of the claim is outlined in Exercise C.1.

Now P is on the graph of the function f, so its coordinates are $(c, f(c))$ for some number c. Similarly, Q has coordinates $(d, f(d))$ for some number d. But by the preceding claim,

d = first coordinate of Q = negative of first coordinate of $P = -c$

$f(d)$ = second coordinate of Q = negative of second coordinate of $P = -f(c)$

Furthermore, since $-c = d$, we must have $f(-c) = f(d)$. By combining these last two facts, we see that

$$f(-c) = f(d) = -f(c)$$

Thus for *any* point $(c, f(c))$ on the graph of f we have $f(-c) = -f(c)$. Consequently, we conclude:

The graph of the function f *is **symmetric with respect to the origin** provided*

$$f(-x) = -f(x)$$

for every number x *in the domain of* f. *Such a function is said to be an **odd function.***

EXAMPLE   The function $f(x) = x^3$ is an odd function since

$$f(-x) = (-x)^3 = -x^3 = -f(x)$$

This is an algebraic verification that the graph of f is indeed symmetric with respect to the origin. This graph is depicted in Figure 4-39 on page 218.

EXERCISES

A.1.   Which of the graphs in Figure 4-48 are symmetric with respect to the origin?

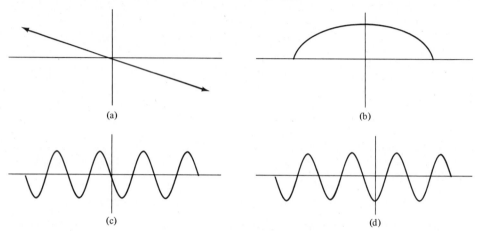

(a)   (b)

(c)   (d)

Figure 4-48

A.2.   Without graphing, decide which of the following functions have graphs that are symmetric with respect to the origin (that is, which functions are *odd*):

(a) $f(x) = 4x$ (e) $y = \sqrt{5 - x^2}$

(b) $g(x) = 4x^3 - 3x$ (f) $g(t) = -t^3 + 1$

(c) $h(u) = |3u|$ (g) $h(x) = \dfrac{1}{x}$

(d) $k(t) = -5t$ (h) $y = x(x^4 - x^2) + 4$

A.3.   Determine which of the functions, whose graphs appear in Figure 4-49, are even; which are odd; and which are neither:

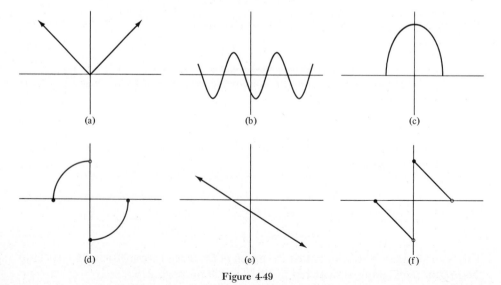

(a)   (b)   (c)

(d)   (e)   (f)

Figure 4-49

B.1. **(a)** Plot the points $(0, 0)$; $(2, 3)$; $(3, 4)$; $(5, 0)$; $(7, -3)$; $(-1, +1)$; $(-4, -1)$; $(-6, 1)$.

(b) Suppose the points in part (a) lie on the graph of an *odd* function f. Plot the points $(-2, f(-2))$; $(-3, f(-3))$; $(-5, f(-5))$; $(-7, f(-7))$; $(1, f(1))$; $(4, f(4))$; $(6, f(6))$.

(c) Draw the graph of an odd function f that includes all the points plotted in parts (a) and (b).°

B.2. Draw the graph of an odd function that includes the points $(-3, 5)$, $(-1, 1)$, $(2, -6)$, $(4, -9)$, and $(5, -5)$.°

B.3. Draw the graph of an odd function that is periodic of period 3.°

C.1. Let r be a fixed positive number and suppose that P and Q are the endpoints of a diameter of the circle $x^2 + y^2 = r^2$ (that is, the circle with radius r and center the origin), as shown in Figure 4-50.

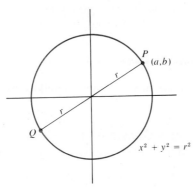

Figure 4-50

Suppose that P has coordinates (a, b). Prove that Q has coordinates $(-a, -b)$ as follows.

(a) Show that the equation of the straight line through P, $(0, 0)$ and Q is $y = \dfrac{b}{a} x$. [*Hint:* (a, b) and $(0, 0)$ are two points on the line.]

(b) Show that $x = a, y = b$ and $x = -a, y = -b$ are the only pairs (x, y) that are solutions of *both* these equations:

$$y = \frac{b}{a} x \quad \text{and} \quad x^2 + y^2 = r^2$$

[*Hint:* Substitute $\dfrac{b}{a} x$ for y in the second equation, then solve for x. Use the fact that $a^2 + b^2 = r^2$ (why?) to show that $x = a$ and $x = -a$ are the only solutions. Finally, substitute these values for x in the equation $y = \dfrac{b}{a} x$ to find the corresponding solutions for y.]

° There are many possible correct answers.

(c) Since P and Q lie on both the straight line $y = \dfrac{b}{a}x$ *and* the circle $x^2 + y^2 = r^2$, their coordinates must be solutions of *both* equations. Since $P = (a, b)$, part (b) shows that Q must have coordinates $(-a, -b)$.

6. NEW GRAPHS FROM OLD

In this section we consider the question:

> If the rule of a function is changed algebraically so as to produce a new function, how is the graph of the new function related to the graph of the original function?

In other words, what do *algebraic* manipulations on "formulas" mean in *geometric* terms? If we know the graph of a particular function f, then the answers to these questions will provide techniques for easily graphing many of the functions whose rules are obtained from the rule of f by various algebraic manipulations.

NEW FUNCTIONS FROM OLD

Here are some common ways in which new functions are constructed algebraically from old ones.

Adding or Subtracting a Constant   If f is a function and c is a positive real number, then we can form two new functions g and h whose rules are:

$$g(x) = f(x) + c \qquad h(x) = f(x) - c$$

EXAMPLE   If $f(x) = x^2$ and $c = 3$, we have the functions

$$g(x) = f(x) + 3 = x^2 + 3 \qquad \text{and} \qquad h(x) = f(x) - 3 = x^2 - 3$$

EXAMPLE   The function $g(x) = x^3 + x^2 + 2$ may be thought of as $f(x) + 2$, where $f(x) = x^3 + x^2$.

Multiplying by a Constant   If f is a function and c is a real number, then a new function g can be formed by the rule

$$g(x) = cf(x)$$

EXAMPLE   If $f(x) = x^2$ and $c = 16$, then we can form the function g whose rule is: $g(x) = 16f(x) = 16x^2$.

EXAMPLE   The function $g(x) = -4x^2 + 8x + 4$ may be considered as $g(x) = (-4)f(x)$, where $f(x) = x^2 - 2x - 1$.

Change of Variable   If f is a function and c is a real number, then we can construct two new functions g and h whose rules are:

$$g(x) = f(x + c) \qquad h(x) = f(x - c)$$

EXAMPLE If $f(x) = x^2$ and $c = 3$, then

$$g(x) = f(x + 3) = (x + 3)^2 = x^2 + 6x + 9 \qquad \text{and}$$
$$h(x) = f(x - 3) = (x - 3)^2 = x^2 - 6x + 9$$

NEW GRAPHS FROM OLD

If you begin with a function f, the methods previously outlined provide numerous ways of constructing new functions from f. As we shall now see, the graph of each of these new functions can easily be obtained from the graph of f by performing some simple geometric procedure.

Adding or Subtracting a Constant Consider, for example, the functions $f(x) = x^2$ and $g(x) = x^2 + 2$. For every number x,

the point (x, x^2) is on the graph of $f(x) = x^2$;

the point $(x, x^2 + 2)$ is on the graph of $g(x) = x^2 + 2 = f(x) + 2$

For instance, when $x = 3$ the point $(3, 9)$ is on the graph of f and $(3, 11)$ is on the graph of g. But the second coordinate of $(x, x^2 + 2)$ is 2 units *larger* than the second coordinate of (x, x^2). So the point $(x, x^2 + 2)$ lies 2 units directly *above* the point (x, x^2), as shown in Figure 4-51.

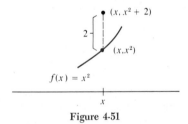

Figure 4-51

Thus for every number x, the graph of $g(x) = x^2 + 2$ lies exactly 2 units above the graph of $f(x) = x^2$. In other words, the graph of $g(x) = x^2 + 2$ (that is, $g(x) = f(x) + 2$) is just the graph of $f(x) = x^2$ *shifted* 2 *units upward*, as shown in Figure 4-52.

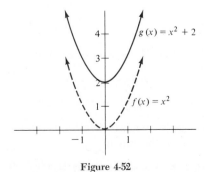

Figure 4-52

Now let's see what happens when you obtain a new function by *subtracting* a constant.

EXAMPLE   Consider the functions $f(x) = x^2$ and $h(x) = x^2 - 3$. For every number x,

the point (x, x^2) is on the graph of $f(x) = x^2$;

the point $(x, x^2 - 3)$ is on the graph of $h(x) = x^2 - 3 = f(x) - 3$

For instance, when $x = 4$ the point $(4, 16)$ is on the graph of $f(x) = x^2$ and the point $(4, 13)$ is on the graph of $h(x) = x^2 - 3$. But the second coordinate of $(x, x^2 - 3)$ is 3 units *smaller* than the second coordinate of (x, x^2). So the point $(x, x^2 - 3)$ lies 3 units directly *below* the point (x, x^2). So the graph of $h(x) = x^2 - 3$ (that is, $h(x) = f(x) - 3$) is just the graph of $f(x) = x^2$ *shifted 3 units downward*, as shown in Figure 4-53.

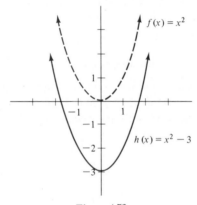

Figure 4-53

The same sort of arguments just used to obtain the graphs of $g(x) = f(x) + 2$ and $h(x) = f(x) - 3$ from the graph of $f(x) = x^2$ can be used with *any* function and any constant c to obtain the graphs of $g(x) = f(x) + c$ and $h(x) = f(x) - c$:

If $c > 0$, then the graph of $g(x) = f(x) + c$ is the graph of f shifted upward c units.

If $c > 0$, then the graph of $h(x) = f(x) - c$ is the graph of f shifted downward c units.

EXAMPLE   The graph of $f(x) = \sqrt{x}$ was determined on page 198. We can now use this graph to find the graphs of the functions

$$g(x) = \sqrt{x} + 5 \qquad h(x) = \sqrt{x} + 1 \qquad k(x) = \sqrt{x} - 3 \qquad r(x) = \sqrt{x} - \tfrac{11}{2}$$

without plotting any points, as shown in Figure 4-54.

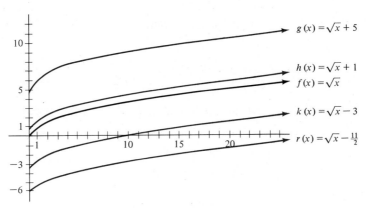

Figure 4-54

Multiplying by a Positive Constant   This situation is most easily understood by considering a specific example. Suppose $f(x) = x^2 - 3$. Then we know what the graph of f looks like (see page 230). Suppose $c = 2$, so that the function $g(x) = cf(x)$ is just the function $g(x) = 2f(x) = 2(x^2 - 3) = 2x^2 - 6$. If $x = 3$, then

$$(3, f(3)) = (3, 6) \text{ is on the graph of } f;$$
$$(3, g(3)) = (3, 12) \text{ is on the graph of } g$$

Observe that $(3, 12)$ lies *directly above* $(3, 6)$ and is *twice as far from the x-axis*, as shown in Figure 4-55.

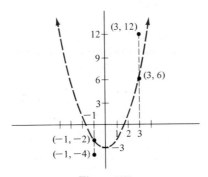

Figure 4-55

Similarly, if $x = -1$, then

$$(-1, f(-1)) = (-1, -2) \text{ is on the graph of } f;$$
$$(-1, g(-1)) = (-1, -4) \text{ is on the graph of } g$$

The point $(-1, -4)$ lies *directly below* $(-1, -2)$ and is *twice as far from the x-axis,* as shown in Figure 4-55. A similar argument for any number x shows that the point $(x, g(x)) = (x, 2f(x))$ on the graph of g lies

> directly above or below,
> on the same side of the x-axis,
> *twice as far* from the x-axis as

the point $(x, f(x))$ on the graph of f. Consequently, the graph of g resembles the one in Figure 4-56.

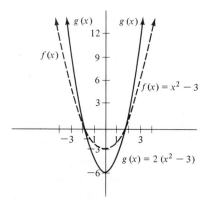

Figure 4-56

Thus the graph of g is the graph of f *stretched vertically away from the x-axis* by a factor of 2.

A similar analysis enables us to obtain the graph of $h(x) = \frac{1}{4}f(x) = \frac{1}{4}(x^2 - 3)$ from the graph of $f(x) = x^2 - 3$. But now the factor is $c = \frac{1}{4}$ instead of $c = 2$. If we plot a few points on both graphs, as shown in Figure 4-57, we can see what happens.

x	$f(x) = x^2 - 3$	$h(x) = \frac{1}{4}(x^2 - 3)$
-3	6	$\frac{1}{4}(6) = \frac{3}{2}$
-1	-2	$\frac{1}{4}(-2) = -\frac{1}{2}$
0	-3	$\frac{1}{4}(-3) = -\frac{3}{4}$
2	1	$\frac{1}{4}(1) = \frac{1}{4}$
3	6	$\frac{1}{4}(6) = \frac{3}{2}$

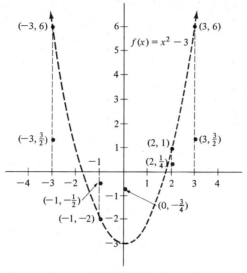

Figure 4-57

In each case we see that the point $(x, h(x)) = (x, \frac{1}{4}f(x))$ on the graph of h lies

> directly above or below,
> on the same side of the x-axis,
> *one-fourth as far from the x-axis* as

the point $(x, f(x))$ on the graph of f. Thus the graph of h is the graph of f *shrunk vertically toward the x-axis* by a factor of $\frac{1}{4}$, as shown in Figure 4-58.

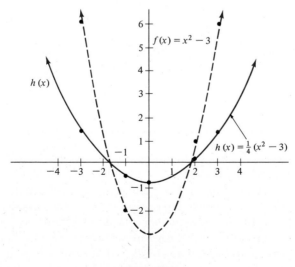

Figure 4-58

Analogous arguments work for any function f and positive real number c:

If $c > 1$, *then the graph of* g(x) $=$ cf(x) *is the graph of* f *stretched vertically away from the* x-*axis by a factor of* c.

If $0 < c < 1$, *then the graph of* h(x) $=$ cf(x) *is the graph of* f *shrunk vertically toward the* x-*axis by a factor of* c.

Multiplying by -1 Consider $f(x) = x^2$ and the function g whose rule is $g(x) = -f(x) = -x^2$. For every number x,

the point (x, x^2) is on the graph of $f(x) = x^2$;

the point $(x, -x^2)$ is on the graph of $g(x) = -x^2 = -f(x)$

For instance, when $x = 2$ the point $(2, 4)$ is on the graph of f and $(2, -4)$ is on the graph of g, as shown in Figure 4-59.

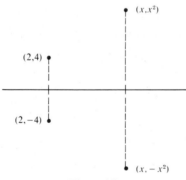

Figure 4-59

Observe that the second coordinates of (x, x^2) and $(x, -x^2)$ are negatives of each other. So the two points lie on the same vertical line on *opposite sides* of the x-axis, the *same distance* from the x-axis. If we fold the plane along the x-axis, the point (x, x^2) will land on the point $(x, -x^2)$. To view this another way, think of the x-axis as a mirror: The points (x, x^2) and $(x, -x^2)$ are mirror images of each other. Consequently, the graph of $g(x) = -x^2$ is just the graph of $f(x) = x^2$ *reflected* in the x-axis (as if the axis were a mirror). See Figure 4-60.

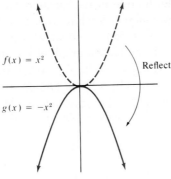

Figure 4-60

EXAMPLE Similar reasoning can be used with the function $f(x) = x^2 - 3$ to obtain the graph of $g(x) = -f(x) = -(x^2 - 3)$. The graph of $f(x) = x^2 - 3$ is shown in Figure 4-58 on page 233. Corresponding to each point $(x, f(x))$ on the graph of f, there is a point $(x, g(x)) = (x, -f(x))$ on the graph of g that lies on the *opposite side* of the x-axis, the *same distance* from the axis. So the graph of g is the reflection of the graph of f in the x-axis, as shown in Figure 4-61.

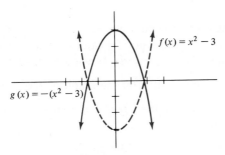

Figure 4-61

Similar arguments can be used with *any* function f and lead to this conclusion:

The graph of $g(x) = -f(x)$ *is the graph of* f *reflected in the x-axis, as shown here.*

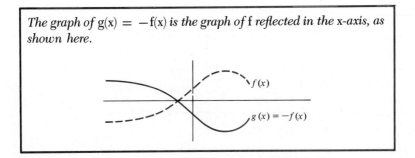

EXAMPLE   If you multiply the rule of the function $f(x) = x^2 - 3$ by the negative constant $-\frac{1}{2}$, you obtain the function h whose rule is $h(x) = -\frac{1}{2}f(x) = -\frac{1}{2}(x^2 - 3)$. The graph of this new function h can be obtained in two steps from the graph of $f(x) = x^2 - 3$. Beginning with the known graph of $f(x) = x^2 - 3$, we first construct the graph of the function $\frac{1}{2}f(x) = \frac{1}{2}(x^2 - 3)$. We have already seen that this is just the graph of f shrunk toward the x axis by a factor of $\frac{1}{2}$, as shown in the center of Figure 4-62. Finally, the graph of $h(x) = -\frac{1}{2}(x^2 - 3) = -\frac{1}{2}f(x)$ is just the reflection of the graph of $\frac{1}{2}f(x) = \frac{1}{2}(x^2 - 3)$ in the x-axis, as shown on the right side of Figure 4-62.

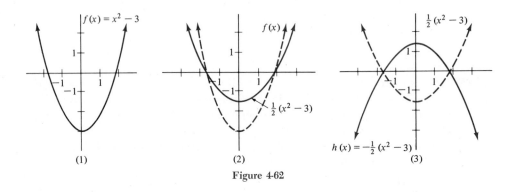

Figure 4-62

Change of Variable   The function $g(x) = (x + 5)^2$ is just the function $f(x + 5)$, where $f(x) = x^2$. To see how the graph of g can be obtained from the graph of f, we consider a specific value of x, say, $x = 2$. When $x = 2$, then $f(x) = 2^2 = 4$ so that

$$\text{the point } (2, 4) \text{ is on the graph of } f(x) = x^2$$

Now look what happens 5 units to the *left* of $x = 2$, at $x = -3$. When $x = -3$, then $g(x) = (-3 + 5)^2 = 4$ so that

$$\text{the point } (-3, 4) \text{ is on the graph of } g(x) = (x + 5)^2$$

Since the points $(2, 4)$ and $(-3, 4)$ have the same second coordinates, they both are the same vertical distance from the x-axis. The first coordinates show that the point $(-3, 4)$ on the graph of g lies 5 units to the *left* of the point $(2, 4)$ on the graph of f, as shown in Figure 4-63.

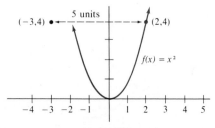

Figure 4-63

Similarly, for any point $(x, f(x))$ on the graph of $f(x) = x^2$ there is a corresponding point on the graph of $g(x) = (x + 5)^2$ that lies exactly 5 units to the *left* of $(x, f(x))$, at the same distance from the x-axis. Consequently, the graph of $g(x) = (x + 5)^2$ is just the graph of $f(x) = x^2$ shifted 5 units to the *left*, as shown in Figure 4-64.

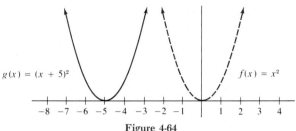

Figure 4-64

Warning Don't get confused about horizontal shifting of graphs. Because of the plus sign in "$x + 5$," many students mistakenly believe that the graph of $g(x) = (x + 5)^2$ really should be 5 units to the right of the graph of $f(x) = x^2$. To see why this is *wrong*, look at the vertex $(0, 0)$ of the parabola $f(x) = x^2$. The point 5 units to the right of $(0, 0)$ is $(5, 0)$. But the point $(5, 0)$ is not on the graph of $g(x) = (x + 5)^2$ since $g(5) = (5 + 5)^2 = 100$. On the other hand, if you go 5 units to the *left* of $(0, 0)$, you come to $(-5, 0)$. Since $g(-5) = (-5 + 5)^2 = 0$, the point $(-5, 0)$ *is* on the graph of g.

The graphs of functions such as $h(x) = (x - 5)^2$ (note the minus sign) can be obtained by analogous arguments. As you might suspect, the graph of $h(x) = (x - 5)^2$ is just the graph of $f(x) = x^2$ shifted 5 units to the *right*. For instance, the point 5 units to the right of $(0, 0)$ on the graph of f is the point $(5, 0)$. When $x = 5$, then $h(5) = (5 - 5)^2 = 0$ so that the point $(5, 0)$ *is* on the graph of $h(x) = (x - 5)^2$. More generally, the following statement is true for any function f.

Let c be a positive constant.

The graph of $g(x) = f(x + c)$ *is the graph of* f *shifted horizontally* c *units to the left.*

The graph of $h(x) = f(x - c)$ *is the graph of* f *shifted horizontally* c *units to the right.*

EXAMPLE   The graph of the function $f(x) = x^3 - 3x$ is shown by the dotted line in Figure 4-65 on the next page. The graph of the function h whose rule is

$$h(x) = f(x - 2) = (x - 2)^3 - 3(x - 2)$$
$$= x^3 - 6x^2 + 9x - 2$$

is just the graph of f shifted 2 units to the right, as shown in Figure 4-65.

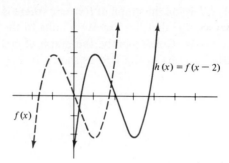

Figure 4-65

A COMPREHENSIVE EXAMPLE

The various techniques developed previously may be used in sequence to graph functions with relatively complicated rules, such as $g(x) = 2(x - 3)^2 - 1$. The key is to note that the rule of g may be obtained in three algebraic steps from the rule of the function $f(x) = x^2$:

$$f(x) = x^2 \xrightarrow{\text{Step 1}} (x - 3)^2 \xrightarrow{\text{Step 2}} 2(x - 3)^2 \xrightarrow{\text{Step 3}} 2(x - 3)^2 - 1 = g(x)$$

Each of these algebraic steps corresponds to one of the graphical changes already studied. Step 1 shifts the graph of f horizontally 3 units to the right. Step 2 then stretches this graph away from the x-axis by a factor of 2. Step 3 shifts this graph 1 unit downward and produces the graph of g, as shown in Figure 4-66.

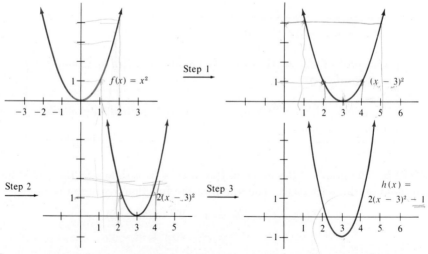

Figure 4-66

With only slightly more work these same techniques can be used to graph *any* quadratic function, such as

$$g(x) = 3x^2 - 2x + 1 \qquad h(x) = -7x^2 + x \qquad k(x) = -4x^2 + 7x - 5$$

For details, see the DO IT YOURSELF! segment at the end of this section.

EXERCISES

A.1. Use the graph of $f(x) = x^2$ to graph each of these functions:
  (a) $g(x) = 4x^2$ (c) $k(x) = -2x^2$ (e) $g(x) = (x + 2)^2$
  (b) $h(x) = \frac{1}{2}x^2$ (d) $t(x) = -\frac{1}{3}x^2$ (f) $h(x) = (x - 4)^2$

A.2. Use the graphs of $g(x) = \sqrt{x}$ and $f(x) = |x|$ (given in Section 3) to graph:
  (a) $h(x) = |x| - 5$ (d) $s(x) = |x - 5|$ (g) $k(x) = \sqrt{x} + 3$
  (b) $k(x) = 3|x|$ (e) $t(x) = |x + 5|$ (h) $r(x) = 5\sqrt{x}$
  (c) $r(u) = \frac{1}{2}|u|$ (f) $h(u) = -4|u|$ (i) $s(x) = -\sqrt{x}$

A.3. Use the graph of $g(x) = x^3$ on page 265 to sketch the graphs of:
  (a) $f(x) = \frac{1}{3}x^3$ (d) $f(x) = -\frac{1}{3}x^3$
  (b) $h(x) = (x - 2)^3$ (e) $h(x) = x^3 + \frac{5}{2}$
  (c) $k(x) = (x + \frac{5}{2})^3$ (f) $y = x^3 - \frac{8}{3}$

A.4. Use the graph of $f(x) = \dfrac{1}{x^2 + 1}$ on page 200 to graph:

  (a) $g(x) = \dfrac{1}{x^2 + 1} + 5$ (b) $h(x) = \dfrac{10}{x^2 + 1}$ (c) $\dfrac{1}{(x - 4)^2 + 1}$

A.5. Graph $f(x) = -g(x)$, where $g(x) = x - [x]$ (see page 204).

A.6. Use the graph of the function f in Figure 4-67 to sketch the graphs of the following functions:
  (a) $g(x) = f(x) + 3$ (e) $g(x) = 5f(x)$ (i) $h(z) = -\frac{1}{3}f(z)$
  (b) $h(x) = f(x) - 1$ (f) $h(x) = \frac{1}{2}f(x)$ (j) $g(x) = f(x - 2)$
  (c) $k(x) = f(x) + \frac{7}{4}$ (g) $k(t) = -f(t)$ (k) $h(x) = f(x + 3)$
  (d) $r(x) = f(x) + \sqrt{2}$ (h) $g(u) = -4f(u)$ (l) $k(x) = f(x - \frac{5}{2})$

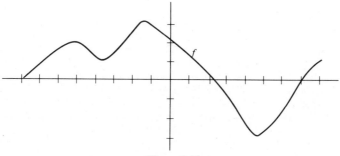

Figure 4-67

Note   In Exercises B.1–B.4 you may need to use several techniques in sequence, as in the comprehensive example on page 238.

B.1.   Use the graph of $f(x) = x^2$ to graph these functions:
  (a) $g(x) = 3x^2 + 1$ (c) $k(x) = 2x^2 - \frac{3}{2}$ (e) $g(x) = -\frac{1}{2}x^2 + \frac{5}{2}$
  (b) $h(x) = -2x^2 + 4$ (d) $p(x) = \frac{1}{2}x^2 + 3$ (f) $h(x) = -2x^2 - 3$

B.2.   Use the graph of $f(x) = x^2$ to graph these functions:
  (a) $g(x) = 2(x + 2)^2$ (e) $g(x) = (x - 1)^2 + 3$
  (b) $h(x) = 2(x + 2)^2 + 2$ (f) $h(x) = -(x + 2)^2 + 4$
  (c) $k(x) = -2(x - 2)^2$ (g) $k(x) = 3(x - 1)^2 + 2$
  (d) $t(x) = -2(x - 2)^2 - 2$ (h) $t(x) = -3(x + 4)^2 - 1$

B.3.   Use the graphs of $g(x) = \sqrt{x}$ and $f(x) = |x|$ (given in Section 3) to graph:
  (a) $h(x) = 3|x| + 5$ (e) $h(x) = -2\sqrt{x} + 3$

  (b) $k(x) = -2|x| - 2$ (f) $r(x) = \dfrac{\sqrt{x}}{2} - 2$

  (c) $r(x) = \frac{1}{3}|x| + \frac{5}{3}$ (g) $k(u) = -\sqrt{u + 1} + 2$

  (d) $h(u) = 2|u - 3|$ (h) $h(x) = 4\sqrt{x - 2} + \frac{3}{2}$

B.4.   Let f be the function whose graph is given in Exercise A.6. Sketch the graphs of
  (a) $g(x) = f(x - 1) + 2$ (c) $g(x) = 3f(x + 1) - 4$
  (b) $h(x) = f(x + 3) - 5$ (d) $h(x) = \frac{1}{2}f(x - 2) + 3$

B.5.   Let h be the function whose graph is given on page 210. Graph:
  (a) $f(x) = 3h(x)$ (d) $f(x) = -2h(x)$
  (b) $g(x) = 3h(x) - 2$ (e) $g(x) = -2h(x - 2)$
  (c) $k(x) = 3h(x + 1) + 2$ (f) $k(x) = -2h(x - 2) - 2$

C.1.   If f is a function and g is the function given by $g(x) = |f(x)|$, then by the definition of absolute value,

$$g(x) = \begin{cases} f(x) & \text{if } f(x) \geq 0 \\ -f(x) & \text{if } f(x) < 0 \end{cases}$$

Therefore the graph of g will be the *same* as the graph of f for all numbers x for which $f(x) \geq 0$. For numbers x with $f(x) < 0$, the graph of g will be the *reflection* of the graph of f in the x-axis. Figure 4-68 is the graph of a function f.

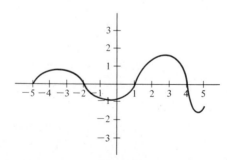

Figure 4-68

Use it to sketch the graphs of the following functions for $-5 \leq x \leq 5$:

(a) $h(x) = -f(x)$ (c) $J(x) = |f(x)| + 2$

(b) $k(x) = |f(x)|$ (d) $R(x) = |f(x - 3)|$

C.2. Graph these functions. (*Hint:* The introduction to Exercise C.1 may be helpful).

(a) $f(x) = |3x|$ (d) $f(x) = |x^2 - 3|$

(b) $g(x) = |x + 5|$ (e) $g(x) = |x^2 + 1| - 5$

(c) $h(x) = |3x - 6|$ (f) $h(x) = |-(x^2 + 1)|$

DO IT YOURSELF!

QUADRATIC FUNCTIONS

A function f whose rule is of the form

$$f(x) = ax^2 + bx + c$$

where a, b, and c are real numbers with $a \neq 0$, is called a *quadratic function*. For example,

$$f(x) = 3x^2 - 2x + 6 \qquad \text{(here } a = 3, b = -2, c = 6\text{)}$$
$$g(x) = 7x^2 - 1 \qquad \text{(here } a = 7, b = 0, c = -1\text{)}$$
$$h(x) = -2x^2 + x \qquad \text{(here } a = -2, b = 1, c = 0\text{)}$$

Sometimes you must do some computation in order to verify that a particular function is actually a quadratic function. For instance, if $f(x) = 2(x - 3)^2 - 1$, then

$$f(x) = 2(x - 3)^2 - 1 = 2(x^2 - 6x + 9) - 1 = 2x^2 - 12x + 17$$

Thus f *is* a quadratic function. The graph of f was found in the comprehensive example on page 238 by using the original form of the rule of f, namely, $f(x) = 2(x - 3)^2 - 1$. We shall now show how the technique of completing the square° can be used to write the rule of *any* quadratic function f in this same general form:

$$f(x) = d(x + k)^2 + s$$

for some real numbers d, k, and s. Later we shall use this form to find the graph of the quadratic function.

EXAMPLE We want to find numbers d, k, and s such that $f(x) = x^2 - 6x + 13$ can be written as $f(x) = d(x + k)^2 + s$. First, we write

$$f(x) = x^2 - 6x + 13 = (x^2 - 6x) + 13$$

The next step is to complete the square in $x^2 - 6x$ by *adding* the square of half the coefficient of x, namely, $(\frac{1}{2}(-6))^2 = (-3)^2 = 9$. But we don't want the rule of the function to change, so we must also *subtract* 9:

$$f(x) = (x^2 - 6x + 9 - 9) + 13 = (x^2 - 6x + 9) - 9 + 13$$

°This technique is discussed on page 51.

Now we factor the term in the parentheses and obtain:

$$f(x) = (x - 3)^2 - 9 + 13 = (x - 3)^2 + 4$$

But $f(x) = (x - 3)^2 + 4$ is in the form $d(x + k)^2 + s$ with $d = 1$, $k = -3$, and $s = 4$.

EXAMPLE   We want to find numbers d, k, and s such that $g(x) = 3x^2 + 30x + 77$ can be written as $g(x) = d(x + k)^2 + s$. First, we write

$$g(x) = 3x^2 + 30x + 77 = 3(x^2 + 10x) + 77$$

The next step is to complete the square in $x^2 + 10x$ by *adding* $(\frac{1}{2} \cdot 10)^2 = 5^2 = 25$ so that $x^2 + 10x + 25 = (x + 5)^2$. But we don't want the rule of the function to change, so we must also *subtract* 25:

$$g(x) = 3(x^2 + 10x) + 77 = 3(x^2 + 10x + 25 - 25) + 77$$

Using the distributive law on the quantity in parenthesis yields:

$$g(x) = 3(x^2 + 10x + 25) - 3 \cdot 25 + 77$$
$$g(x) = 3(x + 5)^2 - 75 + 77 = 3(x + 5)^2 + 2$$

Thus $g(x) = d(x + k)^2 + s$ with $d = 3$, $k = 5$, and $s = 2$.

EXAMPLE   If $f(x) = -4x^2 + 12x - 8$, then $f(x) = -4(x^2 - 3x) - 8$. In order to complete the square in $x^2 - 3x$, we must *add* $(-\frac{3}{2})^2 = \frac{9}{4}$. In order to leave the rule of f unchanged, we must also *subtract* $\frac{9}{4}$:

$$f(x) = -4(x^2 - 3x) - 8 = -4(x^2 - 3x + \tfrac{9}{4} - \tfrac{9}{4}) - 8$$
$$f(x) = -4(x^2 - 3x + \tfrac{9}{4}) - 4(-\tfrac{9}{4}) - 8$$
$$f(x) = -4(x - \tfrac{3}{2})^2 + 9 - 8 = -4(x - \tfrac{3}{2})^2 + 1$$

Thus $f(x) = d(x + k)^2 + s$ with $d = -4$, $k = -\frac{3}{2}$, and $s = 1$.

GRAPHS OF QUADRATIC FUNCTIONS

By using the techniques discussed earlier in this section, the graph of *any* quadratic function can easily be obtained from the graph of $f(x) = x^2$, as illustrated in the following examples.

EXAMPLE   To graph $f(x) = x^2 - 6x + 13$, we first complete the square, as shown in the example on page 241, and rewrite the rule of f in this form: $f(x) = x^2 - 6x + 13 = (x - 3)^2 + 4$. This form of the rule of f can be thought of as being obtained in two algebraic steps from x^2:

$$x^2 \xrightarrow{\text{Step 1}} (x - 3)^2 \xrightarrow{\text{Step 2}} (x - 3)^2 + 4 = f(x)$$

So the graph of f can be obtained by starting with the known graph of $y = x^2$ and performing the geometric operations that correspond to the algebraic operations in Step 1 and Step 2 (see Figure 4-69):

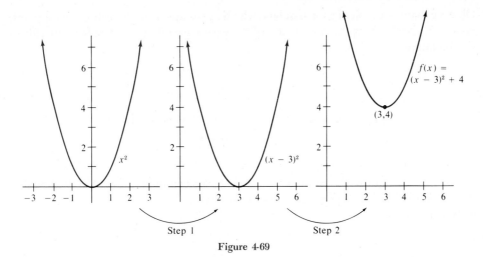

Figure 4-69

Observe that the graph of f is a **parabola** that opens upward. Its **vertex** (lowest point) is $(3, 4)$. Notice how the coordinates of the vertex are related to the algebraic rule of the function:

$$f(x) = (x - 3)^2 + 4 \qquad \text{vertex } (3, 4)$$

same

negatives

EXAMPLE To graph $g(x) = 3x^2 + 30x + 77$, we complete the square, as shown in the first example on page 242, and write $g(x) = 3(x + 5)^2 + 2$ (see Figure 4-70).

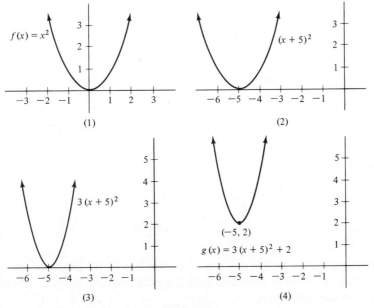

Figure 4-70

Observe that the graph of g is a **parabola** which opens upward. Its **vertex** (lowest point) is $(-5, 2)$. Notice how the coordinates of the vertex are related to the algebraic rule of the function:

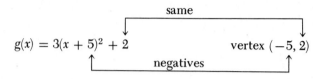

$$g(x) = 3(x + 5)^2 + 2 \qquad \text{vertex } (-5, 2)$$

EXAMPLE To graph $f(x) = -4x^2 + 12x - 8$, we complete the square, as shown in the second example on page 242, and write $f(x) = -4(x - \frac{3}{2})^2 + 1$. The graph is obtained in Figure 4-71.

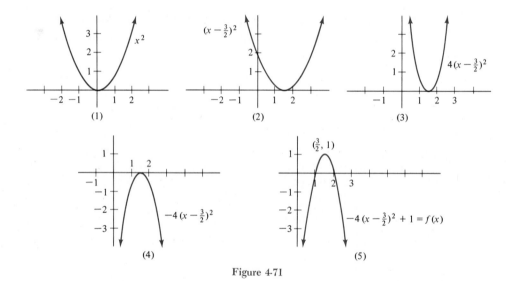

Figure 4-71

The graph of f is a parabola which opens downward. Its vertex (highest point) is $(\frac{3}{2}, 1)$. The coordinates of the vertex are closely related to the graph of the function:

$$f(x) = -4(x - \tfrac{3}{2})^2 + 1 \qquad \text{vertex } (\tfrac{3}{2}, 1)$$

The techniques illustrated above can be used to obtain the graph of *any* quadratic function $f(x) = ax^2 + bx + c$ (with $a \neq 0$) from the graph of $y = x^2$. The preceding examples illustrate these facts:

> *The graph of the quadratic function* $f(x) = ax^2 + bx + c$ *is a parabola; it opens upward if* $a > 0$ *and downward if* $a < 0$. *If the rule of* f *is rewritten in the form* $f(x) = d(x + k)^2 + s$, *then the vertex of the parabola is the point* $(-k, s)$.

APPLICATIONS

If the graph of a quadratic function is a *downward*-opening parabola with vertex $(r, f(r))$, then the number $f(r)$ is the **maximum value** of the function f. In other words, $f(x) \le f(r)$ for every number x. Similarly, if the graph of f opens *upward* and has vertex $(r, f(r))$, then $f(r)$ is the **minimum value** of the function f. In other words, $f(x) \ge f(r)$ for every number x.

EXAMPLE What is the *area* of the largest rectangular field that can be enclosed with 3000 ft of fence and what are its *dimensions* (see Figure 4-72)?

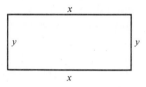

Figure 4-72

Let x denote the length and y the width of the field so that:

$$\text{perimeter} = x + y + x + y = 2x + 2y$$
$$\text{area} = xy$$

But the perimeter is precisely 3000 (the length of the fence), so that $2x + 2y = 3000$ and

$$2y = 3000 - 2x, \qquad \text{and hence} \qquad y = 1500 - x$$

Consequently, the area is

$$A = xy = x(1500 - x) = 1500x - x^2$$

The largest possible area is just the maximum value of the quadratic function $A(x) = 1500x - x^2 = -x^2 + 1500x$. The graph of $A(x)$ is a parabola which opens downward (why?). Its vertex can be found by completing the square:

$$A(x) = -x^2 + 1500x = -1(x^2 - 1500x) = -1(x^2 - 1500x + (750)^2 - (750)^2),$$
$$A(x) = -(x^2 - 1500x + (750)^2) + (750)^2 = -(x - 750)^2 + (750)^2$$

Therefore the vertex is $(750, 750^2)$, as explained in the last box above. This means that the maximum area is $750^2 = 562,000$ sq ft and it occurs when the length $x = 750$. Since the width $y = 1500 - x = 1500 - 750 = 750$, the enclosed area is a square measuring 750 by 750 ft.

EXAMPLE Suppose c and d are real numbers whose difference is 5. What is the smallest possible value for cd and in this case, what are c and d? Since $c - d = 5$, we have $c = 5 + d$. We want the product

$$cd = (5 + d)d = 5d + d^2$$

to be a minimum. Since the graph of $f(d) = d^2 + 5d$ is a parabola which opens upward, the minimum value of $f(d)$ occurs at the vertex of the parabola. To find the vertex we complete the square:

$$f(d) = d^2 + 5d = d^2 + 5d + (\tfrac{5}{2})^2 - (\tfrac{5}{2})^2 = (d^2 + 5d + (\tfrac{5}{2})^2) - (\tfrac{5}{2})^2,$$
$$f(d) = (d + \tfrac{5}{2})^2 - \tfrac{25}{4}$$

Therefore the vertex is $(-\tfrac{5}{2}, -\tfrac{25}{4})$. It occurs when $d = -\tfrac{5}{2}$ and $c = 5 + d = 5 - \tfrac{5}{2} = \tfrac{5}{2}$. The smallest value for $cd = f(d)$ is $-\tfrac{25}{4} = (-\tfrac{5}{2})(\tfrac{5}{2})$.

EXERCISES

A.1. *Without graphing*, determine the vertex of each of the following parabolas and state whether it opens upward or downward.
(a) $f(x) = 3(x - 5)^2 + 2$ (d) $h(x) = -x^2 + 1$
(b) $g(x) = -6(x - 2)^2 - 5$ (e) $y = -\tfrac{3}{2}(x + \tfrac{3}{2})^2 + \tfrac{3}{2}$
(c) $y = -(x - 1)^2 + 2$ (f) $v = 656(t - 590)^2 + 7284$

A.2. Do the same as in Exercise A.1 for these parabolas.
(a) $f(x) = -3x^2 + 4x + 5$ (e) $y = t^2 + t + 1$
(b) $g(x) = 2x^2 - x - 1$ (f) $g(x) = x^2 - 9x$
(c) $y = -x^2 + x$ (g) $h(t) = -2t^2 + 2t - 1$
(d) $h(t) = \tfrac{1}{2}t^2 - \tfrac{3}{2}t + \tfrac{5}{2}$ (h) $y = 3x^2 + x - 4$

A.3. In the example which begins on page 194, $P(x)$ is the weekly profit obtained from selling x widgets. $P(x)$ is given by $P(x) = 1.5x - \dfrac{x^2}{10,000} - 2000$. Find the number x which makes $P(x)$ as large as possible.

B.1. Graph each of these quadratic functions.
(a) $p(x) = x^2 - 4x - 1$ (d) $h(x) = x^2 + 3x + 1$
(b) $q(x) = x^2 + 8x + 6$ (e) $f(x) = 2x^2 - 4x + 1$
(c) $y = x^2 - 10x + 20$ (f) $r(x) = -3x^2 + 9x - 5$

B.2. What must the number b be in order that the vertex of the parabola $y = x^2 + bx + c$ lie on the y-axis?

B.3. For what value of c does the vertex of the parabola $y = x^2 + 8x + c$ lie on the x-axis?

C.1. A ball is thrown upward from the top of a tower. After t sec, its height h above the ground is given by the formula $h = -16t^2 + 80t + 96$. *When* does the ball reach its maximum height and *how high* is it at that time? [*Hint:* consider h as a function of t. To say that a point (a, b) is on the graph of h means that the ball is b ft high at time $t = a$. Thus the maximum height and the time at which it occurs can be determined by finding the highest point on the graph.]

C.2.   A rocket is fired upward from ground level. At t sec after blast-off its height h is $-16t^2 + 1600t$ ft. When does it attain its maximum height and what is it? (See the hint for C.1.)

C.3.   A projectile is fired at an angle of 45° upward. Exactly t sec after firing, its vertical height above the ground is $500t - 16t^2$. What is the greatest height the projectile reaches and at what time does this occur? (See the hint for C.1.)

C.4.   What is the minimum product of two numbers whose difference is 4? What are the numbers?

C.5.   The sum of the height h and base b of a triangle is 30. What height and base will produce a triangle of maximum area?

C.6.   A field bounded on one side by a river is to be fenced on three sides so as to form a rectangular enclosure. If the total amount of fence to be used is 200 ft, what dimensions will yield an enclosure of the largest possible area?

C.7.   A rectangular box (with top) has a square base. The sum of the lengths of its 12 edges is 8 ft. What dimensions should the box have in order, that its surface area be as large as possible?

C.8.   A salesperson finds that her sales average 40 cases per store when she visits 20 stores a week. Each time she visits an additional store per week, the average sales per store decrease by 1 case. How many stores should she visit each week if she wants to maximize her sales?

C.9.   A miniature golf course averages 200 patrons per evening when it charges $2 per person. For each 5-cent increase in the admission price, the average attendance drops by 2 people. What admission price will produce the largest ticket revenue?

C.10.   Find the exact answer to Exercise B.2. (d) on page 196.

7. OPERATIONS ON FUNCTIONS

In this section we explore more ways of creating new functions from given ones. In each case we begin with *two* functions and use them to create a new function. Unlike Section 6, the stress here is primarily on the algebraic aspect of the subject.

COMPOSITION OF FUNCTIONS

Once again we begin in the "real world" with an example of a functional situation (which is numbered 4 to avoid confusion with Examples 1–3 in earlier sections).

EXAMPLE 4—AIR CONDITIONERS   The power company has to estimate the additional load on the system when people start turning on their air conditioners. Such an estimate rests on two basic facts:

Fact 1: As the temperature rises, more air conditioners are turned on.

Fact 2: Weather bureau records of past years provide a reasonably good prediction of what the temperature will be at a specific time on a given day.

To predict the additional load due to air conditioners on a particular day—say, July 24—the power company reasons as follows. On the one hand, the weather bureau predicts the expected temperature T on July 24 at all times of the day. Write $T(h)$ for the expected temperature at h hr after midnight. In other words, the weather bureau furnishes a function $T = T(h)$.

On the other hand, a telephone survey gives an indication of how many people turn on air conditioners when the temperature is 75°, 76°, 77°, and so on. Write $A(T)$ for the number of air conditioners in operation when the temperature is reading $T°$. In other words, the company which conducts the telephone survey provides a function $A(T)$.

In order to find out how many air conditioners are likely to be in operation at 4:00 P.M. (= 16 hr after midnight), the power company

first finds $T(16)$, the temperature at $h = 16$ hr after midnight and, second, finds the value of the function $A(T)$ for the temperature $T = T(16)$.

In short, at 4:00 P.M. the company expects

$$A(T(16))$$

(which is read "A of T of 16") air conditioners to be in operation.

What works for 4:00 P.M. works for any time h:

At h hr, the temperature is expected to be $T(h)$ degrees.
At a temperature of $T(h)$ degrees, there will be $A(T(h))$ air conditioners in operation.

From the two functions $T(h)$ and $A(T)$ we obtain in two steps a new function, namely, the function which assigns to h the number $A(T(h))$. This new function is called the **composite** of the functions $T(h)$ and $A(T)$ because $T(h)$ and $A(T)$ are put together, or "composed," to form a new function. In the language of functions,

> The number of air conditioners operating at h hours is given by the composition $A(T(h))$ of the functions $T(h)$ = temperature at h hours and $A(T)$ = number of air conditioners in operation when the temperature is $T°$

In Example 4 the functions $T(h)$ and $A(T)$ were composed to yield the new function $A(T(h))$. Similarly, given any two functions we can construct a new composite function as follows:

> *Let* f(x) *and* g(t) *be functions. The **composite function** of* f *and* g *is the function which assigns to the number* x, *the number* g(f(x)). *The composite function of* f *and* g *is denoted* g ∘ f.

The symbol $g \circ f$ is read "f followed by g" (note the order carefully). Thus the rule of the composite function may be written

$$(g \circ f)(x) = g(f(x))$$

that is, $(g \circ f)(x)$ and $g(f(x))$ represent the *same* number, the value of the composite function at x.

The domain of the composite function $g \circ f$ is determined by the usual conventions. Since $g(f(x))$ only makes sense when the number x is in the domain of f *and* $f(x)$ is in the domain of g, we have:

> *The domain of the composite function* $g \circ f$ *is the set of all real numbers* x *such that* x *is in the domain of* f *and* f(x) *is in the domain of* g.

EXAMPLE Suppose $f(x) = 4x^2 + 1$ and $g(t) = \dfrac{1}{t + 2}$. Then $(g \circ f)(2)$ is the number

$g(f(2))$. Since $f(2) = 4 \cdot 2^2 + 1 = 17$ and $g(17) = \dfrac{1}{17 + 2} = \dfrac{1}{19}$, we have:

$$(g \circ f)(2) = g(f(2)) = g(17) = \frac{1}{19}$$

Similarly, we can compute $(g \circ f)(x)$ for any number x by evaluating $g(f(x))$. This means that whenever t appears in the formula for $g(t)$, we must replace it by $f(x) = 4x^2 + 1$:

$$(g \circ f)(x) = g(f(x)) = \frac{1}{f(x) + 2} = \frac{1}{(4x^2 + 1) + 2} = \frac{1}{4x^2 + 3}$$

For every real number x, both $f(x) = 4x^2 + 1$ and $g(f(x)) = \dfrac{1}{4x^2 + 3}$ are well defined real numbers. Consequently, the domain of $g \circ f$ is the set of all real numbers.

EXAMPLE If $f(x) = x - 5$ and $g(t) = 3t + \sqrt{t}$, then

$$(g \circ f)(x) = g(f(x)) = 3f(x) + \sqrt{f(x)} = 3(x - 5) + \sqrt{x - 5} = 3x - 15 + \sqrt{x - 5}$$

Thus $(g \circ f)(7) = 3 \cdot 7 - 15 + \sqrt{7 - 5} = 6 + \sqrt{2}$ and $(g \circ f)(9) = 3 \cdot 9 - 15 + \sqrt{9 - 5} = 12 + \sqrt{4} = 14$. Observe that $f(x)$ is defined for every real number x. Since $\sqrt{t}$ is a real number only when $t \geq 0$, the domain of g is the interval $[0, \infty)$. Consequently, $g(f(x))$ will be defined only when $f(x) \geq 0$, that is, when $x - 5 \geq 0$, or equivalently, $x \geq 5$. Therefore the domain of $g \circ f$ is the interval $[5, \infty)$.

In the preceding examples we began with functions f and g and constructed the composite function $g \circ f$. Sometimes it's necessary to reverse this process and write a *given* function as the composite of two others.

EXAMPLE If $h(x) = \sqrt{3x^2 + 1}$, then h may be considered as the composite $g \circ f$, where $f(x) = 3x^2 + 1$ and $g(u) = \sqrt{u}$:

$$(g \circ f)(x) = g(f(x)) = g(3x^2 + 1) = \sqrt{3x^2 + 1} = h(x)$$

EXAMPLE   If $k(x) = (x^2 - 2x + \sqrt{x})^3$, then k is $g \circ f$, where $f(x) = x^2 - 2x + \sqrt{x}$ and $g(t) = t^3$:

$$(g \circ f)(x) = g(f(x)) = g(x^2 - 2x + \sqrt{x}) = (x^2 - 2x + \sqrt{x})^3 = k(x)$$

As you may have noticed, there are two possible ways to form a composite function. If f and g are functions, we can consider either

$$(g \circ f)(x) = g(f(x)), \quad \text{the composite of } f \text{ and } g$$
$$(f \circ g)(x) = f(g(x)), \quad \text{the composite of } g \text{ and } f$$

The *order is important*, as we shall now see:

> g ∘ f *and* f ∘ g *usually are not the same function.*

EXAMPLE   If $f(x) = x^2$ and $g(x) = x + 3$,° then

$$(g \circ f)(x) = g(f(x)) = g(x^2) = x^2 + 3$$

but

$$(f \circ g)(x) = f(g(x)) = f(x + 3) = (x + 3)^2 = x^2 + 6x + 9$$

Obviously, $g \circ f$ and $f \circ g$ are different functions (for example, they have different values at $x = 0$). In other words, $g \circ f \neq f \circ g$.

Although $g \circ f$ and $f \circ g$ are usually different functions, there are some instances where they turn out to be the same function; see Exercise A.6.

ARITHMETIC OPERATIONS ON FUNCTIONS

Although we know how to add, subtract, multiply, and divide *numbers*, we have not yet given a meaning to addition, subtraction, multiplication, and division of *functions*. We do so now, and thus produce several arithmetic ways of creating a new function from two given functions.

Suppose f and g are functions. With one exception, noted below, all of the functions to be constructed will have the same *domain:*

The set of all real numbers x that are in
both the domain of f and the domain of g

The first new function to be constructed is the sum function. The **sum** of f and g is the function h defined by the rule:

$$h(x) = f(x) + g(x)$$

° Up to now we have used different letters in the rules of two functions being composed. Now that you have the idea, we shall use the same letter for the variable in both functions.

EXAMPLE If $f(x) = 3x^2 + 2$ and $g(x) = x^2 + \dfrac{1}{\sqrt{x}} - 5$, then their sum is the function

given by

$$h(x) = f(x) + g(x) = (3x^2 + 2) + \left(x^2 + \frac{1}{\sqrt{x}} - 5\right) = 4x^2 + \frac{1}{\sqrt{x}} - 3$$

Instead of using a different letter h for the sum function of f and g, we shall usually denote the sum function by $f + g$. Thus the sum $f + g$ is defined by the rule:

$$(f + g)(x) = f(x) + g(x)$$

It is important to realize that this rule is *not* just a formal manipulation of symbols. If x is a number, then so are $f(x)$ and $g(x)$. The plus sign in $f(x) + g(x)$ is addition of *numbers*. (The result is a number.) But the plus sign in $f + g$ is addition of *functions*: the result is the function which assigns to the number x the number $f(x) + g(x)$.

The **difference** of two functions f and g is defined similarly. It is the function denoted $f - g$ whose rule is: assign to the number x the number $f(x) - g(x)$. In symbols,

$$(f - g)(x) = f(x) - g(x)$$

The minus sign on the right side indicates subtraction of *numbers*. The minus sign on the left denotes subtraction of *functions*.

EXAMPLE If $f(x) = 3x^2$ and $g(x) = \sqrt{x - 1}$, then $f - g$ is the function given by:

$$(f - g)(x) = f(x) - g(x) = 3x^2 - \sqrt{x - 1}$$

The **product** of two functions f and g is the function denoted fg, whose rule is: assign to the number x the number $f(x)g(x)$. In symbols,

$$(fg)(x) = f(x)g(x)$$

Once again, $f(x)g(x)$ is a product of numbers, while fg is a product of functions.

Warning Do not confuse the *product fg* of f and g with the *composite* function $f \circ g$ (g followed by f). They are *different*. For example, if $f(x) = 2x^2$ and $g(x) = x - 3$, then the product function fg is given by

$$(fg)(x) = f(x)g(x) = 2x^2(x - 3) = 2x^3 - 6x^2$$

But the composite function $f \circ g$ is given by

$$(f \circ g)(x) = f(g(x)) = f(x - 3) = 2(x - 3)^2 = 2(x^2 - 6x + 9) = 2x^2 - 12x + 18$$

The functions fg and $f \circ g$ are clearly different since they take different values at $x = 0$.

EXAMPLE A special case of product functions occurs when one of the functions is a constant function. For instance, suppose $f(x) = x^3 + 2x^2 - 1$ and $g(x) = 6$. In such a situation, we let $6f$ denote the product function gf whose rule is:

$$(6f)(x) = g(x)f(x) = 6f(x) = 6(x^3 + 2x^2 - 1) = 6x^3 + 12x^2 - 6$$

Similarly, for any constant c, the function cf is given by

$$(cf)(x) = cf(x) = c(x^3 + 2x^2 - 1) = cx^3 + 2cx^2 - c$$

Note If f is any function, then the product ff of f with itself is denoted f^2. The product $f(f^2)$ is denoted f^3, and so on.

The **quotient** of two functions f and g is the function denoted f/g. whose rule is

$$\left(\frac{f}{g}\right)(x) = \frac{f(x)}{g(x)}$$

Since $f(x)/g(x)$ is defined only when $g(x) \neq 0$, the domain of f/g is

The set of all numbers x in both the domain
of f and the domain of g with $g(x) \neq 0$

EXAMPLE If $f(x) = \sqrt{x}$ and $g(x) = x^2 - 1$, then f/g is given by the rule

$$\left(\frac{f}{g}\right)(x) = \frac{f(x)}{g(x)} = \frac{\sqrt{x}}{x^2 - 1}$$

The domain of g is the set of all real numbers, and $g(x) = 0$ only when $x = 1$ or $x = -1$. The domain of f is the interval $[0, \infty)$. Consequently, the domain of f/g is the set of all numbers in $[0, \infty)$ *except* $x = 1$.

A COMPREHENSIVE EXAMPLE

The most common way that the operations introduced above are used in calculus is to consider a fairly complicated function as being built up from simple parts. For example, the function $f(x) = \sqrt{\dfrac{3x^2 - 4x + 5}{x^3 + 1}}$ may be considered as the composite $f = g \circ h$, where

$$h(x) = \frac{3x^2 - 4x + 5}{x^3 + 1} \qquad \text{and} \qquad g(x) = \sqrt{x}$$

since

$$(g \circ h)(x) = g(h(x)) = g\left(\frac{3x^2 - 4x + 5}{x^3 + 1}\right) = \sqrt{\frac{3x^2 - 4x + 5}{x^3 + 1}} = f(x)$$

The function $h(x) = \dfrac{3x^2 - 4x + 5}{x^3 + 1}$ is the quotient $\dfrac{p}{q}$, where

$$p(x) = 3x^2 - 4x + 5 \qquad \text{and} \qquad q(x) = x^3 + 1$$

The function $p(x) = 3x^2 - 4x + 5$ may be written $p = k - s + r$, where

$$k(x) = 3x^2, \qquad s(x) = 4x, \qquad r(x) = 5$$

The function k, in turn, can be considered as the product $3I^2$, where I is the identity function [whose rule is $I(x) = x$]:

$$(3I^2)(x) = 3(I^2(x)) = 3(I(x)I(x)) = 3 \cdot x \cdot x = 3x^2 = k(x)$$

Similarly, $s(x) = (4I)(x) = 4I(x) = 4x$. The function $q(x) = x^3 + 1$ may be "decomposed" in the same way.

Thus the complicated function f is just the result of performing suitable operations on the identity function I and various constant functions.

EXERCISES

A.1. Given the functions $g(t) = t^2 - t$ and $f(x) = 1 + |x|$, evaluate the following:
(a) $g(f(0))$ (c) $g(f(2) + 3)$ (e) $(g \circ f)(1 + 2 + 3)$
(b) $(f \circ g)(3)$ (d) $f(2g(1))$ (f) $(f \circ g)(0)$

A.2. In each part, find $(g \circ f)(3)$, $(f \circ g)(1)$, and $(f \circ f)(0)$.
(a) $f(x) = 3x - 2$, $g(x) = x^2$ (d) $f(x) = x$, $g(x) = -3$
(b) $f(x) = -x + 7$, $g(x) = 7x - 1$ (e) $f(x) = [x]$, $g(x) = 2x - 1$
(c) $f(x) = |x + 2|$, $g(x) = -x^2$ (f) $f(x) = x^2 - 1$, $g(x) = \sqrt{x}$

A.3. Let $f(x) = x + 3$ and $g(u) = u^2 - 1$. Find:
(a) $(g \circ f)(x)$ (b) $(f \circ g)(u)$ (c) $(f \circ f)(x)$ (d) $(g \circ g)(u)$

A.4. In each part, find formulas for $(g \circ f)(x)$ and $(f \circ g)(x)$.
(a) $f(x) = 2x^2 + 2x - 1$ (c) $f(x) = -3x + 2$ (e) $f(x) = \sqrt[3]{x}$
     $g(x) = |x - 1| + 2$ $g(x) = x^3$ $g(x) = x^2 - 1$

(b) $f(x) = 4x^2 + x^4$ (d) $f(x) = x^2 + 1$ (f) $f(x) = \dfrac{1}{x}$

     $g(x) = \sqrt{x^2 + 1}$ $g(x) = -5x + \pi$ $g(x) = \sqrt{x}$

A.5. If f is any function and I is the identity function, what are $f \circ I$ and $I \circ f$?

A.6. Verify that in each part below, $f \circ g = I$ and $g \circ f = I$, where I is the identity function. Functions f and g with this property are said to be **inverses** of each other.

(a) $f(x) = 9x + 2$ (d) $f(x) = \sqrt[3]{\dfrac{7 - x}{3}}$
     $g(x) = \dfrac{x - 2}{9}$ $g(x) = 7 - 3x^3$
(b) $f(x) = \sqrt[3]{x - 1}$ (e) $f(x) = \sqrt[3]{x} + 2$
     $g(x) = x^3 + 1$ $g(x) = (x - 2)^3$
(c) $f(x) = 6x + 2$ (f) $f(x) = 2x^3 - 5$
     $g(x) = \dfrac{x}{6} - \dfrac{1}{3}$ $g(x) = \sqrt[3]{\dfrac{x + 5}{2}}$

A.7. In each part of Exercises A.4, find $(f + g)(x)$, $(f - g)(x)$ and $(g - f)(x)$.

A.8. In each part of Exercise A.4, find $(f + g)(x + h)$ and $(fg)(x + h)$ (where h is a fixed constant).

A.9. In each part of Exercise A.4, find $(fg)(x)$, $\left(\dfrac{f}{g}\right)(x)$ and $\left(\dfrac{g}{f}\right)(x)$.

B.1.   Figure 4-73 is the graph of a function f.

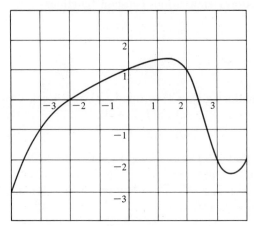

Figure 4-73

Let g be the composite function $f \circ f$ [that is, $g(x) = (f \circ f)(x) = f(f(x))$].
(a)   Use the graph of f to fill in the following table (approximate where necessary).

x	$f(x)$	$g(x) = f(f(x))$
-4		
-3		
-2	0	1
-1		
0		
1		
2		
3		
4		

(b)   Use the information obtained in part (a) to sketch the graph of the function g.

B.2. Here are tables which show the values of functions f and g at certain numbers.

x	$f(x)$
1	3
2	5
3	1
4	2
5	3

t	$g(t)$
1	5
2	4
3	4
4	3
5	2

Fill in each of the following tables.

(a)

x	$(g \circ f)(x)$
1	4
2	
3	5
4	
5	

(b)

t	$(f \circ g)(t)$
1	
2	2
3	
4	
5	

(c)

x	$(f \circ f)(x)$
1	
2	
3	3
4	
5	

(d)

t	$(g \circ g)(t)$
1	
2	
3	
4	4
5	

B.3. Write each of the following functions as the composite of two functions, neither of which is the identity function. (There may be more than one way to do this.)
Example: $f(x) = \sqrt{x^2 + 1}$ can be written $f = g \circ h$ with $g(x) = \sqrt{x}$ and $h(x) = x^2 + 1$.

(a) $f(x) = \sqrt[3]{x^2 + 2}$

(b) $g(x) = \sqrt{x + 3} - \sqrt[3]{x + 3}$

(c) $h(x) = (7x^3 - 10x + 17)^7$

(d) $k(x) = \sqrt[3]{(7x - 3)^2}$

(e) $f(x) = |x^2 - \sqrt{x} + 2|$

(f) $r(t) = (16t^2)^3$

(g) $h(t) = (t + 2)\sqrt{(t + 2)^2 - 5}$

(h) $k(u) = u^2 + 4u + 4$

(i) $f(x) = \dfrac{1}{3x^2 + 5x - 7}$

(j) $g(t) = \dfrac{3}{\sqrt{t - 3}} + 7$

B.4. If $f(x) = x + 1$ and $g(t) = t^2$, then

$$(g \circ f)(x) = g(f(x)) = g(x + 1) = (x + 1)^2 = x^2 + 2x + 1$$

Find two other functions $h(x)$ and $k(t)$ such that $(k \circ h)(x) = x^2 + 2x + 1$.

B.5. Determine whether the functions $f \circ g$ *and* $g \circ f$ are defined. If a composite function *is* defined, find its domain.

(a) $f(x) = x^3$ (c) $f(x) = \sqrt{x + 10}$ (e) $f(x) = \dfrac{1}{x}$

 $g(x) = \sqrt{x}$ $g(x) = 5x$ $g(x) = x^2 + 1$

(b) $f(x) = x^2 + 1$ (d) $f(x) = -x^2$ (f) $f(x) = x^2 + x + 1$

 $g(x) = \sqrt{x}$ $g(x) = \sqrt{x}$ $g(x) = x^3 - x + 2$

B.6. Use the graphs of f and g in Figure 4-74 to sketch the graph of the functions $f + g$ and $f - g$.

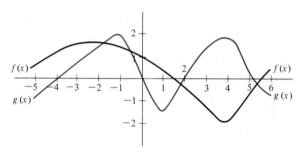

Figure 4-74

B.7. (a) If $f(x) = 2x^3 + 5x - 1$, find $f(x^2)$.

(b) If $f(x) = 2x^3 + 5x - 1$, find $(f(x))^2$.

(c) Are the answers in parts (a) and (b) the same? What can you conclude about $f(x^2)$ and $(f(x))^2$?

B.8. Give an example of a function f such that $f\left(\dfrac{1}{x}\right) \neq \dfrac{1}{f(x)}$.

C.1. This problem deals with the situation described in Example 4 of the text. The telephone survey yields the graph (shown in Figure 4-75), of the number A of air conditioners in operation when the outside temperature is T degrees.

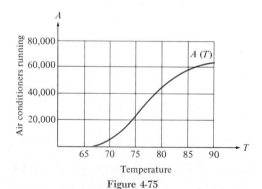

Figure 4-75

On the other hand, on a typical July 24, the graph of the temperature T at h hr after midnight looks like the one in Figure 4-76.

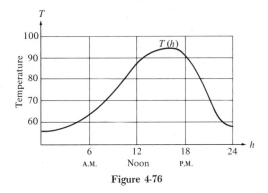

Figure 4-76

(a) Use these graphs to estimate the following quantities: $A(81)$; the temperature at 11:30 A.M.; the number of air conditioners in operation at 4:00 P.M.; $T(8.5)$; $A(T(12))$.

(b) At which time of the day are approximately 21,000 air conditioners in operation? At which time is the number of air conditioners in operation at a maximum?

(c) Find a 2-hr period for which $A(T(h))$ is between 20,000 and 60,000 for all h (in the 2-hr period).

(d) The power company announces a very steep price increase. Sketch into Figure 4-75 what you think the graph of $A(T)$ will look like *after* the rate increase. Sketch the graphs of $A(T(h))$ based on the old and the new power rates.

Polynomial and Rational Functions

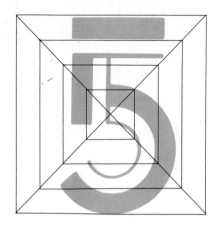

The most frequently seen functions in many parts of mathematics are polynomial functions. Because their values can be computed using only the simple arithmetic operations of addition, subtraction, and multiplication, they are ideally suited for high-speed computers. This fact is crucial since a number of complicated functions that arise in applied mathematics can be approximated by polynomial functions or rational functions (which are just quotients of polynomial functions).

1. POLYNOMIAL FUNCTIONS

A **polynomial function** is a function whose rule is given by a polynomial, such as

$$f(x) = x^2 \qquad g(y) = -y^3 + y + 2 \qquad h(t) = 3t^4 - 6t^3 - 7t + 5$$

Many of the functions studied in Chapter 4 were actually polynomial functions. In this section we shall review and develop some facts about polynomial equations and polynomial arithmetic that will prove useful in dealing with polynomial functions. You should be aware that when dealing with a polynomial function, such as the one whose rule is $f(x) = 7x^3 + 5x^2 - x + 3$, most mathematicians are pretty casual about their language. They may refer to "the polynomial $f(x)$" or "the function $7x^3 + 5x^2 - x + 3$."

We begin by giving a new name to a familiar concept. If $f(x)$ is a polynomial, then a solution of the equation $f(x) = 0$ will be called a **root** (or **zero**) of the polynomial $f(x)$. Thus a number c is a root of $f(x)$, provided that $f(c) = 0$.

EXAMPLE On pages 90 and 91 we saw that the solutions of the equation $x^3 - 4x^2 + 2x + 4 = 0$ are $x = 2$, $x = 1 + \sqrt{3}$, and $x = 1 - \sqrt{3}$. In other words, the numbers 2, $1 + \sqrt{3}$, and $1 - \sqrt{3}$ are the roots of the polynomial $x^3 - 4x^2 + 2x + 4$.

EXAMPLE   The roots of the polynomial $(x - 5)^2(x + \sqrt{3})(x - \frac{9}{4})^7$ are the numbers 5, $-\sqrt{3}$, and $\frac{9}{4}$ since these are the solutions of $(x - 5)^2(x + \sqrt{3})(x - \frac{9}{4})^7 = 0$.

REMAINDERS, FACTORS, AND ROOTS

A useful tool for handling polynomial functions is the following fact, which was discussed on pages 37–39, and is repeated here for convenience:

THE DIVISION ALGORITHM

If a polynomial f(x) *is divided by a nonzero polynomial* h(x), *then there is a quotient polynomial* q(x) *and a remainder polynomial* r(x) *such that*

$$f(x) = h(x)q(x) + r(x)$$

where either r(x) = 0 *or* r(x) *has degree less than the degree of the divisor* h(x).

Consider what happens when a polynomial $f(x)$ is divided by a *first*-degree polynomial of the form $h(x) = x - c$, such as $x - 2$ or $x - (-3) = x + 3$. According to the Division Algorithm, there are quotient and remainder polynomials $q(x)$ and $r(x)$ such that

(°) $f(x) = (x - c)q(x) + r(x)$

where either $r(x) = 0$ or $r(x)$ has smaller degree than the divisor $h(x) = x - c$. But the only polynomials with smaller degree than $x - c$ are the nonzero constants (that is, the polynomials of degree 0). Therefore in all cases the remainder $r(x)$ is just a real number d (possibly 0). So statement (°) above becomes

$$f(x) = (x - c)q(x) + d$$

If we now evaluate the polynomial function $f(x)$ at the number $x = c$, we obtain:

$$f(c) = (c - c)q(c) + d = 0 \cdot q(c) + d = d$$

Thus the remainder d is just the number $f(c)$, the value of $f(x)$ at $x = c$. We have proved

---

THE REMAINDER THEOREM

If a polynomial f(x) *is divided by* x − c, *then the remainder is precisely the number* f(c).

EXAMPLE What is the remainder when $f(x) = 3x^4 - 8x^2 - 11x + 1$ is divided by $x - 2$? Well, $x - 2$ is just $x - c$ with $c = 2$, so the Remainder Theorem states that the remainder is

$$f(c) = f(2) = 3 \cdot 2^4 - 8 \cdot 2^2 - 11 \cdot 2 + 1 = 48 - 32 - 22 + 1 = -5$$

If you have any doubts, look back on page 42 where the entire division of $f(x)$ by $x - 2$ is carried out: The remainder is indeed -5.

EXAMPLE The Remainder Theorem can be used together with synthetic division° to evaluate polynomial functions. For instance, to find $f(6)$ when $f(x) = 8x^5 - 52x^4 + 2x^3 - 198x^2 - 86x + 14$, we need only determine the remainder after division by $x - 6$. This can be done quickly by synthetic division:

6⌋	8	−52	2	−198	−86	14
		48	−24	−132	−1980	−12,396
	8	−4	−22	−330	−2066	−12,382

Therefore $f(6) = $ remainder $= -12{,}382$. The arithmetic involved in the synthetic division here is much easier than that needed to find $f(6)$ by using substitution.

EXAMPLE What is the remainder when $f(x) = x^3 + 4x^2 + 2x - 3$ is divided by $x + 3$? Since $x + 3$ can be written as $x - (-3)$, we can apply the Remainder Theorem with $c = -3$ and conclude that the remainder is

$$f(c) = f(-3) = (-3)^3 + 4(-3)^2 + 2(-3) - 3 = -27 + 36 - 6 - 3 = 0$$

Since the remainder is 0 when $f(x) = x^3 + 4x^2 + 2x - 3$ is divided by $x + 3$, we know that $x + 3$ must be a *factor* of $f(x)$ (as explained in the box on page 39).

The last example illustrates an important special case of the Remainder Theorem—the situation when the remainder is 0. More generally, when a polynomial $f(x)$ is divided by $x - c$, the remainder is the number $f(c)$. This remainder $f(c)$ is 0 exactly when the divisor $x - c$ is a factor of $f(x)$ (as we saw on page 39). But $f(c) = 0$ means that c is a root of the polynomial $f(x)$. In other words,

---

THE FACTOR THEOREM

The number c is a root of the polynomial f(x) *exactly when* x − c *is a factor of* f(x).

The Factor Theorem, stated in slightly different words, and an example showing its use were given on page 90.

MULTIPLICITY AND THE NUMBER OF ROOTS

If $f(x)$ is a polynomial and the number c is a root of $f(x)$, then the Factor Theorem shows that $x - c$ is a factor of $f(x)$. Now it may happen that $(x - c)^2$ or $(x - c)^3$ or

°Synthetic division is explained on pages 42–45. If you are unfamiliar with it, skip this example.

some higher power of $x - c$ is also a factor of $f(x)$. Suppose that the highest power of $x - c$, which is a factor of $f(x)$, is k; that is,

$(x - c)^k$ is a factor of $f(x)$, but $(x - c)^{k+1}$ is not a factor

Then we say that c is a **root of multiplicity k.**

EXAMPLE   Suppose $f(x) = (x^3 + x^2 - 5x + 3)(x + \frac{2}{3})^5$. By multiplying out the right-hand side below, you can verify that $f(x)$ factors as:

$$f(x) = (x - 1)^2(x + 3)(x + \tfrac{2}{3})^5$$

Thus the roots of $f(x)$ are 1, -3, and $-\frac{2}{3}$. Now $(x - 1)^2$ is a factor of $f(x)$, but $(x - 1)^{2+1} = (x - 1)^3$ is not a factor. So 1 is a root of multiplicity 2. The root -3 has multiplicity 1 since $(x - (-3))^1 = (x + 3)$ is a factor of $f(x)$, but $(x - (-3))^2$ is not. Similarly, $-\frac{2}{3}$ is a root of multiplicity 5.

In Section 2 of Chapter 2 we saw that a quadratic equation may have 2, 1, or no real number solutions. Therefore a polynomial of degree 2 (a quadratic polynomial) may have 2, 1, or no **real roots.**° The last example on page 89 shows that the polynomial $x^7 - 7x^5 - 18x^3$ of degree 7 has exactly 3 real roots. These examples illustrate the following useful fact:

> A *polynomial of degree* n *has at most* n *distinct real roots.*

Actually, slightly more is true, as we shall see in Chapter 7. If you count *all* the roots of a polynomial, including the complex ones, and if you count each root the same number of times as its multiplicity, then the total number is precisely the degree of the polynomial.

EXERCISES

A.1.   Which of the given numbers are roots of the given polynomial?
  (a) 7, 3, -7, -3, 2; $f(x) = x^2 - 4x - 21$
  (b) 2, 3, 0, -1; $g(x) = x^4 + 6x^3 - x^2 - 30x$
  (c) 2, -2, 1, 0; $h(x) = x^4 - 16$
  (d) -1, 2, 3; $k(x) = 2x^3 - 3x^2 + 2x - 1$

A.2.   Find the remainder when $f(x)$ is divided by $g(x)$, *without* using long or synthetic division:
  (a) $f(x) = x^{10} + x^8$; $g(x) = x - 1$
  (b) $f(x) = x^6 - 10$; $g(x) = x - 2$
  (c) $f(x) = 3x^4 - 6x^3 + 2x - 1$; $g(x) = x + 1$
  (d) $f(x) = x^5 - 3x^2 + 2x - 1$; $g(x) = x - 2$

° The term "real root" means a root that is a real number.

(e) $f(x) = x^3 - 2x^2 + 5x - 4;$ $g(x) = x + 2$
(f) $f(x) = 10x^{75} - 8x^{65} + 6x^{45} + 4x^{32} - 2x^{15} + 5;$ $g(x) = x - 1$

A.3. Use the Remainder Theorem and synthetic division to find $f(c)$ when:
(a) $f(x) = 2x^5 - 3x^4 + x^3 - 2x^2 + x - 8$ and $c = 10$
(b) $f(x) = x^3 + 8x^2 - 29x + 44$ and $c = -11$
(c) $f(x) = 2x^5 - 3x^4 + 2x^3 - 8x - 8$ and $c = 20$
(d) $f(x) = x^5 - 10x^4 + 20x^3 - 5x - 95$ and $c = -10$
(e) $f(x) = 2x^5 + x^3 - 3x^2 + 4$ and $c = \frac{1}{2}$

A.4. List the roots of these polynomials and state the multiplicity of each root:
(a) $f(x) = x^{54}(x + \frac{4}{5})$
(b) $g(x) = 3(x + \frac{1}{6})(x - \frac{1}{5})(x + \frac{1}{4})$
(c) $h(x) = 2x^{15}(x - \pi)^{14}(x - (\pi + 1))^{13}$
(d) $k(x) = 3(x - \sqrt{7})^7(x - \sqrt{5})^5(2x + 1)$

B.1. Find a polynomial with the given degree n, the given roots, and no other roots:
(a) $n = 3;$ roots $1, 7, -4$ (c) $n = 6;$ roots $1, 2, \pi$
(b) $n = 3;$ roots $1, -1$ (d) $n = 5;$ root 2

B.2. Find a polynomial function f of degree 3 such that $f(10) = 17$ and the roots of $f(x)$ are 0, 5, and 8.

B.3. Do Exercise B.3 on page 94.

B.4. Do Exercise B.4 on page 94.

B.5. Do Exercise B.5 on page 94.

C.1. A favorite topic of science fiction writers is the possibility of animals or humans either shrinking to an incredibly small size or growing enormously large. One reason such stories are scientifically unsound involves a certain polynomial function dealing with heat. Any living thing generates heat as a result of its metabolism. In addition, any animal that is warmer than its surroundings (as is usually the case with mammals) loses heat through its body's surface. In the long run, of course, these two processes must balance out.

Let x be a number measuring the general size of an animal in inches. For a small shrew x might be .1; for a cat x might be 20; for a human, 70; for a hippopotamus, 150. The amount of heat generated by an animal is proportional to the mass of the animal, which is proportional to its volume, which is proportional to x^3. Consequently, the amount of heat generated is given by ax^3, where a is a positive number adjustable within certain bounds by the animal in question. The amount of heat lost is proportional to the amount of body surface and is hence given by bx^2, where b is a positive number that is *fixed* for each animal. Thus the "heat balance formula" for a mammal of size x is given by $h(x) = ax^3 - bx^2$, where a and b must be chosen for each specific mammal. Clearly, if the animal is to survive, x must be a root of $h(x)$, or at least close to a root (so that heat generated, ax^3, will be approximately equal to heat lost, bx^2). Otherwise, the animal will bake itself or freeze to death.
(a) Which type of mammal has the hardest time staying warm in cold weather, very large ones or very small ones? Which type of mammal has the hardest time keeping cool in hot weather?

(b) Do you think that fur should cause more or less heat to be lost through the body surface? Do smaller or larger animals need fur the most? Does this fit the facts of which animals are the furriest? [*Note:* Humans are quite large, as mammals go.]

(c) Suppose that $b = \frac{1}{2}$ for furry mammals and $b = 1$ for mammals with less hair. Suppose that a is given by the fraction of its own weight that an animal eats in a one-day period. For each of the following cases find the function $h(x)$ by inserting the proper values for a and b, and find the root of $h(x)$ to determine what size (in inches) this animal should be.

   (i) A furry creature that eats its own weight in food four times a day.

   (ii) A furry creature that eats its own weight every five days.

   (iii) A nonfurry creature that eats its own weight every 60 days.

(d) If a furry mammal were $x = .001$ inches in size, how often would it have to eat its own weight to stay alive? [*Hint:* Substitute the given values for b and x into the "heat balance formula," set it equal to 0, and solve for a. Then interpret your answer for a.] Is it likely that such a creature could eat this much?

(e) If a hairless mammal were $x = 600$ inches in size, how often would it be allowed to eat its own weight in order to maintain heat balance? Do you think such a creature could survive on this diet? If so, would it be likely to undertake any energetic activities?

(f) As is generally the case when mathematics is applied to a practical situation, many simplifying assumptions have been made in this problem. What are some factors that have been ignored here? Can you think of problems other than diet that a 50-foot mammal might have? [Highly readable discussions of these topics can be found in volume 2 of *The World of Mathematics* (ed. James R. Newman) in the article "On Being the Right Size" by J. B. S. Haldane, and in *The Solar System and Back* by Isaac Asimov in the article "Just Right."]

2. GRAPHS OF POLYNOMIAL FUNCTIONS

As we saw in Section 3 of Chapter 3, the graph of a first-degree polynomial function, such as $f(x) = 3x - 7$ or $g(x) = \frac{7}{3}x + 5$, is just a straight line. The graph of every second degree polynomial is a parabola. For example, see Figure 5-1.

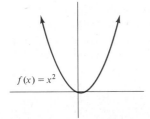
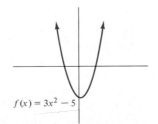
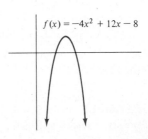

Figure 5-1

A complete discussion of such graphs was given in Section 6 of Chapter 4. If you have not already done so, you may wish to read that section now. However, it is not necessary to read that section in order to understand the material below.

THE FUNCTION $f(x) = x^n$

The simplest kind of higher degree polynomial function is one whose rule is given by a power of x, such as x^3, x^4, x^5, x^6, and so on. The graphs of such functions are easily determined.

EXAMPLE   In order to obtain the graph of $g(x) = x^4$, we plot some points and find that the graph looks like the one in Figure 5-2.

x	$g(x) = x^4$
-3	81
-2	16
-1	1
$-\frac{1}{2}$	$\frac{1}{16}$
0	0
1	1
2	16
3	81

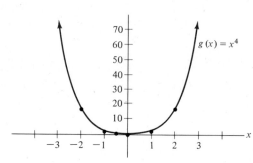

Figure 5-2

This graph is *not* a parabola, but it does have an upward-opening cup shape which is similar to the graph of the parabola $f(x) = x^2$ shown in Figure 5-1. The graphs of $h(x) = x^6$ and other *even* powers of x all have this same general shape. See Exercise A.1 for more details.

EXAMPLE   The graph of $g(x) = x^3$ may be obtained, as usual, by plotting some points. (See Figure 5-3.)

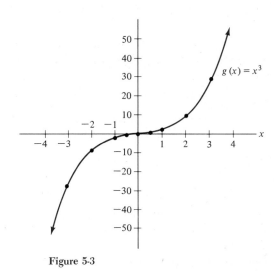

x	$g(x) = x^3$
-4	-64
-3	-27
-2	-8
-1	-1
$-\frac{1}{2}$	$-\frac{1}{8}$
0	0
$\frac{1}{2}$	$\frac{1}{8}$
1	1
2	8
3	27
4	64

Figure 5-3

The graphs of $h(x) = x^5$ and other *odd* powers of x have the same general shape as the graph of $g(x) = x^3$. See Exercise A.2 for more details.

BASIC PROPERTIES OF POLYNOMIAL GRAPHS

For more complicated polynomial functions, the best we can do without calculus is to present some general principles and suggest a basic procedure to follow. We begin with a discussion of certain common properties shared by *all* graphs of polynomial functions.

Extent Since the domain of a polynomial function is always the set of all real numbers, the graph extends on forever both to the left and to the right.

Continuity The graph of a polynomial function is a smooth, unbroken, continuous curve, such as the ones shown in Figure 5-4.

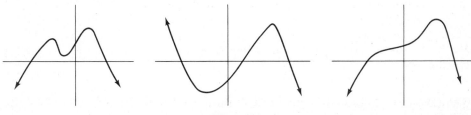

Figure 5-4

There can be no jumps, gaps, holes, or sharp corners on the graph. Thus *none* of the graphs in Figure 5-5 are graphs of polynomial functions.

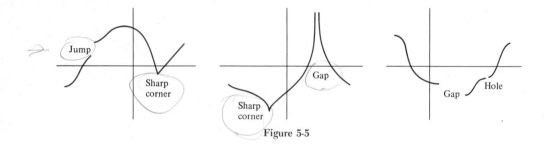

Figure 5-5

We have tacitly assumed these facts in the previous examples where we plotted only a few points and then connected them by a curve.

Behavior When |x| Is Large   When you move very far to the right or very far to the left along the x-axis, the graph of a polynomial function begins to move farther and farther *away* from the x-axis. For example, see Figure 5-6.

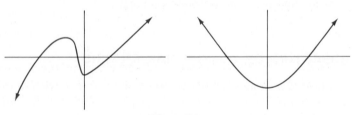

Figure 5-6

Graphs such as the ones in Figure 5-7 *cannot* be the graphs of polynomial functions.

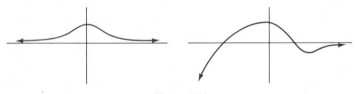

Figure 5-7

The reason why polynomial graphs behave this way is discussed in the DO IT YOURSELF! segment at the end of this section.

Maxima and Minima The graph of a typical polynomial function *may* have several "peaks" and "valleys" as shown in Figure 5-8.

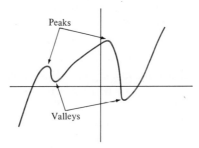

Figure 5-8

The technical term for a peak is a **relative maximum** (plural, maxima). The technical term for a valley is a **relative minimum** (plural, minima). The word "relative" is often omitted. It refers to the fact that a peak or relative maximum is not necessarily the highest point on the entire graph, but only the highest of all nearby points. Similarly, a valley or relative minimum is the lowest point of all the points near it. In calculus it is proved that

> *The total number of relative maxima and minima on the graph of a polynomial function of degree* n *is at most* n − 1.

We have already seen (in Chapter 4) one common example of this fact. The graph of every polynomial of degree 2 is a parabola. As Figure 5-1 shows, every parabola has exactly *one* maximum or exactly *one* minimum. More generally, the graph of the fifth-degree polynomial function $f(x) = x^5 - 6x^4 + 2x^2 + 1$ has a total of at most *four* relative maxima and minima.

Meeting the x-axis The points on the x-axis are precisely the points with second coordinate zero. If a point $(c, f(c))$ on the graph of a function $f(x)$ is also on the x-axis, then the second coordinate of $(c, f(c))$ must be zero; that is, $f(c) = 0$. Thus the graph of a polynomial function meets the x-axis at $x = c$ exactly when c is a *root* of the polynomial. As we saw in Section 1, a polynomial of degree n has at most n real roots. Therefore

> *The graph of a polynomial function of degree* n *meets the x-axis at most* n *times.*

To say that the graph of a function *meets* the x-axis does not necessarily mean that it *crosses* the axis. For instance, the graph of $f(x) = x^2$ shown above meets the x-axis at

$x = 0$ but does not cross the axis. On the other hand, the graph of $g(x) = x^3$ given above does cross the x-axis at $x = 0$. One difference between these two functions is that $x = 0$ is a root of $f(x) = x^2$ of multiplicity 2 (an even number), while $x = 0$ is a root of $g(x) = x^3$ of multiplicity 3 (an odd number). More generally, suppose the number c is a root of a polynomial function:

> *If the multiplicity of the root* c *is an* odd *number, then the graph of the function crosses the* x-axis at x = c.
>
> *If the multiplicity of the root* c *is an* even *number, then the graph of the function meets, but does not cross, the* x-axis at x = c.

The reason why this fact is true will become clear in the examples below. For now we just illustrate some of the possibilities in Figure 5-9.

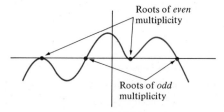

Figure 5-9

Suppose c and d are both roots of the polynomial $f(x)$ and that there are *no* roots *between* c and d. Then the graph of $f(x)$ meets the x-axis at $x = c$ and $x = d$, but *not* at any point in between. Since the graph of $f(x)$ between $x = c$ and $x = d$ is a continuous, unbroken curve that does *not* meet the x-axis, *it must lie entirely on one side of the x-axis*, as illustrated in Figure 5-10.

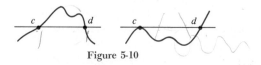

Figure 5-10

This fact is so useful that it's worth repeating:

> *If* c *and* d *are roots of the polynomial function* f, *and* f *has no roots between* x = c *and* x = d, *then the graph of* f *between* x = c *and* x = d *lies either completely above the x-axis or completely below the x-axis.*

GRAPHING A POLYNOMIAL FUNCTION

Until the techniques of calculus are available, we suggest that you use the four-step procedure outlined in the following examples for graphing polynomial functions. It won't work well every time, but will usually be satisfactory whenever the polynomial can be completely factored.

EXAMPLE The *first step in graphing* $f(x) = 2x^3 - x^2 - 15x$ is to *find all its real roots and write $f(x)$ in factored form:*

$$f(x) = 2x^3 - x^2 - 15x = x(2x^2 - x - 15),$$
$$f(x) = x(x - 3)(2x + 5) = x(x - 3)2(x + \tfrac{5}{2}),$$
$$f(x) = 2x(x - 3)(x + \tfrac{5}{2})$$

The roots are obviously $x = 0$, $x = 3$, and $x = -\tfrac{5}{2}$. They divide the x-axis into four intervals, as shown in Figure 5-11.

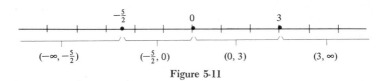

Figure 5-11

We know that in the interval between any two adjacent roots the graph either lies entirely above the x-axis or entirely below it. Likewise, the graph lies entirely on one side of the x-axis over the intervals $(-\infty, -\tfrac{5}{2})$ and $(3, \infty)$, since if it crossed over, there would be another root.

The second step is to determine on which side of the x-axis the graph lies for each of these intervals. To do this, we shall use the fact that the point $(x, f(x))$ lies *above* the x-axis exactly when its second coordinate is *positive;* that is, $f(x) > 0$. Similarly, $(x, f(x))$ lies *below* the x-axis when $f(x) < 0$.

Observe that for each x, $f(x) = 2x(x - 3)(x + \tfrac{5}{2})$ is a product of three factors. The sign of $f(x)$ (positive or negative) is determined by the signs of the three factors. For example, the factor $x + \tfrac{5}{2}$ is positive exactly when

$$x + \tfrac{5}{2} > 0 \qquad \text{or equivalently} \qquad x > -\tfrac{5}{2}$$

Thus $(x + \tfrac{5}{2})$ is positive when x is in any one of the intervals $(-\tfrac{5}{2}, 0)$, $(0, 3)$ or $(3, \infty)$ and $(x + \tfrac{5}{2})$ is negative when x is in the interval $(-\infty, -\tfrac{5}{2})$, as shown in Figure 5-12.

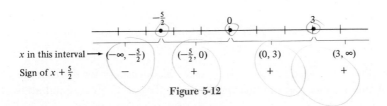

Figure 5-12

Similarly, $2x$ is positive whenever $x \geq 0$, that is, when x is in $(0, 3)$ or $(3, \infty)$. An analogous argument works for the factor $x - 3$, as summarized in the chart shown in Figure 5-13.

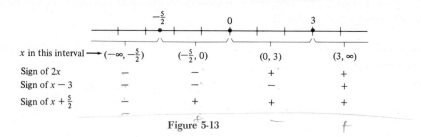

x in this interval →	$(-\infty, -\frac{5}{2})$	$(-\frac{5}{2}, 0)$	$(0, 3)$	$(3, \infty)$
Sign of $2x$	$-$	$-$	$+$	$+$
Sign of $x - 3$	$-$	$-$	$-$	$+$
Sign of $x + \frac{5}{2}$	$-$	$+$	$+$	$+$

Figure 5-13

This chart shows, for example, that in the interval $(-\frac{5}{2}, 0)$, the function $f(x) = 2x(x - 3)(x + \frac{5}{2})$ is a product of one positive and two negative factors, so that $f(x)$ is positive. Similar arguments work in the other intervals, as summarized in the chart shown in Figure 5-14.

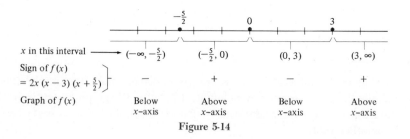

x in this interval →	$(-\infty, -\frac{5}{2})$	$(-\frac{5}{2}, 0)$	$(0, 3)$	$(3, \infty)$
Sign of $f(x)$ = $2x\,(x - 3)\,(x + \frac{5}{2})$	$-$	$+$	$-$	$+$
Graph of $f(x)$	Below x–axis	Above x–axis	Below x–axis	Above x–axis

Figure 5-14

The third step is to use the information above to make a rough sketch of the graph. Since $f(x)$ changes sign at each of its roots, the graph must *cross* the x-axis at each root. (Note that the multiplicity of each root is the odd number 1). So we obtain the rough sketch shown in Figure 5-15.

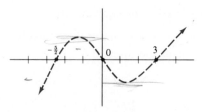

Figure 5-15

We claim that this sketch has the correct basic shape, except for the exact location and height of the maxima and minima (peaks and valleys). For we noted above that the

graph of $f(x)$ is an *unbroken* curve passing through $(-\frac{5}{2}, 0)$ and $(0, 0)$ and lying *above* the
x-axis between these points. Thus it must rise and then fall at least once between these
points as shown in the rough sketch above. Similarly, since the graph passes through
$(0, 0)$ and $(3, 0)$ and lies *below* the x-axis, it must fall, then rise at least once between
these points, as shown in the rough sketch. This accounts for at least one relative
maximum (peak) and one relative minimum (valley). But $f(x) = 2x^3 - x^2 - 15x$ has
degree 3 and therefore has *at most* a total of two relative maxima and minima. Hence
there can be *no more* maxima or minima.

Finally, if $x > 3$ our rough sketch indicates that the graph continues to rise forever.
This must be the case, for if the graph fell even briefly, we would have a situation such
as the one in Figure 5-16.

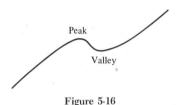

Peak

Valley

Figure 5-16

In this case there would be additional maxima and minima. Similarly, the graph must
always fall as x moves left from $-\frac{5}{2}$. Likewise, there can be no other "wiggles" in the
graph since any wiggle, such as $\sim$, would result in additional maxima or minima.

The fourth step is to sketch the graph accurately. This can often be done by plotting
only 6 to 8 additional points, once you know the correct basic shape of the graph (see
Figure 5-17).

x	$f(x) = 2x^3 - x^2 - 15x$
-3	-18
$-\frac{5}{2}$	0
-2	10
-1	12
0	0
1	-14
2	-18
3	0
4	52

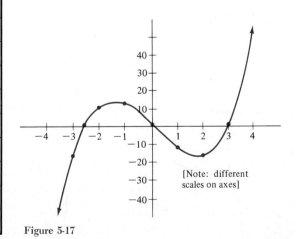

[Note: different scales on axes]

Figure 5-17

One problem with this graph is the location of the maxima and minima. As sketched above, they are very near $(-1, 12)$ and $(2, -18)$, respectively. As you will see in calculus, the actual relative maximum occurs when $x = (1 - \sqrt{91})/6$ [roughly, the point on the graph is $(-1.42, 13.56)$]; the actual relative minimum occurs when $x = (1 + \sqrt{91})/6$ [roughly, the point on the graph is $(1.76, -18.59)$].

EXAMPLE   If the function $g(x) = (x + 3)^2(x^2 - 2)(x - 2)$ were multiplied out, it would be a fifth-degree polynomial. However, it is convenient to leave it as is. *First*, we factor $g(x)$ further:

$$g(x) = (x + 3)^2(x^2 - 2)(x - 2) = (x + 3)^2(x + \sqrt{2})(x - \sqrt{2})(x - 2)$$

The roots of $g(x)$ are -3, $-\sqrt{2}$, $\sqrt{2}$, and 2. They divide the x-axis into five intervals, as shown in Figure 5-18.

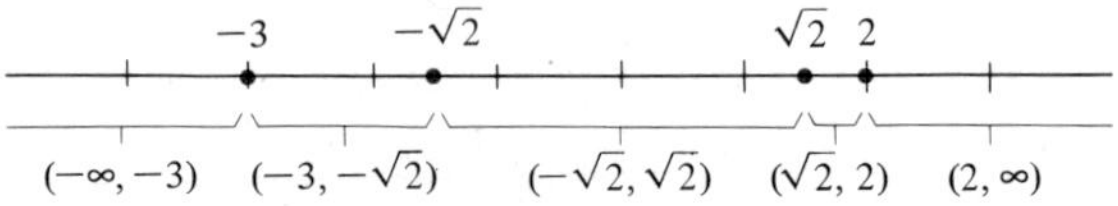

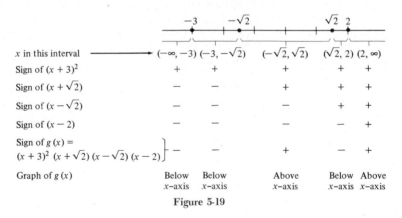

Figure 5-18

Second, we determine whether the graph of g lies above or below the x-axis over each of these intervals by finding the sign of $g(x)$. As above, this is done by examining the sign of each of the factors. Note that for *any* number x, the factor $(x + 3)^2$ is always positive. The signs of the other factors are easily determined, as indicated in Figure 5-19.

x in this interval	$(-\infty, -3)$	$(-3, -\sqrt{2})$	$(-\sqrt{2}, \sqrt{2})$	$(\sqrt{2}, 2)$	$(2, \infty)$
Sign of $(x + 3)^2$	$+$	$+$	$+$	$+$	$+$
Sign of $(x + \sqrt{2})$	$-$	$-$	$+$	$+$	$+$
Sign of $(x - \sqrt{2})$	$-$	$-$	$-$	$+$	$+$
Sign of $(x - 2)$	$-$	$-$	$-$	$-$	$+$
Sign of $g(x) =$ $(x + 3)^2 (x + \sqrt{2})(x - \sqrt{2})(x - 2)$	$-$	$-$	$+$	$-$	$+$
Graph of $g(x)$	Below x-axis	Below x-axis	Above x-axis	Below x-axis	Above x-axis

Figure 5-19

Third, we use this information to make a rough sketch of the graph, as shown in Figure 5-20.

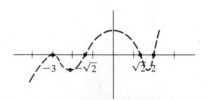

Figure 5-20

This sketch *does* show the correct basic shape since $g(x)$ is a fifth-degree polynomial and thus has at most four relative maxima or minima. Therefore there cannot be additional peaks, valleys, or wiggles in the graph.

The graph does *not* cross the x-axis at $x = -3$ since the analysis above shows that $g(x)$ is negative on *both* sides of $x = -3$. Note that $x = -3$ is a root of *even multiplicity* (2) whereas the roots at which the graph crosses the x-axis (namely, $x = -\sqrt{2}$, $x = \sqrt{2}$, and $x = 2$) are roots of *odd multiplicity* (1).

The *final step* is to plot some additional points to obtain a more accurate sketch of the graph, as shown in Figure 5-21.

x	$g(x) = (x + 3)^2(x^2 - 2)(x - 2)$
-4	-84
-3	0
-2	-8
$-\sqrt{2}$	0
-1	12
0	36
1	16
$\sqrt{2}$	0
1.5	-2.53125
1.8	-5.71392
2	0
3	252

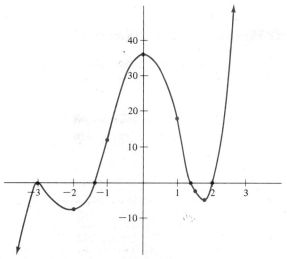

Figure 5-21

If you can't factor a given polynomial completely (that is, you don't know all its roots), then the procedure outlined in the preceding examples may not be of much help. In such cases, all that you can do is to plot a reasonable number of points and use these, together with the basic properties of polynomial functions discussed above, to make an educated guess about the shape of the graph.

EXERCISES

A.1. (a) Sketch careful graphs of $f(x) = x^2$, $\quad g(x) = x^4$, $\quad h(x) = x^6$, $\quad$ for $-3 \leq x \leq 3$ on the same set of coordinate axes.

(b) Use part (a) to estimate what the graph of $k(x) = x^8$ will look like for $-3 \leq x \leq 3$. Sketch the graph of $k(x)$ without plotting any points first.

A.2. (a) Sketch careful graphs of $f(x) = x^3$, $\quad g(x) = x^5$, $\quad h(x) = x^7$, $\quad$ for $-3 \leq x \leq 3$ on the same set of coordinate axes.

(b) Use part (a) to estimate what the graph of $k(x) = x^9$ will look like for $-3 \leq x \leq 3$. Sketch the graph of $k(x)$ without plotting any points first.

A.3. Sketch the graph of these functions. (*Hint:* the quickest way is to use the techniques of Section 6 of Chapter 4 and the graphs on pages 264–265.)

(a) $f(x) = x^3 + 5$ $\qquad$ (c) $h(x) = -x^3 - 3$ $\qquad$ (e) $k(x) = (x - 2)^4$

(b) $g(x) = -2x^3$ $\qquad$ (d) $k(x) = \dfrac{x^3}{2} + 1$ $\qquad$ (f) $f(x) = (x + 5)^3$

A.4. Figure 5-22 shows the graphs of several functions. Which functions are definitely not polynomial functions? Which functions could *possibly* be polynomial functions?

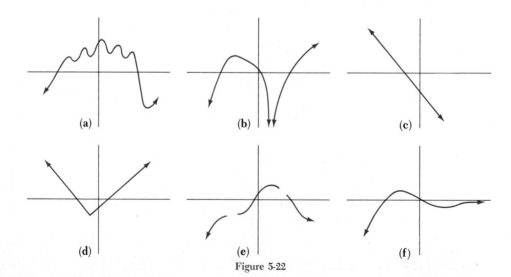

(a) (b) (c)

(d) (e) (f)

Figure 5-22

A.5. Which of the graphs in Figure 5-23 could possibly be the graph of a polynomial function of degree 3? of degree 4? of degree 5?

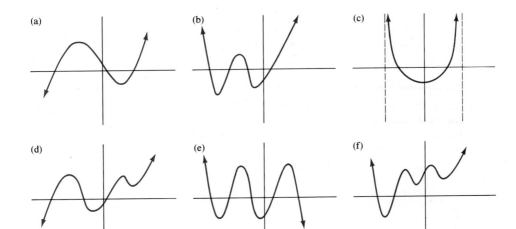

(a)   (b)   (c)

(d)   (e)   (f)

Figure 5-23

B.1. Do a rough sketch of the graph of each of these functions. (Check signs, but don't plot any points except the roots. Then see Exercise B.2.)

    (a) $f(x) = (x - 1)(x + 5)(x + 2)$

    (b) $g(x) = (x - 2)^2(x - 4)$

    (c) $h(x) = -x(x - 3)^2(2x + 3)$

    (d) $k(x) = x^2(x + 1)(3x - 7)$

    (e) $f(x) = \frac{1}{6}(x - 1)(x - 2)(x - 3)(x - 4)$

    (f) $g(x) = -(x - 1)(x + 2)^2x$

B.2. Plot 6–8 points on the graph of each of the functions in Exercise B.1 to see how well the rough sketch you did there corresponds to the actual graph.

B.3. Is the given function increasing (= graph rising from left to right) or decreasing (= graph falling from left to right) on the given interval?

    (a) $f(x) = (x - 1)^2(x + 2)(x - 3)$ on $(3, \infty)$

    (b) $f(x) = (x - 1)^2(x + 2)(x - 3)$ on $(-\infty, -2)$

    (c) $g(x) = (x - 6)(x + 5)^2(x - 3)x$ on $(-\infty, -5)$

    (d) $g(x) = (x - 6)(x + 5)^2(x - 3)x$ on $(6, \infty)$

B.4. (a)   Show that $x^2 - 6x + 7$ is a factor of $x^4 - 6x^3 + 6x^2 + 6x - 7$.

    (b)   Graph the function $f(x) = x^4 - 6x^3 + 6x^2 + 6x - 7$.

B.5. Use the four-step method presented above to sketch a reasonably accurate graph of each of these functions.

(a) $f(x) = -x^3 - x^2 + 2x$ (d) $k(x) = x^4 - 5x^2 + 5$

(b) $g(x) = x^2 - 6x + 5$ (e) $f(x) = x^4 - 6x^2 + 8$

(c) $h(x) = x^3 - 4x$ (f) $g(x) = x^4 - x^2$

B.6. Graph these functions.

(a) $f(x) = x^3 - 3x^2 - 4x$

(b) $g(x) = x^3 - 3x^2 - 4x + 2$ [*Hint:* see part (a) and p. 229.]

(c) $h(x) = x^3 - 3x^2 - 4x - 6$.

B.7. Graph these functions. [*Hint:* in each case, first use the Rational Solutions Test (p. 91) to find all rational roots; then use the Factor Theorem (p. 260) to factor and find the rest of the roots.]

(a) $f(x) = x^3 - 3x^2 - x + 3$ (d) $h(x) = x^4 - 4x^3 + 4x - 1$

(b) $g(x) = x^3 - 3x^2 + x + 1$ (e) $k(x) = x^4 - 3x^3 - 6x^2 + 14x + 12$

(c) $f(x) = x^3 - 4x^2 + 2x + 3$ (f) $g(x) = 4x^4 + 12x^3 - x^2 - 3x$

DO IT YOURSELF!

WHAT HAPPENS FOR LARGE x?

It is important to realize just how *explosive* the growth of the function $f(x) = x^n$ is when $x > 1$. Figure 5-24 shows a combined graph of

$$p(x) = x, \qquad q(x) = x^2, \qquad r(x) = x^3, \qquad s(x) = x^4$$

for positive values of x.

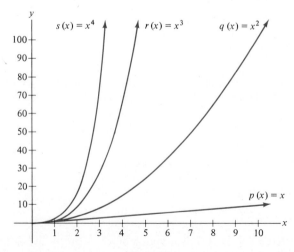

Figure 5-24

The situation only gets worse when x gets still larger. For instance, Figure 5-25 is a combined graph of these same functions from 0 to 100, where the scale has been adjusted to accommodate x^4.

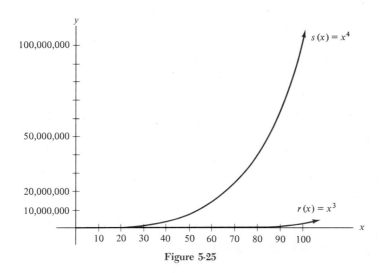

Figure 5-25

Here the values of x^3, x^2 and x are so insignificant in comparison to x^4 that their graphs hardly even show up! We can barely see the graph of x^3 beginning to creep above the x-axis. It would take a microscope to distinguish the graph of x^2 from the x-axis, and an electron microscope to find the graph of $p(x) = x$ on this scale.

The moral here is that each power of x makes lower powers look sickly and is humbled in turn by the next higher power. Thus for large values of x, the highest power of x in a polynomial is extremely important.

Analogous remarks hold when x is a negative number which is large in absolute value. For instance, when $|x|$ is large, then $|x^4|$ is very much larger than $|x^3|$, which is in turn very much larger than $|x^2|$.

EXAMPLE When x is large in absolute value, the graph of $f(x) = x^3 - 3x^2 + 5x + 4$ will be almost the same as that of x^3, turning sharply upwards to the right, sharply downwards to the left. The reason is that when x is large in absolute value, the terms $-3x^2$, $5x$, and 4 will be insignificant *compared* with x^3, as shown in the table.

x	100	500	1,000	$-1,500$
$5x$	500	2,500	5,000	$-7,500$
$-3x^2$	$-30,000$	$-750,000$	$-3,000,000$	$-6,750,000$
x^3	1,000,000	125,000,000	1,000,000,000	$-3,375,000,000$
$f(x) = x^3 - 3x^2 + 5x + 4$	970,504	124,252,504	997,005,004	$-3,381,757,496$

EXERCISES

A.1. **(a)** Make a table of values for the functions $f(x) = x^3$ and $g(x) = 10x^2$ to show that x^3 dominates $10x^2$ for large values of x.

(b) Repeat part (a) for $f(x)$ and $L(x) = 200x^2$. How large (approximately) does x have to go before x^3 exceeds $200x^2$?

(c) Make a table of values for $k(x) = 50x^3$ and $t(x) = \frac{1}{100}x^4$. Which function dominates the other for large values of x? (Make sure you take x large enough to see what's going on.)

A.2. Calculate a table of values for the following polynomials for *large* values of x. Your table should demonstrate that for large values of x, the value of a polynomial of degree n is approximately equal to the value of x^n.

    (a) $x^3 - 7x^2 + 10x - 1$ **(b)** $x^4 + 10x^3 + x^2 - x + 5$ **(c)** $x^5 - x^4 + 1$

B.1. Do the graphs of $f(x) = 10x^2$ and $g(x) = \frac{1}{10}x^3$ cross at any point on the right side of the y-axis? Explain.

3. RATIONAL FUNCTIONS

A **rational function** is a function whose rule is a quotient of two polynomials, such as

$$f(x) = \frac{1}{x}, \qquad g(x) = \frac{4x - 3}{2x + 1}, \qquad h(x) = \frac{5}{x - 3},$$

$$k(x) = \frac{2x^2 + 5x + 2}{2x + 7}, \qquad t(x) = \frac{x^3 - 2}{x - 1}$$

In particular, every polynomial function is also a rational function. For example, $f(x) = x^2 + 3$ can be written as $f(x) = (x^2 + 3)/1$.

Let $f(x) = g(x)/h(x)$ be a rational function [with $g(x)$ and $h(x)$ polynomials]. If c is a real number, then $f(c)$ is a well-defined real number whenever

$$f(c) = \frac{g(c)}{h(c)} \text{ is a real number}$$

The only time $g(c)/h(c)$ is *not* a real number occurs when the denominator $h(c)$ is 0. In other words, $f(c) = g(c)/h(c)$ is not defined when c is a root of the polynomial $h(x)$. Therefore

> The domain of a rational function $f(x) = g(x)/h(x)$ *is the set of all* real numbers *that are* not *roots of the denominator* $h(x)$.

EXAMPLE The domain of the function $k(x) = \dfrac{x - 2}{x^2(x - 3)(x + 1)}$ is the set of all real numbers *except* 0, 3, and -1, the roots of the denominator.

EXAMPLE You are probably accustomed to canceling factors in algebraic expressions, such as

$$\frac{x^2 - 1}{x - 1} = \frac{(x + 1)(x - 1)}{x - 1} = x + 1$$

Nevertheless, the *function* with rule $p(x) = x + 1$ and the *function* with rule $q(x) = \dfrac{x^2 - 1}{x - 1}$ are *not* the same function. The difference occurs when $x = 1$. Then

$$p(1) = 1 + 1 = 2, \quad \text{but} \quad q(1) = \frac{1^2 - 1}{1 - 1} = \frac{0}{0}$$

Thus $q(1)$ is not defined so that the number 1 is *not* in the domain of the function $q(x)$. But 1 *is* in the domain of the function $p(x) = x + 1$. It is true that for any number c *except* 1, the two functions have the same value; for in this case $c - 1 \neq 0$, and the factor $c - 1$ *can* be canceled:

$$q(c) = \frac{c^2 - 1}{c - 1} = \frac{(c + 1)(c - 1)}{c - 1} = c + 1 \quad \text{and} \quad p(c) = c + 1$$

But the difference for $x = 1$ makes $p(x)$ and $q(x)$ *different functions*.

GRAPHS OF LINEAR RATIONAL FUNCTIONS

The simplest rational functions to graph are functions such as

$$f(x) = \frac{5}{x - 3}, \quad g(x) = \frac{4x - 3}{2x + 1}, \quad h(x) = \frac{7}{5}, \quad k(x) = \frac{6x - 9}{3} = 2x - 3$$

in which both numerator and denominator are either first-degree polynomials or constants. Such functions are called **linear rational functions.** We already know that the graphs of linear rational functions such as $h(x)$ and $k(x)$ above are straight lines. The key to graphing other linear rational functions, such as $f(x)$ and $g(x)$ above, is this simple fact from arithmetic:

THE BIG-LITTLE PRINCIPLE

The farther the number c is from 0, the closer the number 1/c is to 0. Conversely, the closer the number c is to 0, the farther the number 1/c is from 0. In less precise but more suggestive terms:

$$\frac{1}{big} = little \quad and \quad \frac{1}{little} = big$$

For example, each of the numbers 100, 750, 1500, and 5000 is bigger (farther from 0) than the preceding one, but each of the numbers

$$\frac{1}{100}, \quad \frac{1}{750}, \quad \frac{1}{1500}, \quad \frac{1}{5000}$$

is smaller (closer to 0) than the preceding one. Similarly, each of the numbers

$$\frac{-2}{10}, \quad \frac{-4}{100}, \quad \frac{-5}{1000}, \quad \frac{-2}{10,000}$$

is closer to 0 (smaller in absolute value) than the preceding one, but each of the numbers

$$\frac{1}{\frac{-2}{10}} = -5, \qquad \frac{1}{\frac{-4}{100}} = -25, \qquad \frac{1}{\frac{-5}{1000}} = -200, \qquad \frac{1}{\frac{-2}{10,000}} = -5000$$

is farther from 0 (bigger in absolute value) than the preceding one.

EXAMPLE In order to graph $f(x) = 5/(x - 3)$, we first observe that there is one *bad point* at which the function is not defined, namely, $x = 3$. It is important to determine what the graph looks like *near* this bad point. When x is a number bigger than 3, but very close to 3, then $x - 3$ is a positive number very close to 0. By the Big-Little Principle $1/(x - 3)$ must be a very large positive number. Thus $f(x) = 5\left(\dfrac{1}{x - 3}\right)$ is also a large positive number. In fact, the closer x is to 3, the smaller $x - 3$ is, so that

$$\text{The closer } x \text{ is to 3, the } \textit{larger } f(x) = \frac{5}{x - 3} \text{ is}$$

In graphical terms this means that the closer x is to 3 on the right side of 3, the farther the point $(x, f(x))$ is above the x-axis. So the graph rises sharply on the right side of $x = 3$, as shown in Figure 5-26.

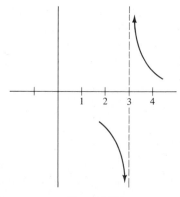

Figure 5-26

Similarly, if x is a bit smaller than 3, but very close to 3, then $x - 3$ is a negative number very close to 0 and $f(x) = 5/(x - 3)$ is a negative number that is very far from 0 (large in absolute value). So the graph of f falls very sharply on the left side of $x = 3$, as shown in Figure 5-26. The graph gets closer and closer to the vertical line $x = 3$, but never touches it. We say that the line $x = 3$ is a **vertical asymptote**° of the graph. Informally, we sometimes say that the graph *"blows up"* at $x = 3$.

Since $f(x) = 5/(x - 3)$ is positive when $x > 3$ and negative when $x < 3$, the graph of f lies above the x-axis to the right of $x = 3$ and below the x-axis to the left of $x = 3$. In order to determine what the graph looks like at the far right and the far left, we must examine $f(x)$ when x is a number very large in absolute value (that is, far from 0). As x gets bigger and bigger in absolute value, so does $x - 3$, and the Big-Little Principle tells us that $1/(x - 3)$ gets closer and closer to 0. Consequently, $f(x) = \dfrac{5}{x - 3} = 5 \cdot \dfrac{1}{x - 3}$ gets closer and closer to 0 as well. Thus the corresponding points $(x, f(x))$ on the graph get closer and closer to the x-axis without touching it, as shown in Figure 5-27.

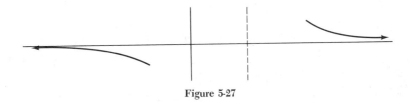

Figure 5-27

We say that the x-axis is a **horizontal asymptote** of the graph.°

By plotting a few points and using the information developed above, we see that the entire graph looks like the one shown in Figure 5-28.

x	$f(x) = \dfrac{5}{x - 3}$
-12	$-\frac{1}{3}$
-2	-1
0	$-\frac{5}{3}$
1	$-\frac{5}{2}$
2	-5
2.5	-10
3.5	10
4	5
6	$\frac{5}{3}$
8	1
13	$\frac{1}{2}$

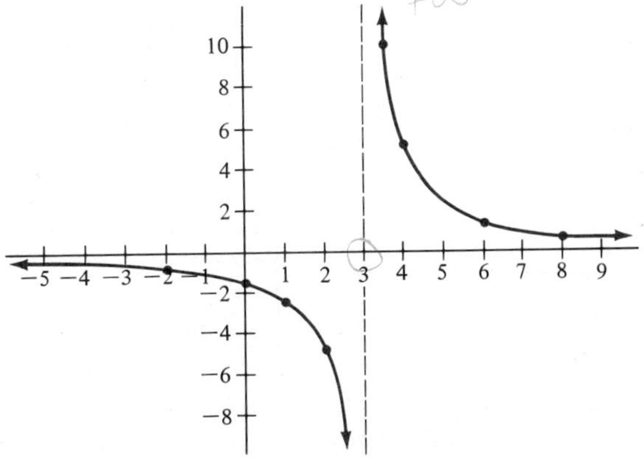

Figure 5-28

°Sometimes we say "asymptote of the function" instead of "asymptote of the graph."

The kind of analysis used in the preceding example works for any rational function of the form $f(x) = b/(cx + d)$ (where b, c, d are fixed real numbers and $c \neq 0$). The graph has a vertical asymptote at the number which is the root of the denominator. The graph lies above the x-axis on one side of the vertical asymptote and below the x-axis on the other side. The x-axis is a horizontal asymptote of the graph. These facts are sufficient to determine the general shape of the graph. A reasonably accurate sketch of the graph can then be obtained by plotting a few points. Some examples are shown in Figure 5-29.

$$f(x) = \frac{1}{x} \quad \text{vertical asymptote } x = 0$$

x	$f(x)$
-3	$-\frac{1}{3}$
-2	$-\frac{1}{2}$
-1	-1
$-\frac{1}{3}$	-3
$\frac{1}{4}$	4
1	1
2	$\frac{1}{2}$
3	$\frac{1}{3}$

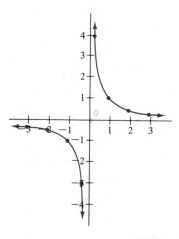

$$k(x) = \frac{-3}{2x + 5} \quad \text{vertical asymptote } x = -\frac{5}{2}$$

x	$k(x)$
-5	$\frac{3}{5}$
-4	1
-3	3
-2	-3
-1	-1
0	$-\frac{3}{5}$
1	$-\frac{3}{7}$

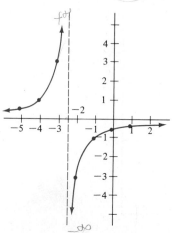

Figure 5-29

EXAMPLE The graph of the function $f(x) = \dfrac{4x - 3}{2x + 1}$ can be obtained by similar techniques. Since $f(x) = \dfrac{4x - 3}{2x + 1} = \dfrac{4x - 3}{2(x + \frac{1}{2})}$, the function is not defined at $x = -\frac{1}{2}$. To determine the shape of the graph near this bad point, note that when x is a number very close to $-\frac{1}{2}$, then the denominator of $f(x) = \dfrac{4x - 3}{2(x + \frac{1}{2})}$ is very close to 0, and the numerator $4x - 3$ is very close to $4(-\frac{1}{2}) - 3 = -5$. By the Big-Little Principle $f(x)$ must be a number that is very large in absolute value (since $\dfrac{-5}{\text{little}}$ must be far from 0). In graphical terms this means that when x is close to $-\frac{1}{2}$, then $f(x)$ is far from the x-axis. As in the previous examples, we must have a vertical asymptote at $x = -\frac{1}{2}$. In order to determine the shape of the graph when $|x|$ is large, we note that for any *nonzero* number x, we can divide both the numerator and denominator of $f(x)$ by x:

$$f(x) = \frac{4x - 3}{2x + 1} = \frac{\dfrac{4x - 3}{x}}{\dfrac{2x + 1}{x}} = \frac{4 - \dfrac{3}{x}}{2 + \dfrac{1}{x}}$$

Now when $|x|$ is large we know by the Big-Little Principle that both $-3/x$ and $1/x$ are very close to 0. Therefore when $|x|$ is large, $f(x) = \dfrac{4 - (3/x)}{2 + (1/x)}$ is very close to $\dfrac{4 - 0}{2 + 0} = 2$. We can see what this means graphically by plotting some points, as shown in Figure 5-30.

x	$f(x) = \dfrac{4x - 3}{2x + 1}$
-5	$\frac{23}{9}$
-3	3
-1	7
0	-3
$\frac{3}{4}$	0
1	$\frac{1}{3}$
2	1
3	$\frac{9}{7}$
5	$\frac{17}{11}$
7	$\frac{5}{3}$

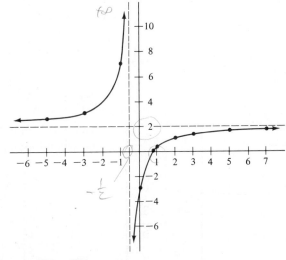

Figure 5-30

As x gets larger and larger in absolute value, the graph of $f(x)$ gets closer and closer to the horizontal line $y = 2$. This line is called a **horizontal asymptote** of the graph.

The kind of analysis used in the preceding example works for any linear rational function of the form

$$f(x) = \frac{ax + b}{cx + d} \quad \text{(where } a, b, c, d \text{ are fixed real numbers and } a \neq 0, c \neq 0)$$

The graph has a vertical asymptote at the number which is a root of the denominator $cx + d$. The horizontal line $y = a/c$ is a horizontal asymptote of the graph since

$$f(x) = \frac{ax + b}{cx + d} = \frac{\dfrac{ax + b}{x}}{\dfrac{cx + d}{x}} = \frac{a + \dfrac{b}{x}}{c + \dfrac{d}{x}} \quad (x \neq 0)$$

so that $f(x)$ is very close to a/c when $|x|$ is large. Some examples are shown in Figure 5-31.

$$f(x) = \frac{-5x + 12}{2x - 4}$$

$$\Rightarrow \quad x = \frac{4 \, f(x) + 12}{2 \, f(x) + 5}$$

vertical asymptote $x = 2$
horizontal asymptote $y = -\frac{5}{2}$

x	$f(x)$
-1	$-\frac{17}{6}$
0	-3
1	$-\frac{7}{2}$
$\frac{12}{5}$	0
3	$-\frac{3}{2}$
4	-2
6	$-2\frac{1}{4}$

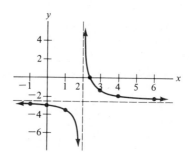

$$k(x) = \frac{3x + 6}{x}$$

vertical asymptote $x = 0$
horizontal asymptote $y = \frac{3}{1} = 3$

x	$k(x)$
-3	1
-2	0
-1	-3
1	9
2	6
3	5
4	$4\frac{1}{2}$

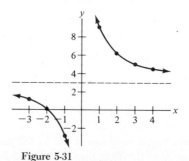

Figure 5-31

BASIC PROPERTIES OF RATIONAL GRAPHS

The graphs of more complicated rational functions share a number of common properties. We summarize them here so that you'll have some idea what to expect when graphing such functions.

Maxima and Minima The graph of a rational function may have some relative maxima and minima (peaks and valleys). The total *number* of relative maxima and minima is much less important for graphing rational functions than it was for graphing polynomial functions.

Roots If the graph of the rational function $f(x) = g(x)/h(x)$ touches the x-axis at $x = c$, then $(c, 0)$ is on the graph. Since the only point on the graph of f with first coordinate c is $(c, f(c))$, we must have $f(c) = 0$. In order for the number $f(c) = g(c)/h(c)$ to be 0, we must have:

$h(c) \neq 0$ (so that the fraction $\dfrac{g(c)}{h(c)}$ is a well-defined real number)

$g(c) = 0$ (since a fraction is 0 only when its numerator is 0)

In other words,

> *The points at which the graph of the rational function* f(x) = g(x)/h(x) *touches the* x-*axis correspond to the numbers that are roots of the numerator* g(x), *but* not *roots of the denominator* h(x).

A number that is a root of the numerator $g(x)$, but not of the denominator $h(x)$, is called a **root of the rational function** $f(x) = g(x)/h(x)$. For example, the numerator of the function $f(x) = \dfrac{x^2 - 1}{x - 1}$ has 1 and -1 as roots. But 1 is also a root of the denominator, so that -1 is the only root of the rational function $f(x)$.

Bad Points The rational function $f(x) = g(x)/h(x)$ is not defined at those numbers that are *roots of the denominator* $h(x)$. If $x = d$ is a root of $h(x)$ that is also a root of $g(x)$, then the graph of $f(x)$ will have either a *hole* or a *vertical asymptote* at $x = d$, as shown in Figure 5-32.

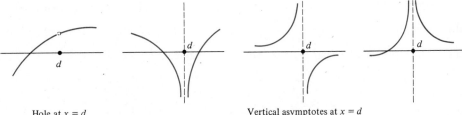

Hole at $x = d$ Vertical asymptotes at $x = d$

Figure 5-32

As we saw above, the function $f(x) = 5/(x - 3)$ has a vertical asymptote at $x = 3$. Observe that $x = 3$ is a root of the denominator $x - 3$ which is *not* a root of the numerator 5. An analogous argument works for any rational function and shows that

---

Whenever x = d *is a root of the denominator* h(x), *but not a root of the numerator* g(x), *then the rational function* f(x) = g(x)/h(x) *has a vertical asymptote at* x = d.

Extent and Continuity As just noted, the graph of a rational function may have several breaks in it (holes or places where there is a vertical asymptote). These occur *only* where the function is not defined. Wherever the function *is* defined, however, its graph is always a continuous, smooth, unbroken curve.

Behavior When $|x|$ Is Large Consider the function $f(x) = \dfrac{3x^4 - 2x}{2x^4 + 5}$ in which the numerator and denominator polynomials have the *same* degree. When $x \neq 0$, we can divide both the numerator and denominator by the highest power of x that occurs, namely, x^4, without affecting the value of $f(x)$:

$$f(x) = \frac{3x^4 - 2x}{2x^4 + 5} = \frac{\dfrac{3x^4 - 2x}{x^4}}{\dfrac{2x^4 + 5}{x^4}} = \frac{3 - \dfrac{2}{x^3}}{2 + \dfrac{5}{x^4}}$$

As $|x|$ gets larger and larger, the terms $2/x^3$ and $5/x^4$ get closer and closer to 0 by the Big-Little Principle. So $f(x)$ gets closer and closer to $\dfrac{3 - 0}{2 + 0} = \dfrac{3}{2}$. Thus as $|x|$ gets larger, the graph of f gets closer and closer to the horizontal line $y = \frac{3}{2}$. Hence this line is a horizontal asymptote of the graph. The same argument works in the general case:

If f(x) = $\dfrac{ax^n + \cdots}{cx^n + \cdots}$ *is a rational function whose numerator and denominator have the same degree* n, *then the line* y = a/c *is a horizontal asymptote of the graph.*

Now suppose f is a rational function in which the denominator has *larger* degree than the numerator, such as $f(x) = \dfrac{x^2 + 7}{x^3 - x^2}$. Dividing both numerator and denominator by the highest power of x that occurs, namely, x^3, shows that for $x \neq 0$

$$f(x) = \frac{x^2 + 7}{x^3 - x^2} = \frac{\dfrac{x^2 + 7}{x^3}}{\dfrac{x^3 - x^2}{x^3}} = \frac{\dfrac{1}{x} + \dfrac{7}{x^3}}{1 - \dfrac{1}{x}}$$

As $|x|$ gets larger and larger, the Big-Little Principle shows that $f(x)$ gets closer and closer to $(0 + 0)/(1 - 0) = 0/1 = 0$. In geometric terms, the graph of f gets closer and closer to the x-axis. So the x-axis is a horizontal asymptote of the graph. This argument also carries over to the general case:

> *If* f(x) = g(x)/h(x) *is a rational function in which the denominator* h(x) *has larger degree than the numerator* g(x), *then the x-axis is a horizontal asymptote of the graph.*

The asymptotes of rational functions in which the degree of the denominator is *less* than the degree of the numerator are somewhat more complicated. Some examples of such functions are discussed at the end of this section.

Change of Sign If the graph of a function f crosses the x-axis at the root $x = c$, then $f(x)$ is a positive number when x is on one side of c and $f(x)$ is a negative number when x is on the other side of c, as shown in Figure 5-33.

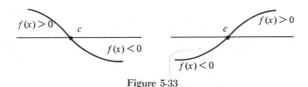

Figure 5-33

We say that f **changes sign** at the root $x = c$. There are two other situations in which a rational function f may possibly change sign. If the graph has a vertical asymptote or a hole on the x-axis at $x = d$, then it *may* happen that $f(x)$ is positive when x is on one side of d and negative when x is on the other side of d, as shown in the examples in Figure 5-34.

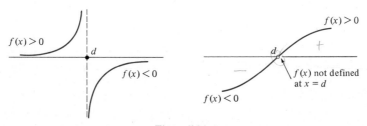

Figure 5-34

Since the graph of a rational function is a continuous, unbroken curve wherever the function *is* defined, it can be proved that

> *A rational function can change sign only at a root, or a vertical asymptote, or a hole on the x-axis.*

This statement does not mean that a rational function *must* change sign at *every* root, vertical asymptote, or hole on the x axis. But *if* it *does* change sign, such a change can occur only at these places.

GRAPHING A RATIONAL FUNCTION

The basic procedure is to examine the behavior of the function near its bad points and roots to obtain an idea of the general shape of the graph. Then plot a few points and obtain a reasonably accurate graph.

EXAMPLE   The first step in graphing $f(x) = \dfrac{x-1}{x^2-x-6}$, is to write $f(x)$ in factored form in order to *find all the real roots and bad points:*

$$f(x) = \frac{x-1}{x^2-x-6} = \frac{x-1}{(x+2)(x-3)}$$

Clearly, $x = 1$ is a root of $f(x)$, and $f(x)$ is not defined when $x = -2$ or $x = 3$. Since neither $x = -2$ nor $x = 3$ is a root of the numerator $x - 1$, the graph must have vertical asymptotes at $x = -2$ and $x = 3$. These asymptotes and the root divide the x-axis into four intervals, as shown in Figure 5-35.

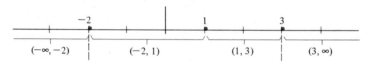

Figure 5-35

Since this rational function can *change* sign only at a root or a vertical asymptote, the sign of $f(x)$ remains the same throughout any one of these intervals. This means that the graph of $f(x)$ must lie *entirely above* the x-axis ($f(x) > 0$) or *entirely below* the x-axis ($f(x) < 0$) on each of these intervals.

   In order to *determine the sign of $f(x)$ on each of the intervals* above, we need only examine the signs of each of the factors $x - 1, x + 2$, and $x - 3$. For example, $x - 1$ is positive exactly when

$$x - 1 > 0 \qquad \text{or equivalently} \qquad x > 1$$

Thus $x - 1$ is positive when x is in the intervals $(1, 3)$ and $(3, \infty)$, and negative when x is in the intervals $(-\infty, -2)$ and $(-2, 1)$. Similar arguments work for the other factors, as summarized in the chart shown in Figure 5-36.

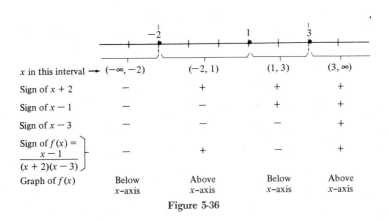

Figure 5-36

Since $f(x)$ changes sign at the root $x = 1$, the graph must cross the x-axis there. Since the numerator of $k(x) = \dfrac{x - 1}{(x + 2)(x - 3)}$ has degree 1 and the denominator $(x + 2)(x - 3) = x^2 - x - 6$ has strictly larger degree 2, the x-axis must be a horizontal asymptote of the graph. Using all the information we now have about roots, asymptotes, and signs, we can make a *rough sketch* of the general shape of most of the graph, as shown in Figure 5-37.

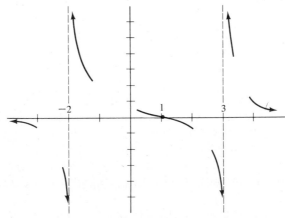

Figure 5-37

It is now easy to plot a few points and obtain a reasonably accurate sketch of the graph, as shown in Figure 5-38.

x	$f(x) = \dfrac{x-1}{x^2-x-6}$
-4	$-\frac{5}{14}$
-3	$-\frac{2}{3}$
-2.2	$-\frac{80}{26} \approx -3.08$
-1.9	$\frac{290}{49} \approx 5.92$
-1	$\frac{1}{2}$
0	$\frac{1}{6}$
1	0
2	$-\frac{1}{4}$
2.8	$-\frac{15}{8} = -1.875$
3.1	$\frac{210}{51} \approx 4.12$
4	$\frac{1}{2}$

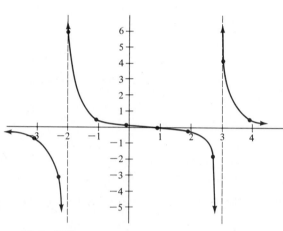

Figure 5-38

EXAMPLE In order to graph $k(x) = \dfrac{x^2 - 3x + 2}{(x^2 - 4)(x - 3)}$ we first factor:

$$k(x) = \frac{x^2 - 3x + 2}{(x^2 - 4)(x - 3)} = \frac{(x - 2)(x - 1)}{(x - 2)(x + 2)(x - 3)}$$

Since $x = 2$ is a root of *both* numerator and denominator, $k(2) = \frac{0}{0}$ is *not* defined. However, for any number x *except* 2, we have $x - 2 \neq 0$ so that

$$k(x) = \frac{(x - 2)(x - 1)}{(x - 2)(x + 2)(x - 3)} = \frac{x - 1}{(x + 2)(x - 3)} \qquad \text{when } x \neq 2$$

Therefore the graph of $k(x)$ looks exactly like the graph of $f(x) = \dfrac{x - 1}{(x + 2)(x - 3)}$ with *one point deleted*, namely, the point where $x = 2$. The graph of $f(x) = \dfrac{x - 1}{(x + 2)(x - 3)}$

was obtained in the preceding example. All we have to do is to delete the point where $x = 2$ in order to get the graph of $k(x)$, as shown in Figure 5-39.

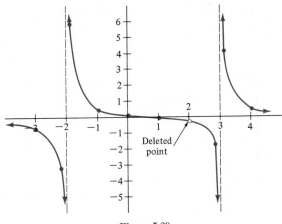

Figure 5-39

Thus the graph of $k(x)$ has a vertical asymptote at $x = -2$ and $x = 3$ and a *hole* at $x = 2$.

EXAMPLE   In order to graph $f(x) = \dfrac{x - 4}{(2x^2 - x - 6)(x - 2)}$ we factor:

$$f(x) = \frac{x - 4}{(2x^2 - x - 6)(x - 2)} = \frac{x - 4}{(2x + 3)(x - 2)(x - 2)} = \frac{x - 4}{2(x + \frac{3}{2})(x - 2)^2}$$

Clearly, $f(x)$ has vertical asymptotes at $x = -\frac{3}{2}$ and $x = 2$ and a root at $x = 4$. The root and asymptotes divide the x-axis into four intervals. We can determine the sign of $f(x)$ when x is in each of these intervals by examining the signs of the factors $2(x + \frac{3}{2})$, $(x - 2)^2$, and $x - 4$, as summarized in the chart shown in Figure 5-40.

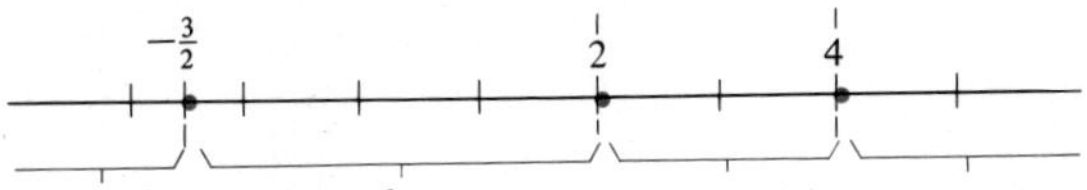

	$\left(-\infty, -\frac{3}{2}\right)$	$\left(-\frac{3}{2}, 2\right)$	$(2, 4)$	$(4, \infty)$
x in this interval $\longrightarrow$				
Sign of $2(x + \frac{3}{2})$	$-$	$+$	$+$	$+$
Sign of $2(x - 2)^2$	$+$	$+$	$+$	$+$
Sign of $x - 4$	$-$	$-$	$-$	$+$
Sign of $f(x) = \dfrac{x - 4}{2(x + \frac{3}{2})(x - 2)^2}$	$+$	$-$	$-$	$+$
Graph of $f(x)$	Above x-axis	Below x-axis	Below x-axis	Above x-axis

Figure 5-40

Since f changes sign at the root $x = 4$, the graph crosses the x-axis there. Note that f does *not* change sign at the asymptote $x = 2$. Since the numerator of $f(x) = \dfrac{x - 4}{(2x^2 - x - 6)(x - 2)}$ has smaller degree than the denominator, the x-axis is a horizontal asymptote of the graph. It is now easy to plot some points and obtain a reasonably accurate sketch of the graph, as shown in Figure 5-41.

x	$f(x) = \dfrac{x - 4}{(2x^2 - x - 6)(x - 2)}$
-3	$\frac{7}{75}$
-2	$\frac{3}{8}$
-1	$-\frac{5}{9}$
0	$-\frac{1}{3}$
1	$-\frac{3}{5}$
1.5	$-\frac{5}{3}$
3	$-\frac{1}{9}$
4	0
5	$\frac{1}{117}$

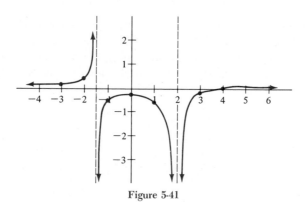

Figure 5-41

Without calculus we can't precisely locate the top of the peak between $x = -\frac{3}{2}$ and $x = 2$ or the tiny peak (molehill?) to the right of $x = 4$. Nor can we guarantee that there aren't some further bends or wiggles in the graph.

In all the examples up to now, the degree of the denominator has always been greater than or equal to the degree of the numerator. We have seen that the graphs of such rational functions have only vertical or horizontal straight lines as asymptotes. But when $f(x) = g(x)/h(x)$ and the degree of the denominator $h(x)$ is strictly less than the degree of $g(x)$, the situation is different. The graph may have oblique asymptotes (that is, straight lines that are neither vertical nor horizontal). Or it may have curves other than straight lines as asymptotes.

EXAMPLE   In order to graph $f(x) = \dfrac{2x^2 + 5x + 2}{2x + 7}$, we first factor:

$$f(x) = \frac{2x^2 + 5x + 2}{2x + 7} = \frac{(2x + 1)(x + 2)}{2x + 7} = \frac{2(x + \frac{1}{2})(x + 2)}{2(x + \frac{7}{2})}$$

We see that $x = -\frac{1}{2}$ and $x = -2$ are roots of f and that there is a vertical asymptote at $x = -\frac{7}{2}$. The usual analysis of signs produces the chart in Figure 5-42.

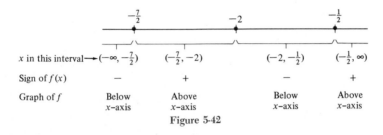

Figure 5-42

By plotting some points we see that near the vertical asymptote and roots the graph looks like the one shown in Figure 5-43.

x	$f(x) = \dfrac{2x^2 + 5x + 2}{2x + 7}$
-4	-14
-3	5
-2	0
-1	$-\frac{1}{5}$
$-\frac{1}{2}$	0
0	$\frac{2}{7}$

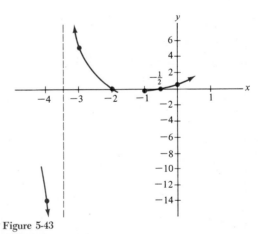

Figure 5-43

In order to determine the rest of the graph, we divide the numerator $2x^2 + 5x + 2$ of $f(x)$ by the denominator $2x + 7$ and find that the quotient is $x - 1$ and the remainder is 9 (verify this!). According to the division algorithm,

$$\text{dividend} = (\text{quotient})(\text{divisor}) + (\text{remainder})$$
$$2x^2 + 5x + 2 = (x - 1)(2x + 7)\ \ + 9$$

Dividing both sides of this last equation by $2x + 7$, we obtain

$$\underbrace{\frac{2x^2 + 5x + 2}{2x + 7}}_{f(x)} = \frac{(x - 1)(2x + 7)}{2x + 7} + \frac{9}{2x + 7}$$

$$= (x - 1) + \frac{9}{2x + 7}$$

Now when $|x|$ is large, the Big-Little Principle tells us that $9/(2x + 7)$ is very close to 0. Therefore when x is large, $f(x) = (x - 1) + \dfrac{9}{2x + 7}$ is very close to $(x - 1) + 0 = x - 1$. Thus for $|x|$ large the graph of f is very close to the graph of $y = x - 1$, as shown in Figure 5-44.

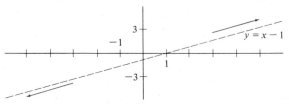

Figure 5-44

The straight line $y = x - 1$ is an **asymptote** of the graph. Note that the graph of f lies above the asymptote $y = x - 1$ when x is a large positive number. The reason is that when x is large positive, $9/(2x + 7)$ is a small positive number, so that $f(x) = (x - 1) + \dfrac{9}{2x + 7}$ is slightly larger than $x - 1$. Similarly, when x is a negative number far to the left of 0, $f(x)$ is slightly smaller than $x - 1$.

We now have enough information to plot a reasonably accurate graph, as shown in Figure 5-45.

x	$f(x) = \dfrac{2x^2 + 5x + 2}{2x + 7}$
-6	$-\frac{44}{5}$
-5	-9
-4	-14
-3	5
-2	0
-1	$-\frac{1}{5}$
$-\frac{1}{2}$	0
0	$\frac{2}{7}$
1	1
2	$\frac{20}{11}$

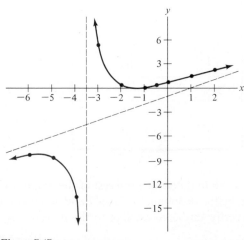

Figure 5-45

Once again, we cannot determine the exact location of the relative maxima and minima (peaks and valleys) without calculus.

EXAMPLE   The graph of $f(x) = \dfrac{x^3 - 2}{x - 1}$ is discussed in Exercise B.6. It has the parabola $y = x^2 + x + 1$ as an asymptote.

EXERCISES

A.1.   State the domain of each of these rational functions.

(a) $f(x) = \dfrac{1}{x + 2}$

(d) $q(x) = \dfrac{x^2 + x + 1}{x^2 - 3}$

(b) $g(x) = \dfrac{x - 3}{x^2 - 4}$

(e) $r(x) = \dfrac{2x^3 - 3x^2 + 1}{x^3 - x}$

(c) $h(x) = \dfrac{x^2 + 5}{x^2 + 2x + 1}$

(f) $f(x) = \dfrac{x^2 - 9}{2x^3 - 5x^2 - 3x}$

A.2.   Give examples of three different rational functions, each of which has as its domain the set of all real numbers except $-\frac{1}{2}$, 1, and 2.

A.3.   Graph these linear rational functions.

(a) $f(x) = \dfrac{1}{x + 5}$

(e) $k(x) = \dfrac{-3}{2x + 5}$

(i) $f(x) = \dfrac{2 - x}{x - 3}$

(b) $q(x) = \dfrac{-7}{x - 6}$

(f) $g(x) = \dfrac{-4}{2 - x}$

(j) $g(x) = \dfrac{3x - 2}{x + 3}$

(c) $g(x) = \dfrac{10}{x + 1}$

(g) $f(x) = \dfrac{3x}{x - 1}$

(k) $q(x) = \dfrac{7x - 3}{-4x + 12}$

(d) $h(x) = \dfrac{2}{3x - 7}$

(h) $p(x) = \dfrac{x - 2}{x}$

(l) $f(x) = \dfrac{-5x + 1}{-2x - 1}$

A.4.   Find the roots of these rational functions.

(a) $f(x) = \dfrac{x^2 - 5x + 6}{x^2 + 1}$

(d) $q(x) = \dfrac{2x^3 + 3x^2 - x}{x^2 + 5x - 3}$

(b) $g(x) = \dfrac{x^2 + 2x - 3}{x^2 - 1}$

(e) $k(x) = \dfrac{(x^2 - 9)(x^2 + 6x + 9)}{x^2 + x - 6}$

(c) $k(x) = \dfrac{x^2 - 7x + 10}{x^2 + 2x}$

(f) $f(x) = \dfrac{x^3 - 4x^2 + 2x}{x^4 - 8x}$

B.1.   Find at least one linear rational function whose graph passes through the points $(0, 1)$, $(1, 0)$, and $(2, -2)$.

B.2.   Find a linear rational function whose asymptotes are the lines $x = -1$ and $y = 2$ and whose graph contains the point $(1, 3)$.

B.3. Graph these rational functions, in which the degree of the denominator is always greater than the degree of the numerator.

(a) $f(x) = \dfrac{1}{x(x+1)^2}$

(e) $p(x) = \dfrac{x^2 - 9}{(x+3)(x-5)(x+4)}$

(b) $g(x) = \dfrac{x}{2x^2 - 5x - 3}$

(f) $q(x) = \dfrac{x^3 + 3x^2}{x^4 - 4x^2}$

(c) $f(x) = \dfrac{x - 3}{x^2 + x - 2}$

(g) $h(x) = \dfrac{(x^2 + 6x + 5)(x + 5)}{(x+5)^3(x-1)}$

(d) $g(x) = \dfrac{x + 2}{x^2 - 1}$

(h) $f(x) = \dfrac{x^2 - 1}{x^3 - 2x^2 + x}$

B.4. Graph these functions, using the same general procedure as in Exercise B.3. The only difference here is that both numerator and denominator have the same degree. So instead of the x-axis, some other horizontal straight line will be a horizontal asymptote (see the last box on p. 286).

(a) $f(x) = \dfrac{-4x^2 + 1}{x^2}$

(c) $q(x) = \dfrac{x^2 + 2x}{x^2 - 4x - 5}$

(b) $k(x) = \dfrac{x^2 + 1}{x^2 - 1}$

(d) $F(x) = \dfrac{x^2 + x}{x^2 - 2x + 4}$

B.5. Graph these functions. (The next to last example in the text may be helpful as a guide.)

(a) $f(x) = \dfrac{x^2 - x - 6}{x - 2}$

(d) $P(x) = \dfrac{x^2 + 1}{x}$

(b) $k(x) = \dfrac{x^2 + x - 2}{x}$

(e) $Q(x) = \dfrac{4x^2 + 4x - 3}{2x - 5}$

(c) $p(x) = \dfrac{x^2 + 1}{x - 1}$

(f) $K(x) = \dfrac{3x^2 - 12x + 15}{3x + 6}$

B.6. Graph the function $f(x) = \dfrac{x^3 - 2}{x - 1}$ as follows:

(a) Determine the roots, vertical asymptotes, signs, and sign changes as usual.

(b) Divide $x^3 - 2$ by $x - 1$ and use the division algorithm (as in the next to last example in the text) to show that $f(x) = (x^2 + x + 1) + (-1)/(x - 1)$. When $|x|$ is large, $-1/(x - 1)$ is very close to 0 (why?), so that $f(x)$ is very close to $x^2 + x + 1$. Thus the curve $y = x^2 + x + 1$ is an asymptote of the graph of f. (*Note:* $y = x^2 + x + 1$ is a parabola—see box on page 245.)

(c) Plot some points and use parts (a) and (b) to sketch the graph of f.

B.7. Graph these functions. (*Hint:* all have parabolic asymptotes; see Exercise B.6.)

(a) $p(x) = \dfrac{x^3 + 8}{x + 1}$

(c) $f(x) = \dfrac{x^4 - 1}{x^2}$

(b) $q(x) = \dfrac{x^3 - 1}{x - 2}$

(d) $k(x) = \dfrac{(x+1)(x-1)(x+3)}{x + 2}$

B.8. Find the rule of a rational function f which has these properties:
  (i)   the curve $y = x^3 - 8$ is an asymptote of the graph of f.
  (ii) $f(2) = 1$.
  (iii) $x = 1$ is a vertical asymptote of the graph.

C.1. The formula for the gravitational acceleration of an object (relative to the earth) is $g(r) = (4 \cdot 10^{14})/r^2$, where r is the distance of the object from the center of the earth (in meters).
  (a) What is the gravitational acceleration at the earth's surface? [The radius of the earth is approximately $(6.4)(10^6)$ m.]
  (b) Graph the function $g(r)$.
  (c) Does the function $g(r)$ have any roots? Does the gravitational acceleration ever vanish for any value of r? Can you ever "escape the pull of gravity"?

C.2. Graph these functions. [Their graphs are somewhat trickier than those discussed in the text. Some involve peaks and valleys whose existence may not be evident unless you plot many points (or use calculus). Furthermore, you may not be able to find all of the roots of these functions exactly.]
  (a) $k(x) = \dfrac{2x^3 + 1}{x^2 - 1}$
  (c) $f(x) = \dfrac{3x^3 - 11x - 1}{x^2 - 4}$
  (b) $p(x) = \dfrac{(x - 2)(x^2 + 1)}{x^2 - 1}$

Exponential and Logarithmic Functions

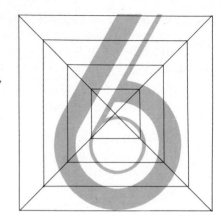

Exponential functions are necessary for the mathematical description of a variety of situations. The exponential function $t(x) = e^x$, which is introduced here, is one of the most important functions for dealing with economic and physical phenomena. The chapter first deals with the technical problem of actually defining the number c^r when the exponent r is *any* real number. Then exponential functions and their characteristic pattern of growth and decay are discussed at length.

Logarithms, which were invented in the seventeenth century as a computational tool, lead to logarithmic functions. These functions are closely related to exponential functions and play an equally important role in applications. In a certain technical sense, explained below, exponential and logarithmic functions are inverses of one another.

Note on Calculators Thus far there have been few opportunities for *efficient* use of calculators. Now, however, we shall deal with functions whose rules are not given by simple algebraic formulas. Evaluating these functions by hand is difficult, except for a few numbers. It will often be necessary to use either tables or calculators. *All the needed tables are provided in this text.* If you do not already have a calculator, there is no need to buy one.

If you *do* have a calculator with appropriate capabilities, you are encouraged to use it. But remember three things:

(i)   A calculator is not a substitute for learning the computational material in this chapter. When computations can be done readily by hand, you will be expected to do them without a calculator.

(ii) In order to use a calculator with maximum efficiency and to interpret certain answers obtained from one, you must have a reasonably complete knowledge of the "theoretical" properties of the functions involved.

(iii) Even with a knowledgeable operator, a calculator often provides rational approximations rather than exactly correct answers. For most practical purposes this restriction causes no difficulty, but you should be aware of it.

1. RATIONAL AND IRRATIONAL EXPONENTS

In this section we shall define the symbol c^r, where c is any positive real number and the exponent r is *any* real number. Although there are some technicalities, most of this section consists simply of *new notation for old ideas*. Most of these "old ideas" were discussed in Section 2 of Chapter 1. You may wish to review that section before reading further.

We know what symbols such as 5^3 or π^{-7} or $(17)^{45}$ or c^9 or c^0 mean. The next step is to extend this exponent notation so that expressions such as $c^{1/2}$ or $c^{9/4}$ or $c^{17/3}$ will have meaning. Our guide for doing this is the basic law of integer exponents: $c^m c^n = c^{m+n}$. We would like this law to remain true when c is a positive real number and m and n are rational numbers. In order for this to happen we should define $c^{1/2}$ in such a way that

$$c^{1/2} c^{1/2} = c^{1/2 + 1/2} = c^1 = c$$

and $c^{1/3}$ so that

$$c^{1/3} c^{1/3} c^{1/3} = c^{1/3 + 1/3 + 1/3} = c^1 = c$$

and so on. In other words, we want

$$(c^{1/2})^2 = c \qquad (c^{1/3})^3 = c \qquad \text{and so on}$$

But for $c \geq 0$ we already know that

$$(\sqrt{c})^2 = c \qquad (\sqrt[3]{c})^3 = c \qquad (\sqrt[4]{c})^4 = c \qquad \text{and so on}$$

Therefore it is reasonable to make the following definition. For any positive number c

$$c^{1/2} \qquad \text{denotes the number} \qquad \sqrt{c}$$
$$c^{1/3} \qquad \text{denotes the number} \qquad \sqrt[3]{c}$$

and in general:

> *For any nonnegative real number c and positive integer k*
> $$c^{1/k} \text{ denotes the number } \sqrt[k]{c}.$$

EXAMPLES $\quad 4^{1/2} = \sqrt{4} = 2; \ 27^{1/3} = \sqrt[3]{27} = 3; \ \left(\dfrac{32}{7}\right)^{1/5} = \sqrt[5]{\dfrac{32}{7}} = \dfrac{\sqrt[5]{32}}{\sqrt[5]{7}} = \dfrac{2}{\sqrt[5]{7}}$

We also want the second law of integer exponents, $(c^m)^n = c^{mn}$, to hold when m and n are *rational*. In particular, since $\dfrac{t}{k} = \left(\dfrac{1}{k}\right)t$ and $\dfrac{t}{k} = t\left(\dfrac{1}{k}\right)$, we want to define $c^{t/k}$ in such a way that

$$c^{t/k} = (c^{1/k})^t = (\sqrt[k]{c})^t \qquad \text{and} \qquad c^{t/k} = (c^t)^{1/k} = \sqrt[k]{c^t}$$

But when c, k, and t are positive, we have

$$(\sqrt[k]{c})^t = \sqrt[k]{c} \cdot \sqrt[k]{c} \cdots \sqrt[k]{c} = \sqrt[k]{c \cdot c \cdots c} = \sqrt[k]{c^t}$$

A similar argument works when t is negative. Therefore for any integers t, k with $k > 0$, and any positive real number c,

$$(\sqrt[k]{c})^t = \sqrt[k]{c^t}$$

It is now reasonable to make this definition:

For every positive real number c *and integers* t *and* k *with* k > 0,

$$c^{t/k} \text{ denotes the number } (\sqrt[k]{c})^t = \sqrt[k]{c^t}$$

EXAMPLES $8^{2/3} = \sqrt[3]{8^2} = \sqrt[3]{64} = 4$ and $(\sqrt{2})^{4/5} = \sqrt[5]{(\sqrt{2})^4}$

$$= \sqrt[5]{(\sqrt{2})^2(\sqrt{2})^2} = \sqrt[5]{4}.$$

EXAMPLE $5^{-2/3} = \sqrt[3]{5^{-2}} = \sqrt[3]{\dfrac{1}{5^2}} = \dfrac{\sqrt[3]{1}}{\sqrt[3]{5^2}} = \dfrac{1}{\sqrt[3]{25}}.$

EXAMPLE   Since every finite decimal is a rational number, expressions such as

$$10^{1.41} \qquad 5^{.3} \qquad \left(\frac{2}{3}\right)^{7.591}$$

now have a meaning. For instance, since $1.41 = 1\dfrac{41}{100} = \dfrac{141}{100}$, we have $10^{1.41} = 10^{141/100} = \sqrt[100]{10^{141}}$. Writing rational exponents in decimal rather than fractional form is especially convenient when using a calculator.

There is a subtle point in the definition of $c^{t/k}$: The same rational number can be expressed many ways. For example,

$$\frac{1}{2} = \frac{2}{4} = \frac{3}{6} = \frac{4}{8} \qquad \frac{2}{3} = \frac{12}{18} = \frac{8}{12} = \frac{10}{15}$$

Consequently, we should verify that if $\dfrac{t}{k} = \dfrac{a}{b}$, then $c^{t/k} = c^{a/b}$. Rather than present a detiled proof, we shall simply illustrate this fact with an example.

EXAMPLE $5^{1/2} = \sqrt{5}$ and $5^{3/6} = \sqrt[6]{5^3} = \sqrt[6]{125} = \sqrt{\sqrt[3]{125}} = \sqrt{5}.$

LAWS OF EXPONENTS

Our definition $c^{t/k} = \sqrt[k]{c^t}$ was motivated by a desire to have the same laws that hold for integer exponents also hold for rational exponents. In making this definition, we guaranteed that some of these exponent laws would hold (such as, $c^{-1}c^1 = 1$ and $(c^{1/k})^k = c$). But we have not yet verified that *all* the exponent laws are valid in *all* possible cases. Because the proofs of these various facts are rather tedious and unenlightening, we shall omit them and simply illustrate each one with some examples.

> If c and d are positive real numbers and r, s are rational numbers, then
>
> (i) $\quad c^r c^s = c^{r+s}$ $\qquad\qquad$ (iv) $\quad (cd)^r = c^r d^r$
>
> (ii) $\quad \dfrac{c^r}{c^s} = c^{r-s}$ $\qquad\qquad$ (v) $\quad \left(\dfrac{c}{d}\right)^r = \dfrac{c^r}{d^r}$
>
> (iii) $\quad (c^r)^s = c^{rs}$ $\qquad\qquad$ (vi) $\quad c^{-r} = \dfrac{1}{c^r}$

EXAMPLE (i) $(8^{2/3})(8^{1/3}) = 8^{(2/3)+(1/3)} = 8^1$ since

$$(8^{2/3})(8^{1/3}) = (\sqrt[3]{8^2})(\sqrt[3]{8}) = (\sqrt[3]{64})(2) = 4 \cdot 2 = 8.$$

Similarly, $(4^{3/2})(4^{-1/2}) = 4^{(3/2)+(-1/2)} = 4^1$ since

$$(4^{3/2})(4^{-1/2}) = \sqrt{4^3}\sqrt{4^{-1}} = \sqrt{64}\sqrt{\frac{1}{4}} = 8 \cdot \frac{1}{2} = 4.$$

EXAMPLE (ii) $\dfrac{3^{-2}}{3^{3/2}} = 3^{-2-(3/2)} = 3^{-7/2}$ since

$$\frac{3^{-2}}{3^{3/2}} = \frac{1/3^2}{\sqrt{3^3}} = \frac{1}{3^2} \cdot \frac{1}{\sqrt{27}} = \frac{1}{9} \cdot \frac{1}{3\sqrt{3}} = \frac{1}{27\sqrt{3}}$$

and

$$3^{-7/2} = \sqrt{3^{-7}} = \sqrt{\frac{1}{3^7}} = \frac{1}{\sqrt{3^6}\sqrt{3}} = \frac{1}{3^3\sqrt{3}} = \frac{1}{27\sqrt{3}}.$$

EXAMPLE (iii) $(4^{3/2})^2 = (\sqrt{4^3})^2 = (\sqrt{64})^2 = 64$ and
$4^{(3/2)2} = 4^3 = 64$, so $(4^{3/2})^2 = 4^{(3/2)2}$.

EXAMPLE (iv) $(8 \cdot 27)^{2/3} = \sqrt[3]{(8 \cdot 27)^2} = \sqrt[3]{8^2 \cdot 27^2} = \sqrt[3]{8^2}\sqrt[3]{27^2} = (8^{2/3})(27^{2/3}).$

EXAMPLE (v) $\left(\dfrac{7}{3}\right)^{1/5} = \sqrt[5]{\dfrac{7}{3}} = \dfrac{\sqrt[5]{7}}{\sqrt[5]{3}} = \dfrac{7^{1/5}}{3^{1/5}}.$

EXAMPLE (vi) $3^{-2/5} = \sqrt[5]{3^{-2}} = \sqrt[5]{\dfrac{1}{3^2}} = \dfrac{\sqrt[5]{1}}{\sqrt[5]{3^2}} = \dfrac{1}{3^{2/5}}.$

The exponent laws listed above can often be used to simplify complicated expressions, as illustrated in the following examples.

EXAMPLE Let k be a positive rational number and express $\sqrt[10]{c^{5k}}\sqrt{(c^{-k})^{1/2}}$ without radicals, using only positive exponents:

$$\sqrt[10]{c^{5k}}\sqrt{(c^{-k})^{1/2}} = (c^{5k})^{1/10}[(c^{-k})^{1/2}]^{1/2} = c^{k/2}c^{-k/4} = c^{2k/4}c^{-k/4} = c^{k/4}$$

EXAMPLE Express $\sqrt[5]{\dfrac{\sqrt[4]{7^3 \cdot x^5}}{\sqrt[3]{7^2 y^4}}}$ without radicals:

$$\sqrt[5]{\frac{\sqrt[4]{7^3 \cdot x^5}}{\sqrt[3]{7^2 \cdot y^4}}} = \left(\frac{(7^3 \cdot x^5)^{1/4}}{(7^2 \cdot y^4)^{1/3}}\right)^{1/5} = \frac{[(7^3 \cdot x^5)^{1/4}]^{1/5}}{[(7^2 y^4)^{1/3}]^{1/5}} = \frac{(7^3 \cdot x^5)^{1/20}}{(7^2 \cdot y^4)^{1/15}} = \frac{7^{3/20} x^{5/20}}{7^{2/15} y^{4/15}}$$

$$= \frac{7^{3/20 - 2/15} x^{1/4}}{y^{4/15}} = \frac{7^{1/60} x^{1/4}}{y^{4/15}}$$

IRRATIONAL EXPONENTS

The expression c^r now has a meaning whenever r is a rational number. Defining c^t when t is an *irrational* number, however, is not so simple. Without resorting to limits and other topics covered in calculus, it is impossible to give a precise definition of c^t. All we can do at this stage is to make it *plausible* that for each positive real number c and each irrational number t, there is a well-defined real number denoted c^t.

The general idea can best be understood in a specific example. Suppose $c = 10$ and we wish to define $10^{\sqrt{2}}$. The key fact is that *every irrational number*, such as $\sqrt{2}$, *has an infinite decimal expansion.*[*] For instance,

$$\sqrt{2} = 1.4142135623 \cdots$$

Consequently, every irrational number may be approximated to any desired degree of accuracy by a suitable finite decimal (that is, a rational number). For instance, there is an infinite list of decimal approximations of $\sqrt{2}$, each more accurate than the preceding:

$$1.4 \qquad 1.41 \qquad 1.414 \qquad 1.4142 \qquad 1.41421 \qquad 1.414213 \qquad \cdots$$

Each of these rational numbers is slightly larger than the preceding one, and *all* of them lie between 1.4 and 1.5.

We know how to raise 10 to each of the rational powers: $10^{1.4} = 10^{14/10}$, $10^{1.41} = 10^{141/100}$, and so on. It seems *reasonable*, therefore, that $10^{\sqrt{2}}$ be defined to be the real number for which the numbers

$$10^{1.4} \qquad 10^{1.41} \qquad 10^{1.414} \qquad 10^{1.4142} \qquad 10^{1.41421} \qquad 10^{1.414213} \qquad \cdots$$

are better and better approximations. Using a calculator, we find that[**]

$$10^{1.4} \approx 25.1189$$
$$10^{1.41} \approx 25.7040$$
$$10^{1.414} \approx 25.9418$$
$$10^{1.4142} \approx 25.9537$$
$$10^{1.41421} \approx 25.9543$$
$$10^{1.414213} \approx 25.9545$$
$$\vdots$$

[*] See pages 13–15 for more details.
[**] $\approx$ means "approximately equal."

It appears that $10^{1.4}$, $10^{1.41}$, and so on are better and better approximations of a specific real number whose infinite decimal expansion begins $25.954 \cdots$. This number is defined to be $10^{\sqrt{2}}$.

A similar procedure can be used to define c^t for any positive real number c and any irrational exponent t. Although a proof is beyond the scope of this book, we shall assume this and also use the fact that:

The exponent laws are valid for *all* real exponents, rational or irrational.

EXERCISES

A.1. Compute (without a calculator):
  (a) $(.001)^{-5/3}$ (c) $(\frac{4}{49})^{-3/2}$ (e) $(1000)^{5/3}$
  (b) $2^{3/2}$ (d) $16^{-5/4}$ (f) $(1,000,000)^{5/6}$

A.2. Express the given number as a power of 2:
  (a) $\sqrt[3]{16}$ (c) $\sqrt[3]{256}$ (e) $\sqrt{32}/(\sqrt[3]{64})$
  (b) $\sqrt[4]{8}$ (d) $\sqrt{8}/(\sqrt[3]{4})$ (f) $\sqrt{1024}/(\sqrt[4]{64})$

A.3. Express without radicals:
  (a) $\sqrt[3]{a^2 + b^2}$ (c) $\sqrt{\sqrt[4]{a^3}}$ (e) $\sqrt[5]{t}\sqrt{16t^5}$
  (b) $\sqrt[4]{a^3 - b^3}$ (d) $\sqrt{\sqrt[3]{a^3b^4}}$ (f) $\sqrt{x}\sqrt[3]{x^2}\sqrt[4]{x^3}$

B.1. Compute and simplify your answer as much as possible. (Assume x and y are positive real numbers).
  (a) $x^{1/2}(x^{2/3} - x^{4/3})$ (d) $(x^{1/3} + y^{1/2})(2x^{1/3} - y^{3/2})$
  (b) $x^{1/2}(3x^{3/2} + 2x^{-1/2})$ (e) $(x + y)^{1/2}[(x + y)^{1/2} - (x + y)]$
  (c) $(x^{1/2} + y^{1/2})(x^{1/2} - y^{1/2})$ (f) $(x^{1/3} + y^{1/3})(x^{2/3} - x^{1/3}y^{1/3} + y^{2/3})$

B.2. Factor these expressions. [For example, $x - x^{1/2} - 2 = (x^{1/2} - 2)(x^{1/2} + 1)$.]
  (a) $x^{2/3} + x^{1/3} - 6$ (d) $x^{1/3} + 7x^{1/6} + 10$
  (b) $x^{2/5} + 11x^{1/5} + 30$ (e) $x^{4/5} - 81$
  (c) $x + 4x^{1/2} + 3$ (f) $x^{2/3} - 6x^{1/3} + 9$

B.3. Simplify the following expressions. (Assume a, b, n, t, x, y are positive rational numbers.)

  (a) $\dfrac{2^{11} \cdot 2^{-7} \cdot 2^{-5}}{2^3 \cdot 2^{-3}}$ (d) $(x^{1/2}y^3)(x^0y^7)^{-2}$ (g) $(a^{x^2})^{1/x}$

  (b) $\sqrt{x^7} \cdot x^{5/2} \cdot x^{-3/2}$ (e) $\dfrac{(7a)^2(5b)^3}{(5a)^3(7b)^4}$ (h) $\dfrac{(x^2y^7)^{-2}}{x^{-3}y^4}$

  (c) $\dfrac{(3^2)^{-1/2}(9^4)^{-1}}{27^{-3}}$ (f) $\sqrt[5]{t} \cdot 16t^4$ (i) $\sqrt[6]{b^{3x}}\sqrt{(b^{-x})^{1/2}}$

B.4. Express without radicals, using only positive exponents:
  (a) $(\sqrt[3]{xy^2})^{-3/5}$ (b) $(\sqrt[4]{r^{14}s^{-21/5}})^{-3/7}$

(c) $\dfrac{c}{(c^{5/6})^{42}(c^{51})^{-2/3}}$

(e) $(c^{5/6} - c^{-5/6})^2$

(d) $\sqrt[5]{\dfrac{(ab^2)^{-10/3}}{(a^2b)^{-15/7}}}$

(f) $(\sqrt{a} + b^{-1/3})^{-2}$

B.5. Use a calculator to find a two-place decimal approximation of each of these numbers. (See also Exercise B.6.)

(a) $\sqrt[5]{176}$

(d) $(\sqrt{6})^{4/5}$

(b) $(\tfrac{3}{2})^{7.56}$

(e) $(\sqrt[3]{17})^{5/7}$

(c) $(\tfrac{2}{3})^{.65}$

(f) $2^{936/125}$

B.6. Use a calculator to find a *six*-place decimal approximation of $(311)^{-4.2}$. Explain why your answer cannot possibly *be* the number $(311)^{-4.2}$. What goes wrong?

B.7. Solve these equations using the methods of Section 4 in Chapter 2:

(a) $(x + 1)^{2/3} = 4$

(c) $(x^2 - 8x + 20)^{1/4} = 2^{3/4}$

(b) $(x^2 + 6x + 9)^{3/2} = 5$

(d) $x^{2/5} + x^{1/5} - 6 = 0$

2. EXPONENTIAL FUNCTIONS

Exponential functions have numerous applications (some of which are discussed below) and will play an important role in calculus. In this section we carefully examine the graphs and general behavior of such functions.

As we saw in Section 1: for every positive real number a and every real number x,

$$a^x \text{ is a well-defined real number}$$

Consequently, for *each* positive real number a, there is a function (called an **exponential function**) whose rule is: $f(x) = a^x$. For example, there are the exponential functions

$$f(x) = 10^x, \qquad g(x) = 2^x, \qquad h(x) = (\tfrac{1}{2})^x, \qquad k(x) = (\tfrac{3}{7})^x, \qquad r(x) = \pi^x$$

GRAPH OF $f(x) = a^x$ WHEN $a > 1$

When $a > 1$, all the various exponential functions $f(x) = a^x$ have similar graphs, as the following examples illustrate.

EXAMPLE Let $a = 10$. In order to sketch the graph of $f(x) = 10^x$, we use a calculator or tables to compute the value of the function at various numbers:

$x =$	-3	-2	-1	$-.5$	0	$.5$	1	1.5	2	2.125	3
$10^x \approx$	$.001$	$.01$	$.1$	$.316$	1	3.16	10	31.6	100	133.4	1000

Next we plot the corresponding points and make a reasonable guess as to the shape of the graph (see Figure 6-1).

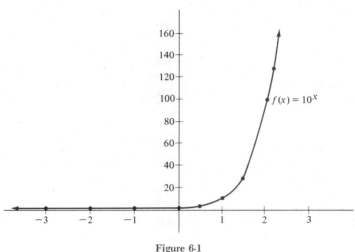

Figure 6-1

EXAMPLE   In order to sketch the graphs of the exponential functions

$$g(x) = (\tfrac{3}{2})^x, \qquad h(x) = 2^x, \qquad k(x) = 3^x$$

we first evaluate the functions at various numbers (using a calculator when necessary).

x	-3	-2	-1	$-.5$	0	$.5$	1	2	2.5	3	4	5
$g(x) = (\tfrac{3}{2})^x$	$\tfrac{8}{27}$	$\tfrac{4}{9}$	$\tfrac{2}{3}$	.82	1	1.22	1.5	2.25	2.76	3.38	5.06	7.59
$h(x) = 2^x$	$\tfrac{1}{8}$	$\tfrac{1}{4}$	$\tfrac{1}{2}$	.71	1	1.41	2	4	5.66	8	16	32
$k(x) = 3^x$	$\tfrac{1}{27}$	$\tfrac{1}{9}$	$\tfrac{1}{3}$	.58	1	1.73	3	9	15.59	27	81	243

Now we plot the points corresponding to the values on the table and sketch the graphs on the same set of coordinate axes (see Figure 6-2 on the next page). For comparison purposes, the graph of $f(x) = 10^x$ from the previous example is also included.

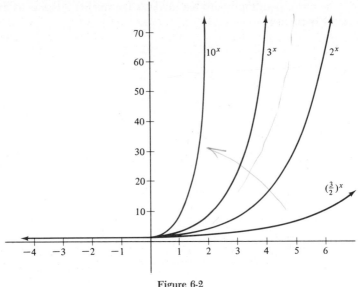

Figure 6-2

Notice that *all of the graphs* in the preceding examples have the same general shape. The principal difference between them is that

> If $b > a > 1$, *then the graph of* $f(x) = b^x$ *rises more steeply than the graph of* $g(x) = a^x$.

For instance, $10 > \frac{3}{2}$ and the graph of $f(x) = 10^x$ rises more steeply than the graph of $g(x) = (\frac{3}{2})^x$. Furthermore, observe that $\frac{3}{2} < 2 < 3$ and the graph of $h(x) = 2^x$ lies *between* the graph of $g(x) = (\frac{3}{2})^x$ and $k(x) = 3^x$. In general,

> If $1 < a < b < c$, *then the graph of* $h(x) = b^x$ *lies between the graph of* $g(x) = a^x$ *and* $k(x) = c^x$.

EXAMPLE There is a certain irrational number that plays an important role in calculus. It is denoted e. The infinite decimal expansion of e begins $e = 2.71828\ldots$.

One example of how the number e arises is given in the DO IT YOURSELF! segment on page 316. The exponential function $t(x) = e^x$ occurs frequently in various applications. Since $2 < e < 3$, we know that the graph of $t(x) = e^x$ lies between the graphs of $h(x) = 2^x$ and $k(x) = 3^x$. Using a calculator, we can sketch a reasonably accurate graph of the function t, as shown in Figure 6-3.

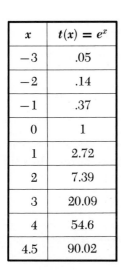

x	$t(x) = e^x$
-3	.05
-2	.14
-1	.37
0	1
1	2.72
2	7.39
3	20.09
4	54.6
4.5	90.02

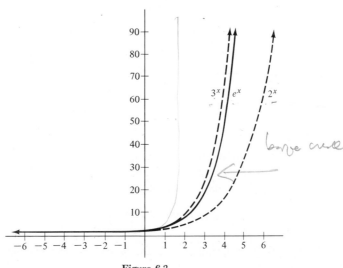

Figure 6-3

GRAPH OF $f(x) = a^x$ WHEN $0 < a < 1$

When $0 < a < 1$, the graph of $f(x) = a^x$ has a different shape, as we now see.

EXAMPLE In order to sketch the graph of $s(x) = (\frac{1}{2})^x$, we use a calculator to determine some values of the function.

x	-5	-4.5	-4	-3.5	-3	-2.5	-2	-1	$-.5$	0	.5	1	2	3
$(\frac{1}{2})^x$	32	22.63	16	11.31	8	5.66	4	2	1.41	1	.707	.5	.25	.125

By plotting the corresponding points, we see that the graph of $s(x) = (\frac{1}{2})^x$ is as shown in Figure 6-4 on the next page. [The graph of $h(x) = 2^x$ is included for comparison purposes.]

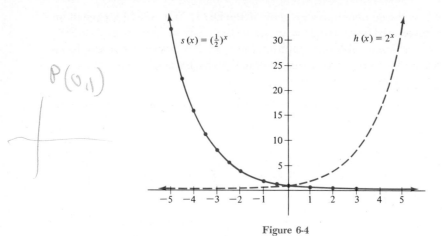

Figure 6-4

If you compare the graph of $h(x) = 2^x$ with the graph of $s(x) = (\frac{1}{2})^x = 1/2^x$, you will see that they are mirror images of each other (with the y-axis as mirror). In a similar manner, the graphs of the exponential functions

$$r(x) = (\tfrac{2}{3})^x = \left(\frac{1}{3/2}\right)^x, \qquad s(x) = (\tfrac{1}{3})^x, \qquad w(x) = (\tfrac{1}{10})^x$$

are just mirror images (in the y-axis) of the graphs of $g(x) = (\frac{3}{2})^x$, $k(x) = 3^x$, and $f(x) = 10^x$, respectively.

Here is a summary of some of the properties illustrated in the preceding examples.

BASIC PROPERTIES OF EXPONENTIAL FUNCTIONS

(*i*) $f(x) = a^x$ *is always positive. The entire graph of* f *lies* above *the x-axis and crosses the y-axis at* $y = 1$.

(*ii*)   *If* a > 1, *then* $f(x) = a^x$ *is an* increasing *function; that is, the graph of* f *is always rising from left to right (see p. 218).*

(*iii*)   *If* $0 < a < 1$, *then* $f(x) = a^x$ *is a* decreasing *function; that is, the graph of* f *is always falling from left to right (see p. 219).*

EXPONENTIAL GROWTH AND DECAY

We have seen that when $a > 1$ and x takes increasing positive values, the corresponding values of the function $f(x) = a^x$ increase sharply. In other words, the graph of $f(x) = a^x$ rises steeply to the right. In order to get an idea of just *how* greatly the values of the function increase, it is instructive to compare the graph of $g(x) = 2^x$, for instance, with the graph of the polynomial function $f(x) = x^4$. The graph of $f(x) = x^4$ on page 276 rises steeply as x takes larger and larger positive values. Indeed, for $0 \leq x \leq 16$ the graph of $f(x) = x^4$ lies considerably *above* the graph of $g(x) = 2^x$. But for larger values of x, the story is quite different, as we see from the following table.

x	16	17	18	19	20	21	22	35
$g(x) = 2^x$	65,536	131,072	262,144	524,288	1,048,576	2,097,152	4,194,304	34,359,738,368
$f(x) = x^4$	65,536	83,521	104,976	130,321	160,000	194,481	234,256	1,500,625

If we choose appropriate scales for the axes and sketch the graphs for $16 \leq x \leq 22$, the difference in steepness becomes dramatically apparent, as shown in Figure 6-5.

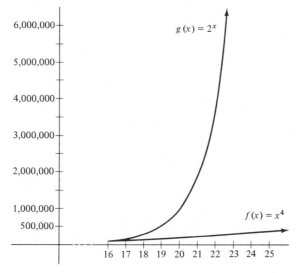

Figure 6-5

If we keep the same scale on the axes and try to extend the graph of $g(x) = 2^x$ just to $x = 50$, we would need a sheet of paper over 6,600 miles long!

The phenomenon of **exponential growth,** as demonstrated by the graph of $f(x) = a^x$ with $a > 1$, is explored further (via real-life examples) in the DO IT YOURSELF! segment at the end of this section. If the preceding discussion has left you wondering about how exponential functions arise in real life and what they *really* mean, you might find the discussion interesting.

When $a < 1$, then the function $f(x) = a^x$ dies out toward 0 as x increases. This phenomenon is sometimes described by the term **exponential decay.** To get an idea of the rate of such decay, it is instructive to compare the exponential function $s(x) = (\frac{1}{2})^x = 1/2^x$ and the rational function $f(x) = 1/x^2$ (with $x > 0$). As x takes larger and larger positive values, both graphs remain positive but die out toward zero. But $s(x) = 1/2^x$ dies out much faster. Using a calculator, we find that

$$\text{if } x = 10, \quad \text{then } \frac{1}{x^2} = .01, \quad \text{but } \frac{1}{2^x} = \frac{1}{1024} < \frac{1}{1000} = .001$$

$$\text{if } x = 100, \quad \text{then } \frac{1}{x^2} = \frac{1}{10^4}, \quad \text{but } \frac{1}{2^x} < \frac{1}{10^{30}}$$

EXERCISES

Note Unless advised otherwise, feel free to use a calculator for any of the computations involved in these problems.

A.1. Find a value of x (with $x > 1$) for which $2^x > x^{10}$.

A.2. Let h and k be the functions given by $h(x) = 2^x$ and $k(x) = 3^x$. Evaluate:
(a) $(h \circ k)(2)$ (c) $(h \circ k)(0)$ (e) $(k \circ h)(-2)$
(b) $(k \circ h)(1)$ (d) $(k \circ h)(-1)$ (f) $(h \circ k)(1)$

A.3. Graph these functions for the given values of x.
(a) $f(x) = 4^x \ (-2 \le x \le 2)$ (d) $k(x) = (\frac{2}{5})^x \ (-3 \le x \le 3)$
(b) $g(x) = 5^x \ (-2 \le x \le 2)$ (e) $f(x) = (1.2)^x \ (-6 \le x \le 12)$
(c) $h(x) = (\frac{3}{4})^x \ (-8 \le x \le 4)$ (f) $g(x) = (.8)^x \ (-10 \le x \le 5)$

A.4. For each of the following functions, compute the difference quotient $\dfrac{f(x + \Delta x) - f(x)}{\Delta x}$. (See Exercises B.7 and B.8 on p. 191.)
(a) $f(x) = 10^x$ (c) $h(x) = 3^{-x}$ (e) $f(x) = 2^x + 2^{-x}$
(b) $g(x) = 2^x$ (d) $k(x) = 5^{x^2}$ (f) $g(x) = 3^x - 3^{-x}$

A.5. For each pair of functions f and g, compute the rule of the product function fg. For example, if $f(x) = e^{2x}$ and $g(x) = e^{-x+2}$, then $(fg)(x) = f(x)g(x) = e^{2x}e^{-x+2} = e^{2x-x+2} = e^{x+2}$.
(a) $f(x) = e^x; \ g(x) = e^{2x+1}$ (c) $f(x) = 5^x + 5^{-x}; \ g(x) = 5^x - 5^{-x}$
(b) $f(x) = e^{x+1}; \ g(x) = e^{-2x-3}$ (d) $f(x) = \dfrac{2^x + 2^{-x}}{2^x - 2^{-x}}; \ g(x) = \dfrac{2^x + 2^{-x}}{2}$

B.1. Observe that $a^{-x} = 1/a^x = (1/a)^x$. Use this fact to graph these functions.
(a) $f(x) = 4^{-x}$ (c) $f(x) = (\frac{4}{3})^{-x}$ (e) $f(x) = (.8)^{-x}$
(b) $f(x) = 5^{-x}$ (d) $f(x) = (\frac{5}{2})^{-x}$ (f) $f(x) = (1.5)^{-x}$

B.2. Carefully graph $h(x) = 2^x$. Then use this graph to graph each of the functions below *without* plotting points. (*Hint:* Section 6 of Chapter 4 should be helpful here.)
(a) $f(x) = 2^x - 5$ (d) $g(x) = 2^{x-1}$ [*Hint:* $h(x - 1) = g(x)$.]
(b) $g(x) = -(2^x)$ (e) $k(x) = 2^{x+2}$
(c) $k(x) = 3(2^x)$ (f) $r(x) = 4(2^{x-5})$

B.3.   Graph each of these functions.

(a) $f(x) = 2^{3x}$ (d) $k(x) = 3^{-2x}$ (g) $f(x) = 2^{3-x^2}$

(b) $g(x) = 3^{x/2}$ (e) $k(x) = 2^{-3x}$ (h) $h(x) = 3^x - 2^x$

(c) $h(x) = 2^{x/3}$ (f) $q(x) = 2^{-x^2}$ (i) $p(x) = 2^x - 2^{-x}$

B.4.   Use your knowledge of the behavior of the function $t(x) = e^x$ (not a calculator) to answer these questions.

(a) When $|x|$ is large and x is positive, is $f(x) = e^x + e^{-x}$ positive or negative? Is $|e^x + e^{-x}|$ large or small?

(b) Answer (a) for the function $g(x) = e^x - e^{-x}$.

B.5.   Use Exercise B.4, together with a calculator to plot a few points, to graph these functions.

(a) $h(x) = \dfrac{e^x + e^{-x}}{2}$ (b) $k(x) = \dfrac{e^x - e^{-x}}{2}$

B.6.   Determine whether each of these functions is even, odd, or neither (see pp. 216 and 225 for definitions).

(a) $f(x) = 10^x$ (c) $h(x) = 3^x + 3^{-x}$ (e) $f(x) = \dfrac{e^x + e^{-x}}{2}$

(b) $g(x) = 2^{-x}$ (d) $k(x) = 5^x - 5^{-x}$ (f) $h(x) = \dfrac{e^x - e^{-x}}{2}$

B.7.   Show graphically that the equation $2^x = x$ has *no* solutions.

B.8.   Oil is piped into a storage tank that already contains some oil in such a way that the volume of the oil in the tank doubles every hour and it takes 15 hr to fill the tank. How long does it take for the tank to become one-fourth full?

B.9.   If you begin with k mg of radium, then the amount $M(t)$ of radium remaining after t years is given by $M(t) = k2^{-t/1600}$. If you begin with 100 mg of radium, how much is left after 800 years? after 1600 years? after 3200 years?

B.10.   Water and salt are continuously added to a tank in such a way that the number of kilograms of salt in the tank at time t min is $200 - 100e^{-t/20}$.

(a) How much salt is in the tank at the beginning (that is, when $t = 0$)?

(b) How much salt is in the tank after 10 min? after 20 min? after 40 min?

B.11.   The number of bacteria in a certain culture at time t is given by the function $B(t) = (5000)3^t$, where the time t is measured in *hours* after 4:00 P.M.

(a) What is the initial number of bacteria at 4:00 P.M. (that is, when $t = 0$)?

(b) What is the number of bacteria at 4:10 P.M.? at 4:30 P.M.? at 5 P.M.? at 5:15 P.M.? at 6:20 P.M.?

C.1.   (a) Find a function $f(x)$ with the property $f(r + s) = f(r)f(s)$ for all real numbers r and s. (*Hint:* think exponential.)

(b) Find a function $g(x)$ with the property $g(2x) = (g(x))^2$ for every real number x.

C.2.   **(a)**   Graph each of the following on the same set of axes for the indicated values of x.

      (i) $g(x) = 2^x$ (ii) $h(x) = (.1)2^x$ (iii) $k(x) = 2^{x/4}$

        $(-5 \le x \le 5)$ $(-8 \le x \le 8)$ $(-20 \le x \le 20)$

Based on your results in part (a), answer the following questions (in which $a > 1$ and x is positive).

    (b)   If c is a fixed real number greater than 1, does $g(x) = a^{cx}$ increase faster or slower than $f(x) = a^x$?

    (c)   If $c < 1$, does $g(x) = a^{cx}$ increase faster or slower than $f(x) = a^x$?

    (d)   Under what circumstances does $h(x) = ka^x$ (k a fixed real number) increase *faster* than $f(x) = a^x$?

    (e)   Suppose $k < 1$ and $c < 1$. How does the growth of $t(x) = ka^{cx}$ compare with that of $f(x) = a^x$?

C.3.   Look back at Section 2 of Chapter 5 where the basic properties of graphs of polynomial functions were listed. Then review the basic properties of the graph of $f(x) = a^x$ discussed in this section. Using these various properties, give an argument to show that for any fixed positive number $a(\neq 1)$, it is *not* possible to find a polynomial function $g(x) = c_n x^n + \cdots + c_1 x + c_0$ such that $a^x = g(x)$ for *all* numbers x. In other words, *no exponential function is a polynomial function.*

C.4.   An eccentric billionaire offers you a job for the month of September. She says that she will pay you 2¢ on the first day, 4¢ on the second day, 8¢ on the third day, and so on, doubling your pay on each successive day.

    (a)   Let $P(x)$ denote your salary in *dollars* on day x. Find the rule of the function P.

    (b)   Would you be better off financially if instead you were paid \$10,000 per day? [*Hint:* consider $P(30)$.]

DO IT YOURSELF!

EXPONENTIAL GROWTH

Thus far we have discussed only the function $f(x) = a^x$. There are many other functions, loosely labeled exponential, which behave similarly. For instance,

$$f(x) = 67a^x, \qquad h(x) = a^{x/10}, \qquad T(x) = (\tfrac{1}{50})3^{x-1}, \qquad S(x) = 15(4^{77x})$$

Such variations on the basic exponential theme occur quite often in real life situations, as the following examples illustrate. We begin with a subject close to all of us these days, *money*.

COMPOUND INTEREST

You are probably familiar with compound interest. You put some money in the bank. At the end of some time period (a year, quarter, month, or day, depending on the bank), the bank pays interest on the amount you deposited. At the end of the next time period, the bank pays interest on the original amount *and* on the interest earned in the first time period (this is what is meant by *compounding* the interest). And so it goes.

Suppose you deposit P dollars at $r\%$ interest. If you leave your money in the bank, then at the end of one time period you will have your original amount, P dollars, *plus* the interest it has earned. The interest earned by P dollars at $r\%$ per time period is just ($r\%$ of P) dollars. As is the usual custom, we think of r as a decimal and just write rP for $r\%$ of P. For instance,

$$5\% \text{ of } P \text{ is } .05P, \qquad 17\% \text{ of } P \text{ is } .17P, \qquad \text{and so on}$$

Therefore after one time period at $r\%$ interest, your P dollars grow to

$$P + rP \text{ dollars} = P(1 + r) \text{ dollars}$$

If you leave this money in the bank for a *second* period, you will then have $P(1 + r)$ dollars *plus* the interest this amount has earned. The interest on $P(1 + r)$ dollars for one period is

$$r\% \text{ of } P(1 + r), \text{ that is, } r[P(1 + r)]$$

Consequently, after two periods at $r\%$ interest, you will have

$$P(1 + r) + r[P(1 + r)] = P(1 + r)[1 + r] = P(1 + r)^2 \text{ dollars}$$

Similarly, at the end of the *third* time period, you will have the amount you started the period with, $P(1 + r)^2$, *plus* the interest on this amount, $r[P(1 + r)^2]$, for a total of

$$P(1 + r)^2 + r[P(1 + r)^2] = P(1 + r)^2[1 + r] = P(1 + r)^3$$

This pattern continues on for each time period, and leads to this conclusion:

THE BASIC FORMULA FOR COMPOUND INTEREST

If P *dollars are invested at* r% *interest per time period, then after* x *time periods, you will have*

$$P(1 + r)^x \text{ dollars}$$

In many banks interest is paid from day of deposit to day of withdrawal, regardless of the time period used for compounding interest, so that this formula is used even when x is not an integer. For instance, if the interest rate is $r\%$ per *year* and you leave your money there for 6 years and 5 months, then $x = 6\frac{5}{12} = \frac{77}{12}$ years, and your total amount is $P(1 + r)^{77/12}$. Hereafter we assume we are dealing with such a bank, so that in the basic formula x is allowed to be any positive real number.

If the interest rate r stays fixed, then $1 + r$ is a constant, as is the original amount P. If we denote $1 + r$ by a, then the basic formula for total amount becomes

$$T = P(1 + r)^x = Pa^x$$

In other words, the total amount T is an *exponential function* of the number of periods x you leave the money in the bank. In functional notation, $T(x) = Pa^x$.

Since $a = 1 + r > 1$, our experience with exponential functions tells us that as x gets larger, $T(x) = Pa^x$ becomes *enormous*. Translated into money, this means that if you leave your money in the bank *long enough* (x is large), you or your descendants will end up *rich* ($T(x) = Pa^x$ is enormous).

EXAMPLE° Suppose the interest rate is 10% per year, and a father invests a thousand dollars on the day his daughter is born. Then $a = 1 + r = 1 + .1 = 1.1$ and the total amount available after x years is given by the function $T(x) = Pa^x = 1000(1.1)^x$. Here are some possible values for x and $T(x)$:

x	10	30	50	65	75	100
$T(x) = 1000(1.1)^x$	$2594	$17,449	$117,391	$490,371	$1,271,895	$13,780,612

Thus the daughter could retire at age 65 with almost *half a million* dollars in the bank, or wait until age 75 and collect over a *million* dollars. If the daughter doesn't touch the money and lives to the ripe old age of 100, then *her* children (and the tax man) will inherit more than *13 million* dollars.

The most common method of paying interest by banks is to pay an *annual rate* of interest *compounded quarterly*, or monthly, or even daily. What this means is explained in the next example.

EXAMPLE Suppose you invest P dollars for 1 year at 5% per year, compounded quarterly. The annual interest rate is .05, so the interest for one quarter ($= \frac{1}{4}$ year) is $\frac{1}{4}$ of the interest for a full year, that is, .05/4. In the basic formula

$$T(x) = P(1 + r)^x$$

the time period is a quarter year, the interest rate r per quarter is .05/4, and the number x of time periods to total 1 year is 4. Hence at the end of a year you will have

$$P\left(1 + \frac{.05}{4}\right)^4 = P(1 + .0125)^4 = P(1.0125)^4 = P(1.05095)$$

whereas at a straight 5% per year you would have only

$$P + .05P = P(1.05)$$

Thus 5% compounded quarterly yields a slightly better return than 5% compounded annually.

As a general rule, the more often your interest is compounded, the better off you are. But there is, alas, a limit to how well you can do, as the following example illustrates.

° In this example and all the ones below, we have used either tables or a calculator to perform the necessary calculations.

EXAMPLE You have \$1 to invest for 1 year. The Exponential Bank offers to pay you 100% interest° per year, compounded n times per year. "But what number is n?" you ask. The banker replies, "Oh, you can pick any value you want for n. Of course, all interest amounts are rounded off to the nearest penny."

Question: can you choose n so large that at the end of the year, your dollar will have grown to some huge amount?

To answer this question we use the basic formula with $P = 1$:

$$T(x) = P(1 + r)^x = (1 + r)^x$$

Since the interest rate is 100% $(= 1.00)$ compounded n times per year, then for a time period of $1/n$ year, the interest rate is $\frac{1}{n}(1.00) = \frac{1}{n}$ and the number of time periods to total 1 year is n. Thus $T(n) = \left(1 + \frac{1}{n}\right)^n$ is the amount \$1 will grow to if 100% interest is compounded n times per year. Let's see what happens for various values of n.

Interest is Compounded	$n =$	$\left(1 + \dfrac{1}{n}\right)^n = $ °°
Annually	1	$(1 + \frac{1}{1})^1 = 2$
Semiannually	2	$(1 + \frac{1}{2})^2 = 2.25$
Quarterly	4	$(1 + \frac{1}{4})^4 \approx 2.4414$
Monthly	12	$(1 + \frac{1}{12})^{12} \approx 2.6130$
Daily	365	$(1 + \frac{1}{365})^{365} \approx 2.71457$
Every 12 hr	$2 \cdot 365 = 730$	$(1 + \frac{1}{730})^{730} \approx 2.71642$
Every 2 hr	$12 \cdot 365 = 4380$	$(1 + \frac{1}{4380})^{4380} \approx 2.71797$
Hourly	$24 \cdot 365 = 8760$	$(1 + \frac{1}{8760})^{8760} \approx 2.718127$
Half-hourly	$2 \cdot 8{,}760 = 17{,}520$	$(1 + \frac{1}{17{,}520})^{17{,}520} \approx 2.718204$
Every 15 min	$2 \cdot 17{,}520 = 35{,}040$	$(1 + \frac{1}{35{,}040})^{35{,}040} \approx 2.718243$
Every minute	$15 \cdot 35{,}040 = 525{,}600$	$(1 + \frac{1}{525{,}600})^{525{,}600} \approx 2.7182792$
Every 30 sec	$2 \cdot 525{,}600 = 1{,}051{,}200$	$(1 + \frac{1}{1{,}051{,}200})^{1{,}051{,}200} \approx 2.7182805$
Every second	$30 \cdot 1{,}051{,}200 = 31{,}536{,}000$	$(1 + \frac{1}{31{,}536{,}000})^{31{,}536{,}000} \approx 2.7182818$

° The number 100 is chosen for computational convenience. Essentially the same point can be made with a more realistic interest rate.

°° The calculations in this table were made on a large computer, using double precision. The results are accurate, except possibly for rounding off in the last digit. A hand calculator is quite likely to compute $(1 + \frac{1}{n})^n$ inaccurately when n is large. (Can you figure out why?)

The bank rounds off all amounts to the nearest penny. Consequently, once n is 730 or larger, the number of times the bank compounds doesn't make any difference. Your investment is worth \$2.72 at the end of the year no matter how big n is

THE NUMBER e

The calculations in the preceding example suggest that as n takes larger and larger values, then the corresponding values of $(1 + 1/n)^n$ get closer and closer to a specific real number, whose decimal expansion begins $2.71828 \cdots$. This is indeed the case, as will be shown in calculus.

The real number $2.71828 \cdots$ is denoted e. It is an irrational number and appears (more or less naturally, as it did here) in several different mathematical contexts. When mathematicians or scientists speak of *the* exponential function, they mean the function $t(x) = e^x$. Its graph was given on page 307.

THE POPULATION EXPLOSION

If we neglect special inhibiting or stimulating factors, a population normally grows at a rate proportional to its size. This means that the ratio

$$\frac{\text{current rate of growth of population}}{\text{current size of population}}$$

is a fixed number at all times. Bacteria colonies grow this way, provided they have a normal environment. The same is true of human populations.

Let $S(t)$ denote the *size* of the population at time t and let k denote the constant ratio of growth rate to size of population. In calculus it is shown that

$$S(t) = ce^{kt}$$

where c is the original population [that is, $S(0)$] and e is the irrational number just introduced. If $k = 1$ and $c = 1$, then the population size at time t is given by the exponential function $S(t) = e^t$, whose graph is on page 307. It increases extremely rapidly, even more rapidly than the function $g(x) = 2^x$ discussed above.

If the constants c and k are small, then $S(t) = ce^{kt}$ grows more slowly than does e^t, as we saw in Exercise C.2 on page 312. But even in such a case, as time goes on (t gets larger), the value of $S(t)$ soon becomes *huge*. This is what the "population explosion" is all about.

RADIOACTIVE DECAY AND RADIOCARBON DATING

The **half-life** of a radioactive element is the time in which a given quantity decays to one-half of its original mass. Denote the mass of the element at time t by $M(t)$. It is shown in calculus that

$$M(t) = k2^{-t/h} = k(\tfrac{1}{2})^{t/h}$$

where h is the half-life and k is the original mass of the element [that is, $k = M(0)$, the mass at starting time $t = 0$].

The radioactive isotope carbon-14 is present in all living organisms. When the organism dies, its carbon-14 begins to decay. Since the half-life of carbon-14 is 5730 years, we have the function

$$M(t) = k2^{-t/5730} = k(\tfrac{1}{2})^{t/5730}$$

This function is used by archaeologists and paleontologists to determine the age of various artifacts and fossils up to 50,000 years old. Here is how they do it.

Suppose you have a sample of some organic matter whose age is to be determined. For instance, the sample might be part of a fossilized tree knocked over by a glacier, or some charcoal from the hearth of some prehistoric family, or an object immersed in lava during a volcanic eruption. In each case time t is measured from the death of the organism, when its carbon-14 began decaying. If the object is 7000 yr old, for example, then the present value of t is 7000. We don't know the present value of t for our sample, but we *can* find the present value of $M(t)$, by measuring the amount of carbon-14 now present in the sample. This is done via radioactive emissions and a Geiger counter.

It is also possible to determine the original amount k of carbon-14 in our sample. The details of this determination need not concern us here. We simply note for the record that they depend on measuring both the carbon-12 and the carbon-14 in a present-day sample of the same material and the fact that the ratio of carbon-14 to carbon-12 is essentially constant over a 50,000-yr period.

Consequently, in the functional relationship for our sample

$$M(t) = k2^{-t/5730}$$

we know both $M(t)$ and k. *If* we can solve the resulting exponential equation for t, then we have the age of the sample.

EXAMPLE The present mass of the carbon-14 in a sample is .5470. Its original mass is determined to have been 1.273. How old is the sample? Substituting $M(t) = .547$ and $k = 1.273$ into the basic decay equation for carbon-14 yields

$$M(t) = k2^{-t/5730}$$
$$.547 = (1.273)2^{-t/5730}$$

As we shall see later in this chapter, this equation can be easily solved. It turns out that $t = 6982.69$. Thus the sample is approximately 6983 years old.

EXERCISES

Note Use a calculator when necessary. Most of these exercises require the use of one of the formulas developed in the text, such as the basic formula for compound interest. In some cases, it may also be necessary to solve exponential equations, such as $(1.12)^x = 2$. The methods for doing this precisely are discussed later in this chapter. For now, just experiment and find an approximate answer. For example, $(1.12)^6 \approx 1.97$ and $(1.12)^{6.2} \approx 2.02$, so the solution of $(1.12)^x = 2$ is approximately $x = 6.1$.

A.1. The half-life of radium is approximately 1660 yr. If the original mass of a sample of radium is 1 gram, how much radium is left after 830 yr?

A.2.   The half-life of a certain element is 1.4 days. If you begin with 2 grams, how much is left after 1 week? after 30 days?

A.3.   If you put $500 in a savings account that pays interest at 5% per year, how much will you have at the end of 10 years if
   (a)   interest is compounded annually?
   (b)   interest is compounded quarterly?
   (c)   interest is compounded twice a day?

B.1.   Bankers have a rule of thumb that tells you *approximately* how many years it will take you to double your money if you leave it in the bank at a fixed interest rate, compounded annually. Find this rule of thumb by using the basic formula for compound interest and some experimentation as follows.
   (a)   Determine how many years (rounded to the nearest year) it takes to double your money at *each* of these interest rates: 3%, 6%, 8%, 10%, 12%, 18%, 24%, and 36%.
   (b)   Compare the answers in (a) to the numbers $\frac{72}{3}$, $\frac{72}{6}$, $\frac{72}{8}$, $\frac{72}{10}$, and so on.

B.2.   At what annual rate of interest should $1000 be invested so that it will double in 10 yr if interest is compounded quarterly?

B.3.   How long does it take $500 to triple if it is invested at 6% compounded annually? compounded quarterly? compounded daily?

B.4.   Any quantity of uranium decays to two-thirds of its original mass in .26 billion yr. Find the half-life of uranium.

3. LOGARITHMS

The invention of logarithms in the seventeenth century was a major advance in the technique of numerical calculation. For over two centuries logarithms were the only effective tool for doing complicated computations in astronomy, chemistry, physics, and other fields. Today, of course, such calculations can be quickly and easily performed by computers or hand calculators.

Despite their decline as computational tools, logarithms still play an important role in mathematics. Several areas of calculus and the sciences require a good understanding of the concept and basic properties of logarithms and logarithmic functions.

COMMON LOGARITHMS

The graph of the function $f(x) = 10^x$, which is shown in Figure 6-6 on the next page, has a crucial geometric property:

> A horizontal straight line that lies above the x-axis
> intersects the graph of $f(x) = 10^x$ at exactly one point

Translated into algebraic terms, this geometric property is just the statement:

> For each positive number v, there is one
> and only one number u such that $10^u = v$

A typical example is shown in Figure 6-6.

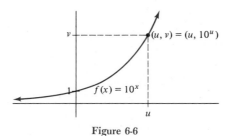

Figure 6-6

The unique u such that $10^u = v$ is called the **logarithm of v to the base 10** (or the **common logarithm** of v) and is denoted by the symbol $\log v$. Thus

> *For each positive number* v, log v *is the unique number such that*
> $10^{\log v} = $ v.

In other words,

$\log v$ is the exponent to which 10 must be raised to produce v

Keep this fact in mind. *A logarithm is just a particular kind of exponent,* so we won't really be saying anything new here. We'll just be restating known facts about exponents in the language and symbolism of logarithms.

EXAMPLE   What is $\log 100$? Answer: $\log 100$ is the exponent to which 10 must be raised to produce 100. Since $10^2 = 100$, we see that $\log 100 = 2$.

EXAMPLE   What is $\log .001$? Answer: $\log .001$ is the exponent to which 10 must be raised to produce .001. But $.001 = \frac{1}{1000} = 1/10^3 = 10^{-3}$, so that $\log .001 = -3$.

EXAMPLE $\log \sqrt{10}$ is the exponent to which 10 must be raised to produce $\sqrt{10}$. Since $\sqrt{10} = 10^{1/2}$, we have $\log \sqrt{10} = \frac{1}{2}$.

Just as in the preceding examples, the logarithm of any power of 10 can be easily found. For any real number k, $\log 10^k$ is the exponent to which 10 must be raised to produce 10^k. Obviously, this exponent is just k itself. Therefore

$$\boxed{log \ 10^k = k \ for \ every \ real \ number \ k.}$$

This fact is true whether k has simple or complicated form. For instance,

$$\log 1 = \log 10^0 = 0 \qquad \text{(here } k = 0\text{)}$$
$$\log 10^{(3-\sqrt{2})} = 3 - \sqrt{2} \qquad \text{(here } k = 3 - \sqrt{2}\text{)}$$
$$\log 10^{2x+1} = 2x + 1 \qquad \text{(here } k = 2x + 1\text{)}$$

Computing $\log v$ when v is not an obvious power of 10 can be quite time-consuming. Fortunately, these computations have already been made for us and are available in various tables of logarithms. (In this context, you can think of a calculator as a pushbutton logarithm table.)

But even without a table, it is possible to make some rough estimates of the logarithms of various number by using our knowledge of the exponential function $f(x) = 10^x$. It's a good idea to be adept at such estimates, since they will warn you of any gross errors that you might make in reading a table or using a calculator.

EXAMPLE   In order to estimate $\log 225$, we first note that $10^2 = 100$ and $10^3 = 1000$. Since 225 lies between 10^2 and 10^3, the exponent to which 10 must be raised to produce 225 (namely, $\log 225$) must be a number between 2 and 3; that is, $2 < \log 225 < 3$. Since 225 is quite a bit closer to $100 = 10^2$ than to $1000 = 10^3$, the exponent $\log 225$ probably lies closer to 2 than to 3. A rough estimate might be that $2 < \log 225 < 2.5$.

EXAMPLE   To estimate $\log(-5)$, you must answer the question: to what exponent must 10 be raised to produce -5? But as we know, *every* power of 10 is *positive* (the graph of 10^x always lies above the x-axis). It is *impossible* to have some power of 10 equal to -5. Therefore $\log(-5)$, or the logarithm of any negative number, is *not defined*.

Since logarithms are just exponents, a table of common logarithms is nothing more than a table of powers of 10. In order to emphasize this fact, the following sample logarithm table is written in both logarithmic and exponential language. (Most logarithm tables assume that you know logarithms are exponents and don't mention exponents.) You can use this table to check the accuracy of our estimate of $\log 225$ in the preceding example.

Logarithmic Statement	Equivalent Exponential Statement	Logarithmic Statement	Equivalent Exponential Statement
$\log 0.1 = -1.$	$10^{-1} = .1$	$\log 45.1 = 1.6542$	$10^{1.6542} = 45.1$
$\log 0.2 = -.6990$	$10^{-.6990} = .2$	$\log 45.2 = 1.6551$	$10^{1.6551} = 45.2$
$\log 0.4 = -.3979$	$10^{-.3979} = .4$	$\log 45.3 = 1.6561$	$10^{1.6561} = 45.3$
$\log 0.6 = -.2218$	$10^{-.2218} = .6$	$\log 45.4 = 1.6571$	$10^{1.6571} = 45.4$
$\log 0.8 = -.0969$	$10^{-.0969} = .8$	$\log 45.5 = 1.6580$	$10^{1.6580} = 45.5$
$\log 1 = 0$	$10^0 = 1$	$\log 220 = 2.3424$	$10^{2.3424} = 220$
$\log 2 = .3010$	$10^{.3010} = 2$	$\log 222.5 = 2.3473$	$10^{2.3473} = 222.5$
$\log 3 = .4771$	$10^{.4771} = 3$	$\log 225 = 2.3522$	$10^{2.3522} = 225$
$\log 4 = .6021$	$10^{.6021} = 4$	$\log 227.5 = 2.3570$	$10^{2.3570} = 227.5$
$\log 5 = .6990$	$10^{.6990} = 5$	$\log 230 = 2.3617$	$10^{2.3617} = 230$

Since most logarithms are actually irrational numbers, most of the entries in this table (as in any logarithm table) are rational number *approximations*. For example, $10^{.6990}$ actually works out to $5.00034535 \cdots$ rather than 5. But for most purposes such approximations are adequate, so it is customary to write $\log 5 = .6990$ and $10^{.6990} = 5$ rather than the more accurate statements $\log 5 \approx .6990$ and $10^{.6990} \approx 5.$° Although a typical calculator computes logarithms to a greater degree of accuracy (for instance, $\log 5 \approx .698970004$), it too provides only rational approximations in most cases.

LOGARITHMS TO OTHER BASES

The definition and discussion of logarithms above depended only on the properties of the exponential function $f(x) = 10^x$. If b is any real number greater than 1, then the exponential function $g(x) = b^x$ has the same basic properties as does $f(x) = 10^x$. Consequently, it is possible to define logarithms in terms of the base b in the same way that logarithms to the base 10 were defined above. We shall do this now, since logarithms to bases other than 10 are often needed.

Let b be a fixed real number with $b > 1$. The graph of the function $g(x) = b^x$ has the same general shape as the graph of $f(x) = 10^x$, as shown in Figure 6-7 on the next page. Furthermore, the function g has the same crucial property:

> For each positive real number v, there is
> one and only one number u such that $b^u = v$

° $\approx$ means "approximately equal."

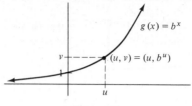

Figure 6-7

The unique number u such that $b^u = v$ is called the **logarithm of v to the base b** and is denoted by the symbol $\log_b v$.° Thus

> *For each positive number v, $\log_b v$ is the unique number such that* $b^{\log_b v} = v$.

In other words,

$\log_b v$ **is the exponent to which b must be raised to produce** v.

EXAMPLE $\log_2 16$ is the exponent to which 2 must be raised in order to produce 16. Since $2^4 = 16$, we see that $\log_2 16 = 4$. Similarly,

$$\log_2 1 = 0 \qquad \text{since } 2^0 = 1$$
$$\log_2 32 = 5 \qquad \text{since } 2^5 = 32$$
$$\log_2(\tfrac{1}{16}) = -4 \qquad \text{since } 2^{-4} = \tfrac{1}{16}$$
$$\log_2 \sqrt{2} = \tfrac{1}{2} \qquad \text{since } 2^{1/2} = \sqrt{2}$$

EXAMPLE Here are some examples of logarithms to various bases. Since logarithms are exponents, each of these logarithmic statements can be translated into a statement in exponential language.

Logarithmic Statement	Equivalent Exponential Statement
$\log_3 81 = 4$	$3^4 = 81$
$\log_4 64 = 3$	$4^3 = 64$
$\log_{125} 5 = \tfrac{1}{3}$	$125^{1/3} = 5$ (since $125^{1/3} = \sqrt[3]{125} = 5$)
$\log_4(\tfrac{1}{16}) = -2$	$4^{-2} = \tfrac{1}{16}$
$\log_8(\tfrac{1}{4}) = -\tfrac{2}{3}$	$8^{-2/3} = \tfrac{1}{4}$ (Verify!)

° If the base b happens to be the number 10, we shall often write $\log v$ as above instead of $\log_{10} v$.

As the preceding examples illustrate, the logarithm of any power of the base b is easily found. For any base b and any real number u, $\log_b(b^u)$ is the exponent to which b must be raised to produce the number b^u. This exponent is just u itself:

$$\log_b(b^u) = u \text{ for every real number } u.$$

NATURAL LOGARITHMS

The irrational number e whose decimal expansion begins $2.71828 \cdots$ was introduced on page 306. Logarithms to the base e are called **natural logarithms** and are frequently used in many scientific contexts. (The reason why this is so will become apparent in calculus.) In some books and on most calculators the natural logarithm of the number v is denoted by the symbol $\ln v$ instead of $\log_e v$. But no matter what notation is used, the basic fact is the same:

$\log_e v$ (or $\ln v$) **is the exponent to which e must be raised to produce** v

Except for obvious cases, such as $\log_e(e^u) = u$, it is necessary to use either tables or a calculator to determine $\log_e v$.

EXAMPLE Find $\log_e 81$. Now $\log_e 81$ is the exponent to which e must be raised to produce 81. Since $e \approx 2.72$ and since $3^4 = 81$, it seems likely that $\log_e 81$ is a number a bit bigger than 4. A calculator shows that $\log_e 81 \approx 4.3944$; that is, $e^{4.3944} \approx 81$.

BASIC PROPERTIES OF LOGARITHMS

Although the following discussion applies equally well to logarithms to any base, the most important cases occur when the base is either 10 or e. So if you want to keep the discussion concrete, just read "10" or "e" whenever you see "b."

Let b be a fixed real number with $b > 1$. The first basic property of logarithms to the base b is just the definition:

$$b^{\log_b v} = v \text{ for every positive real number } v.$$

The second basic property is the fact discussed above:

$$\log_b(b^u) = u \text{ for every real number } u.$$

The remaining properties of logarithms are essentially restatements in logarithmic language of well-known properties of exponents. For instance, the first law of exponents states that $b^m b^n = b^{m+n}$, or in words

The exponent of a product is the sum of the exponents of the factors

Since logarithms are just particular kinds of exponents, this statement translates as

The logarithm of a product is the sum of the logarithms of the factors

We now write this statement in formal symbolic language:

FIRST LAW OF LOGARITHMS

$log_b(vw) = log_b v + log_b w$ *for all positive real numbers* v, w.

PROOF The definition of logarithms (second box on the preceding page) tells us that

$$b^{\log_b v} = v \quad \text{and} \quad b^{\log_b w} = w$$

Therefore by the first law of exponents (with $m = \log_b v$ and $n = \log_b w$),

$$vw = (b^{\log_b v})(b^{\log_b w}) = b^{\log_b v + \log_b w}$$

Thus raising b to the exponent $(\log_b v + \log_b w)$ produces the number vw. But the exponent to which b must be raised to produce vw is precisely $\log_b(vw)$. Therefore

$$\log_b(vw) = \log_b v + \log_b w$$

This completes the proof.

EXAMPLE Suppose $b = 10$. From the table on page 321 we know that $\log_{10} 3 \approx .4771$ and $\log_{10} 4 \approx .6021$. Consequently, by the logarithm property just proved,

$$\log_{10} 12 = \log_{10}(3 \cdot 4) = \log_{10} 3 + \log_{10} 4 \approx .4771 + .6021 = 1.0792$$

Warning Be sure to use the first law of logarithms correctly. Avoid this well-known error: $\log_b 5 + \log_b 9 = \log_b(5 + 9) = \log_b 14$. The correct statement in this situation is $\log_b 5 + \log_b 9 = \log_b(5 \cdot 9) = \log_b 45$.

The second law of exponents—namely, $b^m / b^n = b^{m-n}$—can be roughly stated in words as:

The exponent of the quotient is the difference of the exponents.

If the exponents happen to be logarithms, this statement says:

The logarithm of a quotient is the difference of the logarithms.

In formal and more accurate terminology we have the

SECOND LAW OF LOGARITHMS

$$log_b\left(\frac{v}{w}\right) = log_b v - log_b w \qquad \textit{for all positive real numbers } v, w.$$

PROOF The definition of logarithms states that

$$v = b^{\log_b v} \qquad \text{and} \qquad w = b^{\log_b w}$$

Therefore by the second law of exponents (with $m = \log_b v$ and $n = \log_b w$),

$$\frac{v}{w} = \frac{b^{\log_b v}}{b^{\log_b w}} = b^{\log_b v - \log_b w}$$

Thus if b is raised to the exponent $(\log_b v - \log_b w)$, the result is the number v/w. But the exponent to which b must be raised to produce v/w is precisely $\log_b(v/w)$. Therefore

$$\log_b\left(\frac{v}{w}\right) = \log_b v - \log_b w$$

and the proof is complete.

EXAMPLE Using the table on page 321 we see that

$$\log_{10}\left(\frac{230}{45.3}\right) = \log_{10}230 - \log_{10}45.3 \approx 2.3617 - 1.6561 = .7056$$

EXAMPLE $\log_e\left(\frac{17}{44}\right) = \log_e 17 - \log_e 44.$

Warning Do not confuse $\log_b(v/w)$ with $\log_b v/\log_b w$. They are *different* numbers. For instance,

$$\log_{10}\left(\frac{1000}{100}\right) = \log_{10}10 = 1 \qquad \text{but} \qquad \frac{\log_{10}1000}{\log_{10}100} = \frac{3}{2}$$

Consequently, statements such as these are *false:*

$$\frac{\log_2 32}{\log_2 4} = \log_2\left(\frac{32}{4}\right) \qquad \text{and} \qquad \frac{\log_2 32}{\log_2 4} = \log_2 32 - \log_2 4$$

The third law of exponents—namely, $(b^m)^n = b^{mn}$—is rather awkward to state in words, but it too can be translated into logarithmic language:

THIRD LAW OF LOGARITHMS

$log_b(v^k) = k(log_b v)$ *for all real numbers* k *and* v *with* v > 0.

PROOF Since $v = b^{\log_b v}$ by the definition of logarithms, the third law of exponents (with $m = \log_b v$ and $n = k$) shows that

$$v^k = (b^{\log_b v})^k = b^{(\log_b v)k} = b^{k(\log_b v)}$$

Thus raising b to the exponent $k(\log_b v)$ produces the number v^k. But the exponent to which b must be raised to produce v^k is precisely the number $\log_b(v^k)$. Therefore $\log_b(v^k) = k(\log_b v)$, and the proof is complete.

EXAMPLE Is 5^9 larger than 1 million? Using the table on page 321 we see that

$$\log_{10} 5^9 = 9(\log_{10} 5) \approx 9(.6990) = 6.291$$

So that $10^{6.291} \approx 5^9$. Since $10^{6.291} > 10^6$ and $10^6 = 1,000,000$, we see that 5^9 must be larger than 1,000,000.

EXAMPLE What is $\log_{10} \sqrt{5}$? Using the table on page 321 and the fact that $\sqrt{5} = 5^{1/2}$ we have

$$\log_{10} \sqrt{5} = \log_{10}(5^{1/2}) = \tfrac{1}{2}(\log_{10} 5) \approx \tfrac{1}{2}(.6990) = .3495$$

that is, $10^{.3495} \approx \sqrt{5}$. Observe that this answer is consistent with our intuition, since $\sqrt{5}$ is a number slightly larger than 2 and the table shows that $2 = 10^{.3010}$.

EXAMPLE For any base b and positive number v we have

$$\log_b\left(\frac{1}{v}\right) = \log_b(v^{-1}) = (-1)(\log_b v) = -\log_b v$$

For instance, we saw above that $\log_e 81 \approx 4.3944$. Therefore $\log_e(\tfrac{1}{81}) \approx -4.3944$.

EXAMPLE $\log \sqrt[5]{(\tfrac{7}{39})^4} = \log(\tfrac{7}{39})^{4/5} = \tfrac{4}{5}(\log \tfrac{7}{39})$
$$= \tfrac{4}{5}(\log 7 - \log 39) = \tfrac{4}{5}\log 7 - \tfrac{4}{5}\log 39.$$

THE RELATIONSHIP OF LOGARITHMS TO DIFFERENT BASES

A given positive number has many different logarithms, depending on the base that is used. For example,

$$\log_{10} 220, \quad \log_e 220, \quad \log_4 220, \quad \log_{75} 220$$

are four different numbers. We can use the table on page 321 to find the approximation

$log_{10}220 \approx 2.3424$ and a calculator to find the approximation $log_e 220 \approx 5.3936$. Just how are these two numbers related? And how do you find $log_4 220$ and $log_{75}220$? Surprisingly enough, the answer to both these questions is quite easy. The logarithm to any base b of a given number w can be found directly from its base 10 logarithm by this formula:

$$\text{If } b > 1, \text{ then for any positive number } w,$$
$$log_b w = \frac{log_{10}w}{log_{10}b} = \left(\frac{1}{log_{10}b}\right) log_{10}w$$

We shall prove this statement. But first, you should note carefully what it says. For a fixed base b, the number $1/log_{10}b$ is a *constant*. The statement in the box says that $log_b w$ *can be obtained from* $log_{10}w$ *simply by multiplying by this constant*. In other words, logarithms to the base b are proportional to logarithms to base 10. Once you have an accurate table of logarithms to base 10, you can find logarithms to any base.

EXAMPLE   In order to find logarithms to the base e (remember $e \approx 2.71828 \cdots$), we use the formula in the box above with $b = e$ and the fact that $log_{10}e \approx .4343$. Then the constant multiplier is the number

$$\frac{1}{log_{10}b} = \frac{1}{log_{10}e} \approx \frac{1}{.4343} \approx 2.3026°$$

Using the table of common logarithms on page 321 we have

Number w	$log_{10}w$	(Multiply by $\dfrac{1}{log_{10}e} \approx 2.3026$) $\longrightarrow log_e w$
3	.4771	$(.4771)(2.3026) \approx 1.0986$
45.2	1.6551	$(1.6551)(2.3026) \approx 3.8110$
220	2.3424	$(2.3424)(2.3026) \approx 5.3936$

Now that its meaning is clear, here is a proof of the statement in the preceding box. For any base b and positive number w, we have $b^{log_b w} = w$. If we rewrite the number b as a power of 10, namely, $b = 10^{log_{10}b}$, then the preceding equation becomes

$$(10^{log_{10}b})^{log_b w} = w$$
$$10^{(log_{10}b)(log_b w)} = w$$

Thus if 10 is raised to the exponent $(log_{10}b)(log_b w)$, the result is the number w. But the exponent to which 10 must be raised to produce w is precisely the number $log_{10}w$. Therefore

$$(log_{10}b)(log_b w) = log_{10}w$$

° All logarithms and other numbers have been rounded off to four decimal places, so all results are approximate.

Dividing both sides of this equation by the nonzero number $\log_{10}b$ yields

$$\log_b w = \frac{\log_{10}w}{\log_{10}b} = \left(\frac{1}{\log_{10}b}\right)\log_{10}w$$

which is what we wanted to prove.

LOGARITHMIC EQUATIONS

The various properties of logarithms can be used to solve equations involving logarithms, as illustrated in the following examples.

EXAMPLE   Here is a step-by-step solution of the equation

$$\log(x - 15) = 2 - \log x$$

$$\log(x - 15) + \log x = 2 \qquad \text{(add } \log x \text{ to both sides)}$$

$$\log(x - 15)x = 2 \qquad \text{(first law of logarithms)}$$

$$\log(x^2 - 15x) = 2 \qquad \text{(multiply out left side)}$$

This last equation states that the exponent to which 10 must be raised in order to produce the number $x^2 - 15x$ is 2, that is,

$$x^2 - 15x = 10^2$$

$$x^2 - 15x - 100 = 0 \qquad \text{(subtract } 10^2 = 100 \text{ from both sides)}$$

$$(x - 20)(x + 5) = 0 \qquad \text{(factor left side)}$$

$$x - 20 = 0 \qquad \text{or} \qquad x + 5 = 0$$
$$x = 20 \qquad\qquad\qquad x = -5$$

Therefore the only *possible* solutions of the original equations are $x = 20$ and $x = -5$. We now must check to see if either of these numbers actually *is* a solution. To do this it is convenient to write the original equation in the equivalent form

$$\log(x - 15) + \log x = 2$$

Substituting $x = 20$ in the left side of this equation and using the first law of logarithms yields:

$$\log(20 - 15) + \log 20 = \log 5 + \log 20 = \log(5 \cdot 20) = \log 100 = 2$$

Therefore $x = 20$ is a solution. However, substitution of $x = -5$ in the equation yields

$$\log(-5 - 15) + \log(-5) = 2$$

This is impossible since logarithms of negative numbers are not defined. Therefore $x = -5$ is *not* a solution.

EXAMPLE   In order to solve the equation

$$\log_3(x + 3) - \log_3(x - 5) = 2$$

we apply the second law of logarithms to obtain:

$$\log_3\left(\frac{x + 3}{x - 5}\right) = 2$$

This equation states that the exponent to which 3 must be raised to produce the number $(x + 3)/(x - 5)$ is the number 2, that is,

$$\frac{x + 3}{x - 5} = 3^2$$

$$\frac{x + 3}{x - 5} - 9 = 0 \qquad \text{(subtract 9 from both sides)}$$

$$\frac{(x + 3) - 9(x - 5)}{x - 5} = 0 \qquad \text{(put left side over common denominator)}$$

$$\frac{-8x + 48}{x - 5} = 0 \qquad \text{(simplify left side)}$$

Since the only way that a fraction can be zero is to have its denominator nonzero and its numerator zero, we must have $x \neq 5$ and

$$-8x + 48 = 0$$
$$-8x = -48$$
$$x = 6$$

We can check whether or not $x = 6$ actually is a solution by substituting it in the original equation:

$$\log_3(6 + 3) - \log_3(6 - 5) = \log_3 9 - \log_3 1 = 2 - 0 = 2$$

Therefore $x = 6$ checks and is the solution of the equation.

EXERCISES

A.1.   Find the common (base 10) logarithm of:

(a)   10,000

(c)   1,000,000

(e) $\sqrt[3]{.01}$

(g) $\dfrac{10^5}{.01}$

(b)   .001

(d)   .01

(f) $\sqrt[5]{1000}$

(h) $\dfrac{\sqrt{10}}{1000}$

A.2.   Find the logarithm to base 2 of:

(a)   16

(c) $\dfrac{1}{2\sqrt{2}}$

(e) $\frac{1}{64}$

(g) $\frac{1}{256}$

(b) $\sqrt[3]{256}$

(d)   128

(f) $\dfrac{1}{(\sqrt[3]{2})^5}$

(h)   4096

A.3. Translate each of these exponential statements into an equivalent logarithmic statement:

(a) $10^{-2} = .01$ (d) $10^{.4771} \approx 3$ (g) $10^{7k} = r$

(b) $10^3 = 1000$ (e) $10^{1.4367} \approx 27.3$ (h) $10^{(a+b)} = c$

(c) $\sqrt[3]{10} = 10^{1/3}$ (f) $10^{3.9488} \approx 8888$ (i) $10^{x^2+2} = y$

A.4. Translate each of these exponential statements into an equivalent logarithmic statement:

(a) $5^4 = 625$ (d) $3^{-2} = \frac{1}{9}$ (g) $e^{-4} \approx .0183$

(b) $7^8 = 5{,}764{,}801$ (e) $b^{14} = 3379$ (h) $e^{12/7} \approx 5.553$

(c) $2^{-3} = \frac{1}{8}$ (f) $e^{3.25} \approx 25.79$ (i) $a^{-b} = c$

A.5. Translate each of these logarithmic statements into an equivalent exponential statement (remember $\log v$ means $\log_{10} v$):

(a) $\log 10{,}000 = 4$ (d) $\log 500 \approx 2.699$ (g) $\log a = b$

(b) $\log .001 = -3$ (e) $\log (.8) \approx -.097$ (h) $\log (a + c) = d$

(c) $\log 750 \approx 2.86$ (f) $\log (.005) \approx -2.3$ (i) $\log (x^2 + 2y) = z + w$

A.6. Translate each of these logarithmic statements into an equivalent exponential statement:

(a) $\log_2 \sqrt{2} = \frac{1}{2}$ (c) $\log_8(\frac{1}{4}) = -\frac{2}{3}$ (e) $\log_e 3 \approx 1.099$

(b) $\log_5 125 = 3$ (d) $\log_2(\frac{1}{4}) = -2$ (f) $\log_e 10 \approx 2.303$

A.7. Simplify each of these expressions. For example, $\log_e(e^{17,737}) = 17{,}737$.

(a) $\log 10^{\sqrt{43}}$ (d) $\log_{17}(17^{17})$ (g) $\log_{k+1}(k + 1)^{14}$

(b) $\log 10^{\sqrt{49}}$ (e) $\log 10^{\sqrt{x^2+y^2}}$ (h) $10^{\log 57.3}$

(c) $\log_5(5^{4.7})$ (f) $\log_{3.5}(3.5^{(x^2-1)})$ (i) $e^{\log_e 931}$

A.8. Evaluate each of the following. *Examples:* $\log_{\sqrt{2}} 8 = 6$ since $(\sqrt{2})^6 = 8$ and $\log_{27} 9 = \frac{2}{3}$ since $27^{2/3} = \sqrt[3]{27^2} = \sqrt[3]{3^6} = 3^2 = 9$.

(a) $\log (.0001)$ (d) $\log_{16} 4$ (g) $\log_{16} 32$

(b) $\log 100{,}000$ (e) $\log_e \left(\dfrac{1}{e}\right)$ (h) $\log_8 4$

(c) $\log_2 64$ (f) $\log_{\sqrt{3}}(27)$ (i) $\log_{\sqrt{3}}(\frac{1}{9})$

A.9. In each of these statements, replace u, b, or v by a number, so that the resulting statement is true.

(a) $\log_3 81 = u$ (c) $\log_{81} 27 = u$ (e) $\log (10 \sqrt{10}) = u$

(b) $\log_{27} v = \frac{1}{3}$ (d) $\log_5 v = -4$ (f) $\log_b(\frac{1}{9}) = -\frac{2}{3}$

A.10. Suppose b is a fixed number >1 and that $\log_b 2 = .13$, $\log_b 3 = .2$, and $\log_b 5 = .3$. Use the laws of logarithms to calculate each of the following. For example, $\log_b 6 = \log_b(2 \cdot 3) = \log_b 2 + \log_b 3 = .13 + .2 = .33$.

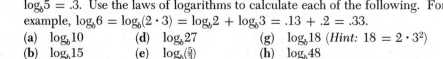

(a) $\log_b 10$ (d) $\log_b 27$ (g) $\log_b 18$ (*Hint:* $18 = 2 \cdot 3^2$)

(b) $\log_b 15$ (e) $\log_b(\frac{5}{3})$ (h) $\log_b 48$

(c) $\log_b 4$ (f) $\log_b(\frac{3}{2})$ (i) $\log_b 45$

A.11. Use the laws of logarithms to express each of the following as a single logarithm. For example, $\log x + 2(\log y) = \log x + \log y^2 = \log (xy^2)$.

(a) $\log_e x^2 + 3 \log_e y$

(b) $\log 2x + 2(\log x) - \log 3y$

(c) $\log_e(x^2 - 9) - \log_e(x + 3)$

(d) $\log_e 3x - 2(\log_e x - \log_e(2 + y))$

(e) $2(\log_e x) - 3(\log_e x^2 + \log_e x)$

(f) $\log_e \left(\dfrac{e}{\sqrt{x}} \right) - \log_e \sqrt{ex}$

A.12. If $\log_b 12 = 7.4$ and $\log_b 8.86 = 19.61$, then what is $\log_b 8.86 / \log_b 12$?

B.1. Use the following approximations and the table on page 321 to find the logarithms below.

$$\log_{10}(\tfrac{14}{3}) \approx \tfrac{2}{3}, \qquad \log_{10}(18) \approx 1.25, \qquad \log_{10}(317) \approx 2.5, \qquad \log_{10}(465) \approx \tfrac{8}{3}$$

(a) $\log_{317}(.8)$

(b) $\log_{18}(.2)$

(c) $\log_{14/3}(.4)$

(d) $\log_{465}(3)$

(e) $\log_{18}(45.1)$

(f) $\log_{14/3}(225)$

(g) $\log_{465}(220)$

(h) $\log_{317}(5)$

(i) $\log_{18}(230)$

B.2. Answer true or false, and give reasons for your answers. Assume all letters represent positive numbers.

(a) $\log_b \left(\dfrac{r}{5} \right) = \log_b r - \log_b 5$

(b) $\dfrac{\log_b a}{\log_b c} = \log_b \left(\dfrac{a}{c} \right)$

(c) $\dfrac{\log_b r}{t} = \log_b(r)^{1/t}$

(d) $\log_b(cd) = \log_b c + \log_b d$

(e) $\log_5(5x) = 5(\log_5 x)$

(f) $\log_b(ab)^t = t \log_b a + t$

(g) $\dfrac{\log_e 10}{\log_e 5} = \log_e 2$

(h) $\log_e(r^e) = r$

B.3. Suppose $\log_b x = 3$. What is $\log_{1/b} x$?

B.4. Solve these equations.

(a) $\log x + \log (x - 3) = 1$

(b) $\log (x - 1) + \log (x + 2) = 1$

(c) $\log_5(x + 3) = 1 - \log_5(x - 1)$

(d) $\log_4(x - 5) = 2 - \log_4(x + 1)$

(e) $\log (x + 9) - \log x = 1$

(f) $\log (2x + 1) = 1 + \log (x - 2)$

(g) $\log (x + 1) + \log (x - 1) = -2$

(h) $\log x = \log (x + 3) - 1$

B.5. Solve these equations.

(a) $\log \sqrt{x^2 - 1} = 2$

(b) $\log \sqrt[3]{x^2 + 21x} = \tfrac{2}{3}$

(c) $\log (x + 2) - \log (4x + 3) = \log \left(\dfrac{1}{x} \right)$

(d) $\log (x + 1) = \tfrac{1}{2} + \log x$

(e) $\log (x^2 + 1) - \log (x - 1) = 1 + \log (x + 1)$

(f) $\dfrac{\log (x + 1)}{\log (x - 1)} = 2$

B.6.   Solve these equations.

(a) $(\log x)^2 = \log x^2$ [*Hint:* let $u = \log x$; then $\log x^2 = 2(\log x) = 2u$, so that the equation becomes $u^2 = 2u$. Solve for u; then find x.]

(b) $\log x^4 = (\log x)^3$ (d) $(\log x)^2 - \log x^5 = -6$

(c) $(\log x)^2 - \log x^2 = 3$ (e) $(\log_5 x)^2 = 5 + \log_5 x^4$

B.7.   Suppose $b > 1$ and that x and v are positive numbers such that $\log_b x = \frac{1}{2}\log_b v + 3$. Show that $x = (b^3)\sqrt{v}$.

B.8.   In chemistry, the concentration of hydrogen ions in a given substance is denoted [H$^+$] and is measured in moles per liter. The pH of the substance is defined to be the number

$$pH = -\log_{10}[H^+]$$

For example, for bananas [H$^+$] is 3×10^{-5} moles/liter, so that pH $= -\log(3 \times 10^{-5}) = -(\log 3 + \log 10^{-5}) = -((\log 3) - 5) = -\log 3 + 5 \approx -.4771 + 5 = 4.5229$. For each substance listed below, the value of [H$^+$] is given. Use the logarithm table on page 321 and the logarithm laws to determine the corresponding pH.

(a)   beer, [H$^+$] $= .8 \times 10^{-4}$ (d)   beets, [H$^+$] $= .4 \times 10^{-5}$

(b)   wine, [H$^+$] $= 4 \times 10^{-4}$ (e)   wheat flour, [H$^+$] $= 2 \times 10^{-6}$

(c)   hominy, [H$^+$] $= 5 \times 10^{-8}$

B.9.   Which is larger: 97^{98} or 98^{97}? [*Hint:* log 97 ≈ 1.9868 and log 98 ≈ 1.9912 and $f(x) = 10^x$ is an increasing function.]

DO IT YOURSELF!

LOGARITHM TABLES

Throughout this discussion *we deal only with common logarithms (base 10).* Obviously, there can't be a table listing the logarithm of *every* real number. A typical logarithm table (such as the one at the end of this book) lists the logarithms of all two-place decimals from 1 to 10 (that is, 1, 1.01, 1.02, 1.03, . . . , 9.97, 9.98. 9.99, 10). Since the logarithm of a decimal need not be a rational number, the entries in a logarithm table are decimal approximations of the actual logarithms. In the table in this book all logarithms are approximated to four decimal places.

LOGARITHMS OF NUMBERS BETWEEN 1 AND 10

For convenience, we reproduce here a portion of the logarithm table at the back of the book. It will be used in the next eleven examples.

x	0	1	2	3	4	5....
5.5	.7404	.7412	.7419	.7427	.7435	.7443 ...
5.6	.7482	.7490	.7497	.7505	.7513	.7520 ...
5.7	.7559	.7556	.7574	.7582	.7589	.7597 ...
.						
.						
.			.			

EXAMPLE In order to find the logarithm of 5.63, we first look in the *left*-hand column for the first two digits of our number, namely, 5.6. Now on the same line as 5.6 we look at the entry in the column labeled 3; it is .7505. So the logarithm of 5.63 is approximately .7505.

EXAMPLE To find the logarithm of 5.7 = 5.70, look in the first column for 5.7 and then across the same line to the entry in the column labeled 0. It is .7559, so $\log 5.7 \approx .7559$.

INTERPOLATION

When the number whose logarithm is wanted does not appear in the table, we must do some approximating.

EXAMPLE We cannot find log 5.527 immediately since our table does *not* include 5.527. However, the table does include 5.52 = 5.520 and 5.53 = 5.530 and

$$5.520 < 5.527 < 5.530$$

Since 27 lies $\frac{7}{10}$ of the way from 20 to 30, we see that 5.527 lies $\frac{7}{10}$ of the way from 5.520 to 5.530. Therefore it seems reasonable that log 5.527 lies approximately $\frac{7}{10}$ of the way from log 5.520 to log 5.530. Using the table, we find that

$$\log 5.530 = \log 5.53 \approx .7427$$
$$\text{difference } .0008$$
$$\log 5.520 = \log 5.52 \approx .7419$$

Therefore log 5.527 lies $\frac{7}{10}$ of the way between .7419 and .7427. The distance from .7419 to .7427 is .0008 and $\frac{7}{10}$ of this distance is $(.7)(.0008) = .00056$. Since we are using four-place logarithms, we round off this number to four places: $.00056 \approx .0006$. Then we have:

$$\log 5.527 \approx \log 5.52 + .0006 \approx .7419 + .0006 = .7425$$

The process used to find log 5.527 in the preceding example is called **linear interpolation**. Due to the approximating involved there may be a slight error in the results. But for most purposes this error is insignificant. The entire process will be justified (in a more general setting) in calculus and the size of the possible error will be discussed.

EXAMPLE In order to find log 5.732 we first find log 5.73 and log 5.74 in the table:

$$\log 5.74 \approx .7589$$
$$\text{difference } .0007$$
$$\log 5.73 \approx .7582$$

Since 5.732 lies $\frac{2}{10}$ of the way between $5.73 = 5.730$ and $5.74 = 5.740$, it seems likely that log 5.732 lies $\frac{2}{10}$ of the way from $\log 5.73 = .7582$ to $\log 5.74 = .7589$. The distance from .7582 to .7589 is .0007 and $\frac{2}{10}(.0007) = .2(.0007) = .00014$. Rounding this number to four decimal places gives .0001, so that

$$\log 5.732 \approx \log 5.73 + .0001 \approx .7582 + .0001 = .7583$$

LOGARITHMS OF OTHER NUMBERS

Once you know how to find logarithms of numbers from 1 to 10, it is easy to find the logarithm of any positive real number. The key is to write the number in scientific notation. (Scientific notation was explained on page 18.)

EXAMPLE In order to find the logarithm of 573.2, we note that

$$573.2 = 5.732 \times 10^2$$

Consequently,

$$\log 573.2 = \log (10^2 \cdot 5.732) = \log 10^2 + \log 5.732$$

But $\log 10^2 = 2$ and 5.732 is a number between 1 and 10. Use the tables to find log 5.732. We actually did this in the preceding example and found that $\log 5.732 \approx .7583$. Therefore

$$\log 573.2 = \log 10^2 + \log 5.732 \approx 2 + .7583 = 2.7583$$

EXAMPLE   In order to find log .00563, we write .00563 in scientific notation:

$$.00563 = 5.63 \times .001 = 5.63 \times 10^{-3}$$

Consequently,

$$\log .00563 = \log (10^{-3} \cdot 5.63) = \log 10^{-3} + \log 5.63$$

We know that $\log 10^{-3} = -3$. Using the tables in the first example above, we found that $\log 5.63 \approx .7505$. Therefore,

$$\log .00563 = \log 10^{-3} + \log 5.63 \approx -3 + .7505$$

   Warning   Be careful here: $-3 + .7505$ is *not* the number -3.7505. If you do your arithmetic carefully, you see that $-3 + .7505 = -2.2495$. However, we shall soon see that for purposes of computation, it will be more convenient to write $\log .00563 \approx -3 + .7505$ rather than -2.2495.

   The preceding examples show that

> **The logarithm of any positive number can always be approximated by the sum of an integer and a number between 0 and 1**

For instance, $\log 5.75 \approx .7597 = 0 + .7597$ and $\log 573.2 \approx 2.7583 = 2 + .7583$ and $\log .000563 \approx -3 + .7505$. A logarithm written in this way is said to be in **standard form**. The integer part of a logarithm in standard form is called the **characteristic**. The decimal fraction part of a logarithm in standard form (that is, the number between 0 and 1) is called the **mantissa**.

ANTILOGARITHMS

We now know how to find the logarithm of a given number. Equally important is the ability to reverse this process:

> Given a logarithm, find the number which has this logarithm

The number whose logarithm is u is called the **antilogarithm** of u, so what we are dealing with here is just the problem: given a number u, find the antilogarithm of u.
   Finding antilogarithms is quite simple, in theory. You just use the basic property of logarithms discussed on page 320.

> $\log 10^u = u$ for every real number u

This property is just another way of saying that the number whose logarithm is u is precisely 10^u, that is,

> The antilogarithm of u is 10^u

The practical problem of determining the antilogarithm of u (that is, computing 10^u) is easily handled if you have a calculator equipped with either a 10^x or a y^x key. Antilogarithms can be found without a calculator by using the logarithm tables "in reverse," as illustrated in the following examples.

EXAMPLE The antilogarithm of .7435 is the number y such that $\log y = .7435$. In order to find y, look through the logarithm table until you find the entry .7435. As shown on page 333, this entry lies on the same line as 5.5 (left column) and in the column labeled 4 at the top. This means that $\log 5.54 \approx .7435$, so that $y \approx 5.54$. Thus the antilogarithm of .7435 is 5.54. But we already know that the antilogarithm of any number u is 10^u. So what we have also shown here is that

$$5.54 \approx \text{antilogarithm of } .7435 = 10^{.7435}$$

EXAMPLE Suppose $\log y = .7495$. In order to find y (that is, the antilogarithm of .7495), we look through the logarithm table for the entry .7495. But it isn't there. The entries closest in value to .7495 are .7490 and .7497. Reading from the table on page 333 we see that

$$\log 5.62 \approx .7497$$
$$\log 5.61 \approx .7490$$
$$\text{difference } .0007$$

Since .7495 lies $\frac{5}{7}$ of the way from .7490 to .7497, it seems reasonable that the number y with $\log y = .7495$ lies $\frac{5}{7}$ of the way from 5.61 to 5.62. Since the distance from 5.61 to 5.62 is .01, and since $\frac{5}{7} \approx .7143$, the distance from 5.61 to the number y is approximately

$$\tfrac{5}{7}(.01) = (.7143)(.01) = .007143$$

Rounding this number to four decimal places gives .0071, so that

$$y \approx 5.61 + .0071 = 5.6171$$

Therefore 5.6171 is the antilogarithm of .7495. Since 10^u is known to be the antilogarithm of u, we can now conclude that $10^{.7495} \approx 5.6171$.

EXAMPLE As we have seen, all logarithms in the table are numbers between 0 and 1. So the antilogarithm of 2.7435 (that is, the number x with $\log x = 2.7435$) cannot be found directly from the tables. But we know that the antilogarithm of any number u is just 10^u. Therefore the antilogarithm of 2.7435 is just $10^{2.7435}$. Simple arithmetic and the laws of exponents show that

$$10^{2.7435} = 10^{2+.7435} = (10^2)(10^{.7435})$$

Now $10^{.7435}$ is just the antilogarithm of .7435. So once we know this number, we can multiply by $10^2 = 100$ to get the antilogarithm of 2.7435. But .7435 *is* a number between 0 and 1 and we have just seen how to use the tables to find antilogarithms of such numbers. In fact, in an example above we found that

$$10^{.7435} = \text{antilogarithm of } .7435 \approx 5.54$$

Therefore the antilogarithm of 2.7435 is just

$$10^2(\text{antilogarithm of } .7435) \approx 10^2(5.54) = 100(5.54) = 554$$

EXAMPLE   Suppose $\log x = -3.2505$. In order to use the table to find x, it is first necessary to write $\log x = -3.2505$ in standard form (that is, as the sum of an integer and a number between 0 and 1). Be careful—it is *not* true that $-3.2505 = -3 + .2505$. It is true that $-3.2505 = -3 - .2505$, but $-.2505$ does not lie between 0 and 1. Here's how to write -3.2505 in standard form:

$$\log x = -3.2505 = (-4 + 4) - 3.2505 = -4 + (4 - 3.2505) = -4 + .7495$$

Now we can proceed as before. Since the antilogarithm of -3.2505 is known to be $10^{-3.2505}$ and since

$$10^{-3.2505} = 10^{-4+.7495} = (10^{-4})(10^{.7495})$$

we need only find $10^{.7495}$, the antilogarithm of .7495. For once we have this, we just multiply by $10^{-4} = .0001$ to obtain the antilogarithm of $-4 + .7495 = -3.2505$. Since .7495 lies between 0 and 1, this can be done via tables. In fact, it was done in the second example on page 336, where we found that

$$10^{.7495} = \text{antilogarithm of } .7495 \approx 5.6171$$

Therefore the antilogarithm of $-3.2505 = -4 + .7495$ is

$$10^{-4}(\text{antilogarithm of } .7495) \approx (10^{-4})(5.6171) = (.0001)(5.6171) = .00056171$$

Here is a summary of the procedure used in the preceding examples to find antilogarithms.

GIVEN *u*, FIND THE ANTILOGARITHM OF *u* AS FOLLOWS:

   (*i*)   Write u *in standard form, as the sum of an integer* k *and a number* v *between 0 and 1:* u = k + v. (Note: k *may be positive, negative, or zero.*)

   (*ii*) Use the tables (and interpolation, if necessary) to find the antilogarithm of v (that is, the number y with log y = v).

   (*iii*) Then the antilogarithm of u is $(10^k)y$.

COMPUTATIONS WITH LOGARITHMS

Now that you know how to use the tables to find both logarithms and antilogarithms, it is relatively easy to compute with logarithms.

EXAMPLE   Find the product $(24.86)(.01392)(1.787)$. Let x denote this product. Using the First Law of Logarithms, we see that

$$\log x = \log [(24.86)(.01392)(1.787)]$$
$$= \log 24.86 + \log .01392 + \log 1.787$$

We now use the logarithm tables and simple addition to calculate the right-hand side of this equation. Note that all logarithms are written in standard form, as the sum of an integer (characteristic) and a number between 0 and 1 (mantissa). When the characteristic is negative, it is usually written after the mantissa:

$$
\begin{aligned}
\log 24.86 &\approx 1.3955 \\
\log .01392 &\approx .1436 - 2 \\
\underline{\log 1.787} &\approx .2521 \\
\text{sum: } &\approx 1.7912 - 2 = .7912 - 1
\end{aligned}
$$

Therefore the equation becomes:

$$\log x \approx .7912 - 1$$

According to the procedure for finding antilogarithms, we know that $x \approx (10^{-1})y$, where $\log y = .7912$. Using the logarithm tables and interpolation, we find that $y \approx 6.183$. Consequently,

$$x \approx (10^{-1})y \approx (.1)(6.183) = .6183, \text{ that is, } (24.86)(.01392)(1.787) \approx .6183$$

Note that our answer is only carried out to four decimal places, whereas the actual product involves ten decimal places. The missing places in our answer represent part of the relatively small error in our approximation.

EXAMPLE In order to compute $(2.4)^{37.8}$, let $x = (2.4)^{37.8}$. Then by the third law of logarithms

$$\log x = \log [(2.4)^{37.8}] = (37.8)(\log 2.4)$$

The logarithm tables show that $\log 2.4 \approx .3802$, so that

$$\log x = (37.8)(\log 2.4) \approx (37.8)(.3802) = 14.37156 \approx 14.3716$$

The antilogarithm procedure shows that $x \approx (10^{14})y$, where $\log y = .3716$. Using the logarithm tables and interpolation, we find that $y \approx 2.353$, so that

$$x \approx (10^{14})y \approx (10^{14})(2.353), \text{ that is, } (2.4)^{37.8} \approx (10^{14})(2.353)$$

It is worth noting that this last example, unlike the preceding one, cannot be worked out by hand or, for that matter, on many simple calculators. Here is another such example.

EXAMPLE In order to compute $\sqrt[7]{2.4/3780}$, let $x = \sqrt[7]{2.4/3780}$ and use the second and third laws of logarithms:

$$\log x = \log \sqrt[7]{\frac{2.4}{3780}} = \log \left(\frac{2.4}{3780}\right)^{1/7} = \frac{1}{7}\left(\log \frac{2.4}{3780}\right) = \frac{1}{7}(\log 2.4 - \log 3780)$$

The logarithm tables show that $\log 2.4 \approx .3802$ and $\log 3780 \approx 3.5775$ so that

$$\log x = \tfrac{1}{7}(\log 2.4 - \log 3780) \approx \tfrac{1}{7}(.3802 - 3.5775) = \tfrac{1}{7}(-3.1973) \approx -.4568$$

In order to find x, we must write $\log x \approx -.4568$ in standard form:

$$\log x \approx -.4568 = (1 - 1) - .4568 = (1 - .4568) - 1 = .5432 - 1$$

Now the antilogarithm procedure shows that $x \approx (10^{-1})y$, where $\log y = .5432$. Using the logarithm tables and interpolation we find that $y \approx 3.493$. Therefore

$$\sqrt[7]{\frac{2.4}{3780}} = x \approx (10^{-1})y \approx (.1)(3.493) = .3493$$

Note It is customary to write an equal sign ($=$) where we have written an "approximately equal" sign ($\approx$). For instance, $\log 2.4 = .3802$ instead of $\log 2.4 \approx .3802$. Since everyone familiar with logarithms *knows* that the entries given in the tables or by calculators are rational approximations, this inaccuracy causes no difficulty in practice.

EXERCISES

A.1. Use the logarithm table at the end of this book to find the following logarithms. Write each logarithm in standard form and label the characteristic.

(a) $\log(1.01)$ (d) $\log(666)$ (g) $\log(.000915)$
(b) $\log(3.79)$ (e) $\log(7880)$ (h) $\log(.0000327)$
(c) $\log(45.6)$ (f) $\log(.00842)$ (i) $\log(57{,}300{,}000)$

A.2. Use the logarithm table and interpolation to find each of these logarithms. Write each one in standard form.

(a) $\log(2.345)$ (d) $\log(.07171)$ (g) $\log(.7631)$
(b) $\log(34.73)$ (e) $\log(.0008463)$ (h) $\log(492{,}700)$
(c) $\log(467.9)$ (f) $\log(.009752)$ (i) $\log(5{,}324{,}000)$

A.3. Use the logarithm tables to find the antilogarithms of these numbers. Remember to put negative numbers in standard form.

(a) .3464   (c) 1.9528   (e) -1.1791
(b) .6937   (d) $-.6126$ (f) -3.8729

A.4. Use the tables and interpolation to find the antilogarithms of

(a) .8776   (c) 5.2955   (e) -4.2608
(b) 2.3797   (d) -1.1247 (f) -2.2705

A.5. Use tables and interpolation, if necessary, to solve each equation.

(a) $\log x = 2.6415$ (c) $\log x = 1.4735$ (e) $\log z = -1.6328$
(b) $\log y = -2.0357$ (d) $\log x = 3.9196$ (f) $\log y = -.1293$

A.6. Use the logarithm table to approximate the following numbers.

(a) $(256)(.0123)$ (d) $(3.94)^{12}$ (g) $\sqrt{93.7}$

(b) $(493)(3.41)(.0412)$ (e) $(7.25)^8(1.26)^5$ (h) $\dfrac{7.98}{(314)(6.12)}$

(c) $\frac{934}{727}$ (f) $\sqrt[3]{756}$

B.1.   Use the logarithm tables to approximate the following.

(a) $(3.841)(710.2)$ (c) $\dfrac{7.981}{(127.6)(8.054)}$ (e) $\sqrt[9]{\dfrac{413}{(.072)^7}}$

(b) $\dfrac{.7812}{.01204}$ (d) $(32.7)^{14.1}$

4. LOGARITHMIC FUNCTIONS

The concept of logarithm leads to a new family of functions. Since logarithms are just exponents, it isn't surprising that these logarithmic functions are closely related to the exponential functions studied in Section 2. What may be surprising, however, is the fact that a variety of physical and other phenomena can be mathematically described by logarithmic functions. Consequently, logarithmic functions play an important role in calculus and certain other branches of mathematics.

Let b be a fixed real number, greater than 1. Each positive number x has a logarithm to the base b. Let f be the function whose domain is the set of all positive real numbers and whose rule is:

$$f(x) = \log_b x$$

The function f is called a **logarithmic function.**

For each base b there is a different logarithmic function. For instance, corresponding to the bases 10, 2, and e ($\approx 2.71828 \cdots$), we have the three functions whose rules are:

$$g(x) = \log x,^\circ \qquad h(x) = \log_2 x, \qquad f(x) = \log_e x$$

By using an appropriate table or a calculator if necessary, we can compute the value of each of these functions for various positive numbers:

$$g(4) = \log 4 \approx .6021, \qquad h(4) = \log_2 4 = 2,$$
$$g(1000) = \log 1000 = 3, \qquad h(1000) = \log_2 1000 \approx 9.9658,$$
$$g(1) = \log 1 = 0, \qquad h(1) = \log_2 1 = 0,$$
$$f(4) = \log_e 4 \approx 1.3863,$$
$$f(1000) = \log_e 1000 \approx 6.9078,$$
$$f(1) = \log_e 1 = 0$$

Although there is a different logarithm function for each base b, all of these functions are very closely related. As we saw in the last section, logarithms to the base b are just constant multiples of logarithms to the base 10. More specifically,

---

$^\circ$ As usual for base 10, we write $\log x$ instead of $\log_{10} x$.

$$\log_b x = \left(\frac{1}{\log b}\right)(\log x)$$

Consequently,

> The logarithmic function $f(x) = \log_b x$ is a constant multiple of the common logarithm function $g(x) = \log x$. The constant multiplier is $1/\log b$.

For example, if $f(x) = \log_e x$, then

$$f(x) = \left(\frac{1}{\log e}\right)g(x) \approx (2.3026)g(x)$$

since $1/\log e \approx 1/.4343 \approx 2.3026$.

As we saw in the last section, logarithms to any base b satisfy the laws of logarithms. If we translate these laws into functional notation, we see that the logarithmic function $f(x) = \log_b x$ has several interesting algebraic properties:

Logarithm Law	Equivalent Functional Statement
$\log_b(vw) = \log_b v + \log_b w$	$f(vw) = f(v) + f(w)$
$\log_b\left(\dfrac{v}{w}\right) = \log_b v - \log_b w$	$f\left(\dfrac{v}{w}\right) = f(v) - f(w)$
$\log_b(v^k) = k(\log_b v)$	$f(v^k) = k \cdot f(v)$

For example, $f(150) = f(3 \cdot 50) = f(3) + f(50)$ and $f(16) = f(2^4) = 4 \cdot f(2)$.

GRAPHS OF LOGARITHMIC FUNCTIONS

Once we have the graph of the common logarithm function $g(x) = \log x$, the graphs of other logarithmic functions can be easily determined.

EXAMPLE Using the properties of logarithms and the table at the end of the book, we first plot some points on the graph of the function $g(x) = \log x$. It then seems that the graph of g looks like the one in Figure 6-8 on the next page.

x	$g(x) = \log x$
10^{-300}	-300
.001	-3
.01	-2
.1	-1
1	0
3	.48
5	.70
10	1
15	1.18
50	1.70
100	2
1,000	3
100,000	5

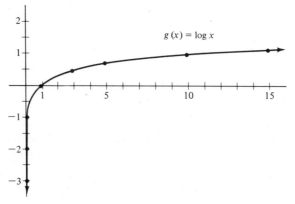

Figure 6-8

Observe that as x moves to the *left* from 1 to 0, the graph falls very sharply and gets closer and closer to the y-axis. The graph never touches the y-axis since the function is not defined when $x = 0$. Thus in the negative direction, the y-axis is a vertical asymptote of the graph. As x moves to the *right* from $x = 1$, the graph continually rises, but extremely slowly. At $x = 100,000$, the height of the graph over the x-axis is only 5 units.

EXAMPLE   One way to graph the logarithmic function $f(x) = \log_e x$ is to plot a number of points. A faster way to graph f is to use the relationship between f and the common logarithm function $g(x) = \log x$ given in the box on page 327:

$f(x)$ is a constant multiple of $g(x)$; specifically,

$$f(x) = \left(\frac{1}{\log e}\right)g(x) \approx (2.3026)g(x)$$

Therefore, as we saw on page 234,° the graph of f is just the graph of g stretched away from the x-axis by a factor of $1/(\log e) \approx 2.3026$ as shown in Figure 6-9.

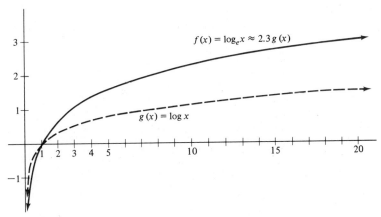

$$f(x) = \log_e x \approx 2.3\, g(x)$$

$$g(x) = \log x$$

Figure 6-9

For any base $b > 1$, the graph of the logarithmic function $f(x) = \log_b x$ may be obtained from the graph of $g(x) = \log x$ as in the preceding example. It will have the same basic shape as the graph of g.

EXAMPLE The term "logarithmic" is often applied to any function whose rule involves logarithms, such as $h(x) = \log (100/x^3 \sqrt{x})$. It is sometimes possible to use the algebraic properties of logarithms to rewrite the rule of such a function and to find its graph.°° We have:

$$h(x) = \log \frac{100}{x^3 \sqrt{x}} = \log 100 - \log (x^3) \sqrt{x} = \log 100 - (\log x^3 + \log \sqrt{x})$$

$$= \log 100 - \log x^3 - \log x^{1/2} = 2 - 3(\log x) - \tfrac{1}{2}(\log x) = 2 - \tfrac{7}{2}(\log x)$$

Now let f be the function given by $f(x) = \log x$. As we saw in Section 6 of Chapter 4, the graph of the function h is just the graph of the function f stretched away from the x-axis by a factor of $\tfrac{7}{2}$, reflected in the x-axis, and moved 2 units upward, as shown in Figure 6-10 on the next page.

° If you have not read this material before, you may prefer to obtain the graph of f by plotting points instead.
°° If you have not read Section 6 of Chapter 4, you may wish to omit this example.

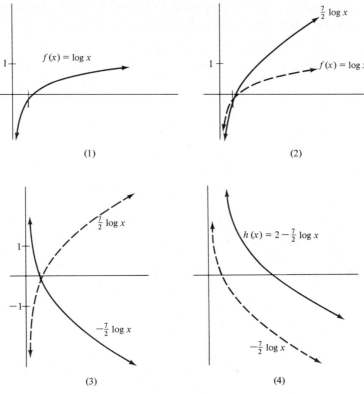

Figure 6-10

Warning   Since the logarithm laws deal only with positive numbers, you must be careful when applying them to logarithmic functions. There wasn't any difficulty in the preceding example since both of the functions $\log(100/x^3\sqrt{x})$ and $2 - \frac{7}{2}(\log x)$ are defined only when x is positive. But this isn't always the case. For instance, the third law of logarithms guarantees that

$$\log x^2 = 2(\log x) \qquad \text{for every } positive \text{ real number } x$$

But the functions

$$g(x) = \log x^2 \qquad \text{and} \qquad h(x) = 2(\log x)$$

are *not* the same function since they have *different domains*. For whenever x is nonzero, the number x^2 is positive, so that $g(x) = \log x^2$ is defined. In particular, $g(x)$ is defined for every *negative* real number. But $h(x) = 2(\log x)$ is only defined when x is *positive*.

EXERCISES

A.1. In each case assume that the given point lies on the graph of the function $f(x) = \log_b x$. Then find b.
(a) $(100, 2)$ (b) $(8, 3)$ (c) $(\sqrt{8}, \frac{3}{2})$ (d) $(\sqrt[3]{(125)^2}, 2)$

A.2. Find the domain of each of the functions below (where, as usual, the domain is the largest set of real numbers for which the rule of the function produces well-defined real numbers).
(a) $f(x) = \log(x + 1)$ (f) $r(x) = \log_e(-x - 3) - 10$
(b) $g(x) = \log_e(x + 2)$ (g) $k(x) = \log(x^2 - 1)$
(c) $h(x) = \log(-x)$ (h) $f(x) = \log_2 x - \log_2(x + 1)$
(d) $k(x) = \log_3(-x + 2)$ (i) $g(x) = \log_e x + \log_e(x - 2)$
(e) $f(x) = (\log x) - 10$

A.3. Use the graph of $g(x) = \log x$ on page 342 and the fact that every logarithmic function is a constant multiple of g to sketch the graph of these functions, without plotting points. (The logarithm table on p. 321 may be helpful.)
(a) $f(x) = \log_4 x$ (b) $p(x) = \log_{225} x$ (c) $k(x) = \log_{45.2} x$

B.1. In Section 2 we saw that if $1 < a < b$, then the graph of the exponential function $f(x) = b^x$ rose much faster than the graph of $g(x) = a^x$. What can be said about the growth of the graphs of $h(x) = \log_a x$ and $k(x) = \log_b x$ when $1 < a < b$ and $x > 0$?

B.2. For each pair of functions f and g, determine the values of x for which $f(x) = g(x)$. [*Example:* if $f(x) = \log x^4$ and $g(x) = 4(\log x)$, then $f(x) = g(x)$ for all positive x.]
(a) $f(x) = \log x^4$; $g(x) = 2(\log x^2)$
(b) $f(x) = \log \sqrt{x + 1}$; $g(x) = \frac{1}{2}(\log(x + 1))$
(c) $f(x) = (\log x^3) + 1$; $g(x) = 3(\log x) + 1$
(d) $f(x) = \log x^4$; $g(x) = 2(\log x) + \log x^2$
(e) $f(x) = \log\left(\dfrac{x}{x - 1}\right)$; $g(x) = \log x - \log(x - 1)$
(f) $f(x) = \log(x\sqrt{x - 2})$; $g(x) = \log x + \frac{1}{2}(\log(x - 2))$

B.3. Use the logarithm laws and the techniques of Section 6 of Chapter 4 to obtain the graph of each of the following functions from the graph of $g(x) = \log x$ without plotting very many points.
(a) $f(x) = \log(5x)$ (c) $k(x) = \log(x - 4)$ (e) $h(x) = \log\left(\dfrac{1}{x^3}\right)$
(b) $h(x) = (\log x) - 7$ (d) $f(x) = \log x^3$ (f) $k(x) = \log x\sqrt{x}$

B.4. Graph the following functions. Whenever possible use algebraic techniques to determine the shape of the graph, rather than plotting points. If the domain of the function includes negative numbers, be careful.
(a) $g(x) = \log x^2$ (c) $f(x) = \log|x|$ (e) $p(x) = \log x + \log x^2$
(b) $h(x) = \log x^4$ (d) $k(x) = |\log x|$ (f) $h(x) = \log x - \log \sqrt{x}$

B.5. **(a)** Graph the function $f(x) = 1/\log x$.

(b) How does the graph of f compare to the graph of $h(x) = \log(1/x)$?

B.6. If $1 < b < 10$, does the graph of $f(x) = \log_b x$ rise at a faster or slower rate than that of $g(x) = \log x$? Why? What's the answer when $b > 10$?

B.7. Suppose $f(x) = A \log x + B$, where A and B are constants. If $f(1) = 10$ and $f(10) = 1$, then find A and B.

C.1. **(a)** By how much must x be increased in order that the graph of $g(x) = \log_2 x$ rise 1 unit?

(b) If you turn the volume of your HiFi up and down, the "loudness" of the music changes. The output of the HiFi can be exactly measured in watts. The law of Weber-Fechner states that the relationship between output x in watts and loudness L at output x is given by the function

$$L(x) = \log_2 x$$

You are accustomed to listening to your HiFi at the level $L = 4$. After some time you develop callous ears, and you turn up the volume to $L = 5$. This goes on and eventually your turn it up from $L = 19$ to $L = 20$. Now whenever you increase the loudness L, you use more watts of power and your power bill increases. By how much does your power bill increase when you go from $L = 4$ to $L = 5$? from $L = 8$ to $L = 9$? from $L = 12$ to $L = 13$? from $L = 19$ to $L = 20$? Can you state a general rule for the increase when L goes from k to $k + 1$? [*Hint:* part (a) may shed some light on this.]

(c) If power costs $\frac{1}{2}¢$ per watt per hr, by how many *dollars* does your bill for 1 hr of power increase when you go from $L = 4$ to $L = 5$? from $L = 8$ to $L = 9$? from $L = 12$ to $L = 13$? from $L = 19$ to $L = 20$?

DO IT YOURSELF!

LOGARITHMIC GROWTH

In order to have a better feeling for the rate at which the graph of a logarithmic function rises when x is large, it is useful to consider the common logarithm function $f(x) = \log x$. By the properties of logarithms, we know that for any positive number v,

$$f(10v) = \log(10v) = \log 10 + \log v = 1 + \log v = 1 + f(v)$$

Therefore the y-coordinate of the point $(10v, f(10v))$ on the graph of f is just the number $f(v) + 1$. This means that the vertical distance between the points

$$(v, f(v)) \quad \text{and} \quad (10v, f(10v)) = (10v, f(v) + 1)$$

is just 1 unit, as shown in Figure 6-11.

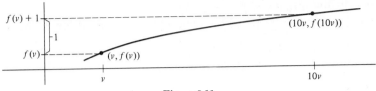

Figure 6-11

In other words, in order for the graph of $f(x) = \log x$ to rise just 1 unit, x must be increased *10 times*. Thus from $x = 5$ to $x = 10 \cdot 5 = 50$ (a horizontal distance of 45 units), the graph rises just 1 unit. Similarly, from $x = 750{,}000$ to $x = 10 \cdot 750{,}000 = 7{,}500{,}000$ (a horizontal distance of 6.75 *million units*), the graph rises only *1 unit*.

More generally, for any number k,

$$f(10^k v) = \log (10^k v) = \log 10^k + \log v = k + \log v = k + f(v)$$

Therefore

> *Changing the value of* x *by a factor of* 10^k *changes the value of* f(x) = log x *by just* k *units.*

The implications of this fact can best be seen in an example from the real world, such as the following one.

EXAMPLE The magnitude of an earthquake is measured on the Richter scale. A mild quake that does little damage might register 3.2 on the Richter scale, whereas the great San Francisco earthquake of 1906 registered 8.4. As we shall now see, magnitude on the Richter scale is determined by a certain logarithmic function.

At the time the Richter scale was invented, the smallest earthquake recorded up to that time was chosen as the "zero earthquake" to which all other quakes would be compared. The magnitude $R(i)$ on the Richter scale of a given earthquake is defined to be

$$R(i) = \log \frac{i}{i_0}$$

where i is the amplitude of the ground motion of the quake (as measured by a seismograph at a fixed distance from the epicenter of the quake) and i_0 is the amplitude of the ground motion of the zero earthquake (as measured by a seismograph at the same fixed distance from the epicenter). Observe that the magnitude of the zero earthquake is in fact 0 since

$$R(i_0) = \log \frac{i_0}{i_0} = \log 1 = 0$$

Since the Richter magnitude $R(i)$ is given by a logarithmic function, the comments above about logarithmic growth are applicable here. In particular,

The value of i must be increased by a factor of 10^k in order
for the magnitude $R(i)$ to increase by just k units

For example, the zero quake has magnitude 0 and a quake that has a thousand times as much ground motion as the zero quake (that is, $i = 1000i_0 = 10^3i_0$) has magnitude 3 since

$$R(10^3i_0) = \log \frac{10^3i_0}{i_0} = \log 10^3 = 3$$

Similarly, if the Richter magnitude of two earthquakes differs by 5, then one quake is 100,000 ($= 10^5$) times stronger than the other. To see this, suppose one quake has magnitude $R(k) = 8$ and the other has magnitude $R(j) = 3$. Then

$$5 = R(k) - R(j) = \log \frac{k}{i_0} - \log \frac{j}{i_0}$$
$$5 = (\log k - \log i_0) - (\log j - \log i_0)$$
$$5 = \log k - \log j$$
$$5 = \log \left(\frac{k}{j} \right)$$

Since $10^{\log x} = x$ for every positive number x, we have:

$$10^5 = 10^{\log (k/j)} = \frac{k}{j}$$

so that $k = 10^5 j$, as claimed.

Other applications of logarithmic functions include physical phenomena, such as sound, and psychological phenomena, such as the rate at which people forget learned information. See the exercises below.

EXERCISES

A.1. What is the magnitude on the Richter scale of an earthquake that is
  (a) 100 times stronger than the zero quake.
  (b) $10^{4.7}$ times stronger than the zero quake.
  (c) 350 times stronger than the zero quake.
  (d) 2500 times stronger than the zero quake.

A.2. The energy intensity i of a sound is related to the loudness of the sound by the function

$$L(i) = 10 \log \left(\frac{i}{i_0} \right)$$

where i_0 is the minimum intensity detectable by the human ear (the threshold of hearing) and $L(i)$ is measured in decibels. [If $L(i)$ is to be measured in bels (1 bel = 10 decibels), then the function is $L(i) = \log(i/i_0)$.]

(a) The intensity of the sound of a ticking watch is approximately 100 times the minimum intensity i_0. What is the decibel measure of the loudness of the watch?

(b) The intensity of soft music is 10,000 times greater than the minimum intensity i_0. How many decibels of loudness is this?

(c) The sound of the Victoria Falls in Africa is 10 billion times more intense than the minimum sound. How many decibels is this?

B.1. Students in a calculus class were given a final exam. Each month thereafter, they took an equivalent exam, to test how much they remembered. The class average on an exam taken after t months is given by the "forgetting function"

$$F(t) = 82 - 18 \log(t + 1)$$

Thus the average on the original exam $(t = 0)$ was $F(0) = 82 - 18 \log(0 + 1)$ $= 82 - 18 \log 1 = 82 - 0 = 82$. After 2 months, the average was $F(2) = 82 - 18 \log 3 \approx 82 - 8.5878 = 73.4122$.

(a) What was the class average at the end of 3 months? 6 months? 9 months? 1 year?

(b) How many months will it take until the class average falls below 60?

B.2. Third graders are taught the elements of Sanskrit. At the end of the instruction period they are tested, and then tested at weekly intervals thereafter. The average score on the exam given after t weeks is given by the function

$$G(t) = 77 - 24 \log(t + 1)$$

(a) What was the average score on the original exam (that is, when $t = 0$)?

(b) What was the average score at the end of 2 weeks? 5 weeks? 10 weeks?

(c) How long will it take for the average score to drop below 50? below 40? below 30?

B.3. How much stronger was the San Francisco earthquake of 1906 (8.4 on the Richter scale) than the Seattle earthquake of 1964 (6.1 on the Richter scale)? How much stronger than the 1964 Alaska quake (7.5 on the Richter scale)?

B.4. (a) Using Exercises B.1 and B.2 as a model, construct a forgetting function $H(t)$ satisfying these conditions: (i) $H(t)$ is the class average on an exam given t months after the instruction period in a certain subject has ended. (ii) The class average immediately after the instruction period was 90. (iii) The class average after 9 months was 75.

(b) Using the function $H(t)$ constructed in part (a), determine the class average after 5 months, 15 months, and 20 months.

B.5. Refer to Exercise A.2 for the loudness function $L(i)$. The sound of freeway traffic measures 85 decibels, while the sound of traffic on a quiet residential street measures 45 decibels. How many times more intense is the sound of the freeway traffic? [*Hint:* If j denotes the sound intensity of freeway traffic and k the intensity of residential traffic, then $L(j) = 85$ and $L(k) = 45$ so that $L(j) - L(k) = 40$.]

5. INVERSE FUNCTIONS

The exponential function $f(x) = 10^x$ and the common logarithm function $g(x) = \log x$ have a very close relationship, as is clear from the two basic properties of logarithms:

$$10^{\log x} = x \qquad \text{for every positive real number } x$$

$$\log 10^x = x \qquad \text{for every real number } x$$

These basic properties can be interpreted as statements about the composite functions°
$f \circ g$ and $g \circ f$:

$$(f \circ g)(x) = f(g(x)) = f(\log x) = 10^{\log x} = x \qquad \text{for every positive real number } x$$

$$(g \circ f)(x) = g(f(x)) = g(10^x) = \log 10^x = x \qquad \text{for every real number } x$$

Since the domain of the function $g(x) = \log x$ is the set of all positive real numbers and the domain of $f(x) = 10^x$ is the set of all real numbers, the two statements above say that the functions f and g have this property:

$$(f \circ g)(x) = x \qquad \text{for every number } x \text{ in the domain of } g$$

$$(g \circ f)(x) = x \qquad \text{for every number } x \text{ in the domain of } f$$

This property may be paraphrased by saying that "f undoes what g does" and "g undoes what f does." A calculator equipped with a log key and a 10^x key will provide a visual demonstration of this. For instance, to evaluate the composite function $f \circ g$ at a given number:

Enter the number . . . . . . Press the log key . . . . . . Press the 10^x key

$$x \qquad\qquad\qquad g(x) \qquad\qquad\qquad f(g(x)) = (f \circ g)(x)$$

The final display will be the number x with which you started,°° thus demonstrating that f does indeed undo what g does; that is, $(f \circ g)(x) = x$. Similar remarks apply to the function $g \circ f$.

More generally, let f and g be *any* functions. We say that g is the **inverse** of f (or that f is the inverse of g, or that f and g are **inverse functions**), provided that

$$(f \circ g)(x) = x \qquad \text{for every number } x \text{ in the domain of } g$$

$$(g \circ f)(x) = x \qquad \text{for every number } x \text{ in the domain of } f$$

As we have just seen $f(x) = 10^x$ and $g(x) = \log x$ are inverse functions. Here is another example.

EXAMPLE Let $f(x) = -2x + 1$ and $g(x) = \dfrac{x - 1}{-2}$. Both these functions have the set of all real numbers as domain. For any number x we have:

$$(f \circ g)(x) = f(g(x)) \qquad\qquad\qquad (\text{definition of } f \circ g)$$

° Composite functions were discussed in Section 7 of Chapter 4.
°° Since all calculators round off after a certain number of digits, there may be a slight error so that the final display sometimes differs slightly from the original number.

$$= f\left(\frac{x-1}{-2}\right) \qquad \text{(definition of } g\text{)}$$

$$= -2\left(\frac{x-1}{-2}\right) + 1 = x \qquad \text{(definition of } f \text{ and arithmetic)}$$

On the other hand,

$$(g \circ f)(x) = g(f(x)) \qquad \text{(definition of } g \circ f\text{)}$$

$$= g(-2x + 1) \qquad \text{(definition of } f\text{)}$$

$$= \frac{(-2x + 1) - 1}{-2} = x \qquad \text{(definition of } g \text{ and arithmetic)}$$

Therefore f and g are inverse functions.

As we shall soon see, it is *not* true that every function has an inverse. Therefore the problem that frequently occurs is this: Given a function f, determine whether or not f has an inverse function, and if so, find the rule of the inverse function. In order to solve the first part of this problem, look at the graphs of the two preceding functions that *do* have inverses (Figure 6-12):

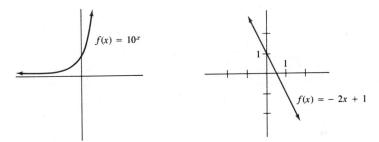

Figure 6-12

Each of these functions is either *increasing* (graph always rising from left to right) or *decreasing* (graph always falling from left to right). Furthermore, the inverse of each of these functions has the same property. For instance, $f(x) = 10^x$ is an increasing function and so is $g(x) = \log x$ (its graph is on page 342). Consequently, the following fact should seem plausible.

> *If f is either an increasing or a decreasing function, then f has an inverse function with the same property.*

A proof of this fact is given in the DO IT YOURSELF! segment at the end of this section. We shall assume it for now.

FINDING THE RULE OF AN INVERSE FUNCTION

Once we know that a given function *f has* an inverse function g, we can often find the rule of g by using algebra. An analogy may be helpful, in order to understand this method. When getting dressed, you first put on your socks and then your shoes. But when you get undressed you have to reverse the order: First take off your shoes and then your socks. Thus to "undo" the dressing process, you must not only reverse each step (take the shoes off instead of putting them on) but you must also reverse the order in which the steps were originally performed (shoes, socks instead of socks, shoes).

EXAMPLE   The graph of the function $f(x) = 3x - 2$ is a straight line with slope 3. Thus the graph is always rising and we know that *f* has an inverse function g. This function g must "undo what *f* does." But the rule of *f* tells us exactly what *f* does to a number:

Multiply it by 3 and then subtract 2

In order to undo what *f* does, we must reverse each step and do so in the opposite order (remember the shoes and socks). In other words, we must first

Add 2 (the reverse of subtracting 2)

and then

Divide by 3 (the reverse of multiplying by 3)

Thus if we begin with a number y, the rule of the inverse function g is:

Add 2 (producing $y + 2$) and then divide by 3 $\left(\text{producing } \dfrac{y + 2}{3}\right)$

that is, $g(y) = \dfrac{y + 2}{3}$. To see that g really is the inverse of *f*, we simply calculate the composite functions $g \circ f$ and $f \circ g$:

$$(g \circ f)(x) = g(f(x)) = g(3x - 2) = \frac{(3x - 2) + 2}{3} = x \qquad \text{for every number } x$$

$$(f \circ g)(y) = f(g(y)) = f\left(\frac{y + 2}{3}\right) = 3\left(\frac{y + 2}{3}\right) - 2 = y \qquad \text{for every number } y$$

Therefore g is the inverse function of *f*. The verbal reasoning used to find the rule of g is equivalent to the following algebraic method. The function *f* is given by the equation

$$y = f(x); \qquad \text{that is, } y = 3x - 2$$

Solving this equation for x, we obtain:

$$3x - 2 = y$$

$$3x = y + 2 \qquad \text{(add 2 to both sides)}$$

$$x = \frac{y + 2}{3} \qquad \text{(divide both sides by 3)}$$

Note that the steps used to solve this equation for x are precisely those used previously to construct the rule of the inverse function g (add 2, and then divide by 3). So it is not surprising that the right-hand side of the last equation is just the rule of the function g. In other words, g is given by the equation

$$x = g(y); \qquad \text{that is, } x = \frac{y + 2}{3}$$

Therefore now we have two equivalent ways of finding the rule of g: the verbal reasoning method used first and the equation method used here. (One final remark: We have used the letter y to denote the variable of the function g so that we would not get confused when solving the equation. But the letter used to describe the variable of a function doesn't matter. So once the rule of g is determined, we can, if we wish, use x as the variable and write $g(x) = \dfrac{x + 2}{3}$.$\Big)$

EXAMPLE The inverse of the function $f(x) = x^3 + 5$ can be found by solving for x in the equation $y = f(x)$; that is, $y = x^3 + 5$:

$$x^3 + 5 = y$$
$$x^3 = y - 5 \qquad \text{(subtract 5 from both sides)}$$
$$x = \sqrt[3]{y - 5} \qquad \text{(take cube root of both sides)}$$

So the function $g(y) = x$; that is, $g(y) = \sqrt[3]{y - 5}$ is the inverse of f. You can check this by computing $f \circ g$ and $g \circ f$:

$$(f \circ g)(y) = f(g(y)) = f(\sqrt[3]{y - 5}) = (\sqrt[3]{y - 5})^3 + 5 = y \qquad \text{for every number } y$$
$$(g \circ f)(x) = g(f(x)) = g(x^3 + 5) = \sqrt[3]{(x^3 + 5) - 5} = x \qquad \text{for every number } x$$

EXAMPLE The domain of the function $f(x) = x^2 - 2$ is the set of all real numbers. The graph of f in Figure 6-13 shows that f is neither increasing nor decreasing (the graph isn't *always* rising or *always* falling).

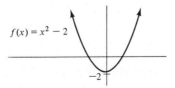

Figure 6-13

The function f does *not* have an inverse (see the DO IT YOURSELF! segment at the end of this section for the reason). However, it is often possible in such cases to find a function closely related to f that does have an inverse. You can see one way to do this by looking at the graph of f: When $x \geq 0$, the graph is always rising. So consider a new function h that has the same rule as f (namely, $h(x) = x^2 - 2$) but a *different domain* (namely, all *nonnegative* real numbers, instead of all real numbers). We say that h is obtained by **restricting the domain** of f. The graph of the function h is just the right half of the graph of f, which is always rising. So h has an inverse function. We can find this inverse by solving for x in the equation $y = h(x)$; that is, $y = x^2 - 2$:

$$x^2 - 2 = y$$
$$x^2 = y + 2$$

Now this equation has two solutions: $x = \sqrt{y + 2}$ and $x = -\sqrt{y + 2}$. But in this case x is in the domain of the function h so that $x \geq 0$. Hence we must have:

$$x = \sqrt{y + 2}$$

Let g be the function whose rule is $g(y) = \sqrt{y + 2}$. Since $\sqrt{y + 2}$ is only defined when $y + 2 \geq 0$, the domain of g is the set of all real numbers y with $y \geq -2$. For every number y in the domain of g we have:

$$(h \circ g)(y) = h(g(y)) = h(\sqrt{y + 2}) = (\sqrt{y + 2})^2 - 2 = (y + 2) - 2 = y$$

On the other hand, if x is in the domain of h (that is, $x \geq 0$), then

$$(g \circ h)(x) = g(h(x)) = g(x^2 - 2) = \sqrt{(x^2 - 2) + 2} = \sqrt{x^2}$$

But when $x \geq 0$, we know that $\sqrt{x^2} = x$. Consequently,

$$(g \circ h)(x) = \sqrt{x^2} = x \qquad \text{for every number } x \text{ in the domain of } h$$

Therefore g is the inverse function of h. Or more completely, g is the inverse of the function obtained by restricting the domain of the function $f(x) = x^2 - 2$ to the interval $[0, \infty)$. Once again, we note that the function g can also be described by the rule $g(x) = \sqrt{x + 2}$ because the letter used for the variable of a function doesn't matter.

GRAPHS OF INVERSE FUNCTIONS

All the functions and inverse functions in the preceding examples were those whose graphs were known or easily obtained by plotting some points. You can always graph inverse functions by plotting points, but sometimes there is a faster way. If f is a function that has an inverse g and the graph of f is known, then the graph of g can be obtained by using this fact:

> *If* f *and* g *are inverse functions, then the point* (u, v) *is on the graph of* f *exactly when the point* (v, u) *is on the graph of* g.

To prove this fact, let (u, v) be a point on the graph of f so that $v = f(u)$. Applying the inverse function g to v yields:

$$g(v) = g(f(u)) = (g \circ f)(u) = u$$

Therefore $g(v) = u$ so that the point $(v, g(v))$ on the graph of g is just the point (v, u). A similar argument, beginning with a point on the graph of g, completes the proof.

The statement in the box above says that each point on the graph of the inverse function g can be obtained by taking a point on the graph of f and "reversing" its coordinates. A simple geometric way of doing that is to reflect the plane in the line $y = x$ (that is, rotate the plane 180° around the line $y = x$). If you do this, the positive vertical axis ends in the positive horizontal position and the positive horizontal axis ends in the positive vertical position, as shown in Figure 6-14. Consequently, the point whose original coordinates were (u, v) now has first coordinate v and second coordinate u.

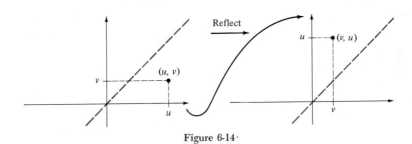

Figure 6-14

Thus reflecting the plane in the line $y = x$ moves each point (u, v) on the graph of f on to the point (v, u) on the graph of g. In summary:

> *If g is the inverse function of f, then the graph of g can be obtained by reflecting the graph of f in the line y = x.*

An informal way of thinking of this fact is this: The graph of g is the mirror image of the graph of f, with the line $y = x$ being the mirror.

Using this reflection method, we can easily obtain the graphs of the inverses of various functions previously discussed, as shown in Figure 6-15 on the next page.°

° Although it may be confusing at first, we have followed the usual custom of labeling all function variables, and hence all horizontal axes, as x.

Graph of Function f   **Graph of Inverse Function g**

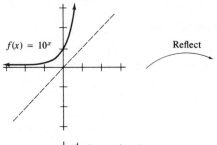

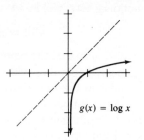

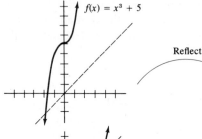

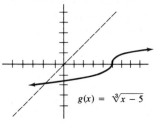

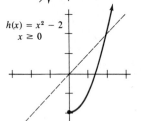

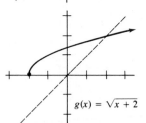

Figure 6-15

EXERCISES

A.1. Verify that each of these pairs are inverse functions by calculating $f \circ g$ and $g \circ f$.

(a) $f(x) = x + 1;$ $\quad$ $g(x) = x - 1$ $\qquad$ (e) $f(x) = x^5;$ $\quad$ $g(x) = \sqrt[5]{x}$

(b) $f(x) = 2x - 6;$ $\quad$ $g(x) = \dfrac{x}{2} + 3$ $\qquad$ (f) $f(x) = x^3 - 1;$ $\quad$ $g(x) = \sqrt[3]{x + 1}$

(c) $f(x) = \dfrac{1}{x + 1};$ $\quad$ $g(x) = \dfrac{1 - x}{x}$ $\qquad$ (g) $f(x) = e^x;$ $\quad$ $g(x) = \log_e x$

(d) $f(x) = \dfrac{-3}{2x + 5};$ $\quad$ $g(x) = \dfrac{-3 - 5x}{2x}$ $\quad$ (h) $f(x) = e^{x-1};$ $\quad$ $g(x) = \log_e x + 1$

B.1. Use the verbal reasoning method (as in the first example on page 352) to find the inverse g of the function f:

(a) $f(x) = 5x + 1$ $\qquad\qquad\qquad$ (d) $f(x) = (x + 4)^3$

(b) $f(x) = \dfrac{x}{2} + 2$ $\qquad\qquad\qquad$ (e) $f(x) = 2(x + 4)^3 - 1$

(c) $f(x) = x^3$ $\qquad\qquad\qquad\qquad$ (f) $f(x) = \dfrac{2(x + 4)^3 - 1}{5}$

B.2. Use algebra to find the inverse of the given function:

(a) $f(x) = -x$ (d) $h(x) = \sqrt[5]{x} + 1$ (g) $f(x) = \sqrt{4x - 7}$

(b) $g(x) = -x + 1$ (e) $f(x) = \dfrac{1}{2x + 1}$ (h) $g(x) = 5 - 2x^3$

(c) $f(x) = (x^5 + 1)^3$ (f) $g(x) = \dfrac{x}{x + 1}$

B.3. None of the following functions has an inverse. State at least one way of restricting the domain of the given function so that the restricted function has an inverse. Find the rule of the inverse function.

(a) $f(x) = |x|$ (e) $f(x) = \dfrac{x^2 + 6}{2}$

(b) $f(x) = |x - 3|$ (f) $f(x) = \sqrt{4 - x^2}$

(c) $f(x) = -x^2$ (g) $f(x) = \dfrac{1}{x^2 + 1}$

(d) $f(x) = x^2 + 4$ (h) $f(x) = 3(x + 5)^2 + 2$

B.4. Each of these functions has an inverse. Graph the function. Then on the same axes graph its inverse function g without plotting any points. (Reflect carefully.)

(a) $f(x) = \dfrac{x}{3} - 2$ (d) $f(x) = \sqrt{3x - 2}$

(b) $f(x) = \dfrac{x - 5}{7}$ (e) $f(x) = x^3 + 1$

(c) $f(x) = \sqrt{x + 3}$ (f) $f(x) = \sqrt[3]{x + 3}$

B.5. Sketch the graph of the inverse function of each of the functions whose graph appears in Figure 6-16.

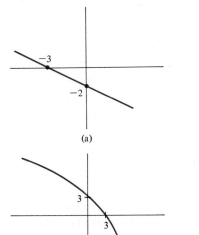

(a)

(b)

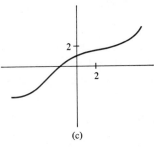

(c)

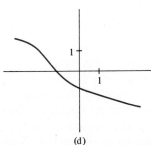

(d)

Figure 6-16

B.6.   Let C be the temperature in degrees Celsius. Then the temperature in degrees Fahrenheit is given by $f(C) = \frac{9}{5}C + 32$. Let g be the function that converts degrees Fahrenheit to degrees Celsius. Show that g is the inverse function of f and find the rule of g.

C.1.   Let m and b be fixed constants with $m \neq 0$. Show that the function $f(x) = mx + b$ has an inverse function g and find the rule of g.

C.2.   We shall use the term *algebraic step* to describe a function that performs a single operation. For instance, the function $f(x) = x + 2$ performs the single operation of "adding 2," the function $g(x) = x/7$ performs the operation of "dividing by 7," the function $h(x) = 1/x$ performs the operation of "taking the reciprocal," and the function $k(x) = x^2$ performs the operation of "squaring." Thus each of these functions is an algebraic step.

(a)   Which of the preceding steps have inverses? We shall say that an algebraic step that does have an inverse is *invertible*.

(b)   Make a list of several algebraic steps that are *not* invertible.

(c)   If the rule of a function consists of a sequence of invertible algebraic steps, we should be able to find the inverse of f by doing the inverse of each algebraic step in reverse order (as in the first example on page 352). This procedure breaks down, however, when some of the algebraic steps in the rule of the function are not invertible. In each part of Exercise B.3 identify the noninvertible step or steps that prevent the function from having an inverse.

(d)   Are either of these functions invertible: $f(x) = (x - 2)^3$ or $g(x) = \sqrt[3]{\log x} + 7$?

DO IT YOURSELF!

WHICH FUNCTIONS HAVE INVERSES?

In answering the question posed in the title, we shall restrict our attention to the type of function that actually occurs in practice, namely, functions whose graphs are smooth, connected, and continuous curves. You should also remember that an increasing function is one whose graph is always rising from left to right and that a decreasing function is one whose graph is always falling from left to right. We claim that:

> *If f is an increasing or decreasing function, then f has an inverse function with the same property.*

In order to prove this statement, we first recall what the range of a function is. If you apply the rule of a function f to every number in its domain, the resulting set of numbers is the range of f. In graphical terms the range of f consists of all numbers that are second coordinates of points on the graph of f. Now suppose that f is an *increasing* function and that v is a number in the range of f. Consider the horizontal line $y = v$ (the line consisting of all points with second coordinate v). For example, the situation might look like the curves in Figure 6-17.

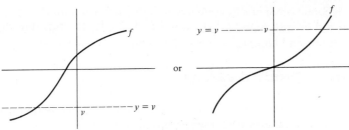

Figure 6-17

Imagine a point moving along the graph of f from left to right. Once the point crosses the horizontal line $y = v$, it keeps moving upward because the graph of f is *always rising*. The point cannot move downward and hence cannot cross the horizontal line $y = v$ again. Thus the graph of an increasing function has this geometric property:

> For each number v in the range of f, the horizontal
> line $y = v$ intersects the graph of f at exactly one point.

This is the same property that was used to construct the logarithm function from the graph of the function $f(x) = 10^x$ on page 318. Since a point (u, v) is on the graph of f exactly when $f(u) = v$, the preceding geometric property is equivalent to this algebraic property:

> For each number v in the range of f, there is exactly
> one number u in the domain of f such that $f(u) = v$.

We can now use this fact to construct an inverse function g for f. Let g be the function whose domain is the same as the range of f and whose rule is:

$$g(v) = u, \text{ where } u \text{ is the unique number such that } f(u) = v$$

Thus for each u in the domain of f and each v in the domain of g:

$$g(v) = u \qquad \text{exactly when} \qquad f(u) = v$$

Therefore

$$(g \circ f)(u) = g(f(u)) = g(v) = u \qquad \text{and} \qquad (f \circ g)(v) = f(g)(v) = f(u) = v$$

This shows that g is the inverse function of f. To see that g is also an increasing function, remember that the graph of the inverse function g is just the reflection of the graph of f in the line $y = x$. It is easy to see geometrically that the reflection of a rising graph (such as the graph of f) is itself a rising graph. For instance, see Figure 6-18.

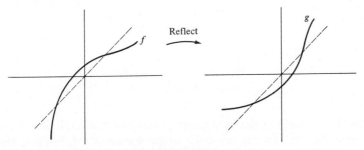

Figure 6-18

A rigorous algebraic proof of this same fact is outlined in Exercise C.1. In any case the result is that the inverse function g is increasing. A similar argument works for decreasing functions and completes the proof of the statement in the preceding box.

FUNCTIONS WITHOUT INVERSES

What can be said about the inverses (if any) of functions that are neither increasing nor decreasing (that is, functions whose graphs are neither *always* rising nor *always* falling)? For example, consider Figure 6-19.

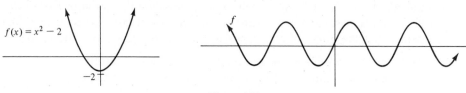

Figure 6-19

Suppose that such a function f did have an inverse g. Then the graph of g would be the reflection of the graph of f in the line $y = x$, as shown in Figure 6-20.

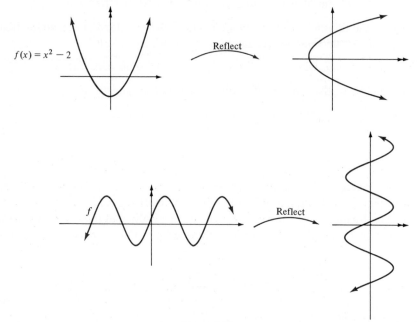

Figure 6-20

But neither of the graphs at the right could possibly be the graph of a *function g*. To see why, remember that for any number v in the domain of a function g, there is only *one* point on the graph of g with first coordinate v, namely, the point $(v, g(v))$ (see Exercise B.7 on page 180 and Exercise B.10 on page 207). But this condition is certainly not satisfied by the right-hand graphs above. For example, there are at least *two* points on each graph with first coordinate 0. Therefore neither of the functions f above has an inverse function. A similar argument works in other cases and shows that:

> *A function with a connected, continuous graph that is neither increasing nor decreasing does* not *have an inverse function.*

Sometimes it is desirable to have some kind of partial inverse for a function that is neither increasing nor decreasing, such as $f(x) = x^2 - 2$. The usual technique is to restrict the domain of f in order to obtain a new function (with the same rule) that is either increasing or decreasing. An inverse can then be found for this restricted function. This was done for $f(x) = x^2 - 2$ in the second example on page 353.

EXERCISES

B.1. (a) Is the function $f(x) = \dfrac{5}{x - 3}$ increasing or decreasing or neither?

(b) Show that the function f does have an inverse function g and find the rule of g. .

(c) Do your answers to parts (a) and (b) contradict the statements in the boxes on pages 358 and 361? Explain.

C.1. On page 219 it is shown that a function f is increasing, provided that

$$\text{whenever } c < d, \quad \text{then } f(c) < f(d)$$

Let g be the inverse function of f, defined by:

$$g(v) = u \quad \text{exactly when} \quad f(u) = v$$

Prove that g is increasing. [*Hint:* Suppose $c < d$ and $g(c) = r$ and $g(d) = s$. We must show that $r < s$. We have $f(r) = c$ and $f(s) = d$. Use the fact that f is increasing to show that $s \leq r$ is impossible.]

C.2. Answer the following questions by presenting examples of your own choice.
(a) Let f be a linear function whose graph is a straight line of slope 2. Is the inverse of f also a linear function? What is its slope?
(b) If f is a linear function whose graph is a line of positive slope, what can you say about the slope of its inverse?
(c) If f is a linear function whose graph is a line of negative slope, what can you say about the slope of its inverse?
(d) How do your answers in parts (b) and (c) relate to the statement in the box on page 358?

6. EXPONENTIAL EQUATIONS AND APPLICATIONS

We now use the information about logarithms and exponents developed earlier in this chapter to solve exponential equations, such as

$$3 \cdot 5^x + 4 = 10, \qquad 2^{x+1} = 3^{x-1}, \qquad 3e^{2x^2-1} - 7 = 17, \qquad 2^x - 3 - 14.2^{-x} = 0$$

The ability to solve such equations will enable us to deal effectively with a number of applications, including compound interest, population growth, atmospheric pressure, and radioactive decay.

EXPONENTIAL EQUATIONS

The key to solving equations such as those just given, in which the unknown appears as an exponent, is to use the third law of logarithms:

$$\log_b(v^k) = k(\log_b v) \qquad \text{for all real numbers } v, k \text{ with } v > 0$$

The following examples show how this fact is used to solve exponential equations.

EXAMPLE Here is a step-by-step solution of the equation:

$$3 \cdot 5^x + 4 = 10$$

$$3 \cdot 5^x = 6 \qquad \text{(subtract 4 from both sides)}$$

$$5^x = 2 \qquad \text{(divide both sides by 3)}$$

Now take the logarithm of each side (to base 10). Since equal numbers have equal logarithms, we obtain:

$$\log 5^x = \log 2$$

$$x(\log 5) = \log 2 \qquad \text{(third law of logarithms)}$$

$$x = \frac{\log 2}{\log 5} \qquad \text{(divide both sides by the number } \log 5\text{)}$$

For many purposes this answer is perfectly adequate. But if a numerical approximation is needed, we can use a calculator or the table on page 321 to find that

$$x = \frac{\log 2}{\log 5} \approx \frac{.3010}{.6990} \approx .4306$$

(Remember $\log 2/\log 5$ is *not* the same as $\log \frac{2}{5}$ or $\log 2 - \log 5$.)

In order to solve the equation $5^x = 2$ in the preceding example, we took logarithms to base 10. If we had used logarithms to some other base, such as e or 5, the solutions would have gone like this:

Base e	Base 5

$$5^x = 2$$
$$\log_e(5^x) = \log_e 2$$
$$x(\log_e 5) = \log_e 2$$
$$x = \frac{\log_e 2}{\log_e 5}$$

$$5^x = 2$$
$$\log_5(5^x) = \log_5 2$$
$$x(\log_5 5) = \log_5 2$$
$$x = \frac{\log_5 2}{\log_5 5} = \frac{\log_5 2}{1} = \log_5 2$$

At first glance, each of these answers seems quite different from the answer above, $x = \log 2/\log 5$. But actually *all three answers are exactly the same number.* As we saw on page 327, logarithms to the base e are just constant multiples of logarithms to base 10, with the constant multiplier being the nonzero number $1/\log e$. Therefore,

$$\frac{\log_e 2}{\log_e 5} = \frac{(1/\log e)(\log 2)}{(1/\log e)(\log 5)} = \frac{\log 2}{\log 5}.$$

Similarly, $\log_5 v = (1/\log 5) \log v$, so that

$$\log_5 2 = \frac{\log_5 2}{1} = \frac{\log_5 2}{\log_5 5} = \frac{(1/\log 5)(\log 2)}{(1/\log 5)(\log 5)} = \frac{\log 2}{\log 5}.$$

Consequently, *when solving exponential equations, you may use logarithms to any base.* If numerical approximations are needed, base 10 is usually the most convenient. But in some cases it may be more helpful to use a different base in order that the answer have a simpler form.

EXAMPLE   To solve $2^{x+1} = 3^{x-1}$, we take logarithms of both sides (base 10):

$$\log 2^{x+1} = \log 3^{x-1}$$

$(x + 1)(\log 2) = (x - 1)(\log 3)$ (third law of logarithms)

$x(\log 2) + \log 2 = x(\log 3) - \log 3$ (multiply out both sides)

$x(\log 2) - x(\log 3) = -\log 2 - \log 3$ (rearrange terms)

$x(\log 2 - \log 3) = -\log 2 - \log 3$ (factor left side)

$x = \dfrac{-\log 2 - \log 3}{\log 2 - \log 3}$ (divide both sides by $(\log 2 - \log 3)$).

A numerical approximation of this answer can be found by using the table on page 321:

$$x = \frac{-\log 2 - \log 3}{\log 2 - \log 3} \approx \frac{-.3010 - .4771}{.3010 - .4771} = \frac{-.7781}{-.1761} \approx 4.4185$$

EXAMPLE   To solve $2^x - 5 - 14 \cdot 2^{-x} = 0$ we begin by multiplying both sides of the equation by 2^x. Since $2^x > 0$ for every x, the resulting equation is equivalent to the original one:

$$2^x 2^x - 5 \cdot 2^x - 14 \cdot 2^{-x} 2^x = 0$$
$$(2^x)^2 - 5 \cdot 2^x - 14 = 0$$

Now let $u = 2^x$ so that the equation becomes

$$u^2 - 5u - 14 = 0$$
$$(u + 2)(u - 7) = 0$$

$$u + 2 = 0 \qquad \text{or} \qquad u - 7 = 0$$
$$u = -2 \qquad\qquad u = 7$$
$$2^x = -2 \qquad\qquad 2^x = 7$$

Since 2^x is always positive, the equation $2^x = -2$ has no solution. To solve $2^x = 7$ we use logarithms to base 10:

$$\log 2^x = \log 7$$
$$x(\log 2) = \log 7$$

$$x = \frac{\log 7}{\log 2} \approx \frac{.8451}{.3010} \approx 2.8076$$

This is the only solution of the original equation.

APPLICATIONS

The necessary background for understanding the following examples was presented on pages 312–317. If you have not already done so, you may wish to read those pages before going further in this section.

EXAMPLE   Three thousand dollars is to be invested at an interest rate of 8% per year, compounded quarterly. How many years will it be until the investment is worth $8750?

According to the basic formula for compound interest (p. 313),

$$T(x) = P(1 + r)^x$$

where P is the original amount invested, r is the interest rate per time period (expressed as a decimal), x is the number of time periods, and $T(x)$ is the value of the investment after x time periods In this case $P = 3000$. Since interest is compounded quarterly, the basic time period is one-fourth of a year. Since the interest rate for the full year is 8% $(= .08)$, the interest rate for a quarter-year is $\frac{1}{4}(.08) = .02$. Therefore after x quarter-years the value of the investment will be

$$T(x) = 3000(1 + .02)^x = 3000(1.02)^x$$

In order to find out when the investment has the value 8750, we must find the value of x for which $T(x) = 8750$. In other words, we must solve the equation

$$3000(1.02)^x = 8750$$

Dividing both sides by 3000 and taking logarithms yields

$$(1.02)^x = \frac{8750}{3000}$$

$$\log (1.02)^x = \log \frac{8750}{3000}$$

By the second and third laws of logarithms, this equation becomes

$$x(\log 1.02) = \log 8750 - \log 3000$$

Dividing both sides by the nonzero number log 1.02 and using a calculator or logarithm table, we find that

$$x = \frac{\log 8750 - \log 3000}{\log 1.02} \approx \frac{3.9420 - 3.4771}{.0086} = \frac{.4649}{.0086} \approx 54.0581$$

Since x is the number of quarter-years, we must divide by 4 to find the number of years: $54.0581/4 = 13.514525$.

EXAMPLE A biologist observes that a culture contains 1000 of a certain type of bacteria. Seven hours later there are 5000 bacteria in the culture. How many bacteria will there be in 12 hours? in 1 day?

As we saw on page 316, the normal population growth is given by the function $S(t) = ce^{kt}$, where c is the original population, $S(t)$ is the population at time t, and k is a constant. In this case $c = 1000$, so that

$$S(t) = 1000e^{kt}$$

In order to determine the constant k we use the fact that after 7 hr the bacteria population is 5000, that is,

$$S(7) = 5000, \quad \text{or equivalently,} \quad 1000e^{7k} = 5000$$

We need only solve the right-hand equation to find k:

$$1000e^{7k} = 5000$$
$$e^{7k} = 5$$
$$\log_e(e^{7k}) = \log_e 5$$
$$7k = \log_e 5$$
$$k = \frac{\log_e 5}{7} \approx \frac{1.609}{7} \approx .2299 \approx .23$$

Therefore the function describing the growth of this bacteria population is given by $S(t) \approx 1000e^{.23t}$. After 12 hours, the number of bacteria is

$$S(12) \approx 1000e^{(.23)12} = 1000e^{.76} \approx 1000(5.8)^\circ = 15,800$$

After 1 day ($t = 24$ hours) the number of bacteria is

$$S(24) \approx 1000e^{(.23)24} = 1000e^{5.52} \approx 1000(249.635)^\circ = 249,635,000$$

EXAMPLE The skeleton of a mastodon has been found. Analysis shows that the bones have lost 58% of the carbon-14 that was present when the mastodon died. How old is the skeleton?

° A calculator was used to evaluate $e^{2.76}$ and $e^{5.52}$.

As we saw on page 316, the basic formula for radioactive decay is $M(t) = k2^{-t/h}$, where k is the original mass of the element, h is its half-life, and $M(t)$ is the mass of the element at time t. In this case the element is carbon-14, which has a half-life of 5730 years. If time is measured from the death of the mastodon, then we want to find the value of t corresponding to the present time. We know that the present mass of carbon-14 is .58 less than the original mass k. Therefore the present mass is $k - .58k = .42k$, and we have

$$M(t) = k2^{-t/h}$$
$$.42k = k2^{-t/5730}$$

The solution of this equation is the desired value of t, that is, the age of the skeleton. Dividing both sides by k and taking logarithms yields

$$.42 = 2^{-t/5730}$$
$$\log(.42) = \log(2^{-t/5730})$$
$$\log(.42) = \left(\frac{-t}{5730}\right)(\log 2) = -\frac{t(\log 2)}{5730}$$

Multiplying both sides by $-5730/\log 2$ shows that

$$t = -\frac{5730}{\log 2}(\log .42) \approx -\frac{5730(-.3768)}{.301} = \frac{2159.064}{.301} = 7172.9701$$

Therefore the skeleton is approximately 7173 years old.

EXERCISES

A.1. Solve these equations.

(a) $3^x = 81$ (d) $2^{(2x+1)} = \frac{1}{8}$ (g) $3^{5x} \cdot 9^{x^2} = 27$

(b) $3^x + 3 = 30$ (e) $3^{(x-1)} = 9^{5x}$ (h) $2^{(x^2+5x)} = \frac{1}{16}$

(c) $2^{5-x} = 16$ (f) $4^{5x} = 16^{(2x-1)}$ (i) $9^{x^2} = 3^{(-5x-2)}$

A.2. Explain why none of the final answers in Exercise A.1 involves any logarithms.

In Exercises A.3–A.5, solve the given equations. Express your answers in terms of common logarithms [for instance, $x = (2 + \log 5)/(\log 3)$] unless directed otherwise. If you have a calculator, find a rational approximation for each answer [for instance, $x = (2 + \log 5)/\log 3 \approx 5.6568$].

A.3. (a) $3^x = 5$ (c) $10^x = 2$ (e) $4 \cdot 7^x + 1 = 21$

(b) $5^x = 4$ (d) $(\frac{1}{3})^x = 3000$ (f) $5 \cdot 2^x - 3 = 27$

A.4. (a) $2^x = 3^{x-1}$ (c) $3^{1-2x} = 5^{x+5}$ (e) $2^{1-3x} = 3^{x+1}$

(b) $4^{x+2} = 2^{x-1}$ (d) $4^{3x-1} = 3^{x-2}$ (f) $3^{x+3} = 2^x$

A.5. (a) $9^x - 4 \cdot 3^x + 3 = 0$ [*Hint:* note that $9^x = (3^2)^x = (3^x)^2$ and use the substitution $u = 3^x$.]

(b) $4^x - 6 \cdot 2^x = -8$ (d) $7^x - 6 \cdot 7^{-x} = 1$ (f) $5^x + 3 = 10 \cdot 5^{-x}$

(c) $2^x - 2 + 2^{-x} = 0$ (e) $4^x + 6 \cdot 4^{-x} = 5$ (g) $2^x + 5 = 6(\sqrt{2})^x$

B.1. Use logarithms to base 5 to solve each of these equations for x.

(a) $\dfrac{5^x + 5^{-x}}{2} = 3$ (*Hint:* use an appropriate multiplication and substitution, as in Exercise A.5, to obtain a quadratic equation; solve this equation via the quadratic formula.)

(b) $\dfrac{5^x - 5^{-x}}{2} = 2$ (c) $\dfrac{5^x + 5^{-x}}{2} = t$

B.2. Use natural logarithms to solve each of these equations for x. (Compare Exercise B.1.)

(a) $\dfrac{e^x + e^{-x}}{2} = 2$ (b) $\dfrac{e^x - e^{-x}}{2} = t$ (c) $\dfrac{e^x + e^{-x}}{e^x - e^{-x}} = t$

In Exercises B.3–B.12, set up each problem and find the answers in terms of either common or natural logarithms, as appropriate. If you have a calculator (or are willing to use logarithm tables), find a rational approximation for each answer.

B.3. (a) How many years will it take for an investment of $2000 to double its value when interest is compounded annually at a rate of 7%?

(b) How long will it take for the investment in part (a) to double its value if the 7% interest is compounded monthly instead of annually?

(c) What is the "doubling time" in part (a) if 7% interest is compounded daily? (Use 365 days per year for every year, including leap year.)

B.4. (a) Find a formula which tells how many years it will take for an investment of k dollars to double at an interest rate of 7% per year, compounded annually.

(b) Do part (a) with 7% replaced by r% (r constant).

B.5. (a) How long will it take to triple your money if you invest $500 at a rate of 5% per year, compounded annually?

(b) How long will it take if the 5% interest is compounded quarterly?

B.6. At what rate of interest (compounded annually) should you invest $500 if you want to have $1500 in 12 years?

B.7. How much money should be invested in a bank that pays 5% interest (compounded quarterly) so that 9 years later the balance will be $5000?

B.8. Under normal conditions, the atmospheric pressure (in millibars) at height h feet above sea level is given by $P(h) = 1015e^{-kh}$, where k is a positive constant.

(a) Assume that the pressure at 18,000 ft is half the pressure at sea level and find k.

(b) Using the information from part (a), determine the atmospheric pressure at these heights: 1000 ft, 5000 ft, 15,000 ft.

B.9. How old is a piece of ivory that has lost 36% of its carbon-14?

B.10. A certain radioactive substance loses one-third of its original mass in 5 days. Find its half-life.

B.11. The half-life of a certain substance is 3.6 days. How long will it take for 20 grams of the substance to decay to 3 grams?

B.12. In 1960 the population of the United States was 179 million, and in 1970 it was 203 million.
  (a) Use the population growth function to predict the population in 1990.
  (b) In what year will the population reach 416 million?
  (c) If you have a reasonably reliable estimate of the U.S. population for the current year, compare it to the number predicted by the growth function. How far apart are the two figures? What could account for the difference?

B.13. How old is a mummy that has lost 49 percent of its carbon-14?

B.14. An experiment is conducted with a certain culture. One hour after the experiment begins the number of bacteria in the culture is 100. Two hours after the experiment starts the number is 500. Assume that the time needed for the number of bacteria to double does not depend on the original number of bacteria at the beginning of the experiment.
  (a) Find the number of bacteria at the beginning of the experiment and the number 3 hours later.
  (b) How long does it take for the number of bacteria to double?

B.15. (a) Do Exercise B.3. on page 318.
  (b) Do Exercise B.4. on page 318.

The Complex Numbers

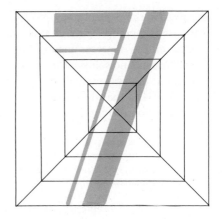

A new number system called the complex number system is introduced here. It contains the familiar real numbers, as well as solutions for equations such as $x^2 = -1$ which cannot be solved in the real number system. Although we shall consider only the mathematical properties of complex numbers, they have many practical applications in electrical engineering and other fields. Sections 2 and 3 both depend on Section 1, but Section 3 can be read before Section 2 if you wish.

1. THE COMPLEX NUMBER SYSTEM

When you began to study arithmetic in grade school, the only numbers you knew or used were the nonnegative integers. At the fifth grade level or thereabouts, fractions (that is, positive rational numbers) were introduced. In later grades other real numbers, such as π and $\sqrt{2}$ made their appearance. The number system was enlarged again in high school when negative numbers were introduced. At the beginning of this book, or even before, the entire real number system was presented.

Each time the number system is enlarged, it becomes possible to solve problems that were impossible in the original number system. For instance, a third grader, whose number system contains only integers, will tell you that the equation $7x = 19$ has no solution.° But a fifth grader, whose number system contains all positive rationals, will easily solve this equation.° Similarly, the equation $x^2 = 2$ has no solution in the system of rational numbers (see p. 2) but does have solutions in the real number system, namely, $x = \sqrt{2}$ and $x = -\sqrt{2}$.

Thus the idea of enlarging the number system in order to solve a problem that can't

---

° Of course, the equation would usually be presented to a third or fifth grader in somewhat different language, such as "Fill the box with a number that makes the sentence true: $7 \times \square = 19$."

be solved in the present number system is a perfectly natural one. You have been doing it for years, perhaps without even realizing it. And now we are about to do it again.

One of the shortcomings of the real number system is that some very simple equations have no solutions in this system. In particular, the equation $x^2 = -1$ has no solution in the real number system since the square of every real number is nonnegative. We claim that there is a larger number system that includes all the real numbers *and* a solution for the equation $x^2 = -1$. More specifically,

---

There is a number system, called the **complex number system,** *with these properties:*

 (i) *The complex number system contains the real number system.*

 (ii) *Addition, subtraction, multiplication, and division are defined in the complex number system and obey the same rules of arithmetic that hold in the real number system (as summarized in the boxes on pp. 5–7).*

 (iii) *The complex number system contains a number (usually denoted by* i) *such that* $i^2 = -1$.

 (iv) *Every complex number can be written in the standard form*

$$a + bi$$

where a *and* b *are real numbers and* $i^2 = -1$.°

 (v) *Two complex numbers* a + bi *and* c + di *are equal exactly when* a = c *and* b = d.

In view of our past experience with enlarging the number system, this claim *ought* to appear plausible. Nevertheless, we are so accustomed to saying that no negative number has a square root that it may seem strange to deal with a "number" i such that $i^2 = -1$, that is, such that $i = \sqrt{-1}$. This feeling of strangeness bothered many mathematicians in the seventeenth and eighteenth centuries when the complex number system was first developed. They showed their uneasiness by the terminology they chose, terminology that is still used today. The number i and multiples of it, such as

$$5i, \quad -\tfrac{3}{5}i, \quad \sqrt{7}i, \quad \text{and more generally,} \quad bi \quad (b \text{ any real number})$$

were called **imaginary numbers.** The old familiar numbers (the integers, rationals, and irrationals) were called **real numbers.** Sums of real and imaginary numbers, such as $7 + 5i$, $\sqrt{2} - \tfrac{3}{5}i$, $-6 + \tfrac{4}{9}i$ and more generally

$$a + bi \quad (a, b \text{ any real numbers})$$

were then called **complex numbers.**

° Hereafter, whenever we write $a + bi$ or $c + di$, it is assumed without explicit mention that a, b, c, d are real numbers and $i^2 = -1$.

Despite their name, imaginary numbers are no more "unreal" than rational or irrational numbers. Complex numbers are just as valid mathematical entities as are real numbers. The actual construction of the complex number system and the proof that it has the properties claimed in the box above are outlined in Exercise C.5. For now, we shall simply accept the existence of this new system and explore the arithmetic of complex numbers.

ARITHMETIC OF COMPLEX NUMBERS

According to property (iv) in the box above, the complex numbers consist of all sums $a + bi$ with a, b real numbers and $i^2 = -1$. In particular, when a is any real number and $b = 0$, the number $a + 0i$ is a complex number. But $a + 0i$ is just the real number a since

$$a + 0i = a + 0 = a°$$

For example, $3 = 3 + 0i$ and $-\sqrt{2} = -\sqrt{2} + 0i$. This shows exactly how the complex numbers contain the real numbers. Similarly, every imaginary number bi (with b real) is also a complex number since $bi = 0 + bi$. For instance, $7i = 0 + 7i$ and $-\frac{2}{3}i = 0 + (-\frac{2}{3})i$.

When performing arithmetic with complex numbers, you should usually put your answer in the standard form $a + bi$. Ordinarily this is quite easy, since the usual laws of arithmetic are valid.

EXAMPLE $(1 + i) + (3 - 7i) = 1 + i + 3 - 7i = (1 + 3) + (i - 7i) = 4 - 6i$.

EXAMPLE $(\frac{3}{2} + 6i) - (\frac{7}{2} + 2i) = \frac{3}{2} + 6i - \frac{7}{2} - 2i = (\frac{3}{2} - \frac{7}{2}) + (6i - 2i) = -\frac{4}{2} + 4i = -2 + 4i$.

EXAMPLE $4i(2 + \frac{3}{2}i) = 4i(2) + 4i(\frac{3}{2}i) = 8i + 4(\frac{3}{2})i^2 = 8i + 6i^2 = 8i + 6(-1) = -6 + 8i$.

EXAMPLE $(2 + i)(3 - 4i) = 2 \cdot 3 + 3i - 2 \cdot 4i - 4i^2 = 6 + 3i - 8i - 4(-1) = (6 + 4) + (3i - 8i) = 10 - 5i$.

As these examples demonstrate, you can *treat all symbols just as if they were real numbers providing that you replace i^2 by -1*. In particular, all of the multiplication and factoring patterns for real numbers, such as

$$(x + y)^2 = x^2 + 2xy + y^2 \quad \text{and} \quad (x + y)(x - y) = x^2 - y^2$$

are also valid for complex numbers.

EXAMPLE $(3 + 2i)(3 - 2i) = 3^2 - (2i)^2 = 9 - 4i^2 = 9 - 4(-1) = 9 + 4 = 13$. In this case, the product of two complex numbers turns out to be a positive real number.

° Remember that the usual rules of arithmetic still apply so that $z + 0 = z$ and $0z = 0$ for *every* number z.

The laws of exponents, such as $r^m r^n = r^{m+n}$ and $(r^m)^n = r^{mn}$ also hold for complex numbers.

EXAMPLE Find i^{54}. We begin with low powers of i:

$$i^2 = -1, \qquad i^3 = i^2 i = (-1)i = -i, \qquad i^4 = i^2 i^2 = (-1)(-1) = 1$$

Since $i^4 = 1$, we see that $i^8 = (i^4)^2 = 1^2 = 1$, $i^{12} = (i^4)^3 = 1^3 = 1$, and similarly, $i^{16} = 1$, $i^{20} = 1$, and so on. Now observe that $54 = 52 + 2 = 4 \cdot 13 + 2$, so that

$$i^{54} = i^{52+2} = i^{52} i^2 = i^{4 \cdot 13} i^2 = (i^4)^{13} i^2 = (1)^{13}(-1) = -1$$

CONJUGATES AND DIVISION

The **conjugate** of the complex number $a + bi$ is defined to be the number $a - bi$, and the conjugate of $a - bi$ is defined to be $a + bi$.

EXAMPLE The conjugate of $3 + 4i$ is $3 - 4i$. Since $3i = 0 + 3i$, the conjugate of $3i$ is $-3i$. The conjugate of $-5 - 2i$ is $-5 + 2i$. Since $17 = 17 + 0i = 17 - 0i$, the conjugate of 17 is 17 itself.

Here is a useful property of conjugates; other properties are discussed below:

> *The product of a complex number and its conjugate is a nonnegative real number.*

For example, we saw above that $(3 + 2i)(3 - 2i) = 9 - 4i^2 = 13$. More generally,

$$(a + bi)(a - bi) = a^2 - (bi)^2 = a^2 - b^2 i^2 = a^2 - b^2(-1) = a^2 + b^2$$

Since a^2 and b^2 are nonnegative real numbers, so is $a^2 + b^2$. This property of conjugates is very convenient when dividing complex numbers.

EXAMPLE Divide $3 + 4i$ by $1 + 2i$. As usual, we can write the answers as a fraction $(3 + 4i)/(1 + 2i)$. In order to express this fraction in the form $a + bi$, the first step is to *take the conjugate of the denominator*, namely, $1 - 2i$. Since $(1 - 2i)/(1 - 2i) = 1$, we have

$$\frac{3 + 4i}{1 + 2i} = \frac{3 + 4i}{1 + 2i} \cdot 1 = \frac{3 + 4i}{1 + 2i} \cdot \frac{1 - 2i}{1 - 2i} = \frac{(3 + 4i)(1 - 2i)}{(1 + 2i)(1 - 2i)}$$

$$= \frac{3 + 4i - 6i - 8i^2}{1^2 - (2i)^2} = \frac{3 + 4i - 6i - 8(-1)}{1 - 4i^2} = \frac{11 - 2i}{1 - 4(-1)}$$

$$= \frac{11 - 2i}{5} = \frac{11}{5} - \frac{2}{5}i$$

Thus we have expressed $(3 + 4i)/(1 + 2i)$ in the form $a + bi$, with $a = \frac{11}{5}$ and $b = -\frac{2}{5}$. This technique always works since the product of the denominator and its conjugate always gives a real number for the denominator of the quotient.

EXAMPLE To find $\dfrac{i}{2 + i} + \dfrac{3 + i}{1 - i}$, we first express everything in terms of a common denominator, namely, $(2 + i)(1 - i)$:

$$\frac{i}{2 + i} + \frac{3 + i}{1 - i} = \frac{i(1 - i)}{(2 + i)(1 - i)} + \frac{(2 + i)(3 + i)}{(2 + i)(1 - i)} = \frac{i(1 - i) + (2 + i)(3 + i)}{(2 + i)(1 - i)}$$

$$= \frac{i - i^2 + 6 + 3i + 2i + i^2}{2 + i - 2i - i^2} = \frac{6 + 6i}{3 - i}$$

Finally, we express this quotient in the form $a + bi$ as above:

$$\frac{i}{2 + i} + \frac{3 + i}{1 - i} = \frac{6 + 6i}{3 - i} = \frac{6 + 6i}{3 - i} \cdot \frac{3 + i}{3 + i} = \frac{18 + 18i + 6i + 6i^2}{9 - i^2}$$

$$= \frac{12 + 24i}{10} = \frac{12}{10} + \frac{24}{10}i = \frac{6}{5} + \frac{12}{5}i$$

PROPERTIES OF COMPLEX CONJUGATES

It is sometimes convenient to denote the complex number $a + bi$ by a single letter. If z is a complex number, then its conjugate is denoted by $\bar{z}$. Thus if $z = a + bi$, then $\bar{z} = a - bi$. Complex conjugation has these basic properties:

(i)   *For any complex number* z, *both* $z\bar{z}$ *and* $z + \bar{z}$ *are real numbers.*

(ii) *For any complex numbers* z *and* w,

$$\overline{z + w} = \bar{z} + \bar{w}, \qquad \overline{zw} = \bar{z} \cdot \bar{w}, \qquad \overline{\left(\frac{z}{w}\right)} = \frac{\bar{z}}{\bar{w}} \quad (w \neq 0)$$

(iii) $z = \bar{z}$ *exactly when* z *is a real number.*

The first part of statement (i) was proved on page 372. The other proofs are equally straightforward (see Exercise C.3), so we shall only illustrate them with some examples.

EXAMPLE (i) Suppose $z = 2 + 3i$ so that $\bar{z} = 2 - 3i$. Then

$$z + \bar{z} = (2 + 3i) + (2 - 3i) = 4$$

EXAMPLE (ii) Suppose $z = 2 + 3i$ as above and $w = 5 - i$. Then

$$zw = (2 + 3i)(5 - i) = 10 + 15i - 2i - 3i^2 = 13 + 13i$$

so that $\overline{zw} = 13 - 13i$. But

$$\bar{z} \cdot \bar{w} = (2 - 3i)(5 + i) = 10 - 15i + 2i - 3i^2 = 13 - 13i$$

Hence $\overline{zw} = \bar{z} \cdot \bar{w}$.

EXAMPLE (iii) $2 = 2 + 0i$ is a real number and $\bar{2} = 2 - 0i = 2$. Thus $2 = \bar{2}$.

ABSOLUTE VALUE

The **absolute value** of the complex number $a + bi$ is denoted $|a + bi|$ and is defined to be the real number $\sqrt{a^2 + b^2}$.

EXAMPLE $|3 + 2i| = \sqrt{3^2 + 2^2} = \sqrt{13}$. Similarly, $|4 - 5i| = \sqrt{4^2 + (-5)^2} = \sqrt{41}$.

The concept of absolute value for real numbers is just a special case of absolute value for complex numbers. Remember that for every real number c, we have $\sqrt{c^2} = |c|$ and $c = c + 0i$.

EXAMPLE $|5 + 0i| = \sqrt{5^2 + 0^2} = \sqrt{5^2} = |5|$ and $|-3 + 0i| = \sqrt{(-3)^2 + 0^2} = \sqrt{(-3)^2} = |-3|$.

The properties of absolute value for complex numbers are discussed in Exercise C.4 and include these:

For any complex numbers z *and* w:

$$|z| = |\bar{z}|, \qquad |z|^2 = z\bar{z}, \qquad |zw| = |z| \cdot |w|,$$

$$\left| \frac{z}{w} \right| = \frac{|z|}{|w|} \quad (w \neq 0)$$

THE COMPLEX PLANE

The real number system can be represented geometrically by a straight line. Each point on such a number line corresponds to a real number, and vice versa. In an analogous fashion the complex number system can be represented geometrically by the ordinary coordinate plane:

The complex number $a + bi$ corresponds to the point (a, b) on the plane

In other words, the point (a, b) is labeled by the complex number $a + bi$. For example, see Figure 7-1.

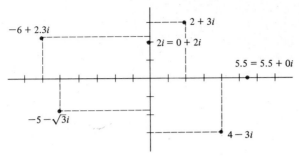

Figure 7-1

When the coordinate plane is labeled by complex numbers in this way, it is called the **complex plane.** Each real number $a = a + 0i$ corresponds to the point $(a, 0)$ on the horizontal axis. Consequently, the horizontal axis is called the **real axis.** Similarly, since each imaginary number $bi = 0 + bi$ corresponds to the point $(0, b)$, the vertical axis is called the **imaginary axis.**

Recall that the absolute value of the complex number $a + bi$ is defined to be the real number $|a + bi| = \sqrt{a^2 + b^2}$. Absolute values have a convenient geometric interpretation:

> The distance from a + bi to 0 in the complex plane is |a + bi|,

For the distance from $a + bi$ to 0 is just the distance from the point (a, b) to the point $(0, 0)$. It is given by the distance formula:

$$\sqrt{(a - 0)^2 + (b - 0)^2} = \sqrt{a^2 + b^2} = |a + bi|$$

Addition of complex numbers has an interesting geometric interpretation. For details, see Exercise C.6.

EXERCISES

Directions Express all numerical answers in the form $a + bi$ (a, b real numbers).

A.1. Perform the indicated addition or subtraction.
 (a) $(2 + 3i) + (6 - i)$
 (b) $(-5 + 7i) + (14 + 3i)$

 (c) $(2 - 8i) - (4 + 2i)$

 (d) $(3 + 5i) - (3 - 7i)$

 (e) $\frac{5}{4} - (\frac{7}{4} + 2i)$
 (f) $(\sqrt{3} + i) + (\sqrt{5} - 2i)$

 (g) $\left(\dfrac{\sqrt{2}}{2} + i\right) - \left(\dfrac{\sqrt{3}}{2} - i\right)$

 (h) $\left(\dfrac{1}{2} + \dfrac{\sqrt{3}i}{2}\right) + \left(\dfrac{3}{4} - \dfrac{5\sqrt{3}i}{2}\right)$

A.2. Multiply.

(a) $(2 + i)(3 + 5i)$

(b) $(2 - i)(5 + 2i)$

(c) $(-3 + 2i)(4 - i)$

(d) $(4 + 3i)(4 - 3i)$

(e) $(2 - 5i)^2$

(f) $(1 + i)(2 - i)i$

(g) $(\sqrt{3} + i)(\sqrt{3} - i)$

(h) $(\frac{1}{2} - i)(\frac{1}{4} + 2i)$

A.3. Multiply.

(a) i^{15} (b) i^{26} (c) i^{33} (d) $(-i)^{53}$ (e) $(-i)^{107}$

A.4. Find $\bar{z}$, $\bar{w}$, and $\overline{zw}$.

(a) $z = 1 + i$; $w = 2i$

(b) $z = -2 - 2i$; $w = 3i$

(c) $z = 4 - 5i$; $w = 2 - 3i$

(d) $z = (1 + i)^2$; $w = 1 - 2i$

A.5. Plot the point in the complex plane corresponding to each of these numbers:

(a) $3 + 2i$

(b) $-7 + 6i$

(c) $-\frac{8}{3} - \frac{5}{3}i$

(d) $\sqrt{2} - 7i$

(e) $(1 + i)(1 - i)$

(f) $(2 + i)(1 - 2i)$

(g) $(2i)(3 - \frac{5}{2}i)$

(h) $(\frac{4}{3}i)(-6 - 3i)$

B.1. Divide.

(a) $\dfrac{1}{5 - 2i}$

(b) $\dfrac{1}{i}$

(c) $\dfrac{1}{3i}$

(d) $\dfrac{i}{2 + i}$

(e) $\dfrac{3}{4 + 5i}$

(f) $\dfrac{2 + 3i}{i}$

(g) $\dfrac{7 - 4i}{2i}$

(h) $\dfrac{2 + 3i}{1 + i}$

B.2. Divide. (*Hint*: first multiply out the denominator.)

(a) $\dfrac{1}{i(4 + 5i)}$

(b) $\dfrac{1}{(2 - i)(2 + i)}$

(c) $\dfrac{2 + 3i}{i(4 + i)}$

(d) $\dfrac{2}{(2 + 3i)(4 + i)}$

(e) $\dfrac{2 + 3i}{(3 + 2i)(3 - i)}$

(f) $\dfrac{5 - 3i}{(2 - 4i)^2}$

B.3. Compute:

(a) $\dfrac{2 + i}{1 - i} + \dfrac{1}{1 + 2i}$

(b) $\dfrac{1}{2 - i} + \dfrac{3 + i}{2 + 3i}$

(c) $\dfrac{i}{3 + i} - \dfrac{3 + i}{4 + i}$

(d) $6 + \dfrac{2i}{3 + i}$

(e) $\dfrac{1 - i}{4 + 3i} - 2i$

(f) $\dfrac{1}{(1 - i)(2 + 3i)} + \dfrac{2 + 3i}{i + 5}$

B.4. Give an example of complex numbers, z and w, such that $|z + w| \neq |z| + |w|$.

B.5. Find these absolute values.

(a) $|5 - 12i|$

(b) $|2i|$

(c) $|1 + \sqrt{2}i|$

(d) $|2 - 3i|$

(e) $|-12i|$

(f) $|i^7|$

(g) $|i(3 + i)| + |3 - i|$

(h) $|3 + 2i| - |1 + 2i|$

(i) $\left| \dfrac{1 + i}{3 - 5i} \right|$

B.6. Simplify: $i + i^2 + i^3 + \cdots + i^{15}$.

B.7. Solve for x and y. (*Example:* $2x + 3i = 4 + yi$. Remember that $a + bi = c + di$ exactly when $a = c$ and $b = d$. Hence $2x + 3i = 4 + yi$ exactly when $2x = 4$ and $3 = y$. Thus $x = 2$ and $y = 3$ are the solutions.)

(a) $3x - 4i = 6 + 2yi$

(b) $8 - 2yi = 4x + 12i$

(c) $3 + 4xi = 2y - 3i$

(d) $8 - xi = \frac{1}{2}y + 2i$

B.8. Sketch the graph of these equations in the complex plane (z denotes a complex number):

(a) $|z| = 4$

(b) $|z| = 1$

(c) $\text{Re}(z) = -5$ (See Exercise C.1.)

(d) $\text{Im}(z) = 2$

C.1. The **real part** of the complex number $z = a + bi$ is defined to be the number a and is denoted $\text{Re}(z)$. The **imaginary part** of $z = a + bi$ is defined to be the number b (*not* bi) and is denoted $\text{Im}(z)$.

(a) Show that $\text{Re}(z) = \dfrac{z + \bar{z}}{2}$

(b) Show that $\text{Im}(z) = \dfrac{z - \bar{z}}{2i}$

C.2. If $z = a + bi$ (a, b fixed real numbers), find $\dfrac{1}{z}$.

C.3. Let $z = a + bi$ and $w = c + di$ (a, b, c, d fixed real numbers).

(a) Find $\bar{z}$ and $z + \bar{z}$. Verify that $z + \bar{z}$ is a real number.

(b) Find $z + w$ and $\overline{z + w}$.

(c) Find $\bar{w}$ and $\bar{z} + \bar{w}$. Verify that $\overline{z + w} = \bar{z} + \bar{w}$.

(d) Show that $\overline{zw} = \bar{z} \cdot \bar{w}$.

C.4. Let $z = a + bi$ and $w = c + di$ (a, b, c, d fixed real numbers).

(a) Find $\bar{z}$, $|\bar{z}|$ and $|z|$. Verify that $|z| = |\bar{z}|$.

(b) Show that $|z|^2 = z\bar{z}$.

(c) Find zw and $|zw|$.

(d) Find $|w|$ and $|z| \cdot |w|$. Verify that $|zw| = |z| \cdot |w|$ [see part (c)].

(e) Assume $w \neq 0$. Find $\dfrac{z}{w}$ and $\left|\dfrac{z}{w}\right|$.

(f) Find $\dfrac{|z|}{|w|}$ and verify that $\left|\dfrac{z}{w}\right| = \dfrac{|z|}{|w|}$.

C.5. **Construction of the Complex Numbers.** We assume that the real number system is known. In order to construct a new number system with the desired properties, we must do the following:

(i) Define a set C (whose elements will be called complex numbers).

(ii) The set C must contain the real numbers, or at least a copy of them.

(iii) Define addition and multiplication in the set C in such a way that the usual laws of arithmetic are valid.

(iv) Show that C has the other properties listed in the box on page 370.

We begin by defining C to be the set of all ordered pairs of real numbers. Thus $(1, 5), (-6, 0), (\frac{4}{3}, -17)$, and $(\sqrt{2}, \frac{12}{5})$ are some of the elements of the set C. More generally, a complex number ($=$ element of C) is any pair (a, b) where a and b

are real numbers. By definition, two complex numbers are *equal* exactly when they have the same first and the same second coordinate.

(a)   *Addition in C* is defined by this rule:

$$(a, b) + (c, d) = (a + c, b + d)$$

For example, $(3, 2) + (5, 4) = (3 + 5, 2 + 4) = (8, 6)$. Similarly, $(-1, 2) + (3, -5) = ((-1) + 3, 2 + (-5)) = (2, -3)$. Verify that this addition has the following properties. For any complex numbers $(a, b), (c, d), (e, f)$ in C:

(i) $(a, b) + (c, d) = (c, d) + (a, b)$
(ii) $((a, b) + (c, d)) + (e, f) = (a, b) + ((c, d) + (e, f))$
(iii) $(a, b) + (0, 0) = (a, b)$
(iv) $(a, b) + (-a, -b) = (0, 0)$

(b)   *Multiplication in C* is defined by this rule:

$$(a, b)(c, d) = (ac - bd, bc + ad)$$

For example, $(3, 2)(4, 5) = (3 \cdot 4 - 2 \cdot 5, 2 \cdot 4 + 3 \cdot 5) = (12 - 10, 8 + 15) = (2, 23)$. Similarly, $(\frac{1}{2}, 1)(-2, 1) = (\frac{1}{2}(-2) - 1 \cdot 1, 1(-2) + \frac{1}{2} \cdot 1) = (-2, -\frac{3}{2})$. Verify that this multiplication has the following properties. For any complex numbers $(a, b), (c, d), (e, f)$ in C:

(i) $(a, b)(c, d) = (c, d)(a, b)$
(ii) $((a, b)(c, d))(e, f) = (a, b)((c, d)(e, f))$
(iii) $(a, b)(1, 0) = (a, b)$
(iv) $(a, b)(0, 0) = (0, 0)$

(c)   Since C consists of ordered pairs, we can think of C as being the set of points in the coordinate plane. Verify that for any two points on the x-axis (that is, any elements of C with second coordinate zero):

(i) $(a, 0) + (c, 0) = (a + c, 0)$
(ii) $(a, 0)(c, 0) = (ac, 0)$

Now consider the x-axis as a number line in the usual way: *identify* $(t, 0)$ on the x-axis with the real number t. Statements (i) and (ii) show that when addition or multiplication in C is performed on two real numbers (that is, points on the x-axis), the result is the usual sum or product of real numbers. Thus C contains (a copy of) the real number system.

(d)   *New Notation.* Since we are identifying the complex number $(a, 0)$ with the real number a, we shall hereafter denote $(a, 0)$ simply by the symbol a. Also, let i denote the complex number $(0, 1)$.

(i)   Show that $i^2 = -1$ [that is, $(0, 1)(0, 1) = (-1, 0)$].

(ii)   Show that for any complex number $(0, b)$, $(0, b) = bi$ [that is, $(0, b) = (b, 0)(0, 1)$].

(iii) Show that any complex number (a, b) can be written: $(a, b) = a + bi$ [that is, $(a, b) = (a, 0) + (b, 0)(0, 1)$].

In this new notation, every complex number is of the form $a + bi$ with a, b real and $i^2 = -1$, and our construction is finished.

C.6.   The sum of two distinct complex numbers, $a + bi$ and $c + ci$, can be found geometrically by means of the so-called **parallelogram rule:** plot the points $a + bi$ and $c + di$ in the complex plane and form the parallelogram three of whose vertices are 0, $a + bi$, and $c + di$; for example, see Figure 7-2.

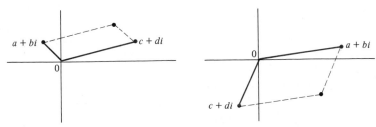

Figure 7-2

Then the fourth vertex of the parallelogram is the point whose coordinate is the sum $(a + bi) + (c + di) = (a + c) + (b + d)i$. Here is a *proof* of the parallelogram rule when $a \neq 0$ and $c \neq 0$.

(a)   Find the *slope* of the line K from 0 to $a + bi$. [*Hint:* K contains the points $(0, 0)$ and (a, b).]

(b)   Find the *slope* of the line N from 0 to $c + di$.

(c)   Find the *equation* of the line L, through $a + bi$ and parallel to line N of part (b). [*Hint:* the point (a, b) is on L; find the slope of L by using (b) and facts about the slopes of parallel lines.]

(d)   Find the *equation* of the line M, through $c + di$ and parallel to line K. [*Hint:* part (a) may be helpful.]

(e)   Label the lines K, L, M, N in Figure 7-2.

(f)   Show by substitution that the point $(a + c, b + d)$ satisfies both the equation of line L and the equation of line M. Therefore $(a + c, b + d)$ lies on both L and M. Since the only point on both L and M is the fourth vertex of the parallelogram (see Figure 7-2), this vertex must be $(a + c, b + d)$. Hence this vertex has coordinate $(a + c) + (b + d)i = (a + bi) + (c + di)$.

2. EQUATIONS AND COMPLEX NUMBERS

The system of complex numbers was constructed in order to obtain a solution for the equation $x^2 = -1$. In this section we shall see that the complex numbers contain solutions for many other equations as well.

SQUARE ROOTS

Since $i^2 = -1$, it seems reasonable to say that i is the square root of -1 and to write $i = \sqrt{-1}$. Similarly, since $(5i)^2 = 5^2 i^2 = 25(-1) = -25$, we define $\sqrt{-25}$ to be the complex number $5i$. More generally, any *positive* real number b has a real square root $\sqrt{b}$ and

$$(\sqrt{b}\,i)^2 = (\sqrt{b^2})i^2 = b(-1) = -b$$

Consequently $\sqrt{-b}$ is defined to be the complex number $\sqrt{b}\,i$. Thus

> *Every real number (in particular, every negative one) has a square root in the complex number system.*

EXAMPLE $\sqrt{-3} = \sqrt{3}i$ since $(\sqrt{3}i)^2 = (\sqrt{3})^2 i^2 = 3(-1) = -3$. Similarly, $\sqrt{-\frac{81}{4}} = \frac{9}{2}i$ since $\sqrt{\frac{81}{4}} = \frac{9}{2}$ and $(\frac{9}{2}i)^2 = (\frac{9}{2})^2 i^2 = \frac{81}{4}(-1) = -\frac{81}{4}$.

Many expressions that are not defined in the real number system now make sense in the complex number system.

EXAMPLE $\dfrac{1 + \sqrt{-3}}{2} = \dfrac{1 + \sqrt{3}i}{2} = \dfrac{1}{2} + \dfrac{\sqrt{3}}{2}i$.

EXAMPLE $\sqrt{-20}\,\sqrt{-5} = (\sqrt{20}i)(\sqrt{5}i) = \sqrt{20}\,\sqrt{5}i^2 = \sqrt{100}i^2 = 10(-1) = -10$.

Warning The property of radicals $\sqrt{cd} = \sqrt{c}\,\sqrt{d}$, which is valid for positive real numbers, *does not hold* when both c and d are negative. For instance, suppose $c = -20$ and $d = -5$. The preceding example shows that $\sqrt{c}\,\sqrt{d} = \sqrt{-20}\,\sqrt{-5} = -10$. But $\sqrt{cd} = \sqrt{(-20)(-5)} = \sqrt{100} = 10$. So $\sqrt{c}\,\sqrt{d} \neq \sqrt{cd}$. To avoid difficulty, always write square roots of negative numbers in terms of i *before* doing any simplifying.

POLYNOMIAL EQUATIONS WITH REAL COEFFICIENTS

Since every negative real number has a square root in the complex number system, we can now find complex solutions for equations that have no real solutions. For example, the solutions of $x^2 = -25$ are $x = \pm\sqrt{-25} = \pm 5i$ and the solutions of $x^2 = -3$ are $x = \pm\sqrt{-3} = \pm\sqrt{3}i$. In fact, the examples below show that

> *Every quadratic equation with real coefficients has solutions in the complex number system.*

EXAMPLE To solve the equation $2x^2 + x + 3 = 0$, we apply the quadratic formula:

$$x = \frac{-1 \pm \sqrt{1^2 - 4 \cdot 2 \cdot 3}}{2 \cdot 2} = \frac{-1 \pm \sqrt{-23}}{4}$$

Since $\sqrt{-23}$ is not a real number, this equation has no real number solutions. But $\sqrt{-23}$ *is* a complex number, namely, $\sqrt{-23} = \sqrt{23}i$. Thus the equation does have solutions in the complex number system:

$$x = \frac{-1 \pm \sqrt{-23}}{4} = \frac{-1 \pm \sqrt{23}i}{4} = -\frac{1}{4} \pm \frac{\sqrt{23}}{4}i$$

Note that the two solutions, $-\frac{1}{4} + \frac{\sqrt{23}}{4}i$ and $-\frac{1}{4} - \frac{\sqrt{23}}{4}i$, are conjugates of each other.

EXAMPLE To find *all* solutions of $x^3 = 1$, we rewrite the equation and factor:

$$x^3 = 1$$
$$x^3 - 1 = 0$$
$$(x - 1)(x^2 + x + 1) = 0$$
$$x - 1 = 0 \quad \text{or} \quad x^2 + x + 1 = 0$$

The solution of the first equation is $x = 1$. The solutions of the second can be obtained from the quadratic formula:

$$x = \frac{-1 \pm \sqrt{1^2 - 4 \cdot 1 \cdot 1}}{2 \cdot 1} = \frac{-1 \pm \sqrt{-3}}{2} = \frac{-1 \pm \sqrt{3}i}{2} = \frac{-1}{2} \pm \frac{\sqrt{3}}{2}i$$

Therefore the equation $x^3 = 1$ has one real solution ($x = 1$) and two complex solutions $[x = -\frac{1}{2} + (\sqrt{3}/2)i$ and $x = -\frac{1}{2} - (\sqrt{3}/2)i]$. Each of these solutions is said to be a **cube root of one** or a **cube root of unity**. Observe that the two complex cube roots of unity are conjugates of each other.

The preceding examples illustrate this useful fact:

> *Let* f(x) *be a polynomial with real coefficients. If a complex number* z *is a root of* f(x), *then its conjugate* $\bar{z}$ *is also a root of* f(x).

A formal proof is outlined in Exercise C.1. Before giving examples of how this fact is used, we must first introduce polynomials whose coefficients are complex numbers, such as:

$$x + 5i, \quad x - (3 + i), \quad 3x^2 + (1 + 2i)x + (i - 1), \quad (1 - 7i)x^4 + 5ix^3 + (2 + i)x - 8$$

The discussion of polynomials with real coefficients on pp. 35–39 and 258–261 depends only on the fact that the arithmetic of real numbers obeys certain rules. Since the arithmetic of complex numbers obeys the same basic rules, *the entire discussion is also valid for polynomials with complex coefficients.* In particular, the Division Algorithm, the Remainder Theorem, and the Factor Theorem are true for such polynomials.

EXAMPLE Find a polynomial with *real* coefficients whose roots include the numbers 2 and $3 + i$. Since $3 + i$ is to be a root, the fact in the box above shows that its conjugate $3 - i$ must also be a root. Since a product is 0 in the complex number system only when one of its factors is 0, the polynomial

$$f(x) = (x - 2)(x - (3 + i))(x - (3 - i))$$

obviously has roots 2, $3 + i$, and $3 - i$. Now this polynomial *appears* to have nonreal coefficients. However, multiplying out and simplifying yields:

$$\begin{aligned}
f(x) &= (x - 2)(x - (3 + i))(x - (3 - i)) \\
&= (x - 2)(x^2 - (3 + i)x - (3 - i)x + (3 + i)(3 - i)) \\
&= (x - 2)(x^2 - 3x - ix - 3x + ix + (3^2 - i^2)) \\
&= (x - 2)(x^2 - 6x + 10) = x^3 - 8x^2 + 22x - 20
\end{aligned}$$

Thus $f(x) = x^3 - 8x^2 + 22x - 20$ is a polynomial with real coefficients whose roots are 2, $3 + i$, and $3 - i$.

EXAMPLE Given that $z = 1 + i$ is a root of the polynomial $f(x) = x^4 - 2x^3 - x^2 + 6x - 6$, find all of its roots. According to the fact in the box above, the conjugate $\overline{z} = 1 - i$ must also be a root of $f(x)$. By the Factor Theorem (p. 260), both $x - z$ and $x - \overline{z}$ are factors of $f(x)$. Therefore the product $(x - z)(x - \overline{z})$ is a factor of $f(x)$. But

$$\begin{aligned}
(x - z)(x - \overline{z}) &= (x - (1 + i))(x - (1 - i)) \\
&= x^2 - (1 + i)x - (1 - i)x + (1 + i)(1 - i) \\
&= x^2 - x - ix - x + ix + (1 - i^2) \\
&= x^2 - 2x + 2
\end{aligned}$$

Thus $x^2 - 2x + 2$ is a factor of $f(x)$. Long division shows that the other factor is $x^2 - 3$. Consequently, $f(x) = x^4 - 2x^3 - x^2 + 6x - 6 = (x^2 - 2x + 2)(x^2 - 3)$ and its roots are easily found:

$$x^4 - 2x^3 - x^2 + 6x - 6 = 0$$
$$(x^2 - 2x + 2)(x^2 - 3) = 0$$
$$x^2 - 2x + 2 = 0 \quad \text{or} \quad x^2 - 3 = 0$$

The solutions of the first equation are $1 + i$ and $1 - i$, as can be seen from our work above or from the quadratic formula. The solutions of $x^2 - 3 = 0$ are obviously $x = \pm\sqrt{3}$. Therefore $f(x)$ has roots $1 + i$, $1 - i$, $\sqrt{3}$, and $-\sqrt{3}$.

THE FUNDAMENTAL THEOREM OF ALGEBRA

The complex numbers were constructed in order to obtain a solution for the equation $x^2 = -1$. As we have just seen, they contain a good deal more—solutions for every quadratic equation with real coefficients. A natural question now arises:

> Do the complex numbers contain solutions for *every* polynomial equation with real or complex coefficients?

If the answer to this question were no, it would be necessary to enlarge the complex number system (perhaps many times) in order to obtain solutions for complicated high-degree polynomial equations. Fortunately, and perhaps surprisingly, the answer to the question turns out to be yes. Since every real number is also a complex number and since solving polynomial equations is equivalent to finding the roots of certain polynomials, the formal answer to the question is usually phrased like this:

THE FUNDAMENTAL THEOREM OF ALGEBRA

Every nonconstant polynomial with complex coefficients has a root in the complex number system.

Although this is obviously a powerful result, neither the Fundamental Theorem nor its proof provide a practical method for actually *finding* a root of a given polynomial.° The proof of the Fundamental Theorem will be omitted since it involves mathematical concepts beyond the scope of this book. But we shall explore some of the theorem's implications, which are sometimes useful for understanding and analyzing various problems.

Here is one consequence of the Fundamental Theorem:

Suppose $f(x)$ *is a polynomial with complex coefficients with degree* $n > 0$ *and leading coefficient* d. *Then there are (not necessarily distinct) complex numbers* $c_1, c_2, c_3, \ldots, c_n$ *such that*

$$f(x) = d(x - c_1)(x - c_2)(x - c_3) \cdots (x - c_n)$$

This statement is proved below. To understand its meaning, we consider a specific example. Suppose

$$f(x) = 5x^3 - (10 + 10i)x^2 + (-5 + 20i)x + 10$$

° It may seem strange that it is possible to prove that a root exists without actually exhibiting one. But such "existence theorems" are quite common in mathematics. A very rough analogy is the situation that occurs when a person walking the street is killed by a sniper's bullet. The police know that there *is* a killer, but actually *finding* the killer may be difficult or even impossible.

In this case, $n = 3$, the degree of $f(x)$, and $d = 5$, the leading coefficient of $f(x)$. By multiplying out the right side below, you will see that $f(x)$ factors as:

$$f(x) = 5(x - 2)(x - i)(x - i)$$

so that $c_1 = 2$, $c_2 = i$, and $c_3 = i$.

In order to prove the statement in the box above, suppose $f(x)$ is a polynomial of positive degree n with complex coefficients. According to the Fundamental Theorem, $f(x)$ has a root in the complex number system—call it c_1. Consequently, by the Factor Theorem (p. 260), $x - c_1$ is a factor of $f(x)$. Thus

$$f(x) = (x - c_1)g(x)$$

for some polynomial $g(x)$. Since $g(x)$ is the quotient when $f(x)$ is divided by the first-degree polynomial $x - c_1$, the degree of $g(x)$ must be one less than the degree of $f(x)$. Now the Fundamental Theorem also applies to the polynomial $g(x)$: if $g(x)$ is not a constant, it must have a root in the complex number system—call this root c_2. The Factor Theorem shows that $x - c_2$ is a factor of $g(x)$, so that $g(x) = (x - c_2)h(x)$ for some polynomial $h(x)$. Just as before, $h(x)$ has degree one less than the degree of $g(x)$. Thus

$$f(x) = (x - c_1)g(x) = (x - c_1)(x - c_2)h(x)$$

If $h(x)$ is not a constant, it must have a root—call it c_3—and the same argument can be applied again. As long as the last factor is not constant, we can keep repeating the argument. At each step the degree of the last factor goes down by one. Since $f(x)$ has degree n, we see that after n steps the last factor will have degree 0. In other words, the last factor will be a nonzero constant—call it d. At this point, we have $f(x)$ factored in the desired form:

$$f(x) = (x - c_1)(x - c_2)(x - c_3) \cdots (x - c_n)d$$

Multiplying out the right side of this equation shows that

$$f(x) = dx^n + \text{lower degree terms}$$

Thus the constant d is actually the leading coefficient of $f(x)$. This completes the proof.

When a polynomial $f(x)$ of degree $n > 0$ is written in factored form as

$$f(x) = d(x - c_1)(x - c_2) \cdots (x - c)_n \quad (d \neq 0)$$

it is easy to see that the numbers $c_1, c_2, \ldots, c_n$ are roots of $f(x)$. Furthermore, every root of $f(x)$ must be one of these numbers. For if k is any root of $f(x)$, then

$$0 = f(k) = d(k - c_1)(k - c_2) \cdots (k - c_n) \quad (d \neq 0)$$

The product on the right is 0 only when one of the factors is 0, that is, when

$$k - c_1 = 0 \quad \text{or} \quad k - c_2 = 0 \quad \text{or} \quad \cdots \quad k - c_n = 0$$
$$k = c_1 \quad \text{or} \quad k = c_2 \quad \text{or} \quad \cdots \quad k = c_n$$

Therefore k is indeed one of the c's. Since there may be some repetitions in the list of roots $c_1, c_1, \ldots, c_n$ we conclude that:

> *Every polynomial of degree* n > 0 *with complex coefficients has at most* n *distinct roots in the complex number system.*

Suppose a number c is a root of a polynomial $f(x)$ of degree $n > 0$. If $f(x)$ is written in factored form as above, then c appears one or more times on the list of roots c_1, $c_2, \ldots, c_n$. If c appears *exactly* k times on the list, then $f(x)$ has exactly k factors of the form $x - c$. Hence $(x - c)^k$ is a factor of $f(x)$ and no higher power of $x - c$ is a factor of $f(x)$. Therefore c is a root of *multiplicity* k (as defined on p. 261) and we see that

> *A polynomial of degree* n > 0 *with complex coefficients has exactly* n *roots in the complex number system, provided that each root is counted as many times as its multiplicity.*

EXERCISES

Directions   Express all complex answers in the form $a + bi$ unless directed otherwise.

A.1.   Express in terms of i:
    (a) $\sqrt{-36}$ **(c)** $\sqrt{-14}$ **(e)** $-\sqrt{-16}$
    (b) $\sqrt{-81}$ **(d)** $\sqrt{-50}$ **(f)** $-\sqrt{-12}$

A.2.   Express in terms of i and simplify:
    (a) $\sqrt{-16} + \sqrt{-49}$ **(d)** $\sqrt{-12}\sqrt{-3}$ **(g)** $\sqrt{-16}/\sqrt{-36}$
    (b) $\sqrt{-25} - \sqrt{-9}$ **(e)** $\sqrt{-8}\sqrt{-6}$ **(h)** $-\sqrt{-64}/\sqrt{-4}$
    (c) $\sqrt{-15} - \sqrt{-18}$ **(f)** $-\sqrt{-10}\sqrt{-6}$

A.3.   Simplify:
    (a) $(\sqrt{-25} + 2)(\sqrt{-49} - 3)$ **(e)** $\sqrt{-2}(\sqrt{2} + \sqrt{-2})$
    (b) $(5 - \sqrt{-3})(-1 + \sqrt{-9})$ **(f)** $(5 - \sqrt{-1})(3 + \sqrt{-2})$
    (c) $(2 + \sqrt{-5})(1 - \sqrt{-10})$ **(g)** $1/(1 + \sqrt{-2})$
    (d) $\sqrt{-3}(3 - \sqrt{-27})$ **(h)** $(1 + \sqrt{-4})/(3 - \sqrt{-9})$

B.1.   Solve these equations:
    (a) $x^2 - 2x + 5 = 0$ **(c)** $5x^2 + 2x + 1 = 0$ **(e)** $x + 6 = 2x^2$
    (b) $x^2 - 4x + 13 = 0$ **(d)** $x^2 + 5x = -12$ **(f)** $5x^2 + 3 = 2x$

B.2.   Solve these equations. (Hint: factor first.)
    (a) $x^3 - 27 = 0$ **(c)** $x^3 = -8$ **(e)** $x^4 - 1 = 0$
    (b) $x^3 + 125 = 0$ **(d)** $x^6 - 64 = 0$ **(f)** $x^4 - x^2 - 6 = 0$

B.3. Find a polynomial with *real* coefficients whose roots include the given numbers.
(a) $2 + i$, $2 - i$ (c) 2, $2 + i$ (e) -1, i
(b) $1 + 3i$, $1 - 3i$ (d) i, $2i$ (f) -3, $1 - i$, $1 + 2i$

B.4. Find all roots of the given polynomial. In each case, one root is given.
(a) $x^4 - x^3 - 5x^2 - x - 6$;   root i
(b) $x^3 + x^2 + x + 1$;   root i
(c) $x^4 - 4x^3 + 6x^2 - 4x + 5$;   root $2 - i$
(d) $x^4 - 5x^3 + 10x^2 - 20x + 24$;   root $2i$

B.5. Find a polynomial with *real* coefficients having the given degree and roots:
(a) degree 2;   roots $1 + 2i$ and $1 - 2i$
(b) degree 4;   roots $3i$ and $-3i$, each of multiplicity 2
(c) degree 6;   0 is a root of multiplicity 3;   and 3, $1 + i$, and $1 - i$ are each roots of multiplicity 1.

Note: Exercises B.6–B.8 deal with polynomial equations with *complex* coefficients. The techniques for solving such equations are essentially the same ones used with real coefficients.

B.6. Solve these equations. [*Hint:* first collect all terms involving the unknown x on the left side and the other terms on the right. For example, $x - 4i = 3 - 2ix$ becomes $x + 2ix = 3 + 4i$ so that $(1 + 2i)x = 3 + 4i$. Dividing both sides by $1 + 2i$ shows that $x = (3 + 4i)/(1 + 2i)$. The final step is to express this solution in the form $a + bi$.]
(a) $3x = 2 + ix$
(b) $2ix = 1 - ix$
(c) $(7 + i)x - 3 = 2i + ix$
(d) $3x + (4 + 2i) + ix = (5 + i)x$
(e) $(3 + 2i)x + (3 + 2i) = (2 + i)x - (4 + 2i)$
(f) $2 + 3ix - (4 + 5i) = (4i - 3)x - 5i$
(g) $(5 - 3i)x + 4x - 1 = (1 - 4i)x + 7x - i$
(h) $(4 + 6i)x - 7 + i = (3 + 4i)x - (5 + 2i)$

B.7. It can be proved that every complex number has a square root. Assume this fact for now. Since the derivation of the quadratic formula depends only on the existence of square roots and the usual rules of arithmetic, the quadratic formula may be used to solve $ax^2 + bx + c = 0$, even when a, b, c are complex numbers. Solve the equations below, leaving square roots of complex numbers in the form $\sqrt{a + bi}$.
(a) $x^2 + ix - (2 + 3i) = 0$
(b) $x^2 + (1 + i)x - (1 + 2i) = 0$
(c) $ix^2 + (2 - i)x - (1 + i) = 0$
(d) $ix^2 + (1 - 2i)x + (2 + 3i) = 0$
(e) $(1 + i)x^2 + 3ix = 1 - 3i$
(f) $(2 - i)x^2 + (1 + i)x = -2 + 2i$

B.8. Find a polynomial with complex coefficients, having the given degree and given roots.

    (a) degree 2;   roots i and $1 - 2i$

    (b) degree 2;   roots $2i$ and $1 + i$

    (c) degree 3;   roots 3, i, and $2 - i$

    (d) degree 4;   roots $\sqrt{2}$, $-\sqrt{2}$, $1 + i$, and $1 - i$

C.1. Prove that if z is a root of a polynomial with real coefficients and degree 3, then so is $\bar{z}$, as follows. We know that $f(x) = ax^3 + bx^2 + cx + d$ for some fixed real numbers a, b, c, d and that $0 = f(z) = az^3 + bz^2 + cz + d$. Use facts (ii) and (iii) in the box on page 373 to show that:

    (a) $\overline{f(z)} = \bar{0} = 0$.

    (b) $\overline{f(z)} = \overline{az^3} + \overline{bz^2} + \overline{cz} + \bar{d}$.

    (c) $\overline{f(z)} = a\overline{z^3} + b\overline{z^2} + c\bar{z} + d$ [remember that a, b, c, d are real numbers].

    (d) $\overline{f(z)} = a\bar{z}^3 + b\bar{z}^2 + c\bar{z} + d = f(\bar{z})$.

    (e) $\bar{z}$ is a root of $f(x)$. [Use parts (a) and (d).]

    (f) Now suppose $f(x)$ is any polynomial with real coefficients and positive degree. Prove that if z is a root of $f(x)$, then so is $\bar{z}$. (*Hint:* except for notation, the proof is essentially the same as in the case of degree 3 done above.)

C.2. **(a)** Suppose z is a fixed complex number. Show that the polynomial $(x - z)(x - \bar{z})$ has *real* coefficients. [*Hint:* multiply out and use fact (i) in the box on p. 373.]

    (b) Let $f(x)$ be a nonconstant polynomial with real coefficients. By the Fundamental Theorem of Algebra $f(x) = d(x - c_1)(x - c_2) \cdots (x - c_n)$. If one of the roots c_i is complex (and *not* real), then some other root (say, c_j) must be its conjugate, $c_j = \bar{c_i}$ (why?). Use part (a) to show that $f(x)$ has as a factor a quadratic polynomial with *real* coefficients and roots c_i and c_j.

    (c) Prove that every nonconstant polynomial $f(x)$ with *real* coefficients is a product of factors, each of which is either (i) a first-degree polynomial with real coefficients or (ii) a quadratic polynomial with real coefficients and no real roots. [*Hint:* see part (b).]

Topics in Algebra

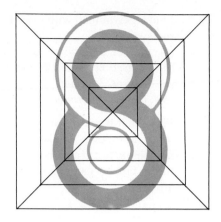

Section 1 deals with systems of linear equations. Such systems lead naturally to a discussion of matrices and determinants in Section 2. The last three sections (*The Binomial Theorem, Combinatorial Algebra, Mathematical Induction*) are independent of the first two sections and of each other. Any one of them can be read at any time.

1. SYSTEMS OF LINEAR EQUATIONS

In this section, we shall consider equations such as

$$2x + 3y = -7, \qquad 5x - y + 3z = 1, \qquad 4x + 2y - 8z + 23w = 0$$

that involve only the first powers of the unknowns and no higher powers (such as x^3, xy, xyz, y^2w, and so on). Such equations are called **linear equations.** Many applications of mathematics involve **systems of linear equations.** For example,

$$
\begin{aligned}
x + 2y &= 3, \\
5x - 4y &= -6,
\end{aligned}
\qquad
\begin{aligned}
2x + 5y + z + w &= 0, \\
2y - 4z + 3w &= 0, \\
2x + 17y - 23z + 41w &= 0,
\end{aligned}
\qquad
\begin{aligned}
x + 2y - 3z &= 1, \\
-3x + 2y + z &= 3, \\
2x + 2y - 5z &= 0
\end{aligned}
$$

two equations in two unknowns	three equations in four unknowns	three equations in three unknowns

A **solution of a system of equations** is a solution that satisfies *all* the equations in the system. For example, in the system of three equations in three unknowns shown at the right above,

$$x = 0, \qquad y = \tfrac{5}{4}, \qquad z = \tfrac{1}{2}$$

is a solution of all three equations (check it out) and hence is a solution for the system.

388

On the other hand,

$$x = \tfrac{1}{2}, \qquad y = \tfrac{7}{4}, \qquad z = 1$$

is a solution of the first two equations in the system, but not of the third one (check it). Therefore this is *not* a solution of the system. It can be shown that

---

For any system of linear equations, exactly one of the following statements is true:

(i)   The system has no solution.
(ii) The system has exactly one solution.
(iii) The system has infinitely many different solutions.

The examples below will illustrate all three possibilities.

THE SUBSTITUTION METHOD

Any system of two equations in two unknowns, as well as some larger systems, can be solved by means of substitution.

EXAMPLE   Any solution of the system

$$x + 2y = 3$$
$$5x - 4y = -6$$

must necessarily be a solution of the first equation. Hence x must satisfy

$$x + 2y = 3, \qquad \text{or equivalently,} \qquad x = 3 - 2y$$

Substituting this value of x in the second equation, we have:

$$5x - 4y = -6$$
$$5(3 - 2y) - 4y = -6$$
$$15 - 10y - 4y = -6$$
$$- 14y = -21$$
$$y = \tfrac{-21}{-14} = \tfrac{3}{2}$$

Therefore every solution of the original system must have $y = \tfrac{3}{2}$. But when $y = \tfrac{3}{2}$, we see from the first equation that:

$$x + 2y = 3$$
$$x + 2(\tfrac{3}{2}) = 3$$
$$x + 3 = 3$$
$$x = 0$$

(We would also have found that $x = 0$ if we had substituted $y = \tfrac{3}{2}$ in the second equation.) Consequently, the original system has exactly one solution: $x = 0$, $y = \tfrac{3}{2}$. This solution could also have been found by solving the first equation for y instead of x and substituting this value in the second equation.

Warning In order to guard against arithmetic mistakes, you should always *check your answers.* We have in fact checked the answers in all the examples. But these checks are omitted to save space.

The solutions of any system of equations in two unknowns can be interpreted geometrically by graphing each of the equations in the system. From Section 3 of Chapter 3, we know that each graph is a straight line. For instance, the graph of the equations in the preceding example is shown in Figure 8-1.

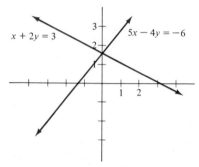

Figure 8-1

Each point on the line $x + 2y = 3$ represents a solution of this equation, and similarly for the line $5x - 4y = -6$. Since there is exactly one point on both lines, there is just one solution of the system of two equations. The geometric statement that the two lines intersect only at the point $(0, \frac{3}{2})$ is equivalent to the algebraic statement that the only solution of the system is $x = 0$, $y = \frac{3}{2}$.

THE ELIMINATION METHOD

In order to develop a systematic way of solving systems with three or more equations and unknowns, we first consider an example of a large system in which the substitution method can be used successfully.

EXAMPLE Any solution of this system of four equations in four unknowns

$$
\begin{aligned}
3x - 3y + 2z + w &= 4 \\
y - 3z + 2w &= -3 \\
z - 4w &= -8 \\
2w &= 6
\end{aligned}
$$

must necessarily be a solution of the last equation. Therefore w must satisfy

$$2w = 6, \quad \text{or equivalently,} \quad w = 3$$

Substituting $w = 3$ in the third equation shows that

$$
\begin{aligned}
z - 4w &= -8 \\
z - 4 \cdot 3 &= -8 \\
z &= -8 + 12 = 4
\end{aligned}
$$

Thus any solution of the original system must have $w = 3$ and $z = 4$. Substituting these values in the second equation yields:

$$y - \quad 3z + \quad 2w = -3$$
$$y - 3 \cdot 4 + 2 \cdot 3 = -3$$
$$y = -3 + 12 - 6 = 3$$

Finally, substituting $y = 3$, $z = 4$, and $w = 3$ in the first equation shows that

$$3x - \quad 3y + \quad 2z + w = 4$$
$$3x - 3 \cdot 3 + 2 \cdot 4 + \quad 3 = 4$$
$$3x = 4 + 9 - 8 - 3 = 2$$
$$x = \tfrac{2}{3}$$

Therefore the original system has just one solution: $x = \tfrac{2}{3}$, $y = 3$, $z = 4$, $w = 3$.

The substitution method works in the preceding example because of the particular form of the system (sometimes called **echelon form**): the unknown x appears in the first equation but not in any subsequent ones; the unknown y appears in the second equation, but not in any subsequent ones; and so on. Consequently, it is possible to begin with the last equation and solve for one unknown at a time.

The fact that a system of equations in echelon form can be solved, as in the example above, suggests a possible line of attack for solving *any* system of equations: replace the given system by another system that has the same solutions *and* is in echelon form. Then solve the new system. We shall now see that this can be accomplished in several steps by changing one or two equations at a time, in such a way that the system obtained by each change has the same solutions as the original system.

One operation that can be used in such a process is to:

> *Interchange any two equations in the system.*

For the order in which the equations are listed obviously doesn't affect their solutions. Another operation is to multiply both sides of an equation in the system by a nonzero constant. It is often convenient to state this operation in different words (but with the same meaning):

> *Replace an equation in the system by a nonzero constant multiple of itself.*

As we have seen before, multiplying an equation by a nonzero constant doesn't change the solutions of the equation. Thus replacing an equation in a system by a nonzero constant multiple of itself must necessarily produce a system with the same solutions as the original system.

A third operation that can be used here is one that we haven't seen before, so we begin with an example. Suppose a system of equations includes these two equations:

$$x + 4y - 3z = 1 \qquad \text{equation A}$$
$$-3x - 6y + \quad z = 3 \qquad \text{equation B}$$

(The system may include other equations as well, and equations A and B may not appear next to each other when the equations of the system are listed.) Any solution of the system is necessarily a solution of both equations A and B, and hence is also a solution of these two equations:

$$3x + 12y - 9z = 3 \qquad \text{3 times equation A}$$
$$-3x - 6y + z = 3 \qquad \text{equation B}$$

Now we know that if equal quantities are added to equal quantities, the sums are equal. Consequently, any solution of the two equations above must also satisfy the sum of those equations:

$$
\begin{array}{ll}
3x + 12y - 9z = 3 & \text{3 times equation A} \\
-3x - 6y + z = 3 & \text{equation B} \\
\hline
6y - 8z = 6 & \text{sum of equation B and 3 times equation A}
\end{array}
$$

Therefore any solution of the original system will also be a solution of the system obtained by

Replacing equation B by the sum of equation B and 3 times equation A

A similar argument now shows that every solution of this new system is also a solution of the original system. Thus the two systems have exactly the same solutions.

The procedures used in this example are valid in any system of equations, with any constant in place of 3; that is, you can:

> *Replace an equation in the system by the sum of itself and a constant multiple of another equation in the system.*

The same argument used in the example shows that the system obtained by this replacement will have the same solutions as the original system. You should note two important special cases of this operation. If the constant multiplier is the number 1, then the operation is:

Replace an equation in the system by the sum
of itself and another equation in the system

Since for any quantities A and B, we know that $A + (-1)B$ is just $A - B$, we see that when the constant multiplier is -1, the operation is:

Replace an equation in the system by the difference
of itself and another equation in the system

Although there are other operations that could be used, those listed above are sufficient. We can now summarize the basic plan:

THE ELIMINATION METHOD

Any system of linear equations can be transformed into a system in echelon form with the same solutions, by using a finite number of operations of these three types:

(*i*) *Interchange any two equations in the system.*

(*ii*) *Replace an equation in the system by a nonzero constant multiple of itself.*

(*iii*) *Replace an equation in the system by the sum of itself and a constant multiple of another equation in the system.*

The resulting echelon form system can then be easily solved.

The preceding discussion showed that these three types of operations do not change the solutions of a system. The following examples will show how to use these operations to transform a given system into one in echelon form.

EXAMPLE In order to transform the system

$$
\begin{aligned}
x + 4y - 3z &= 1 \qquad \text{equation A} \\
-3x - 6y + z &= 3 \qquad \text{equation B} \\
2x + 11y - 5z &= 0 \qquad \text{equation C}
\end{aligned}
$$

into a system in echelon form, the first step is to replace the second and third equations by equations that do not involve x. We begin by replacing equation B by the sum of itself and 3 times equation A (this was done in detail in the example on p. 392):

$$
\begin{aligned}
(*) \qquad x + 4y - 3z &= 1 \qquad \text{equation A} \\
6y - 8z &= 6 \qquad \text{sum of equation B and 3 times equation A} \\
2x + 11y - 5z &= 0 \qquad \text{equation C}
\end{aligned}
$$

In order to eliminate the x term in equation C, we form a new equation, the sum of equation C and -2 times equation A:

$$
\begin{array}{ll}
-2x - 8y + 6z = -2 & \quad -2 \text{ times equation A} \\
\underline{2x + 11y - 5z = 0} & \quad \text{equation C} \\
 3y + z = -2 & \quad \text{sum of equation C and } -2 \text{ times equation A}
\end{array}
$$

Now in the system (*) above, replace equation C by this new equation:

$$
\begin{aligned}
x + 4y - 3z &= 1 \qquad \text{equation A} \\
6y - 8z &= 6 \\
3y + z &= -2 \qquad \text{sum of equation C and } -2 \text{ times equation A}
\end{aligned}
$$

The next step is to eliminate the y term in one of the last two equations. This can be done by replacing the second equation by the sum of itself and -2 times the third equation:

$$x + 4y - 3z = 1$$
$$- 10z = 10 \qquad \text{sum of second equation and } -2 \text{ times third equation}$$
$$3y + z = -2$$

Finally, interchange the last two equations:

$$x + 4y - 3z = 1$$
$$3y + z = -2$$
$$- 10z = 10$$

We now have a system in echelon form. Since it was obtained by using only the types of transformations discussed above, we know that it has the same solutions as the system we started with. So we can find the solutions of that original system by solving this one. Beginning with the last equation, we see that

$$-10z = 10, \qquad \text{or equivalently,} \qquad z = -1$$

Substituting $z = -1$ in the second equation shows that

$$3y + z = -2$$
$$3y + (-1) = -2$$
$$3y = -1$$
$$y = -\tfrac{1}{3}$$

Substituting $y = -\tfrac{1}{3}$ and $z = -1$ in the first equation yields:

$$x + 4y - 3z = 1$$
$$x + 4(-\tfrac{1}{3}) - 3(-1) = 1$$
$$x = 1 + \tfrac{4}{3} - 3 = -\tfrac{2}{3}$$

Therefore the original system has just one solution: $x = -\tfrac{2}{3}$, $y = -\tfrac{1}{3}$, $z = -1$.

EXAMPLE The first step in solving the system

$$x + 2y + 3z = -2$$
$$2x + 6y + z = 2$$
$$3x + 3y + 10z = -2$$

is to eliminate the x terms from the last two equations by performing suitable operations:

$$x + 2y + 3z = -2$$
$$2y - 5z = 6 \qquad \text{sum of second equation and } -2 \text{ times first equation}$$
$$3x + 3y + 10z = -2$$

$$x + 2y + 3z = -2$$
$$2y - 5z = 6$$
$$- 3y + z = 4 \qquad \text{sum of third equation and } -3 \text{ times first equation}$$

In order to eliminate the y term in the last equation, we first arrange for y to have coefficient 1 in the second equation:

$$x + 2y + 3z = -2$$
$$y - \tfrac{5}{2}z = 3 \qquad \text{second equation multiplied by } \tfrac{1}{2}$$
$$- 3y + z = 4$$

Now it is easy to eliminate the y term in the last equation:

$$x + 2y + 3z = -2$$
$$y - \tfrac{5}{2}z = 3$$
$$- \tfrac{13}{2}z = 13 \qquad \text{sum of third equation and 3 times second equation}$$

This last system is in echelon form and we can solve the third equation: $z = 13(-\tfrac{2}{13}) = -2$. Substituting $z = -2$ in the second equation shows that

$$y - \tfrac{5}{2}(-2) = 3$$
$$y = 3 - 5 = -2$$

Substituting $y = -2$ and $z = -2$ in the first equation yields

$$x + 2(-2) + 3(-2) = -2$$
$$x = -2 + 4 + 6 = 8$$

Therefore the only solution of the original system is $x = 8$, $y = -2$, $z = -2$.

EXAMPLE   A system such as this one

$$2x + 5y + z + 3w = 0$$
$$2y - 4z + 3w = 0$$
$$2x + 17y - 23z + 41w = 0$$

in which all the constants on the right side are zero is called a **homogeneous system.** It obviously has at least one solution, namely, $x = 0$, $y = 0$, $z = 0$, $w = 0$. This solution is called the **trivial solution.** In order to see if there are any nontrivial solutions, we shall put the system into echelon form. The x term in the third equation can be eliminated by replacing the third equation by the sum of itself and -1 times the first equation:

$$2x + 5y + z + 3w = 0$$
$$2y - 4z + 3w = 0$$
$$12y - 24z + 38w = 0$$

Now we replace the third equation by the sum of itself and -6 times the second equation:

$$2x + 5y + z + 3w = 0$$
$$2y - 4z + 3w = 0$$
$$20w = 0$$

This echelon form system can now be solved. The last equation shows that $w = 0$. Substituting $w = 0$ in the second equation yields:

$$2y - 4z = 0$$
$$2y = 4z$$
$$y = 2z$$

This equation obviously has an infinite number of solutions. For example, $z = 1$, $y = 2$ is a solution and $z = -\tfrac{5}{2}$, $y = -5$ is a solution. More generally, for each real number t, $z = t$ and $y = 2t$ is a solution of the second equation. Substituting $w = 0$, $z = t$, $y = 2t$ in the first equation shows that

$$2x + 5(2t) + t + 3(0) = 0$$
$$2x = -11t$$
$$x = \frac{-11t}{2}$$

Therefore this echelon form system, and hence the original system, has an infinite number of different solutions, one for each real number t:

$$x = \frac{-11t}{2}, \qquad y = 2t, \qquad z = t, \qquad w = 0$$

For example, if $t = 2$, we have the solution

$$x = \frac{-11(2)}{2} = -11, \qquad y = 2(2) = 4, \qquad z = 2, \qquad w = 0$$

If $t = -3$, we have the solution $x = \frac{33}{2}$, $y = -6$, $z = -3$, $w = 0$; and so on.

The homogeneous system of equations in the preceding example has an infinite number of solutions. It is also quite possible for a nonhomogeneous system to have infinitely many solutions (see Exercise B.4). A system with infinitely many solutions is said to be a **dependent system.**

EXAMPLE   To solve the system

$$2x - 3y = 5$$
$$4x - 6y = 1$$

we replace the second equation by the sum of itself and -2 times the first equation:

$$2x - 3y = \quad 5$$
$$0x + 0y = -9$$

But the left side of the equation $0x + 0y = -9$ is always 0, no matter what x and y are. Since $0 = -9$ is always false, the equation $0x + 0y = -9$ has *no solutions.* Therefore the original system cannot possibly have any solutions. This fact can be seen geometrically by graphing the two equations of the original system. The graphs are parallel lines, so there is no point which is on both graphs—that is, no solution which satisfies *both* equations in the system.

The phenomenon observed in the preceding example may occur in any size system. During the process of transforming a given system of equations into echelon form you may obtain an equation in which all the unknowns have coefficients 0, but the constant on the right side is nonzero. In this case, the system has no solutions. Such a system is called an **inconsistent system.**

SHORTCUTS

Most computer programs for solving systems of linear equations are based on the elimination method. But when you are working by hand there often are more conven- ient ways to find the solutions of certain systems, especially systems of two equations in two unknowns. Some of these other methods are illustrated in the examples below. You will see that they are just combinations of the substitution method and some special cases of the elimination method, in which all the steps are not written out in full. Feel free to use such shortcuts. But when in doubt, remember that the elimination method *always* works, even though it may take a bit longer.

EXAMPLE   Any solution of the system

$$4x - 3y = 8$$
$$2x + 3y = -2$$

must also satisfy the equation obtained by adding these two equations:

$$
\begin{array}{r}
4x - 3y = 8 \\
2x + 3y = -2 \\
\hline
6x = 6
\end{array}
$$

Solving this last equation shows that $x = 1$. Substituting $x = 1$ in one of the original equations—say, the first one—shows that

$$4 - 3y = 8$$
$$-3y = 4$$
$$y = -\tfrac{4}{3}$$

Therefore the solution of the original system is $x = 1$, $y = -\tfrac{4}{3}$.

EXAMPLE   Any solution of the system

$$2x - 2y = 1$$
$$3x - 5y = 2$$

must also be a solution of this system:

$$6x - 6y = 3 \qquad \text{first equation multiplied by 3}$$
$$6x - 10y = 4 \qquad \text{second equation multiplied by 2}$$

(The multipliers 3 and 2 were chosen so that the coefficient of x would be the same in both new equations.) Consequently, any solution of this system must be a solution of the equation obtained by subtracting the second equation from the first:

$$
\begin{array}{r}
6x - 6y = 3 \\
6x - 10y = 4 \\
\hline
4y = -1°
\end{array}
$$

Solving this last equation, we see that we must have $y = -\tfrac{1}{4}$. Substituting this value in either of the original equations—say, the first one—shows that

$$2x - 2(-\tfrac{1}{4}) = 1$$
$$2x = 1 - \tfrac{1}{2} = \tfrac{1}{2}$$
$$x = \tfrac{1}{4}$$

° If this subtraction is confusing, write it out horizontally. For instance, $-6y - (-10y) = -6y + 10y = 4y$.

EXERCISES

A.1. Which of these systems have $x = 2$, $y = -1$ as a solution?

(a) $\begin{aligned} 3x - 5y &= 11 \\ x + 8y &= 6 \end{aligned}$ (b) $\begin{aligned} 2x + 3y &= 1 \\ x - 5y &= 7 \end{aligned}$ (c) $\begin{aligned} \tfrac{1}{2}x + \tfrac{1}{3}y &= \tfrac{2}{3} \\ \tfrac{1}{3}x + \tfrac{1}{2}y &= \tfrac{1}{6} \end{aligned}$

A.2. Which of these systems have $x = \tfrac{1}{2}$, $y = 3$, $z = -1$ as a solution?

(a) $\begin{aligned} 2x - y + 4z &= -6 \\ 3y + 3z &= 6 \\ 2z &= 2 \end{aligned}$ (b) $\begin{aligned} \tfrac{1}{2}x + 3y - z &= \tfrac{41}{4} \\ 2x - 2y + 2z &= -7 \\ \tfrac{3}{2}x + \tfrac{2}{3}y - 4z &= 9 \end{aligned}$

B.1. Solve these systems by the substitution method.

(a) $\begin{aligned} x - 2y &= 5 \\ 2x + y &= 3 \end{aligned}$ (c) $\begin{aligned} 3x - y &= 1 \\ -x + 2y &= 4 \end{aligned}$ (e) $\begin{aligned} -5x + 2y &= 5 \\ 2x - 4y &= -3 \end{aligned}$

(b) $\begin{aligned} 3x - 2y &= 4 \\ 2x + y &= -1 \end{aligned}$ (d) $\begin{aligned} 2x - 3y &= 5 \\ 6x + 2y &= 2 \end{aligned}$ (f) $\begin{aligned} \tfrac{1}{2}x + \tfrac{5}{2}y &= \tfrac{3}{4} \\ 2x - \tfrac{3}{2}y &= 1 \end{aligned}$

B.2. Solve these systems. (*Hint:* first write each equation in the form $ax + by = c$.)

(a) $\begin{aligned} \frac{x+y}{4} - \frac{x-y}{3} &= 1 \\[4pt] \frac{x+y}{4} + \frac{x-y}{2} &= 9 \end{aligned}$ (c) $\begin{aligned} \frac{x-y}{4} + \frac{x+y}{3} &= 1 \\[4pt] \frac{x+2y}{3} + \frac{3x-y}{2} &= -2 \end{aligned}$

(b) $\begin{aligned} \frac{y-x}{3} + \frac{x+y}{2} &= 0 \\[4pt] \frac{x+y}{4} + \frac{x+y}{3} &= 0 \end{aligned}$ (d) $\begin{aligned} \frac{2x-y}{3} - \frac{3x+y}{2} &= 1 \\[4pt] \frac{2x+2y}{3} + \frac{x-3y}{2} &= -2 \end{aligned}$

B.3. Solve these systems, each of which has exactly one solution.

(a) $\begin{aligned} x + y &= 5 \\ -x + 2z &= 0 \\ 2x + y - z &= 7 \end{aligned}$ (d) $\begin{aligned} 2x - 2y + z &= -6 \\ 3x + y + 2z &= 2 \\ x + y - 2z &= 0 \end{aligned}$

(b) $\begin{aligned} x + 2y + 4z &= 3 \\ x + 2z &= 0 \\ 2x + 4y + z &= 3 \end{aligned}$ (e) $\begin{aligned} -x + 3y + 2z &= 0 \\ 2x - y - z &= 3 \\ x + 2y + 3z &= 0 \end{aligned}$

(c) $\begin{aligned} 2x + y - z &= 4 \\ x + 2z &= 9 \\ -3x - y + 2z &= 9 \end{aligned}$ (f) $\begin{aligned} 3x + 7y + 9z &= 0 \\ x + 2y + 3z &= 2 \\ x + 4y + z &= 2 \end{aligned}$
(*Hint:* begin by interchanging the first and second equations.)

B.4. Solve these dependent systems.

(a) $\begin{aligned} x + y + z &= 1 \\ x - 2y + 2z &= 4 \\ 2x - y + 3z &= 5 \end{aligned}$ (c) $\begin{aligned} 11x + 10y + 9z &= 5 \\ x + 2y + 3z &= 1 \\ 3x + 2y + z &= 1 \end{aligned}$

(b) $\begin{aligned} 2x - y + z &= 1 \\ 3x + y + z &= 0 \\ 7x - y + 3z &= 2 \end{aligned}$ (d) $\begin{aligned} -x + 2y - 3z + 4w &= 8 \\ 2x - 4y + z + 2w &= -3 \\ 5x - 4y + z + 2w &= -3 \end{aligned}$

B.5. Solve these systems.

(a) $\begin{aligned} x + y &= 3 \\ 5x - y &= 3 \\ 9x - 4y &= 1 \end{aligned}$

(b) $\begin{aligned} 2x - y + 2z &= 3 \\ -x + 2y - z &= 0 \\ x + y - z &= 1 \end{aligned}$

(c) $\begin{aligned} 2x - y + z &= 1 \\ x + y - z &= 2 \\ -x - y + z &= 0 \end{aligned}$

(d) $\begin{aligned} x + 2y + 3z &= 4 \\ 2x - y + z &= 3 \\ 3x + y + 4z &= 7 \end{aligned}$

(e) $\begin{aligned} x + y &= 3 \\ -x + 2y &= 3 \\ 2x - y &= 3 \end{aligned}$

(f) $\begin{aligned} 3x + y - 2z &= 4 \\ -5x + 2z &= 5 \\ -7x - y + 3z &= -2 \end{aligned}$

B.6. Carry out the elimination method far enough to determine whether the given system is dependent or inconsistent. (It isn't necessary to solve the dependent systems.)

(a) $\begin{aligned} x + 2y &= 0 \\ y - z &= 2 \\ x + y + z &= -2 \end{aligned}$

(b) $\begin{aligned} x + 2y + z &= 0 \\ y + 2z &= 0 \\ x + y - z &= 0 \end{aligned}$

(c) $\begin{aligned} x + 2y + 4z &= 6 \\ y + z &= 1 \\ x + 3y + 5z &= 10 \end{aligned}$

(d) $\begin{aligned} x + y + 2z + 3w &= 1 \\ 2x + y + 3z + 4w &= 1 \\ 3x + y + 4z + 5w &= 2 \end{aligned}$

(e) $\begin{aligned} x + 2y &= 1 \\ -x + y &= 0 \\ 2x + 4y &= 3 \end{aligned}$

(f) $\begin{aligned} x + 2y + 3z &= 1 \\ 3x + 2y + 4z &= -1 \\ 2x + 6y + 8z + w &= 3 \\ 2x + 2z - 2w &= 3 \end{aligned}$

B.7. Solve these systems:

(a) $\begin{aligned} x + y + z + w &= 10 \\ x + y + 2z &= 11 \\ x - 3y + w &= -14 \\ y + 3z - w &= 7 \end{aligned}$

(b) $\begin{aligned} 2x + y + z &= 3 \\ y + z + w &= 5 \\ 4x + z + w &= 0 \\ 3y - 2z - w &= 6 \end{aligned}$

(c) $\begin{aligned} 2x - 4y + 5z &= 1 \\ x - 3z &= 2 \\ 5x - 8y + 7z &= 6 \\ 3x - 4y + 2z &= 3 \\ x - 4y + 8z &= -1 \end{aligned}$

(d) $\begin{aligned} 4x + z + 2w + 24v &= 0 \\ 2x + y + 12v &= 0 \\ 3x + z + 2w + 18v &= 0 \\ 4x - y + w + 24v &= 0 \\ 7x - y + z + 3w + 42v &= 0 \end{aligned}$

B.8. Solve these systems:

(a) $\dfrac{1}{x} - \dfrac{3}{y} = 2$ (*Hint:* let $u = 1/x$ and $v = 1/y$ so that the system becomes

$\dfrac{2}{x} + \dfrac{1}{y} = 3$

$$u - 3v = 2$$
$$2u + v = 3$$

Solve for u and v; then determine x and y.)

(b) $\dfrac{5}{x} + \dfrac{2}{y} = 0$

$\dfrac{6}{x} - \dfrac{4}{y} = 3$

(e) $\dfrac{1}{x+1} - \dfrac{2}{y-3} + \dfrac{3}{z-2} = 4$

$\dfrac{5}{y-3} - \dfrac{10}{z-2} = -5$

(c) $\dfrac{3}{x} - \dfrac{1}{y} + \dfrac{4}{z} = -13$

$\dfrac{-3}{x+1} + \dfrac{4}{y-3} - \dfrac{1}{z-2} = -2$

$\dfrac{1}{x} + \dfrac{2}{y} - \dfrac{1}{z} = 12$

$\dfrac{4}{x} - \dfrac{1}{y} + \dfrac{3}{z} = -7$

(d) $\dfrac{3}{x+1} - \dfrac{4}{y-2} = 2$

$\dfrac{1}{x+1} + \dfrac{4}{y-2} = 5$ $\left(\textit{Hint: let } u = \dfrac{1}{x+1}, \ v = \dfrac{1}{y-2}.\right)$

B.9. (a) Consider this system:

$$x + y + 4z - w = 1$$
$$y - 2z + 3w = 0$$

Verify that for each *pair* of real numbers, s and t, the system has a solution:

$$w = s, \quad z = t, \quad y = 2t - 3s, \quad x = 1 - (2t - 3s) - 4t + s = 1 - 6t + 4s$$

With this model in mind, solve these dependent systems by the elimination method.

(b)
$$x - y + 2z + 3w = 0$$
$$x + z + w = 0$$
$$3x - 2y + 5z + 7w = 0$$

(d)
$$x + y + z - w = 0$$
$$2x - 4y - 4z + w = 0$$
$$4x - 2y + 2z - 3w = 0$$
$$7x - y - z - 3w = 0$$

(c)
$$x + 2y + z + 4w = 1$$
$$y + 3z - w = 2$$
$$x + 4y + 7z - 2w = 5$$
$$3x + 7y + 6z + 11w = 5$$

(e)
$$x + 2y + 3z + 4v = 0$$
$$2x + 4y + 6z + w + 9v = 0$$
$$x + 2y + 3z + w + 5v = 0$$

B.10. Solve these systems by using the same methods as used above together with a calculator.

(a) $3.25x - 2.18y = 1.96$
$1.92x + 6.77y = -3.87$

(b) $463x - 801y = 946$
$.0375x + .912y = -1.003$

B.11. Find constants a, b, c, such that the three points $(-3, 2)$, $(1, 1)$, and $(2, -1)$ all lie on the graph of the quadratic function $f(x) = ax^2 + bx + c$. [*Hint:* since $(-3, 2)$ is to be on the graph, we must have $a(-3)^2 + b(-3) + c = 2$, that is, $9a - 3b + c = 2$. In a similar manner, the other two points lead to *linear* equations in a, b, c. Solve this system of three equations for a, b, c.]

B.12.   In each part, find a quadratic function whose graph includes the three given points. (*Hint:* see Exercise B.11.)
(a) $(1, -2)$, $(3, 1)$, $(4, -1)$ (c) $(1, 1)$, $(0, 0)$, $(-1, 2)$
(b) $(1, -4)$, $(-1, 6)$, $(2, -9)$ (d) $(-1, 6)$, $(-2, 16)$, $(1, 4)$

B.13.   The substitution method can sometimes be used to solve systems of nonlinear equations.
(a)   Solve the system

$$
\begin{aligned}
x^2 - y &= 0 \\
2x - y &= -3
\end{aligned}
$$

by solving one of the equations for y, substituting this answer in other equation, and solving it.
(b)   Graph the two equations in part (a). The points where the graphs intersect are precisely the solutions of the *system* in part (a). Why?

B.14.   Solve each of these systems by substitution. Then exhibit the solutions geometrically by graphing the equations in each system. (See Exercise B.13.)
(a) $2x + y = -1$ (e) $x^2 + y^2 + 4x - 2y = 5$
      $x^2 - y = 4$ $x + y = 1$
(b) $x^2 - y = -1$ (*Hint:* to graph the first equation,
      $2x + y = 4$ complete the square in x and y; see
(c) $x^2 + y^2 = 25$ p. 159.)
      $x^2 + y = 19$
(d) $x^2 + y^2 = 20$ (f) $4x^2 - y^2 = -4$
      $3x - y = -2$ $16x^2 + 9y^2 = 244$

B.15.   Find two integers whose sum is 32 and whose difference is 6. (*Hint:* if x and y denote the two integers, then x and y must satisfy $x + y = 32$ *and* $x - y = 6$.)

B.16.   Find two integers whose sum is -9 and whose difference is 45. (See Exercise B.15.)

B.17.   Are there two *integers* whose sum is 29 and whose difference is 8? (See Exercise B.15.)

B.18.   A collection of nickels and dimes totals $3.05. If there are 38 coins altogether, how many are nickels and how many are dimes? (*Hint:* if x is the number of nickels and y the number of dimes, then $.05x + .10y = 3.05$. Use the other given information to obtain a second linear equation, then solve the resulting system for x and y.)

B.19.   A collection of nickels, dimes, and quarters totals $6.00. If there are 52 coins altogether and twice as many dimes as nickels, how many of each kind of coin are there? (See Exercise B.18.)

B.20.   At a certain store, cashews cost $4.40/lb and peanuts $1.20/lb. If you want to buy exactly 3 lb of nuts for $6.00, how many pounds of each kind of nuts should you buy? (Let x be the pounds of cashews and y the pounds of peanuts you must buy. Then $x + y = 3$. Find another linear equation satisfied by x and y and solve the resulting system.)

B.21. A plane flies 3000 miles from San Francisco to Boston at a constant speed in 5 hr, flying *with* the wind all the way. The return trip, against the wind, takes 6 hr. Find the speed of the plane and the speed of the wind. [*Hint:* if x is the plane's speed and y the wind speed, then on the trip to Boston (*with* the wind), the plane travels at speed $x + y$ for 5 hr. Since it goes a distance of 3000 mi, we have $5(x + y) = 3000$. Find another equation in x and y and solve the resulting system.]

B.22. A boat travels at a constant speed a distance of 57 km downstream in 3 hours, then turns around and travels 55 km upstream in 5 hours. What is the speed of the boat and of the current? (see Exercise B.21.)

B.23. A winemaker has two large casks of wine. One wine is 8% alcohol and the other 18% alcohol. How many liters of each wine should be mixed to produce 30 liters of wine that is 12% alcohol?

B.24. If Tom, Dick, and Harry work together they can paint a large room in 4 hours. When only Dick and Harry work together, it takes 8 hours to paint the room. Tom and Dick, working together, take 6 hours to paint the room. How long would it take each of them to paint the room alone? [*Hint:* If x is the amount of the room painted in 1 hour by Tom, y the amount painted by Dick and z the amount painted by Harry, then $x + y + z = \frac{1}{4}$.]

B.25. Pipes R, S, T are connected to the same tank. When all three pipes are running, they can fill the tank in 2 hours. When only pipes S and T are running, they can fill the tank in 4 hours. When only R and T are running, they can fill the tank in 2.4 hours. How long would it take each pipe running alone to fill the tank?

2. MATRICES AND DETERMINANTS

Matrices and determinants are two different but related concepts that arise naturally in the study of systems of linear equations. The definitions and use of matrices and determinants in solving systems of equations are discussed here. Both matrices and determinants have many other applications in mathematics. Many of these are beyond the scope of this book, but a few are presented in the exercises at the end of the section.

MATRIX METHODS FOR SOLVING SYSTEMS OF LINEAR EQUATIONS

Once you have solved several systems of linear equations by the elimination method, one fact becomes clear. The symbols used for the unknowns play no real role in the solution process, and a lot of time is wasted copying the x's, y's, z's, and so on, at each stage of the process. This fact suggests a shorthand system for representing a system of equations.

EXAMPLE   This system of equations

$$
\begin{aligned}
x + 2y - z - 3w &= 2 \\
6y + 3z - 4w &= 0 \\
6x + 12y - 3z - 16w &= 3 \\
-5x + 2y + 15z + 10w &= -21
\end{aligned}
$$

can be represented by the following rectangular array of numbers, consisting of the coefficients of the unknowns and the constants on the right side, arranged in the same order they appear in the system:

$$
\left(
\begin{array}{cccc|c}
1 & 2 & -1 & -3 & 2 \\
0 & 6 & 3 & -4 & 0 \\
6 & 12 & -3 & -16 & 3 \\
-5 & 2 & 15 & 10 & -21
\end{array}
\right)
$$

This array is called the **augmented matrix**° of the system. Note that the second equation above has no x term, meaning that x has coefficient 0 in the equation. This is indicated in the matrix by the 0 at the beginning of the second row.

To solve this system by the elimination method, we begin by eliminating the x term in the third equation. We replace the third equation by the sum of itself and -6 times the first equation, namely, $3z + 2y = -9$. In the matrix shorthand, where a horizontal row represents an equation, this operation is carried out on the rows of the matrix.

-6	-12	6	18	-12	-6 times the first row
6	12	-3	-16	3	third row
0	0	3	2	-9	sum of the third row and -6 times the first row

Replacing the third row of the original matrix by this row yields the matrix

$$
\left(
\begin{array}{cccc|c}
1 & 2 & -1 & -3 & 2 \\
0 & 6 & 3 & -4 & 0 \\
0 & 0 & 3 & 2 & -9 \\
-5 & 2 & 15 & 10 & -21
\end{array}
\right)
$$

We continue the solution process in the same manner, using the matrix shorthand to represent the system of equations. Replace the fourth row of the last matrix above by the sum of itself and 5 times the first row (this amounts to eliminating the x term from the last equation):

$$
\left(
\begin{array}{cccc|c}
1 & 2 & -1 & -3 & 2 \\
0 & 6 & 3 & -4 & 0 \\
0 & 0 & 3 & 2 & -9 \\
0 & 12 & 10 & -5 & -11
\end{array}
\right)
$$

° The plural of "matrix" is "matrices."

Next we must make various entries in the last row 0. (This amounts to eliminating the y and z term from the last equation.)

$$\begin{pmatrix} 1 & 2 & -1 & -3 & | & 2 \\ 0 & 6 & 3 & -4 & | & 0 \\ 0 & 0 & 3 & 2 & | & -9 \\ 0 & 0 & 4 & 3 & | & -11 \end{pmatrix}$$

replace fourth row by the sum of itself and -2 times the second row

$$\begin{pmatrix} 1 & 2 & -1 & -3 & | & 2 \\ 0 & 6 & 3 & -4 & | & 0 \\ 0 & 0 & 1 & \frac{2}{3} & | & -3 \\ 0 & 0 & 4 & 3 & | & -11 \end{pmatrix}$$

multiply third row by $\frac{1}{3}$

$$\begin{pmatrix} 1 & 2 & -1 & -3 & | & 2 \\ 0 & 6 & 3 & -4 & | & 0 \\ 0 & 0 & 1 & \frac{2}{3} & | & -3 \\ 0 & 0 & 0 & \frac{1}{3} & | & 1 \end{pmatrix}$$

replace fourth row by the sum of itself and -4 times the third row

This last matrix is just shorthand notation for this echelon form system:

$$\begin{aligned} x + 2y - z - 3w &= 2 \\ 6y + 3z - 4w &= 0 \\ z + \tfrac{2}{3}w &= -3 \\ \tfrac{1}{3}w &= 1 \end{aligned}$$

The solution is now easily found to be $x = -3$, $y = \frac{9}{2}$, $z = -5$, $w = 3$.

The matrix notation in the example above is certainly more convenient than the equation notation. When matrix notation is used, we usually change our language to suit the situation. Instead of speaking of operations on equations in the system (such as multiplying by a nonzero constant), we speak of **row operations** on the matrix. Similarly, the solution process ends when we obtain an **echelon form matrix** (such as the last matrix shown above).

EXAMPLE The homogeneous system

$$\begin{aligned} 4x + 12y - 16z &= 0 \\ 3x + 4y + 3z &= 0 \\ x + 8y - 19z &= 0 \end{aligned}$$

has augmented matrix

$$\begin{pmatrix} 4 & 12 & -16 & | & 0 \\ 3 & 4 & 3 & | & 0 \\ 1 & 8 & -19 & | & 0 \end{pmatrix}$$

The last vertical column of this matrix consists entirely of zeros. Furthermore, any matrix obtained from this one by the usual row operations will have this same property.

For interchanging two rows, or multiplying a row by a constant, or replacing a row by the sum of itself and a constant multiple of another row, will always result in rows with last entry 0. Consequently, when dealing with homogeneous systems such as this, there is no need to write out this last column of zeros at every stage. Instead we need only deal with the **coefficient matrix:**

$$\begin{pmatrix} 4 & 12 & -16 \\ 3 & 4 & 3 \\ 1 & 8 & -19 \end{pmatrix}$$

instead of the augmented matrix of the system given above. Using the matrix of coefficients, we proceed as before to reduce it to echelon form:

$$\begin{pmatrix} 1 & 3 & -4 \\ 3 & 4 & 3 \\ 1 & 8 & -19 \end{pmatrix}$$ multiply first row by $\frac{1}{4}$

$$\begin{pmatrix} 1 & 3 & -4 \\ 0 & -5 & 15 \\ 1 & 8 & -19 \end{pmatrix}$$ replace second row by the sum of itself and -3 times the first row

$$\begin{pmatrix} 1 & 3 & -4 \\ 0 & -5 & 15 \\ 0 & 5 & -15 \end{pmatrix}$$ replace third row by the sum of itself and -1 times the first row

$$\begin{pmatrix} 1 & 3 & -4 \\ 0 & -5 & 15 \\ 0 & 0 & 0 \end{pmatrix}$$ replace third row by the sum of itself and 1 times the second row

This echelon form matrix represents the following homogeneous system:

$$x + 3y - 4z = 0$$
$$- 5y + 15z = 0$$

We don't bother to write out the trivial third equation $0x + 0y + 0z = 0$ since it is satisfied by *all* real numbers. The last equation above is equivalent to $y = 3z$ and hence has infinitely many solutions. For each real number t, there is the solution $z = t$, $y = 3t$. Substituting these values in the first equation shows that $x = -3y + 4z = -9t + 4t = -5t$. Therefore the solutions of the system are given by:

$$x = -5t, \qquad y = 3t, \qquad z = t \qquad (t \text{ any real number})$$

MATRICES

Up to now, we have used matrices only as a convenient shorthand notation for dealing with systems of equations. Matrices have many other uses, most of which have nothing to do with systems of equations. Consequently, matrices are often studied as a subject in their own right (see Exercises B.2–B.5). We shall limit our discussion here to defining some standard terms.

Let m and n be positive integers. An $m \times n$ **matrix** (read "m by n matrix") is a rectangular array of numbers,° with m horizontal rows and n vertical columns. For example,

$$\begin{pmatrix} 3 & 2 & -5 \\ 6 & 1 & 7 \\ -2 & 5 & 0 \end{pmatrix} \qquad \begin{pmatrix} -3 & 4 \\ 2 & 0 \\ 0 & 1 \\ 7 & 3 \\ 1 & -6 \end{pmatrix} \qquad \begin{pmatrix} 3 & 0 & 1 & 0 \\ \sqrt{2} & -\frac{1}{2} & 4 & \frac{8}{3} \\ 10 & 2 & -\frac{3}{4} & 12 \end{pmatrix} \qquad \begin{pmatrix} \sqrt{3} \\ 2 \\ 0 \\ 11 \end{pmatrix}$$

3×3 matrix	5×2 matrix	3×4 matrix	4×1 matrix
3 rows	5 rows	3 rows	4 rows
3 columns	2 columns	4 columns	1 column

In a matrix, the *rows* are horizontal and are numbered from top to bottom. The *columns* are vertical and are numbered from left to right. For example,

$$\begin{pmatrix} 11 & 3 & 14 \\ -2 & 0 & -5 \\ \frac{1}{3} & 6 & 7 \end{pmatrix} \begin{matrix} \longleftarrow \text{ row 1} \\ \longleftarrow \text{ row 2} \\ \longleftarrow \text{ row 3} \end{matrix}$$

$$\uparrow \qquad \uparrow \qquad \uparrow$$
column 1   column 2   column 3

A matrix with the same number of rows and columns is called a **square matrix.** Observe that each entry in a matrix can be exactly located by stating the row and column it appears in. For instance, in the 3×3 matrix above, the entry in row 1, column 2, is the number 3; the entry in row 2, column 2, is the number 0; the entry in row 3, column 1, is $\frac{1}{3}$.

The **main diagonal** of a matrix consists of the entry in row 1, column 1, the entry in row 2, column 2, the entry in row 3, column 3, and so on. For example, this matrix

$$\begin{pmatrix} 1 & 2 & -1 & -3 & 2 \\ 0 & 0 & 3 & -4 & 0 \\ 0 & 0 & -4 & \frac{2}{3} & -3 \\ \frac{4}{5} & -2 & 0 & \frac{1}{3} & 1 \end{pmatrix} \quad \text{has main diagonal} \quad \begin{matrix} 1 \\ 0 \\ -4 \\ \frac{1}{3} \end{matrix}$$

DETERMINANTS

Associated with every square matrix is a certain number, called its determinant. Determinants are used in many areas of mathematics and have applications to systems

° We shall deal only with matrices of real numbers here. But complex numbers can also be used as the entries in a matrix.

of linear equations. The **determinant of the 2 × 2 matrix** $A = \begin{pmatrix} a & b \\ c & d \end{pmatrix}$ is defined to be
the number $ad - bc$. An easy way to remember this definition is to note that $ad - bc$ is
just the difference of the products of diagonally opposite entries: $\begin{smallmatrix} a & b \\ c & d \end{smallmatrix}$.

Here are some examples of 2 × 2 matrices and their determinants:

Matrix	**Determinant**
$\begin{pmatrix} 1 & 2 \\ 6 & 4 \end{pmatrix}$	$1 \cdot 4 - 2 \cdot 6 = 4 - 12 = -8$
$\begin{pmatrix} \frac{1}{2} & 2 \\ 0 & -3 \end{pmatrix}$	$\frac{1}{2}(-3) - 2 \cdot 0 = -\frac{3}{2} - 0 = -\frac{3}{2}$
$\begin{pmatrix} 2 & -4 \\ -3 & 6 \end{pmatrix}$	$2 \cdot 6 - (-4)(-3) = 12 - 12 = 0$

The determinant of the matrix $A = \begin{pmatrix} a & b \\ c & d \end{pmatrix}$ is denoted by any one of these symbols:

$$\det A \quad \text{or} \quad |A| \quad \text{or} \quad \begin{vmatrix} a & b \\ c & d \end{vmatrix}$$

Note the straight vertical lines in this last symbol. They are *not* the same as the curved
parentheses used to denote the matrix. For example,

$$\begin{pmatrix} 3 & 2 \\ 4 & 5 \end{pmatrix} \text{ is a 2 × 2 } matrix,$$

but its determinant $\begin{vmatrix} 3 & 2 \\ 4 & 5 \end{vmatrix}$ is the *number* $3 \cdot 5 - 2 \cdot 4 = 7$

Before defining determinants of 3 × 3 matrices, we must introduce a new concept.
Observe that if you erase one row and one column of a 3 × 3 matrix, the remaining
entries form a 2 × 2 matrix. For example, erasing the first row and second column of
the 3 × 3 matrix

$$\begin{pmatrix} -3 & 4 & -7 \\ 1 & 2 & 0 \\ -4 & 8 & 11 \end{pmatrix} \text{ produces the 2 × 2 matrix } \begin{pmatrix} 1 & 0 \\ -4 & 11 \end{pmatrix}$$

If you now take the determinant of this 2 × 2 matrix, the result is a *number*. The **minor**
of any entry in a 3 × 3 matrix is just such a number, namely, the determinant of the
2 × 2 matrix obtained by erasing the row and column in which the given entry
appears. For instance, in the 3 × 3 matrix

$$\begin{pmatrix} a_1 & b_1 & c_1 \\ a_2 & b_2 & c_2 \\ a_3 & b_3 & c_3 \end{pmatrix}$$

the minor of c_1 is the number $a_2 b_3 - b_2 a_3$, obtained by erasing the row and column in which c_1 appears and taking the determinant of the result:

$$
\begin{pmatrix} a_1 & b_1 & c_1 \\ a_2 & b_2 & c_2 \\ a_3 & b_3 & c_3 \end{pmatrix} \longrightarrow \begin{vmatrix} a_2 & b_2 \\ a_3 & b_3 \end{vmatrix} = a_2 b_3 - b_2 a_3
$$

The **determinant of the 3 × 3 matrix**

$$
A = \begin{pmatrix} a_1 & b_1 & c_1 \\ a_2 & b_2 & c_2 \\ a_3 & b_3 & c_3 \end{pmatrix}
$$

is denoted by any one of these symbols

$$
\det A \quad \text{or} \quad |A| \quad \text{or} \quad \begin{vmatrix} a_1 & b_1 & c_1 \\ a_2 & b_2 & c_2 \\ a_3 & b_3 & c_3 \end{vmatrix}
$$

and is defined to be the *number*

$$
\begin{vmatrix} a_1 & b_1 & c_1 \\ a_2 & b_2 & c_2 \\ a_3 & b_3 & c_3 \end{vmatrix} = a_1 \begin{pmatrix} \text{minor} \\ \text{of } a_1 \end{pmatrix} - b_1 \begin{pmatrix} \text{minor} \\ \text{of } b_1 \end{pmatrix} + c_1 \begin{pmatrix} \text{minor} \\ \text{of } c_1 \end{pmatrix}
$$

$$
= a_1 \begin{vmatrix} b_2 & c_2 \\ b_3 & c_3 \end{vmatrix} - b_1 \begin{vmatrix} a_2 & c_2 \\ a_3 & c_3 \end{vmatrix} + c_1 \begin{vmatrix} a_2 & b_2 \\ a_3 & b_3 \end{vmatrix}
$$

$$
= a_1 (b_2 c_3 - c_2 b_3) - b_1 (a_2 c_3 - c_2 a_3) + c_1 (a_2 b_3 - b_2 a_3)
$$

$$
= a_1 b_2 c_3 - a_1 b_3 c_2 - a_2 b_1 c_3 + a_3 b_1 c_2 + a_2 b_3 c_1 - a_3 b_2 c_1
$$

It isn't necessary to memorize the last line of this formula. Just remember the directions given in the top line: to find $|A|$, multiply each entry in the first row of A by its minor, insert the proper signs $(+, -, +)$, and add up the result.

EXAMPLE The determinant of the matrix

$$
A = \begin{pmatrix} 2 & 4 & 3 \\ 0 & 5 & -1 \\ 1 & -1 & 2 \end{pmatrix}
$$

is just the number -1 since

$$
|A| = 2 \begin{vmatrix} 5 & -1 \\ -1 & 2 \end{vmatrix} - 4 \begin{vmatrix} 0 & -1 \\ 1 & 2 \end{vmatrix} + 3 \begin{vmatrix} 0 & 5 \\ 1 & -1 \end{vmatrix}
$$

$$
= 2(5 \cdot 2 - (-1)(-1)) - 4(0 \cdot 2 - (-1)1) + 3(0(-1) - 5 \cdot 1)
$$

$$
= 2(9) - 4(1) + 3(-5) = 18 - 4 - 15 = -1
$$

When the determinant of a 3 × 3 matrix is defined as above, one says that the determinant is obtained by **expanding along the first row.** Providing that the proper signs are inserted, the determinant can actually be calculated by following an analogous procedure and expanding along any row or column. See Exercise B.8 for details.

DETERMINANTS AND SYSTEMS OF LINEAR EQUATIONS

The connection between determinants and systems of linear equations can be most easily seen by looking at an arbitrary system of two equations in two unknowns. Suppose a, b, c, d, r, s are fixed real numbers. In order to solve the system

$$ax + by = r$$
$$cx + dy = s$$

we eliminate the y terms by multiplying the first equation by d and the second by $-b$:

$$
\begin{array}{ll}
adx + bdy = rd & \text{first equation multiplied by } d \\
-bcx - bdy = -bs & \text{second equation multiplied by } -b \\
\hline
adx - bcx = rd - bs & \text{sum} \\
(ad - bc)x = rd - bs &
\end{array}
$$

Now *if* the number $ad - bc$ is nonzero, we can divide both sides of the last equation by it and conclude that there is only one possible value for x:

$$x = \frac{rd - bs}{ad - bc}$$

Observe that the denominator of x is just the determinant of the **coefficient matrix** $\begin{pmatrix} a & b \\ c & d \end{pmatrix}$, while the numerator is the determinant of the matrix $\begin{pmatrix} r & b \\ s & b \end{pmatrix}$ obtained by replacing the *first* column of the coefficient matrix by the column of constants from the right side of the original equations. Thus when the determinant of the coefficient matrix is nonzero,

$$x = \frac{\begin{vmatrix} r & b \\ s & d \end{vmatrix}}{\begin{vmatrix} a & b \\ c & d \end{vmatrix}}$$

A similar argument shows that when the determinant of the coefficient matrix is nonzero, then there is only one possible value for y:

$$y = \frac{\begin{vmatrix} a & r \\ c & s \end{vmatrix}}{\begin{vmatrix} a & b \\ c & d \end{vmatrix}}$$

Note that the numerator of y is the determinant of the matrix obtained by replacing the *second* column of the coefficient matrix by the column of constants from the right side of the original equations.

EXAMPLE The determinant of the coefficient matrix of the system

$$3x - 4y = 2$$
$$7x + 7y = 3$$

is the nonzero number

$$\begin{vmatrix} 3 & -4 \\ 7 & 7 \end{vmatrix} = 3 \cdot 7 - (-4)7 = 21 + 28 = 49$$

Therefore the system has exactly one solution. It can be found by using the formulas developed above with $a = 3$, $b = -4$, $r = 2$, and $c = 7$, $d = 7$, $s = 3$:

$$x = \frac{\begin{vmatrix} 2 & -4 \\ 3 & 7 \end{vmatrix}}{\begin{vmatrix} 3 & -4 \\ 7 & 7 \end{vmatrix}} = \frac{2 \cdot 7 - (-4)3}{49} = \frac{26}{49} \quad \text{and}$$

$$y = \frac{\begin{vmatrix} 3 & 2 \\ 7 & 3 \end{vmatrix}}{\begin{vmatrix} 3 & -4 \\ 7 & 7 \end{vmatrix}} = \frac{3 \cdot 3 - 2 \cdot 7}{49} = \frac{-5}{49}$$

We have now taken care of the case of two equations in two unknowns. Analogous but more complicated arguments work for larger systems and prove:

CRAMER'S RULE

A system of n linear equations in n unknowns has exactly one solution, if the determinant of the coefficient matrix is nonzero. In this case, the solution of the system is given by a formula similar to the one presented above for the case of two equations.

The last example above shows that solving a system of two equations via Cramer's Rule involves about the same amount of computation as do the various other methods of solving such systems. Solving systems of three equations via Cramer's Rule often (though not always) involves more computation than does the elimination method. The solution of larger systems via Cramer's Rule almost always involves far more computation than does the elimination method. Determinants are grossly inefficient for solving such systems, even if a computer is used. However, there is one situation in which Cramer's Rule can sometimes be used effectively.

EXAMPLE The homogeneous system

$$3x + 2y + z = 0$$
$$7x + 3y + 5z = 0$$
$$-5x + y - z = 0$$

like all homogeneous systems, always has at least one solution, the trivial solution $x = 0$, $y = 0$, $z = 0$. The determinant of the coefficient matrix is

$$\begin{vmatrix} 3 & 2 & 1 \\ 7 & 3 & 5 \\ -5 & 1 & -1 \end{vmatrix} = 3 \begin{vmatrix} 3 & 5 \\ 1 & -1 \end{vmatrix} - 2 \begin{vmatrix} 7 & 5 \\ -5 & -1 \end{vmatrix} + 1 \begin{vmatrix} 7 & 3 \\ -5 & 1 \end{vmatrix}$$

$$= 3(-3 - 5) - 2(-7 + 25) + 1(7 + 15)$$
$$= 3(-8) - 2(18) + 22$$
$$= -24 - 36 + 22 = -38$$

Since this determinant is nonzero, the system has *exactly one* solution by Cramer's Rule. But we already have one solution, namely, $x = 0$, $y = 0$, $z = 0$. Therefore this trivial solution is the *only* solution of the system.

EXERCISES

A.1. Compute these determinants

(a) $\begin{vmatrix} 3 & 5 \\ 7 & 2 \end{vmatrix}$

(d) $\begin{vmatrix} 2 & 5 \\ 1 & \frac{5}{2} \end{vmatrix}$

(g) $\begin{vmatrix} 0 & 2 & 3 \\ 1 & 7 & 9 \\ 0 & -1 & 5 \end{vmatrix}$

(b) $\begin{vmatrix} -2 & 1 \\ 6 & 4 \end{vmatrix}$

(e) $\begin{vmatrix} 1 & 0 & 2 \\ 3 & -1 & 2 \\ 1 & 2 & -3 \end{vmatrix}$

(h) $\begin{vmatrix} 3 & 2 & -3 \\ 1 & 0 & 1 \\ 0 & 4 & 0 \end{vmatrix}$

(c) $\begin{vmatrix} 3 & 5 \\ \frac{5}{2} & 7 \end{vmatrix}$

(f) $\begin{vmatrix} -1 & 2 & 3 \\ 0 & 1 & 2 \\ 4 & 0 & 5 \end{vmatrix}$

(i) $\begin{vmatrix} 3 & 2 & -3 \\ 1 & 0 & 1 \\ 0 & 4 & 1 \end{vmatrix}$

B.1. Use matrix methods to solve these systems.

(a)
$$3x - 2y + 6z = -6$$
$$-3x + 10y + 11z = 13$$
$$x - 2y - z = -3$$

(e)
$$x - y + 2z + 3w = 0$$
$$3x - y + 7z + 7w = 0$$
$$2x - 2y + 5z + 10w = 0$$
$$x - y + 3z + 7w = 0$$

(b)
$$x + 2y - 3z = 9$$
$$3x - y - 4z = 3$$
$$2x - y + 2z = -8$$

(f)
$$x - 3y + 4z + w + 2v = -2$$
$$2x - 2y - z + 2w + 3v = 7$$
$$-x + y - 2z - 2w + v = 0$$
$$-2x - y + 2z + w - v = 5$$
$$2x - 2y + z + 2w + 2v = 3$$

(c)
$$x - y - z = -5$$
$$2x - 3y - 8z = -33$$
$$x - 2y - 8z = -32$$

(g)
$$2x + y + 3z - 2w = -6$$
$$4x + 3y + z - w = -2$$
$$x + y + z + w = -5$$
$$-2x - 2y + 2z + 2w = -10$$

(d)
$$x + 3y + 10z = -8$$
$$-x - 2y - 5z = 3$$
$$2x + 4y + 5z = -6$$

B.2. The sum of two 2×2 matrices is the 2×2 matrix defined by this rule:

$$\begin{pmatrix} a & b \\ c & d \end{pmatrix} + \begin{pmatrix} r & s \\ t & u \end{pmatrix} = \begin{pmatrix} a+r & b+s \\ c+t & d+u \end{pmatrix}$$

For example,

$$\begin{pmatrix} 1 & 2 \\ 3 & 4 \end{pmatrix} + \begin{pmatrix} 5 & -3 \\ 2 & 6 \end{pmatrix} = \begin{pmatrix} 1+5 & 2+(-3) \\ 3+2 & 4+6 \end{pmatrix} = \begin{pmatrix} 6 & -1 \\ 5 & 10 \end{pmatrix}$$

Find these sums:

(a) $\begin{pmatrix} 3 & 2 \\ 5 & 1 \end{pmatrix} + \begin{pmatrix} 7 & -5 \\ -2 & 6 \end{pmatrix}$

(d) $\begin{pmatrix} \frac{3}{4} & 7 \\ 6 & -\frac{5}{4} \end{pmatrix} + \begin{pmatrix} \frac{1}{2} & 3 \\ -5 & \frac{3}{2} \end{pmatrix}$

(b) $\begin{pmatrix} -6 & 2 \\ 7 & -1 \end{pmatrix} + \begin{pmatrix} -8 & 4 \\ 2 & 7 \end{pmatrix}$

(e) $\begin{pmatrix} 0 & 0 \\ 0 & 0 \end{pmatrix} + \begin{pmatrix} 3 & 5 \\ 7 & 9 \end{pmatrix}$

(c) $\begin{pmatrix} \frac{3}{2} & 2 \\ 4 & \frac{7}{2} \end{pmatrix} + \begin{pmatrix} \frac{1}{2} & -\frac{3}{2} \\ \frac{5}{2} & 1 \end{pmatrix}$

(f) $\begin{pmatrix} 1 & -2 \\ -3 & 5 \end{pmatrix} + \begin{pmatrix} -1 & 2 \\ 3 & -5 \end{pmatrix}$

B.3. The product of two 2×2 matrices is the 2×2 matrix defined by this rule:

$$\begin{pmatrix} a & b \\ c & d \end{pmatrix} \begin{pmatrix} r & s \\ t & u \end{pmatrix} = \begin{pmatrix} ar+bt & as+bu \\ cr+dt & cs+du \end{pmatrix}$$

For example,

$$\begin{pmatrix} 2 & 3 \\ -1 & 5 \end{pmatrix} \begin{pmatrix} 4 & -2 \\ 3 & 0 \end{pmatrix} = \begin{pmatrix} 2 \cdot 4 + 3 \cdot 3 & 2(-2) + 3 \cdot 0 \\ (-1)4 + 5 \cdot 3 & (-1)(-2) + 5 \cdot 0 \end{pmatrix} = \begin{pmatrix} 17 & -4 \\ 11 & 2 \end{pmatrix}$$

Find these products:

(a) $\begin{pmatrix} 2 & 3 \\ 1 & 2 \end{pmatrix} \begin{pmatrix} 4 & -3 \\ 2 & 5 \end{pmatrix}$

(d) $\begin{pmatrix} -1 & 2 \\ 3 & -4 \end{pmatrix} \begin{pmatrix} 5 & 2 \\ 3 & -1 \end{pmatrix}$

(b) $\begin{pmatrix} 1 & 0 \\ 0 & 1 \end{pmatrix} \begin{pmatrix} 2 & 3 \\ 5 & 7 \end{pmatrix}$

(e) $\begin{pmatrix} 5 & 2 \\ 3 & -1 \end{pmatrix} \begin{pmatrix} -1 & 2 \\ 3 & -4 \end{pmatrix}$

[compare your answer with (d)]

(c) $\begin{pmatrix} 0 & 1 \\ 1 & 0 \end{pmatrix} \begin{pmatrix} 3 & 5 \\ 7 & 9 \end{pmatrix}$

(f) $\begin{pmatrix} 1 & -1 \\ 2 & -2 \end{pmatrix} \begin{pmatrix} 3 & -1 \\ 3 & -1 \end{pmatrix}$

B.4. Verify that $A(B + C) = AB + AC$ and $(AB)C = A(BC)$ when

$$A = \begin{pmatrix} 1 & 2 \\ 3 & 0 \end{pmatrix}, \quad B = \begin{pmatrix} -1 & 2 \\ 3 & 4 \end{pmatrix}, \quad C = \begin{pmatrix} 2 & 3 \\ 1 & 2 \end{pmatrix}$$

B.5. Multiplication of matrices satisfies *some* of the laws that multiplication of numbers does (Exercise B.4), but *not all* of them. In each case verify that *the given statement is false* for the given matrices.

(a) $AB = BA$; $A = \begin{pmatrix} 1 & 2 \\ 3 & 4 \end{pmatrix}$ and $B = \begin{pmatrix} -1 & 4 \\ 5 & 2 \end{pmatrix}$

(b) If $AB = AC$, then $B = C$; $A = \begin{pmatrix} 1 & 2 \\ 2 & 4 \end{pmatrix}$, $B = \begin{pmatrix} 3 & 6 \\ -\frac{3}{2} & -3 \end{pmatrix}$, $C = \begin{pmatrix} 0 & 0 \\ 0 & 0 \end{pmatrix}$

(c) $A^2 = \begin{pmatrix} 0 & 0 \\ 0 & 0 \end{pmatrix}$ only if $A = \begin{pmatrix} 0 & 0 \\ 0 & 0 \end{pmatrix}$; $A = \begin{pmatrix} 0 & 2 \\ 0 & 0 \end{pmatrix}$

(d) $(A + B)(A - B) = A^2 - B^2$; $A = \begin{pmatrix} 3 & 1 \\ 2 & -4 \end{pmatrix}$ and $B = \begin{pmatrix} 2 & -1 \\ 5 & 3 \end{pmatrix}$

(e) $(A + B)(A + B) = A^2 + 2AB + B^2$; $A = \begin{pmatrix} 2 & -1 \\ 3 & 5 \end{pmatrix}$ and $B = \begin{pmatrix} 1 & 2 \\ -3 & 4 \end{pmatrix}$

B.6. Verify each of these statements by calculating the determinant on the left side, finding the product on the right side, and comparing the two.

(a) $\begin{vmatrix} 1 & x & x^2 \\ 1 & y & y^2 \\ 1 & z & z^2 \end{vmatrix} = (x - y)(y - z)(z - x)$

(b) $\begin{vmatrix} 1 & 1 & 1 \\ u & v & w \\ u^2 & v^2 & w^2 \end{vmatrix} = (u - v)(v - w)(w - u)$

B.7. (a) Compute the determinant

$$\begin{vmatrix} 1 & x & y \\ 1 & a & b \\ 1 & c & d \end{vmatrix}$$

(b) Verify that the equation of the straight line through the distinct points (a, b) and (c, d) is

$$\begin{vmatrix} 1 & x & y \\ 1 & a & b \\ 1 & c & d \end{vmatrix} = 0$$

B.8. Calculation of $|A|$ by expansion along a row or column. Consider the matrix

$$A = \begin{pmatrix} a_1 & b_1 & c_1 \\ a_2 & b_2 & c_2 \\ a_3 & b_3 & c_3 \end{pmatrix}$$

(a) Choose any row or column of the matrix (one or the other, not both). Use the entries in the chosen row or column to compute the following number

$$\pm \begin{pmatrix} \text{first entry} \\ \text{in chosen row} \\ \text{or column} \end{pmatrix} \begin{pmatrix} \text{minor of} \\ \text{this entry} \end{pmatrix} \pm \begin{pmatrix} \text{second entry} \\ \text{in chosen row} \\ \text{or column} \end{pmatrix} \begin{pmatrix} \text{minor of} \\ \text{this entry} \end{pmatrix}$$

$$\pm \begin{pmatrix} \text{third entry} \\ \text{in chosen} \\ \text{row or column} \end{pmatrix} \begin{pmatrix} \text{minor of} \\ \text{this entry} \end{pmatrix}$$

where the sign ($+$ or $-$) of each term is determined by the position of the chosen entry in the matrix, according to the following scheme:

$$\begin{pmatrix} + & - & + \\ - & + & - \\ + & - & + \end{pmatrix}$$

(b) Verify that the number you have computed is precisely the determinant of the matrix A. (Compare your answer with $|A|$ as given on p. 408, where the computation was made using the first row.)

(c) Make this computation five times using successively row 2, row 3, column 1, column 2, and column 3. In each case, verify that the answer is $|A|$.

B.9. Each of the following statements is true for all $n \times n$ matrices and determinants. Give a specific numerical example of each statement, using 3×3 matrices and determinants.

(a) If the matrix B is obtained from the matrix A by interchanging two rows, then $|B| = -|A|$.

(b) If the matrix B is obtained from the matrix A by multiplying a row of A by a constant c, then $|B| = c|A|$.

(c) If the matrix B is obtained from the matrix A by adding a constant multiple of one row to another row, then $|B| = |A|$.

(d) If a matrix A contains a row of zeros, then $|A| = 0$.

(e) Statements (a)–(d) are true with "row" replaced by "column."

B.10. Use Cramer's Rule to solve these systems of equations:

(a) $-3x + 5y = 2$
$2x + 7y = 1$

(c) $\frac{3}{2}x + 2y = \frac{5}{2}$
$5x - 7y = 1$

(e) $7x - 12y = 4$
$3x - 5y = 2$

(b) $7x - 12y = 4$
$3x - 5y = 2$

(d) $x - \frac{5}{3}y = 2$
$6x + \frac{4}{3}y = 1$

(f) $\sqrt{5}x - 2\sqrt{3}y = 2$
$\sqrt{3}x + 2\sqrt{5}y = 3$

B.11. Use Cramer's Rule to determine which of these homogeneous systems have exactly one solution (namely, the trivial one $x = 0$, $y = 0$, $z = 0$).

(a) $2x + y - 2z = 0$
$3x + 2y - z = 0$
$4x + y - 3z = 0$

(c) $2x + 4y + z = 0$
$6x - y + 3z = 0$
$4x + 6y + 2z = 0$

(b) $x + 2y - 3z = 0$
$3x - 5y - 9z = 0$
$2x + 4y - 6z = 0$

(d) $3x + 2y - z = 0$
$2x + y + z = 0$
$5x - 2y - z = 0$

3. THE BINOMIAL THEOREM

The Binomial Theorem provides a formula for calculating the product $(x + y)^n$ for any positive integer n. Before we can state the Binomial Theorem, certain preliminary definitions are needed.

FACTORIALS AND BINOMIAL COEFFICIENTS

Let n be a positive integer. The symbol $n!$ (read **n factorial**) denotes the product of all the integers from 1 to n. For example,

$$2! = 1 \cdot 2 = 2, \quad 3! = 1 \cdot 2 \cdot 3 = 6, \quad 4! = 1 \cdot 2 \cdot 3 \cdot 4 = 24,$$
$$5! = 1 \cdot 2 \cdot 3 \cdot 4 \cdot 5 = 120, \quad 10! = 1 \cdot 2 \cdot 3 \cdot 4 \cdot 5 \cdot 6 \cdot 7 \cdot 8 \cdot 9 \cdot 10 = 3,628,800$$

and in general,

$$n! = 1 \cdot 2 \cdot 3 \cdot 4 \cdots (n - 2)(n - 1)n$$

As you can see, $n!$ may be very large even when n is relatively small. In fact, 15! is larger than a trillion and 20! is larger than $2 \cdot 10^{18}$. It will be convenient for certain calculations later to give a meaning to the symbol 0! (read zero factorial). We *define* 0! to be the number 1.

We now use factorials to define some numbers that will turn out to be quite important.

> *If* r *and* n *are integers with* $0 \leq r \leq n$, *then*
>
> *the symbol* $\binom{n}{r}$ *denotes the number* $\dfrac{n!}{r!(n - r)!}$.
>
> *Each of the numbers* $\binom{n}{r}$ *is called a* **binomial coefficient.**

For example,

$$\binom{5}{3} = \frac{5!}{3!(5 - 3)!} = \frac{5}{3!2!} = \frac{1 \cdot 2 \cdot 3 \cdot 4 \cdot 5}{(1 \cdot 2 \cdot 3)(1 \cdot 2)} = \frac{4 \cdot 5}{2} = 10,$$

$$\binom{4}{2} = \frac{4!}{2!(4 - 2)!} = \frac{4!}{2!2!} = \frac{1 \cdot 2 \cdot 3 \cdot 4}{(1 \cdot 2)(1 \cdot 2)} = \frac{3 \cdot 4}{2} = 6,$$

$$\binom{3}{0} = \frac{3!}{0!(3 - 0)!} = \frac{3!}{0!3!} = \frac{3!}{3!} = 1 \quad \text{and} \quad \binom{3}{3} = \frac{3!}{3!(3 - 3)!} = \frac{3!}{3!0!} = \frac{3!}{3!} = 1$$

More generally, for any nonnegative integer n we have

$$\binom{n}{0} = \frac{n!}{0!(n-0)!} = \frac{n!}{0!n!} = \frac{n!}{n!} = 1 \quad \text{and} \quad \binom{n}{n} = \frac{n!}{n!(n-n)!} = \frac{n!}{n!0!} = \frac{n!}{n!} = 1$$

Therefore

$$\binom{n}{0} = 1 \quad and \quad \binom{n}{n} = 1 \quad for\ each\ integer\ n \geq 0$$

The preceding examples illustrate this important fact about binomial coefficients:

$$Every\ binomial\ coefficient\ \binom{n}{r}\ is\ an\ integer.$$

This fact will be proved in the next section. We shall assume it for now.

If we list the binomial coefficients for each value of n in this manner,

$$n = 0 \qquad \binom{0}{0}$$

$$n = 1 \qquad \binom{1}{0} \qquad \binom{1}{1}$$

$$n = 2 \qquad \binom{2}{0} \qquad \binom{2}{1} \qquad \binom{2}{2}$$

$$n = 3 \qquad \binom{3}{0} \qquad \binom{3}{1} \qquad \binom{3}{2} \qquad \binom{3}{3}$$

$$n = 4 \qquad \binom{4}{0} \qquad \binom{4}{1} \qquad \binom{4}{2} \qquad \binom{4}{3} \qquad \binom{4}{4}$$

$$\vdots$$

and then calculate each of them, we obtain the following array of numbers:

row 0					1				
row 1				1		1			
row 2			1		2		1		
row 3		1		3		3		1	
row 4	1		4		6		4		1

$$\vdots$$

This array is called **Pascal's triangle.** Some of its properties are discussed in Exercise C.1(d).

THE BINOMIAL THEOREM

We want to find a formula for calculating products such as

$$(x + y)^4, \qquad (x + y)^7, \qquad (x + y)^{24}$$

and more generally,

$$(x + y)^n, \qquad n \text{ any nonnegative integer}$$

We begin by calculating these products for small values of n to see if we can find some kind of pattern. Verify that the following computations are accurate:

$$
\begin{array}{lll}
n = 0 & (x + y)^0 = & 1 \\
n = 1 & (x + y)^1 = & x + y \\
n = 2 & (x + y)^2 = & x^2 + 2xy + y^2 \\
n = 3 & (x + y)^3 = & x^3 + 3x^2y + 3xy^2 + y^3 \\
n = 4 & (x + y)^4 = & x^4 + 4x^3y + 6x^2y^2 + 4xy^3 + y^4
\end{array}
$$

For these small values of n, some parts of the pattern are already clear. For each positive n, the first term is x^n and the last term is y^n. Beginning with the second term,

The successive exponents of y are $1, 2, 3, \ldots, n$

In each term before the last one, the exponent of x is 1 less than the preceding term

Suppose this pattern holds true for larger values of n as well. Then for a fixed n, the expansion of $(x + y)^n$ would have first term x^n. In the second term, the exponent of x would be 1 less than n, namely, $n - 1$, and the exponent of y would be 1. So the second term would be of the form $(\text{constant})x^{n-1}y$. In the next term, the exponent of x would be 1 less again, namely, $n - 2$, and the exponent of y would be 2. Continuing in this fashion, we would have

$$(x + y)^n = x^n + (^\circ)x^{n-1}y + (^\circ)x^{n-2}y^2 + (^\circ)x^{n-3}y^3 + \cdots + (^\circ)xy^{n-1} + y^n$$

where the symbols $(^\circ)$ indicate the various constant coefficients.

In order to determine the constant coefficients in the expansion of $(x + y)^n$, we return to the computations made above for $n = 0, 1, 2, 3, 4$. The terms x, y, x^2, y^2, and so on, each have coefficient 1. If we omit the x's and y's and just list the coefficients that appear in the computations above, we obtain this array of numbers:

$$
\begin{array}{ccccccccc}
n = 0 & & & & & 1 & & & \\
n = 1 & & & & 1 & & 1 & & \\
n = 2 & & & 1 & & 2 & & 1 & \\
n = 3 & & 1 & & 3 & & 3 & & 1 \\
n = 4 & 1 & & 4 & & 6 & & 4 & & 1
\end{array}
$$

But this is just the top of Pascal's triangle. In the case $n = 4$, it means that the coefficients of the expansion of $(x + y)^4$ are just the binomial coefficients $\binom{4}{0}, \binom{4}{1}, \binom{4}{2},$

$\binom{4}{3}$, $\binom{4}{4}$; and similarly for the other small values of n. If this pattern holds true for larger n as well, then the coefficients of the expansion of $(x + y)^n$ are just the binomial coefficients

$$\binom{n}{0}, \ \binom{n}{1}, \ \binom{n}{2}, \ \binom{n}{3}, \cdots, \binom{n}{n-1}, \ \binom{n}{n}$$

Since $\binom{n}{0} = 1$ and $\binom{n}{n} = 1$ for every n, the first and last coefficients on this list are 1. This is consistent with the fact that the first and last terms are x^n and y^n.

The preceding discussion suggests that the following result is true:

THE BINOMIAL THEOREM

For each positive integer n,

$$(x + y)^n = x^n + \binom{n}{1}x^{n-1}y + \binom{n}{2}x^{n-2}y^2 +$$

$$\binom{n}{3}x^{n-3}y^3 + \cdots + \binom{n}{n-1}xy^{n-1} + y^n$$

The Binomial Theorem will be proved in Section 5 by means of mathematical induction. We shall assume its truth for now and illustrate some of its uses.

EXAMPLE In order to compute $(x + y)^8$ we apply the Binomial Theorem in the case $n = 8$:

$$(x + y)^8 = x^8 + \binom{8}{1}x^7y + \binom{8}{2}x^6y^2 + \binom{8}{3}x^5y^3$$

$$+ \binom{8}{4}x^4y^4 + \binom{8}{5}x^3y^5 + \binom{8}{6}x^2y^6 + \binom{8}{7}xy^7 + y^8$$

Now verify that

$$\binom{8}{1} = \frac{8!}{1!7!} = 8, \qquad \binom{8}{2} = \frac{8!}{2!6!} = 28, \qquad \binom{8}{3} = \frac{8!}{3!5!} = 56, \qquad \binom{8}{4} = \frac{8!}{4!4!} = 70$$

Using these facts, we see that

$$\binom{8}{5} = \frac{8!}{5!3!} = \binom{8}{3} = 56, \qquad \binom{8}{6} = \frac{8!}{6!2!} = \binom{8}{2} = 28, \qquad \binom{8}{7} = \frac{8!}{7!1!} = \binom{8}{1} = 8$$

Substituting these values in the expansion above, we have

$$(x + y)^8$$
$$= x^8 + 8x^7y + 28x^6y^2 + 56x^5y^3 + 70x^4y^4 + 56x^3y^5 + 28x^2y^6 + 8xy^7 + y^8$$

EXAMPLE To find $(1-z)^6$, we note that $1-z = 1+(-z)$ and apply the Binomial Theorem with $x=1$, $y=-z$, and $n=6$:

$$(1-z)^6$$

$$= 1^6 + \binom{6}{1}1^5(-z) + \binom{6}{2}1^4(-z)^2 + \binom{6}{3}1^3(-z)^3 + \binom{6}{4}1^2(-z)^4 + \binom{6}{5}1(-z)^5 + (-z)^6$$

$$= 1 - \binom{6}{1}z + \binom{6}{2}z^2 - \binom{6}{3}z^3 + \binom{6}{4}z^4 - \binom{6}{5}z^5 + z^6$$

$$= 1 - 6z + 15z^2 - 20z^3 + 15z^4 - 6z^5 + z^6$$

EXAMPLE Show that $(1.001)^{1000} > 2$ without using a calculator. We write 1.001 as $1 + .001$ and apply the Binomial Theorem with $x=1$, $y=.001$, and $n=1000$:

$$(1.001)^{1000} = (1+.001)^{1000} = 1^{1000} + \binom{1000}{1}1^{999}(.001) + \text{other positive terms}$$

$$= 1 + \binom{1000}{1}(.001) + \text{other positive terms}$$

But $\binom{1000}{1} = \dfrac{1000!}{1!999!} = \dfrac{1000 \cdot 999!}{999!} = 1000.$ Therefore $\binom{1000}{1}(.001) = 1,000(.001) = 1$ and

$$(1.001)^{1000} = 1 + 1 + \text{other positive terms} = 2 + \text{other positive terms}$$

Hence $(1.001)^{1000} > 2$.

Sometimes we only need to know one term in the expansion of $(x+y)^n$. If you examine the expansion given by the Binomial Theorem, you will see that in the second term y has exponent 1, in the third term y has exponent 2, and so on. Thus

---

In the binomial expansion of $(x+y)^n$,

> *The exponent of* y *is always one less than the number of the term.*

Furthermore, in each of the middle terms of the expansion,

> *The coefficient of the term containing* y^r *is* $\binom{n}{r}$.

> *The sum of the* x-*exponent and the* y-*exponent is* n.

For instance, in the *ninth* term of the expansion of $(x+y)^{13}$, y has exponent 8, the coefficient is $\binom{13}{8}$ and x must have exponent 5 (since $8+5=13$). Thus the ninth term is $\binom{13}{8}x^5y^8$.

EXAMPLE What is the ninth term of the expansion of $\left(2x^2 + \dfrac{\sqrt[4]{y}}{\sqrt{6}}\right)^{13}$? We shall use

the Binomial Theorem with $n = 13$ and with $2x^2$ in place of x and $\sqrt[4]{y}/\sqrt{6}$ in place of y. The remarks above show that the ninth term is

$$\binom{13}{8}(2x^2)^5 \left(\frac{\sqrt[4]{y}}{\sqrt{6}}\right)^8$$

Since $\sqrt[4]{y} = y^{1/4}$ and $\sqrt{6} = \sqrt{3}\sqrt{2} = 3^{1/2}2^{1/2}$, we can simplify as follows:

$$\binom{13}{8}(2x^2)^5 \left(\frac{\sqrt[4]{y}}{\sqrt{6}}\right)^8 = \binom{13}{8}2^5(x^2)^5 \frac{(y^{1/4})^8}{(3^{1/2})^8(2^{1/2})^8} = \binom{13}{8}2^5 x^{10} \frac{y^2}{3^4 \cdot 2^4}$$

$$= \binom{13}{8}\frac{2}{3^4}x^{10}y^2 = \frac{13 \cdot 12 \cdot 11 \cdot 10 \cdot 9}{5 \cdot 4 \cdot 3 \cdot 2} \cdot \frac{2}{3^4}x^{10}y^2 = \frac{286}{9}x^{10}y^2$$

EXERCISES

A.1. Evaluate:

    (a) $6!$ (b) $\dfrac{11!}{8!}$ (c) $\dfrac{12!}{9!3!}$ (d) $\dfrac{9! - 8!}{7!}$

A.2. Evaluate

    (a) $\dbinom{5}{3} + \dbinom{5}{2} - \dbinom{6}{3}$ (e) $\dbinom{100}{96}$

    (b) $\dbinom{12}{11} - \dbinom{11}{10} + \dbinom{7}{0}$ (f) $\dbinom{75}{72}$

    (c) $\dbinom{6}{0} + \dbinom{6}{1} + \dbinom{6}{2} + \dbinom{6}{3} + \dbinom{6}{4} + \dbinom{6}{5} + \dbinom{6}{6}$

    (d) $\dbinom{6}{0} - \dbinom{6}{1} + \dbinom{6}{2} - \dbinom{6}{3} + \dbinom{6}{4} - \dbinom{6}{5} + \dbinom{6}{6}$

A.3. Expand:
    (a) $(x + y)^5$ (c) $(a - b)^5$ (e) $(2x + y^2)^5$
    (b) $(a + b)^7$ (d) $(c - d)^8$ (f) $(3u - v^3)^6$

B.1. (a) Verify that $\dbinom{9}{1} = 9$ and $\dbinom{9}{8} = 9$.

    (b) Prove that for each positive integer n, $\dbinom{n}{1} = n$ and $\dbinom{n}{n-1} = n$. [*Note:* part (a) is just the case when $n = 9$ and $n - 1 = 8$.]

B.2. Expand and simplify (where possible).
(a) $(\sqrt{x} + 1)^6$ (c) $(1 - c)^{10}$ (e) $(x^{-3} + x)^4$

(b) $(2 - \sqrt{y})^5$ (d) $\left(\sqrt{c} + \dfrac{1}{\sqrt{c}}\right)^7$ (f) $(3x^{-2} - x^2)^6$

B.3. Use the Binomial Theorem to compute:
(a) $(1 + \sqrt{3})^4 + (1 - \sqrt{3})^4$ (c) $(1 + i)^6$, where $i^2 = -1$
(b) $(\sqrt{3} + 1)^6 - (\sqrt{3} - 1)^6$ (d) $(\sqrt{2} - i)^4$, where $i^2 = -1$

B.4. Find the indicated term of the expansion of the given expression.
(a) third, $(x + y)^5$ (d) third, $(a + 2)^8$

(b) fourth, $(a + b)^6$ (e) fourth, $\left(u^{-2} + \dfrac{u}{2}\right)^7$

(c) fifth, $(c - d)^7$ (f) fifth, $(\sqrt{x} - \sqrt{2})^7$

B.5. Find the coefficient of
(a) x^5y^8 in the expansion of $(2x - y^2)^9$
(b) $x^{12}y^6$ in the expansion of $(x^3 - 3y)^{10}$

(c) $\dfrac{1}{x^3}$ in the expansion of $\left(2x + \dfrac{1}{x^2}\right)^6$

B.6. Find the constant term in the expansion of $\left(y - \dfrac{1}{2y}\right)^{10}$.

B.7. (a) Verify that $\dbinom{7}{2} = \dbinom{7}{5}$.

(b) Let r and n be integers with $0 \le r \le n$. Prove that $\dbinom{n}{r} = \dbinom{n}{n - r}$. [*Note:* part (a) is just the case when $n = 7$ and $r = 2$.]

B.8. For any positive integer n,
(a) Prove that $2^n = \dbinom{n}{0} + \dbinom{n}{1} + \dbinom{n}{2} + \cdots + \dbinom{n}{n}$. [*Hint:* $2^n = (1 + 1)^n$.]

(b) Prove that $\dbinom{n}{0} - \dbinom{n}{1} + \dbinom{n}{2} - \dbinom{n}{3} + \dbinom{n}{4} - \cdots + (-1)^k \dbinom{n}{k} + \cdots$
$+ (-1)^n \dbinom{n}{n} = 0$.

B.9. (a) Use the Binomial Theorem with $x = \sin\theta$ and $y = \cos\theta$ to find $(\cos\theta + i\sin\theta)^4$ where $i^2 = -1$.
(b) Use DeMoivre's Theorem to find $(\cos\theta + i\sin\theta)^4$.
(c) Use the fact that the two expressions obtained in parts (a) and (b) must be equal to express $\cos 4\theta$ and $\sin 4\theta$ in terms of $\sin\theta$ and $\cos\theta$.

B.10. (a) Let f be the function given by $f(x) = x^5$. Let h be a nonzero number and compute $f(x + h) - f(x)$ [but leave all binomial coefficients in the form $\binom{5}{r}$ here and below].

(b) Use part (a) to show that h is a factor of $f(x + h) - f(x)$ and find $\dfrac{f(x + h) - f(x)}{h}$.

(c) If h is *very* close to 0, find a simple approximation of the quantity $\dfrac{f(x + h) - f(x)}{h}$. [See part (b).]

(d) Do parts (a)–(c) with $f(x) = x^8$ in place of $f(x) = x^5$.

(e) Do parts (a)–(c) with $f(x) = x^{12}$ in place of $f(x) = x^5$.

(f) Let n be a fixed positive integer. Do parts (a)–(c) with $f(x) = x^n$ in place of $f(x) = x^5$.

C.1. Let r and n be integers such that $0 \le r \le n$.

(a) Verify that $(n - r)! = (n - r)(n - (r + 1))!$

(b) Verify that $(n - r)! = ((n + 1) - (r + 1))!$

(c) Prove that $\binom{n}{r+1} + \binom{n}{r} = \binom{n+1}{r+1}$ for any $r \le n - 1$. [*Hint:* write out the terms on the left side and use parts (a) and (b) to express each of them as a fraction with denominator $(r + 1)!(n - r)!$. Then add these two fractions, simplify the numerator and compare the result with $\binom{n+1}{r+1}$.]

(d) Interpret the result of part (c) as a statement about how the entries of one row of Pascal's triangle are related to the entries in the next row.

(e) Use part (d) to write out rows 2 to 10 of Pascal's triangle *without* computing any binomial coefficients.

C.2. (a) Find these numbers and write them one *below* the next: 11^0, 11^1, 11^2, 11^3, 11^4.

(b) Compare the list in part (a) with rows 0 to 4 of Pascal's triangle. What's the explanation?

(c) What can be said about 11^5 and row 5 of Pascal's triangle?

(d) Calculate all integer powers of 101 from 101^0 to 101^8, list the results one under the other, and compare the list with rows 0 to 8 of Pascal's triangle. What's the explanation? What happens with 101^9?

4. COMBINATORIAL ALGEBRA

The answers to many questions involve systematic counting of all the possibilities that might occur. For instance, how many different three-person subcommittees can be formed from a ten-person committee? How likely is it that a five-card poker hand will contain a pair? How many possible outcomes are there in a four-team tournament? In this section we shall develop the techniques necessary to answer questions such as these.

Warning Factorial notation will be used frequently. If you have not already done so, you should read page 415 (but *not* the rest of Section 3) before going on.

PERMUTATIONS

A **permutation** of a set is an ordering of the elements of the set. To describe a specific permutation you must indicate which element is first, which is second, and so on. One way to do this is to list the elements in order from left to right: first, second, third, and so on. For example, each of the following is a permutation of the first 4 letters of the alphabet:

$$A\ B\ C\ D \qquad C\ A\ B\ D \qquad B\ C\ A\ D \qquad D\ C\ B\ A \qquad A\ C\ D\ B$$

  To solve many problems you need to know the total *number* of permutations of a particular set. To guide us in finding a formula for this number, we shall consider a specific example. We shall determine the total number of permutations of the letters A, B, C, D by systematically listing all the possibilities. There are 4 possibilities for first place: A, B, C, or D. Once first place is filled, there are just 3 possibilities for second place. For instance, if A is first, then the 3 possibilities for second are B, C, D (as shown in the first column below). Continuing in this fashion, we can list all the possibilities for both first and second place:

$$
\begin{array}{llll}
A\ B & B\ A & C\ A & D\ A \\
A\ C & B\ C & C\ B & D\ B \\
A\ D & B\ D & C\ D & D\ C
\end{array}
$$

As you can see, for *each* of the 4 possible first-place entries there are 3 possible second-place entries. So there are a total of $4 \cdot 3 = 12$ possibilities for both first and second place.

  Once the first two places have been determined, there are just 2 possibilities for third place. For example, if A is first and B is second, then the 2 possibilities for third are C and D. Each of these 2 possibilities leads to a different permutation, as shown below. (Note that once third place is determined, there's only one letter left for fourth place.]

$$
\begin{array}{llll}
A\ B\ C\ D & B\ A\ C\ D & C\ A\ B\ D & D\ A\ B\ C \\
A\ B\ D\ C & B\ A\ D\ C & C\ A\ D\ B & D\ A\ C\ B \\
A\ C\ B\ D & B\ C\ A\ D & C\ B\ A\ D & D\ B\ A\ C \\
A\ C\ D\ B & B\ C\ D\ A & C\ B\ D\ A & D\ B\ C\ A \\
A\ D\ B\ C & B\ D\ A\ C & C\ D\ A\ B & D\ C\ A\ B \\
A\ D\ C\ B & B\ D\ C\ A & C\ D\ B\ A & D\ C\ B\ A
\end{array}
$$

Each of the 12 possible orders for first and second place leads to 2 different permutations. So the total number of possible permutations of these four letters is $12 \cdot 2 = 24$.

  We can summarize this discussion by noting that $24 = 4 \cdot 3 \cdot 2 \cdot 1 = 4!$ and observing the role played by the numbers 4, 3, 2, 1 in our calculations:

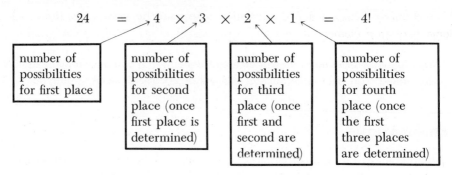

Essentially the same argument just used to show that the total number of permutations of a set of 4 elements is 4! can be used for any finite set. For example, to determine the number of permutations of a 6-element set, we note that there are 6 possibilities for first place and 5 possibilities for second place (once first place is determined). So there are $6 \cdot 5 = 30$ possibilities for both first and second place. Once these are determined, there are 4 possibilities for third place and thus $6 \cdot 5 \cdot 4$ possibilities for the first three places. Continuing in this manner, we see that the total number of permutations of a set of 6 elements is $6 \cdot 5 \cdot 4 \cdot 3 \cdot 2 \cdot 1 = 6! = 720$.

More generally, let n be a fixed positive integer. To determine the total number of permutations of a set of n elements, note that there are n possibilities for first place, $n - 1$ possibilities for second place (once first place is determined), $n - 2$ possibilities for third place (once first and second are determined), and so on until finally there is just 1 possibility for nth place (once the first $n - 1$ places are determined). Consequently,

> *The total number of permutations of a set of*
> n *elements is* $n(n - 1)(n - 2) \cdots 3 \cdot 2 \cdot 1 = n!$

EXAMPLE The number of possible batting orders for a nine-person baseball team (that is, the number of permutations of a 9-element set) is $9! = 362,880$.

EXAMPLE The number of possible ways that a deck of 52 cards can be shuffled (that is, the number of permutations of a 52-element set) is $52!$ (which is approximately equal to 8.066×10^{67}).

PERMUTATIONS OF *n* THINGS TAKEN *r* AT A TIME

A permutation of a set of n elements is a list of the n elements in order. But sometimes we don't want to list *all* of the elements of a set, but just some of them. For instance, in a typical race only the first, second, and third place runners win prizes. If you want to list the possible prize winners (in order of finishing) in an 8-person race, you must list all possible ways of ordering any 3 of the 8 racers.° Each such ordering is called a

---

° We assume that no ties occur.

permutation of 8 things taken 3 at a time. More generally, if $r \leq n$, an ordering of r elements of an n element set is called a **permutation of n things taken r at a time.**

EXAMPLE In how many ways can first, second, and third prizes be awarded in an 8-person race?[°] In other words, what is the total *number* of permutations of 8 things taken 3 at a time? Well, there are 8 possibilities for first place. After first place is determined, there are 7 possibilities for second place. Hence there are $8 \cdot 7 = 56$ possible ways for first and second place to occur. For each one of these 56 possible ways there are 6 possibilities for third place. So there are a total of $56 \cdot 6 = 336$ ways for first, second, and third place prizes to be awarded. Note that $336 = 8 \cdot 7 \cdot 6$.

In the preceding example we saw that the number of permutations of 8 things taken 3 at a time is $8 \cdot 7 \cdot 6$. Note that this number is the product of 3 consecutive integers, beginning with 8 and working down. The number of permutations of 11 things taken 5 at a time can be computed in a similar manner. It is $11 \cdot 10 \cdot 9 \cdot 8 \cdot 7 = 55,540$ since there are 11 possibilities for first place; 10 possibilities for second place; 9, for third; 8, for fourth; and 7 for fifth place. Note that the number $11 \cdot 10 \cdot 9 \cdot 8 \cdot 7$ is the product of 5 consecutive integers, beginning with *11* and working down. The same argument works in the general case and shows that:

> *The number of permutations of* n *things taken* r *at a time is the product of* r *consecutive integers, beginning with* n *and working down. This number is denoted by the symbol* $_nP_r$.

EXAMPLE The number $_9P_4$ of permutations of 9 things taken 4 at a time is the product of 4 consecutive integers, beginning with 9 and working down:

$$_9P_4 = 9 \cdot 8 \cdot 7 \cdot 6 = 3024$$

Similarly,

$$_8P_5 = 8 \cdot 7 \cdot 6 \cdot 5 \cdot 4 = 6720$$

$$\underbrace{}$$
5 consecutive integers beginning with 8

There is another convenient formula for finding $_nP_r$, the number of permutations of n things taken r at a time. For instance, in the preceding example we saw that $_9P_4 = 9 \cdot 8 \cdot 7 \cdot 6$. This number can be rewritten as follows:

$$_9P_4 = 9 \cdot 8 \cdot 7 \cdot 6 = \frac{9 \cdot 8 \cdot 7 \cdot 6}{1} \cdot \frac{5!}{5!} = \frac{9!}{5!} = \frac{9!}{(9-4)!}.$$

A similar argument with n in place of 9 and r in place of 4 shows that

[°] We assume that no ties occur.

> *The number* $_nP_r$ *of permutations of* n *things*
>
> *taken* r *at a time is* $\dfrac{n!}{(n-r)!}$.

EXAMPLE The number $_6P_4$ of permutations of 6 things taken 4 at a time is given by:

$$_6P_4 = \frac{6!}{(6-4)!} = \frac{6!}{2!} = \frac{6 \cdot 5 \cdot 4 \cdot 3 \cdot 2 \cdot 1}{2 \cdot 1} = 6 \cdot 5 \cdot 4 \cdot 3 = 360$$

Similarly,

$$_{20}P_5 = \frac{20!}{(20-5)!} = \frac{20!}{15!} = \frac{(20 \cdot 19 \cdot 18 \cdot 17 \cdot 16)(15!)}{15!} = 20 \cdot 19 \cdot 18 \cdot 17 \cdot 16 = 1{,}860{,}480$$

EXAMPLE The formulas given above are consistent with one another. For instance, the number of permutations of a set of 16 elements is 16!. This is the same as $_{16}P_{16}$, the number of permutations of 16 things taken 16 at a time since

$$_{16}P_{16} = \frac{16!}{(16-16)!} = \frac{16!}{0!} = \frac{16!}{1} = 16!$$

A FUNDAMENTAL COUNTING PRINCIPLE

Almost all the counting techniques in this section are just special cases of one general principle. The statement of this principle will be easy to understand if we first consider one of the examples above from a slightly different point of view. Suppose 8 people participate in a race in which first, second, and third prizes are awarded. Think of the awarding of the first prize as one **event,** the awarding of the second prize as another event, and the awarding of the third prize as still another event. There are 8 possible ways for the first event to occur, depending on which of the 8 runners wins the race. After that there are 7 ways for the next event to occur, depending on which of the 7 other runners comes in second.° Finally, there are 6 ways for the last event to occur, depending on which of the 6 remaining runners finishes third. So the total number of ways that all three events can occur is the product $8 \cdot 7 \cdot 6$. This is just an example of

> ### THE FUNDAMENTAL COUNTING PRINCIPLE
>
> *Consider a list of* k *events. Suppose the first event can occur in* n_1 *ways; the second event can occur in* n_2 *ways (once the first event has occurred); the third event can occur in* n_3 *ways (once the first two events have occurred); and so on. Then the total number of ways that all the events can occur is the product* $n_1 n_2 n_3 \cdots n_k$.

°We assume that no ties occur.

EXAMPLE A committee consisting of 8 Democrats and 6 Republicans must choose a chairperson, a vice-chairperson, a secretary, and a treasurer. The chairperson must be a Democrat and the vice-chairperson, a Republican. The secretary and treasurer may belong to either party. No person may hold more than one office. In how many different ways can these four officers be chosen? Let the first event be the choice of a chairperson. Since any one of the 8 Democrats can be chairperson, this event can occur in 8 ways (in the notation above $n_1 = 8$). Let the second event be the choice of a vice-chairperson. Since any of the 6 Republicans can be vice-chairperson, this event can occur in 6 ways (that is, $n_2 = 6$). Let the third event be the choice of a secretary. After the chairperson and vice-chairperson have been chosen, any of the 12 remaining members may be secretary. So this event can occur in 12 ways [that is, $n_3 = 12$]. Finally, let the fourth and last event be the choice of a treasurer. After the first three officers have been chosen, there are 11 members left as possible treasurers. So this event can occur in 11 ways [in the notation above $k = 4$ and $n_k = n_4 = 11$]. Therefore the total number of ways all four officers can be chosen is the product $n_1 n_2 n_3 n_4 = 8 \cdot 6 \cdot 12 \cdot 11 = 6336$.

EXAMPLE How many license plates are there consisting of 3 letters of the alphabet followed by 3 numerals (using the ten digits 0 through 9), subject to the conditions that no plate begin with A, E, I, O, or U and that the first numeral may not be 0? Since each license plate has six positions, we can think of the filling of each position by a letter or number as an event. The 5 vowels are excluded from the first position, so it may be filled in 21 ways. The second and third positions may each be filled in 26 ways. The fourth position (the first numeral) cannot be 0, so it may be filled in 9 ways. *Each* of the last two positions may be filled in 10 ways. According to the Fundamental Counting Principle, the total number of license plates is the product $21 \cdot 26 \cdot 26 \cdot 9 \cdot 10 \cdot 10 = 12{,}776{,}400$.

DISTINGUISHABLE PERMUTATIONS*

Suppose you have 3 identical red marbles, 3 identical white marbles, and 2 identical blue ones. How many different color patterns can be formed by placing the 8 marbles in a row? Each way of placing the marbles in a row is a permutation and we know that there are 8! permutations of 8 marbles. But the *same* color pattern may result from *different* permutations. To see how this can happen, consider the color pattern

R W B R W B R W

where R indicates red, W white, and B blue. To keep the marbles straight, mentally label the red ones R_1, R_2, R_3, the white ones W_1, W_2, W_3, and the blue ones B_1, B_2. Here are several different permutations of the marbles that all produce the *same* color pattern shown above:

$$R_3 \ W_1 \ B_1 \ R_1 \ W_3 \ B_2 \ R_2 \ W_2; \qquad R_2 \ W_2 \ B_1 \ R_3 \ W_1 \ B_2 \ R_1 \ W_1;$$
$$R_1 \ W_3 \ B_2 \ R_3 \ W_2 \ B_1 \ R_2 \ W_1$$

° This subsection is optional and is not needed to understand the discussion of combinations that begins on page 429.

Permutations that produce the same color pattern, such as the three listed above, are said to be **indistinguishable.** Observe that any one of the three indistinguishable permutations shown above may be obtained from any of the others simply by rearranging the red marbles among themselves, the white marbles among themselves, and the blue marbles among themselves. Permutations that produce different color patterns are said to be **distinguishable.** If two permutations are distinguishable, then one *cannot* be obtained from the other simply by rearranging the marbles of the same color. Finding the total number of different color patterns is the same as finding the total number of distinguishable permutations of the 8 marbles.

In order to find the total number of different color patterns (distinguishable permutations), we shall proceed indirectly. We shall examine the way in which a specific permutation of the marbles is determined. Any permutation of the marbles (for instance, $R_1 \, W_3 \, B_2 \, R_3 \, W_2 \, B_1 \, R_2 \, W_1$) is determined by these four things:

(i)   A color pattern (in the example the pattern R W B R W B R W)
(ii) The order in which the red marbles appear in the red positions of the pattern (in the example, $R_1 \, R_3 \, R_2$), that is, a permutation of the 3 red marbles
(iii) The order in which the white marbles appear in the white positions of the pattern (in the example $W_3 \, W_2 \, W_1$), that is, a permutation of the 3 white marbles
(iv) The order in which the blue marbles appear in the blue positions of the pattern (in the example, $B_2 \, B_1$), that is, a permutation of the 2 blue marbles

A specific choice of one possibility for *each* of items (i) to (iv) will lead to exactly one permutation of the 8 marbles. Conversely, every permutation of the 8 marbles uniquely determines a choice in each one of items (i) to (iv), as shown by the example above. So the total number of permutations of the 8 marbles, namely, 8!, is the same as the total number of ways that items (i) to (iv) can all occur. According to the Fundamental Counting Principle, this number is the product of the numbers of ways each of the four items can occur. Therefore

$$8! = \begin{pmatrix} \text{number of} \\ \text{color} \\ \text{patterns} \end{pmatrix} \times \begin{pmatrix} \text{number of} \\ \text{permutations of} \\ \text{3 red marbles,} \\ \text{namely, 3!} \end{pmatrix} \times \begin{pmatrix} \text{number of} \\ \text{permutations of} \\ \text{3 white marbles,} \\ \text{namely, 3!} \end{pmatrix} \times \begin{pmatrix} \text{number of} \\ \text{permutations of} \\ \text{2 blue marbles,} \\ \text{namely, 2!} \end{pmatrix}$$

If we let N denote the number of color patterns, this statement becomes:

$$8! = N \cdot 3! \cdot 3! \cdot 2!$$

Solving this equation for N we see that

$$N = \frac{8!}{3! \cdot 3! \cdot 2!} = 560$$

So there are 560 different color patterns, or in other words, 560 distinguishable permutations of the 8 marbles.

More generally, suppose that n and $k_1, k_2, \ldots, k_t$ are positive integers such that $n = k_1 + k_2 + \cdots + k_t$. Suppose that a set consists of n objects and that k_1 of these objects are all of one kind (such as red marbles), that k_2 of the objects are all of another kind (such as white marbles), that k_3 of the objects are all of a third kind (such as blue marbles), and so on. We say that two permutations of this set are distinguishable if one cannot be obtained from the other simply by rearranging objects of the same kind. The total number of distinguishable permutations can be found by using the same method that was used to find the total number of color patterns in the marble example above (where we had $n = 8$ and $k_1 = 3$, $k_2 = 3$, $k_3 = 2$):

Given a set of n *objects in which* k_1 *are of one kind,* k_2 *are of a second kind,* k_3 *are of a third kind, and so on, then the number of distinguishable permutations of the set is*

$$\frac{n!}{k_1! \cdot k_2! \cdot k_3! \cdots k_t!}$$

EXAMPLE The number of distinguishable ways that the letters in the word TEN-NESSEE can be arranged is just the number of distinguishable permutations of the set consisting of the 9 symbols T, E, N, N, E, S, S, E, E. There are 4 E's, 2 N's, 2 S's, and 1 T. So we apply the formula in the box above with $n = 9$; $k_1 = 4$; $k_2 = 2$; $k_3 = 2$; $k_4 = 1$; and find that the number of distinguishable permutations is

$$\frac{9!}{4! \; 2! \; 2! \; 1!} = \frac{9 \cdot 8 \cdot 7 \cdot 6 \cdot 5 \cdot 4 \cdot 3 \cdot 2 \cdot 1}{4 \cdot 3 \cdot 2 \cdot 1 \cdot 2 \cdot 1 \cdot 2 \cdot 1 \cdot 1} = 3780$$

COMBINATIONS

A bridge player is interested in the 13 cards in his or her hand but not in the order that these cards were dealt. The same hand can be dealt in many different orders. The bridge player might also be interested in the total number of possible bridge hands, that is, the number of different ways that 13 cards can be selected from a 52-card deck, without regard to the order in which the cards are chosen. In order to find this number, we shall consider an analogous, but more general situation.

Let r be a positive integer. A **combination** of r objects in a set is any collection of r distinct objects in the set (without regard to the order in which the r objects might be chosen). For instance, a bridge hand is a combination of 13 cards in the deck of cards. When the set has n elements, the combination of r objects of the set is sometimes called a **combination of n things taken r at a time.**

EXAMPLE A bridge hand is a combination of 52 things taken 13 at a time. The collection consisting of the 5 letters A, M, P, T, X of the 26-letter alphabet is a combination of 26 things taken 5 at a time.

Warning Be sure you understand the difference between combinations and permutations. A combination is a collection in which order doesn't matter. Consider, for instance, the 26-letter alphabet. *One* combination of these 26 letters taken 3 at a time consists of the letters A, B, C. If we list these letters as B, A, C or C, B, A or B, A, C, we still have the same collection—the *same combination*. But order *does* matter with permutations. There are *six different permutations* of these 3 letters:

$$A\ B\ C \qquad A\ C\ B \qquad B\ A\ C \qquad B\ C\ A \qquad C\ A\ B \qquad C\ B\ A$$

In order to find the total number of combinations of n things taken r at a time, we shall examine the relationship between such combinations (where order doesn't matter) and *permutations* of n things taken r at a time (where order matters). A specific permutation of n things taken r at a time is determined by two factors:

(i)   A choice of r things in the set, that is, a combination of n things taken r at a time

(ii) A specific ordering of these r things, that is, a permutation of r things

Consequently, the total number of permutations of n things taken r at a time, namely, $\dfrac{n!}{(n-r)!}$, is the same as the total number of ways that items (i) and (ii) can both occur. According to the Fundamental Counting Principle, this number is the product of the number of ways item (i) can occur and the number of ways item (ii) can occur. Therefore

$$\frac{n!}{(n-r)!} = \binom{\text{number of combinations of}}{n \text{ things taken } r \text{ at a time}} \times \binom{\text{number of permutations of}}{r \text{ things, namely, } r!}$$

If we temporarily let C denote the number of combinations of n things taken r at a time, then this last statement becomes:

$$\frac{n!}{(n-r)!} = C \cdot r!$$

Dividing both sides of this equation by $r!$ shows that $C = \dfrac{n!}{r!(n-r)!}$. As we saw on page 415, this number is denoted $\dbinom{n}{r}$ and called a binomial coefficient. Therefore

---

The number of combinations of n *things taken* r *at a time is*

$$\binom{n}{r} = \frac{n!}{r!(n-r)!}$$

EXAMPLE   To find the number of 3-person subcommittees that can be formed from a 10-person committee, that is, the number of combinations of 10 things taken 3 at a time, apply the formula in the box with $n = 10$ and $r = 3$:

$$\binom{10}{3} = \frac{10!}{3!(10-3)!} = \frac{10!}{3! \cdot 7!} = \frac{10 \cdot 9 \cdot 8 \cdot 7!}{3 \cdot 2 \cdot 1 \cdot 7!} = \frac{10 \cdot 9 \cdot 8}{3 \cdot 2} = 120$$

EXAMPLE   The number of possible bridge hands; that is, the number of combinations of 52 cards taken 13 at a time is:

$$\binom{52}{13} = \frac{52!}{13!(52-13)!} = \frac{52!}{13! \cdot 39!} = 635{,}013{,}559{,}600$$

EXAMPLE The senate in a certain state legislature consists of 18 Democrats, 20 Republicans, and 7 Independents. In how many ways can you select a committee consisting of 3 Democrats, 4 Republicans, and 2 Independents? The number of ways of choosing 3 of the 18 Democrats is the number $\binom{18}{3}$ of combinations of 18 things taken 3 at a time. The number of ways of choosing 4 of the 20 Republicans is the number $\binom{20}{4}$ of combinations of 20 things taken 4 at a time. Similarly, the number of ways of choosing 2 of the 7 Independents is $\binom{7}{2}$. According to the Fundamental Counting Principle, the number of ways that all these choices can be made is the product

$$\binom{18}{3}\binom{20}{4}\binom{7}{2} = \frac{18!}{3!(18-3)!} \cdot \frac{20!}{4!(20-4)!} \cdot \frac{7!}{2!(7-2)!} = \frac{18!}{3! \cdot 15!} \frac{20!}{4! \cdot 16!} \frac{7!}{2! \cdot 5!}$$
$$= 83{,}023{,}920$$

EXERCISES

A.1. Compute:
  (a) $_4P_3$ (b) $_7P_5$ (c) $_8P_8$ (d) $_5P_1$ (e) $_{12}P_2$ (f) $_{11}P_3$

A.2. Compute:

  (a) $\binom{14}{2}$ (b) $\binom{20}{3}$ (c) $\binom{99}{95}$ (d) $\binom{65}{60}$

B.1. Compute:

  (a) $_nP_2$ (b) $_nP_{n-1}$ (c) $\binom{n}{n-1}$ (d) $\binom{n}{1}$ (e) $\binom{n}{2}$ (f) $_nP_1$

B.2. Find the number n that makes the given statement true:
  (a) $_nP_4 = 8(_nP_3)$ (c) $_nP_6 = 9(_{n-1}P_5)$ (e) $_nP_5 = 21(_{n-1}P_3)$
  (b) $_nP_5 = 7(_nP_4)$ (d) $_nP_7 = 11(_{n-1}P_6)$ (f) $_nP_6 = 30(_{n-2}P_4)$

B.3. In how many different orders can 8 people be seated in a row?

B.4. In how many orders can 6 pictures be arranged in a vertical line?

B.5. How many outcomes are possible in a four-team tournament (in which there are no ties)?

B.6. How many 5-digit numbers can be formed from the numerals 2, 3, 4, 5, 6 if (a) no repeated digits are allowed? (b) repeated digits are allowed?

B.7. In how many ways can the first four people in the batting order of a nine-person baseball team be chosen?

B.8. In how many different ways can first through third prizes be awarded in a ten-person race (assume no ties occur)?

B.9. How many five-letter identification codes can be formed from the first twenty letters of the alphabet if
(a) no repetitions are allowed? (b) repetitions are allowed?

B.10. How many different numbers can be formed from the digits 3, 5, 7, 9 if no repetitions are allowed? [*Hint:* How many one-digit numbers can be formed? How many two-digit ones?]

B.11. How many seven-digit phone numbers can be formed from the numerals 0 through 9 if none of the first three digits can be 0?

B.12. How many batting orders are possible for a nine-player baseball team if the four infielders bat first and the pitcher bats last?

B.13. A man has four pairs of pants, six sports coats, and eight ties. In how many different ways can he wear one of each?

B.14. In how many different ways can an eight-question True–False test be answered?

B.15. An exam consists of ten multiple-choice questions, with four choices for each question. In how many ways can the exam be answered?

B.16. In how many ways can 6 men and 6 women be seated in a row of 12 chairs if the women sit in the even numbered seats?

B.17. In how many distinguishable ways can the letters in the given word be arranged?
(a) LOOK (c) CINCINNATI
(b) MISSISSIPPI (d) BOOKKEEPER

B.18. How many color patterns can be obtained by placing five red, seven black, three white, and four orange discs in a row?

B.19. In how many different ways can you write the algebraic expression $x^4y^2z^3$ without using exponents (no fractions allowed)?

B.20. A professor plans to grade a 22-person class on a curve by giving 2 A's, 6 B's, 11 C's, 2 D's, and 1 F. In how many ways can this be done?

B.21. A student must answer five questions on an eight-question exam. In how many ways can this be done?

B.22. How many different straight lines are determined by 8 points in the plane, no 3 of which lie on the same straight line? (Remember that a line is determined by 2 points.)

B.23. How many games must be played in an eight-team league if each team is to play every other team exactly twice?

B.24. (a) How many different 5-card poker hands are possible from a 52-card deck?

    (b) How many of these are flushes (5 cards of the same suit)? [*Hint:* The number of club flushes is the number of ways 5 cards can be chosen from the 13 clubs.]

B.25. How many eight-digit numbers can be formed using three 6's and five 7's?

B.26. How many different 5-person committees consisting of 3 women and 2 men can be chosen from a group of 10 women and 8 men?

B.27. How many ways can two committees, one of 4 people and one of 3 people, be chosen from a group of 11 people if no person serves on both committees?

B.28. How many six-digit numbers can be formed using only the numerals 5 and 9?

B.29. **(a)** A basketball squad consists of 5 people who can play center or forward and 7 people who can only play guard. In how many ways can a team consisting of a center, 2 forwards, and 2 guards be chosen?
    (b) How many teams are possible if the squad consists of 2 centers, 4 forwards, and 6 people who can play either guard or forward?

B.30. **(a)** How many different pairs are possible from a standard 52-card deck? [*Hint:* how many pairs can be formed from the 4 aces? how many from the 4 kings?]
    (b) How many 5-card poker hands consist of a pair of aces and three other cards none of which are aces?
    (c) How many 5-card poker hands contain at least two aces?
    (d) How many 5-card poker hands are full houses (three of a kind and a pair of another kind)?

C.1. **(a)** In how many different orders can 3 objects be placed around a circle? (Note that ABC, BCA, and CAB are different orders when the three letters are in a line, but the *same* order in a circular arrangement.)
    (b) Do part (a) for 4 objects.
    (c) Do part (a) for 5 objects.
    (d) Let n be a positive integer and do part (a) for n objects.

C.2. In how many ways can six different foods be arranged around the edge of a circular table? (See Exercise **C.1.**)

C.3. In how many different orders could King Arthur and 12 knights be seated at the Round Table? (See Exercise **C.1.**)

C.4. All students at a certain college are required to take economics, mathematics, and history during their first year. The economics classes meet at 9, 11, 1, and 3 o'clock; mathematics classes meet at 10, 12, 2, and 4 o'clock; history classes meet at 8, 10, 12, and 5 o'clock. How many different schedules are possible for a student?

C.5. A promotor wants to make up a program consisting of 10 acts. He has 7 singing acts and 9 instrumental acts available. If singing and instrumental acts are to be alternated, how many different program orders are possible? [*Hint:* First consider the possibilities when a singing act begins the program.]

5. MATHEMATICAL INDUCTION

In earlier parts of this book, we have used several results like the Binomial Theorem that were only verified for small values of n. In these cases, there was usually a clear pattern and it seemed plausible that the results would be valid for all values of n. But at some stage of mathematical development such plausible statements must be backed up by *proof*. We have now reached that stage. In this section, we shall study mathematical induction, which can be used to prove the Binomial Theorem and many other statements, such as

The sum of the first n positive integers is the number $\dfrac{n(n + 1)}{2}$.

$2^n > n$ for every positive integer n.

For each positive integer n, 4 is a factor of $7^n - 3^n$.

All of the statements above have a common property. For example, a statement such as

the sum of the first n *positive integers is the number* $\dfrac{n(n + 1)}{2}$,

or, in symbols,

$$1 + 2 + 3 + \cdots + n = \frac{n(n + 1)}{2}$$

is really an infinite sequence of statements, one for each possible value of n:

$$n = 1: \qquad\qquad 1 = \frac{1(2)}{2}$$

$$n = 2: \qquad\qquad 1 + 2 = \frac{2(3)}{2}$$

$$n = 3: \qquad\qquad 1 + 2 + 3 = \frac{3(4)}{2}$$

$$n = 4: \qquad 1 + 2 + 3 + 4 = \frac{4(5)}{2}$$

and so on. Obviously, there isn't time enough to verify every one of the statements on this list, one at a time. But we can find a workable method of proof by examining how each statement on the list is *related* to the *next* statement on the list.

For instance, for $n = 50$, the statement is:

$$1 + 2 + 3 + \cdots + 50 = \frac{50(51)}{2}$$

At the moment, we don't know whether or not this statement is true. But just *suppose* that it were true. What could then be said about the next statement, the one for $n = 51$:

$$1 + 2 + 3 + \cdots + 50 + 51 = \frac{51(52)}{2}?$$

Well, *if* it is true that

$$1 + 2 + 3 + \cdots + 50 = \frac{50(51)}{2}$$

then adding 51 to both sides and simplifying the right side would yield these equalities:

$$1 + 2 + 3 + \cdots + 50 + 51 = \frac{50(51)}{2} + 51$$

$$1 + 2 + 3 + \cdots + 50 + 51 = \frac{50(51)}{2} + \frac{2(51)}{2} = \frac{50(51) + 2(51)}{2}$$

$$1 + 2 + 3 + \cdots + 50 + 51 = \frac{(50 + 2)51}{2}$$

$$1 + 2 + 3 + \cdots + 50 + 51 = \frac{51(52)}{2}$$

Since this last equality is just the original statement for $n = 51$, we conclude that

If the statement is true for $n = 50$, then it is also true for $n = 51$

We have *not* proved that the statement actually *is* true for $n = 50$, but only that *if* it is, then it is also true for $n = 51$.

We claim that this same conditional relationship holds for any two consecutive values of n. In other words, we claim that for any positive integer k,

(°)   *If the statement is true for $n = k$, then it is also true for $n = k + 1$.*

The proof of this claim is the same argument used above (with k and $k + 1$ in place of 50 and 51): *if* it is true that

$$1 + 2 + 3 + \cdots + k = \frac{k(k + 1)}{2} \qquad \text{(original statement for } n = k),$$

then adding $k + 1$ to both sides and simplifying the right side produces these equalities:

$$1 + 2 + 3 + \cdots + k + (k + 1) = \frac{k(k + 1)}{2} + (k + 1)$$

$$1 + 2 + 3 + \cdots + k + (k + 1) = \frac{k(k + 1)}{2} + \frac{2(k + 1)}{2} = \frac{k(k + 1) + 2(k + 1)}{2}$$

$$1 + 2 + 3 + \cdots + k + (k + 1) = \frac{(k + 2)(k + 1)}{2}$$

$$1 + 2 + 3 + \cdots + k + (k + 1) = \frac{(k + 1)((k + 1) + 1)}{2} \qquad \text{(original statement for } n = k + 1)$$

We have proved that claim (°) is valid for each positive integer k. We have *not* proved that the original statement is true for any value of n, but only that *if* it is true for

$n = k$, then it is also true for $n = k + 1$. Applying this fact when $k = 1, 2, 3, \ldots$, we see that

$$(^{\circ\circ})\begin{cases} \textit{if} \quad \text{the statement is true for } n = 1, \quad \textit{then} \text{ it is also true for } n = 1 + 1 = 2; \\ \textit{if} \quad \text{the statement is true for } n = 2, \quad \textit{then} \text{ it is also true for } n = 2 + 1 = 3; \\ \textit{if} \quad \text{the statement is true for } n = 3, \quad \textit{then} \text{ it is also true for } n = 3 + 1 = 4; \\ \quad \vdots \\ \textit{if} \quad \text{the statement is true for } n = 50, \textit{then} \text{ it is also true for } n = 50 + 1 = 51; \\ \textit{if} \quad \text{the statement is true for } n = 51, \textit{then} \text{ it is also true for } n = 51 + 1 = 52; \\ \quad \vdots \end{cases}$$

and so on.

We are finally in a position to *prove* the original statement: $1 + 2 + 3 + \cdots + n = n(n + 1)/2$. Obviously, it *is true* for $n = 1$ since $1 = 1(2)/2$. Now apply in turn each of the propositions on list $(^{\circ\circ})$ above. Since the statement *is* true for $n = 1$, it must also be true for $n = 2$, and hence for $n = 3$, and hence for $n = 4$, and so on, for every value of n. Therefore the original statement is true for *every* positive integer n.

The preceding proof is an illustration of the following principle:

PRINCIPLE OF MATHEMATICAL INDUCTION

Suppose there is given a statement involving the positive integer n *and that:*

(*i*)   *The statement is true for* n = 1.

(*ii*)   *If the statement is true for* n = k (*where* k *is a positive integer*), *then the statement is also true for* n = k + 1.

Then the statement is true for every *positive integer* n.

Property (i) in this principle is simply a statement of fact. To verify that it holds, you must prove the given statement is true for $n = 1$. This is usually easy, as in the preceding example. Property (ii) is a *conditional* property. It does not assert that the given statement *is* true for $n = k$, but only that *if* it is true for $n = k$, then it is also true for $n = k + 1$. So to verify that property (ii) holds, you need only prove this conditional proposition:

If the statement is true for $n = k$, *then* it is also true for $n = k + 1$

In order to prove this, or any conditional proposition, you must proceed as in the example above: assume the "if" part and use this assumption to prove the "then" part. As we saw above, the same argument will usually work for any possible k. Once this conditional proposition has been proved, you can use it *together with* property (i) to conclude that the given statement is necessarily true for every n, just as in the preceding example.

Thus proof by mathematical induction reduces to two steps:

Step 1:   Prove that the given statement is true for $n = 1$.

Step 2:   Let k be a positive integer. Assume that the given statement is true for $n = k$. Use this assumption to prove that the statement is true for $n = k + 1$.

Step 2 may be performed before step 1 if you wish. Step 2 is sometimes referred to as the **inductive step.** The assumption that the given statement is true for $n = k$ in this inductive step is called the **induction hypothesis.** Here are some more examples of inductive proofs.

EXAMPLE   Here's how mathematical induction is used to prove that

$$2^n > n \quad \text{for every positive integer } n$$

In this case, the statement involving n is: $2^n > n$.

Step 1   When $n = 1$, we have the statement $2^1 > 1$. This is obviously true.

Step 2   Let k be any positive integer. We assume that the statement is true for $n = k$, that is, we assume that $2^k > k$. We shall use this assumption to prove that the statement is true for $n = k + 1$, that is, that $2^{k+1} > k + 1$. We begin with the induction hypothesis:° $2^k > k$. Multiplying both sides of this inequality by 2 yields:

$$2 \cdot 2^k > 2k$$
$$2^{k+1} > 2k$$

Since k is a positive integer, we know that $k \geq 1$. Adding k to each side of the inequality $k \geq 1$, we have

$$k + k \geq k + 1$$
$$2k \geq k + 1$$

Combining this result with inequality (°) above, we see that

$$2^{k+1} > 2k \geq k + 1$$

The first and last terms of this inequality show that $2^{k+1} > k + 1$. Therefore the statement is true for $n = k + 1$. This argument works for any positive integer k. Thus we have completed the inductive step. By the Principle of Mathematical Induction, we conclude that $2^n > n$ for every positive integer n.

EXAMPLE   Simple arithmetic shows that:

$$7^2 - 3^2 = 49 - 9 = 40 = 4 \cdot 10 \quad \text{and} \quad 7^3 - 3^3 = 343 - 27 = 316 = 4 \cdot 79$$

° This is the point at which you usually must do some work. Remember that what follows is the "finished proof." It does not include all the thought, scratch work, false starts, and so on, that were done before this proof was actually found.

In each case, 4 is a factor. These examples suggest that

For each positive integer n, *4 is a factor of* $7^n - 3^n$

This conjecture can be proved by induction as follows.

Step 1 When $n = 1$, the statement is: 4 is a factor of $7^1 - 3^1$. Since $7^1 - 3^1 = 4 = 4 \cdot 1$, the statement is true for $n = 1$.

Step 2 Let k be a positive integer and assume that the statement is true for $n = k$, that is, that 4 is a factor of $7^k - 3^k$. Let us denote the other factor by D, so that the induction hypothesis is: $7^k - 3^k = 4D$. We must use this assumption to prove that the statement is true for $n = k + 1$, that is, that 4 is a factor of $7^{k+1} - 3^{k+1}$. Here is the proof:

$$
\begin{aligned}
7^{k+1} - 3^{k+1} &= 7^{k+1} - 7 \cdot 3^k + 7 \cdot 3^k - 3^{k+1} &&\text{(since } -7 \cdot 3^k + 7 \cdot 3^k = 0) \\
&= 7(7^k - 3^k) + (7 - 3)3^k &&\text{(factor)} \\
&= 7(4D) + (7 - 3)3^k &&\text{(induction hypothesis)} \\
&= 7(4D) + 4 \cdot 3^k &&(7 - 3 = 4) \\
&= 4(7D + 3^k) &&\text{(factor out 4)}
\end{aligned}
$$

From this last line, we see that

$$7^{k+1} - 3^{k+1} = 4(7D + 3^k), \quad \text{that is,} \quad \text{4 is a factor of } 7^{k+1} - 3^{k+1}$$

Thus the statement is true for $n = k + 1$ and the inductive step is complete. Therefore by the Principle of Mathematical Induction the conjecture is actually true for every positive integer n.

Another example of mathematical induction, the proof of the Binomial Theorem, is given at the end of this section.

Sometimes a statement involving the integer n may be false for $n = 1$ and (possibly) other small values of n, but true for all values of n beyond a particular number. For instance, the statement $2^n > n^2$ is false for $n = 1, 2, 3, 4$. But it is true for $n = 5$ and all larger values of n. A variation on the Principle of Mathematical Induction can be used to prove this fact and similar statements. See Exercise B.11 for details.

A COMMON MISTAKE WITH INDUCTION

It is often tempting to omit step 2 of an inductive proof when the given statement can easily be verified for small values of n, especially if a clear pattern seems to be developing. In fact, we have omitted step 2 in earlier sections of this book when presenting plausible results such as DeMoivre's Theorem and the Binomial Theorem. Although this approach simplified the discussion of those results, it may have left some students with the mistaken impression that step 2 is not really *necessary* in such cases. As the next example shows, however, the truth of a statement for many small values of n does *not* guarantee that it is true for every positive integer n. In other words, *omitting step 2 may lead to error.*

EXAMPLE   A positive integer is said to be **prime** if its only positive integer factors are itself and 1. For instance, 11 is prime since its only positive integer factors are 11 and 1. But 15 is not prime since it has factors other than 15 and 1, namely, 3 and 5. For each positive integer n, consider the number

$$f(n) = n^2 - n + 11$$

You can readily verify that

$$f(1) = 11, \quad f(2) = 13, \quad f(3) = 17, \quad f(4) = 23, \quad f(5) = 31$$

and that *each of these numbers is prime*. Furthermore, as n increases there is a clear pattern: the first two numbers differ by 2, the next two differ by 4, the next two differ by 6, the next two by 8, and so on. Based on this evidence, we might make the conjecture:

For each positive integer n, the number $f(n) = n^2 - n + 11$ is prime

We have seen that this conjecture is true for $n = 1, 2, 3, 4, 5$. Unfortunately, however, it is *false* for some values of n. For instance, when $n = 11$,

$$f(11) = 11^2 - 11 + 11 = 11^2 = 121$$

But 121 is obviously *not* prime since it has a factor other than 121 and 1, namely, 11. You can verify that the statement is also false for $n = 12$ but true for $n = 13$.

In the preceding example, the proposition

If the statement is true for $n = k$, then it is true for $n = k + 1$

is false when $k = 10$ and $k + 1 = 11$. If you were not aware of this and tried to complete step 2 of an inductive proof, you would not have been able to find a valid proof for it. Of course, the fact that you can't find a proof of a proposition doesn't always mean that no proof exists. But when you are unable to complete step 2, you are warned that there is a possibility that the given statement may be false for some values of n. This warning should prevent you from drawing any wrong conclusions.

PROOF OF THE BINOMIAL THEOREM (Optional)

We shall use induction to prove that for every positive integer n,

$$(x + y)^n = x^n + \binom{n}{1}x^{n-1}y + \binom{n}{2}x^{n-2}y^2 + \binom{n}{3}x^{n-3}y^3 + \cdots + \binom{n}{n-1}xy^{n-1} + y^n$$

This theorem was discussed and its notation explained in Section 3.

Step 1.   When $n = 1$, there are only two terms on the right side of the equation above and the statement reads $(x + y)^1 = x^1 + y^1$. This is certainly true.

Step 2.   Let k be any positive integer and assume that the theorem is true for $n = k$, that is, that

$$(x + y)^k$$
$$= x^k + \binom{k}{1}x^{k-1}y + \binom{k}{2}x^{k-2}y^2 + \cdots + \binom{k}{r}x^{k-r}y^r + \cdots + \binom{k}{k-1}xy^{k-1} + y^k$$

On the right side above, we have included a typical middle term $\binom{k}{r}x^{k-r}y^r$: the sum of the exponents is k and the bottom part of the binomial coefficient is the same as the y-exponent. We shall use this assumption to prove that the theorem is true for $n = k + 1$, that is, that

$$(x + y)^{k+1}$$
$$= x^{k+1} + \binom{k+1}{1}x^k y + \binom{k+1}{2}x^{k-1}y^2 + \cdots + \binom{k+1}{r+1}x^{k-r}y^{r+1} + \cdots$$
$$+ \binom{k+1}{k}xy^k + y^{k+1}$$

We have simplified some of the terms on the right side; for instance, $(k + 1) - 1 = k$ and $(k + 1) - (r + 1) = k - r$. But this is the correct statement for $n = k + 1$: the coefficients of the middle terms are $\binom{k+1}{1}, \binom{k+1}{2}, \binom{k+1}{3}$, and so on; the sum of the exponents of each middle term is $k + 1$ and the bottom part of each binomial coefficient is the same as the y-exponent.

In order to prove the theorem for $n = k + 1$, we shall need this fact about binomial coefficients: for any integers r and k with $0 \le r < k$,

$(°)$
$$\binom{k}{r+1} + \binom{k}{r} = \binom{k+1}{r+1}$$

A proof of this fact is outlined in Exercise C.1 on page 422.

To prove the theorem for $n = k + 1$, we first note that

$$(x + y)^{k+1} = (x + y)(x + y)^k$$

Applying the induction hypothesis to $(x + y)^k$, we see that

$$(x + y)^{k+1}$$
$$= (x + y)\left[x^k + \binom{k}{1}x^{k-1}y + \binom{k}{2}x^{k-2}y^2 + \cdots + \binom{k}{r}x^{k-r}y^r + \binom{k}{r+1}x^{k-(r+1)}y^{r+1}\right.$$
$$\left. + \cdots + \binom{k}{k-1}xy^{k-1} + y^k\right]$$
$$= x\left[x^k + \binom{k}{1}x^{k-1}y + \cdots + y^k\right] + y\left[x^k + \binom{k}{1}x^{k-1}y + \cdots + y^k\right]$$

Next we multiply out the right-hand side. Remember that multiplying by x increases the x-exponent by 1 and multiplying by y increases the y-exponent by 1.

$$(x + y)^{k+1}$$
$$= \left[x^{k+1} + \binom{k}{1}x^k y + \binom{k}{2}x^{k-1}y^2 + \cdots + \binom{k}{r}x^{k-r+1}y^r + \binom{k}{r+1}x^{k-r}y^{r+1}\right.$$
$$\left. + \cdots + \binom{k}{k-1}x^2 y^{k-1} + xy^k\right] + \left[x^k y + \binom{k}{1}x^{k-1}y^2 + \binom{k}{2}x^{k-2}y^3\right.$$

$$+ \cdots + \binom{k}{r}x^{k-r}y^{r+1} + \binom{k}{r+1}x^{k-(r+1)}y^{r+2} + \cdots$$

$$+ \binom{k}{k-1}xy^k + y^{k+1}\Big]$$

$$= x^{k+1} + \Big[\binom{k}{1} + 1\Big]x^k y + \Big[\binom{k}{2} + \binom{k}{1}\Big]x^{k-1}y^2 + \cdots$$

$$+ \Big[\binom{k}{r+1} + \binom{k}{r}\Big]x^{k-r}y^{r+1} + \cdots + \Big[1 + \binom{k}{k+1}\Big]xy^k + y^{k+1}$$

Now apply statement (°) above to each of the coefficients of the middle terms. For instance, with $r = 1$, statement (°) shows that $\binom{k}{2} + \binom{k}{1} = \binom{k+1}{2}$. Similarly, with $r = 0$, $\binom{k}{1} + 1 = \binom{k}{1} + \binom{k}{0} = \binom{k+1}{1}$; and so on. Then the expression above for $(x + y)^{k+1}$ becomes:

$$(x + y)^{k+1} = x^{k+1} + \binom{k+1}{1}x^k y + \binom{k+1}{2}x^{k-1}y^2$$

$$+ \cdots + \binom{k+1}{r+1}x^{k-r}y^{r+1} + \cdots + \binom{k+1}{k}xy^k + y^{k+1}$$

Since this last statement says the theorem is true for $n = k + 1$, the inductive step is complete. By the Principle of Mathematical Induction the theorem is true for every positive integer n.

EXERCISES

Directions for Exercises B.1–B.7 Use mathematical induction to prove that each of the given statements is true for every positive integer n.

B.1. (a) $1 + 2 + 2^2 + 2^3 + 2^4 + \cdots + 2^{n-1} = 2^n - 1$

(b) $1 + 3 + 3^2 + 3^3 + 3^4 + \cdots + 3^{n-1} = \dfrac{3^n - 1}{2}$

(c) $1 + 3 + 5 + 7 + \cdots + (2n - 1) = n^2$

(d) $2 + 4 + 6 + 8 + \cdots + 2n = n^2 + n$

(e) $1^2 + 2^2 + 3^2 + \cdots + n^2 = \dfrac{n(n + 1)(2n + 1)}{6}$

B.2. (a) $\dfrac{1}{2} + \dfrac{1}{4} + \dfrac{1}{8} + \cdots + \dfrac{1}{2^n} = 1 - \dfrac{1}{2^n}$

(b) $\dfrac{1}{1 \cdot 2} + \dfrac{1}{2 \cdot 3} + \dfrac{1}{3 \cdot 4} + \cdots + \dfrac{1}{n(n + 1)} = \dfrac{n}{n + 1}$

B.3. $\left(1 + \dfrac{1}{1}\right)\left(1 + \dfrac{1}{2}\right)\left(1 + \dfrac{1}{3}\right) \cdots \left(1 + \dfrac{1}{n}\right) = n + 1$

B.4. (a) $n + 2 > n$ (d) $3^n \geq 1 + 2n$
     (b) $2n + 2 > n$ (e) $3n > n + 1$
     (c) $3^n \geq 3n$ (f) $(\frac{3}{2})^n > n$

B.5. Let c and d be fixed real numbers. Prove that $c + (c + d) + (c + 2d) +$

$$(c + 3d) + \cdots + (c + (n - 1)d) = \frac{n(2c + (n - 1)d)}{2}.$$

B.6. Let r be a fixed real number with $r \neq 1$. Prove that $1 + r + r^2 + r^3 +$

$\cdots + r^{n-1} = \dfrac{r^n - 1}{r - 1}$. (Remember that $1 = r^0$; so when $n = 1$ the left side
reduces to $r^0 = 1$.)

B.7. (a) 3 is a factor of $2^{2n+1} + 1$ (c) 64 is a factor of $3^{2n+2} - 8n - 9$
     (b) 5 is a factor of $2^{4n-2} + 1$ (d) 64 is a factor of $9^n - 8n - 1$

B.8. (a) Write *each* of $x^2 - y^2$, $x^3 - y^3$, and $x^4 - y^4$ as a product of $x - y$ and
another factor.
     (b) Make a conjecture as to how $x^n - y^n$ can be written as a product of $x - y$
and another factor. Use induction to prove your conjecture.

B.9. Let $x_1 = \sqrt{2}$; $x_2 = \sqrt{2 + \sqrt{2}}$; $x_3 = \sqrt{2 + \sqrt{2 + \sqrt{2}}}$; and so on. Prove that
$x_n < 2$ for every positive integer n.

B.10. Is the given statement true or false? If it is true, prove it. If it is false, give a
counterexample.
     (a) Every odd positive integer is prime.
     (b) The number $n^2 + n + 17$ is prime for every positive integer n.
     (c) $(n + 1)^2 > n^2 + 1$ for every positive integer n.
     (d) 3 is a factor of the number $n^3 - n + 3$ for every positive integer n.
     (e) 4 is a factor of the number $n^4 - n + 4$ for every positive integer n.

B.11. Let q be a *fixed* integer. Suppose a statement involving the integer n has these
two properties:

    (i) The statement is true for $n = q$.
    (ii) *If* the statement is true for $n = k$ (where k is an integer with $k \geq q$), then
the statement is also true for $n = k + 1$.

Then we can claim that the statement is true for every integer n greater than or
equal to q.

     (a) Give an informal explanation that shows why the claim above should be
valid. Note that when $q = 1$, this claim is precisely the Principle of Mathematical Induction.
     (b) The claim made above will be called the Extended Principle of Mathe-
matical Induction. State the two steps necessary to use this principle to
prove that a given statement is true for all $n \geq q$. (See the discussion on
pages 436–437.)

(c) Use the Extended Principle of Mathematical Induction to prove that $2n - 4 > n$ for every $n \geq 5$. (Use 5 for q here.)

(d) Let r be a fixed real number with $r > 1$. Prove that $(1 + r)^n > 1 + nr$ for every integer $n \geq 2$. (Use 2 for q here.)

In parts (e)–(h) prove that the given statement is true for the indicated integer values of n.

(e) $n^2 > n$ for all $n \geq 2$ (g) $3^n > 2^n + 10n$ for all $n \geq 4$

(f) $2^n > n^2$ for all $n \geq 5$ (h) $2n < n!$ for all $n \geq 4$

C.1. Let n be a positive integer. Suppose that there are three pegs and on one of them n rings are stacked, with each ring being smaller in diameter than the one below it (see Figure 8-2).

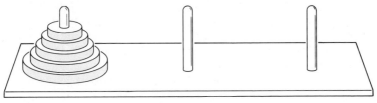

Figure 8-2

We want to transfer the stack of rings to another peg according to these rules: (i) only one ring may be moved at a time; (ii) a ring can be moved to any peg, provided it is never placed on top of a smaller ring; (iii) the final order of the rings on the new peg must be the same as the original order on the first peg.

(a) What is the smallest possible number of moves when $n = 2$? $n = 3$? $n = 4$?

(b) Make a conjecture as to the smallest possible number of moves required for any n. Prove your conjecture by induction.

C.2. The basic formula for compound interest $T(x) = P(1 + r)^x$ was discussed on page 313. Prove by induction that the formula is valid whenever x is a positive integer. (*Note:* P and r are assumed to be constant.)

Geometry Review

The few facts from high school geometry that are needed to read this book are reviewed here. We shall frequently deal with **triangles** such as those shown below. Each triangle has three sides (straight-line segments) and three angles, formed at the points where the various sides meet. When angles are measured in degrees, the sum of the measures of all three angles of a triangle is *always* 180°. For instance, see Figure A-1.

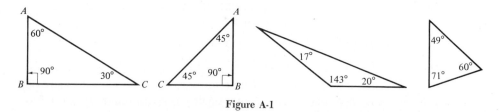

Figure A-1

A **right angle** is an angle that measures 90°. A right triangle is a triangle, one of whose angles is a right angle, such as the first two triangles shown in Figure A-1. The side of a right triangle that lies opposite the right angle is called the **hypotenuse**. In each of the right triangles in Figure A-1, side AC is the hypotenuse. A famous result of antiquity is the following theorem:

PYTHAGOREAN THEOREM

If the sides of a right triangle have lengths a *and* b *and the hypotenuse has length* c, *then*

$$c^2 = a^2 + b^2$$

EXAMPLE Consider the right triangle with sides of lengths 5 and 12, as shown in Figure A-2.

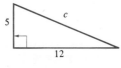

Figure A-2

According to the Pythagorean Theorem the length c of the hypotenuse satisfies the equation: $c^2 = 5^2 + 12^2 = 25 + 144 = 169$. Since $169 = 13^2$, we see that c must be 13.

SPECIAL TRIANGLES

There are two theorems of plane geometry that are often helpful when dealing with right triangles.

THEOREM I

If two angles of a triangle are equal, then the two sides opposite these angles have the same length.

EXAMPLE Suppose the hypotenuse of the right triangle shown in Figure A-3 has length 1 and that angles B and C each measure $45°$.

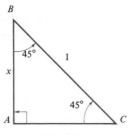

Figure A-3

Then by Theorem I, sides AB and AC have the same length. If x is the length of side AB, then by the Pythagorean Theorem:

$$x^2 + x^2 = 1^2$$
$$2x^2 = 1$$
$$x^2 = \tfrac{1}{2}$$
$$x = \sqrt{\frac{1}{2}} = \frac{1}{\sqrt{2}} = \frac{\sqrt{2}}{2}$$

(We ignore the other solution of this equation, namely, $x = -\sqrt{\frac{1}{2}}$, since x represents a length here and thus must be nonnegative.) Therefore the sides of a 90°-45°-45° triangle with hypotenuse 1 are each of length $\sqrt{2}/2$.

THEOREM II

In a right triangle that has an angle of 30°, the length of the side opposite the 30° angle is one-half the length of the hypotenuse.

EXAMPLE   Suppose that in the right triangle shown in Figure A-4 angle B is 30° and the length of hypotenuse BC is 2.

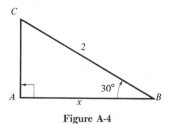

Figure A-4

By Theorem II the side opposite the 30° angle, namely, side AC, has length 1. If x denotes the length of side AB, then by the Pythagorean Theorem:

$$1^2 + x^2 = 2^2$$
$$x^2 = 3$$
$$x = \sqrt{3}$$

EXAMPLE   The right triangle shown in Figure A-5 has a 30° angle at C and side AC has length $\sqrt{3}/2$.

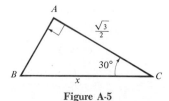

Figure A-5

Let x denote the length of the hypotenuse BC. By Theorem II, side AB has length $\frac{1}{2}x$. By the Pythagorean Theorem:

$$\left(\frac{1}{2}x\right)^2 + \left(\frac{\sqrt{3}}{2}\right)^2 = x^2$$

$$\frac{x^2}{4} + \frac{3}{4} = x^2$$

$$\frac{3}{4} = \frac{3}{4}x^2$$

$$x^2 = 1$$

$$x = 1$$

Therefore the triangle has hypotenuse of length 1 and sides of lengths $1/2$ and $\sqrt{3}/2$.

SIMILAR TRIANGLES

Two triangles, as in Figure A-6,

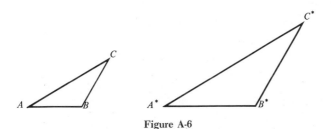

Figure A-6

are said to be **similar** if their corresponding angles are equal (that is, $\angle A = \angle A°$; $\angle B = \angle B°$; and $\angle C = \angle C°$). Thus similar triangles have the same *shape* but not necessarily the same *size*. Here is the key fact about similar triangles:

THEOREM III

Suppose triangle ABC with sides a, b, c *is similar to triangle* A°B°C° *with sides* a°, b°, c° (*that is,* $\angle A = \angle A°$; $\angle B = \angle B°$; $\angle C = \angle C°$).

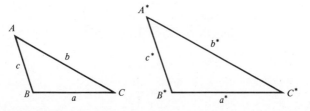

Then

$$\frac{a}{a^\circ} = \frac{b}{b^\circ} = \frac{c}{c^\circ}$$

These equalities are equivalent to:

$$\frac{a}{b} = \frac{a^\circ}{b^\circ}, \qquad \frac{b}{c} = \frac{b^\circ}{c^\circ}, \qquad \frac{a}{c} = \frac{a^\circ}{c^\circ}$$

The equivalence of the equalities in the conclusion of the theorem is easily verified. For example, since

$$\frac{a}{a^\circ} = \frac{b}{b^\circ}$$

we have

$$ab^\circ = a^\circ b$$

Dividing both sides of this equation by bb° yields:

$$\frac{ab^\circ}{bb^\circ} = \frac{a^\circ b}{bb^\circ}$$

$$\frac{a}{b} = \frac{a^\circ}{b^\circ}$$

The other equivalences are proved similarly.

EXAMPLE   Suppose the triangles in Figure A-7

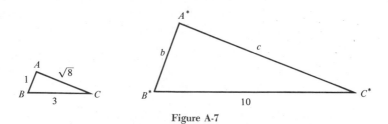

Figure A-7

are similar and that the sides have the lengths indicated. Then by Theorem III,

$$\frac{\text{length } AC}{\text{length } A^\circ C^\circ} = \frac{\text{length } BC}{\text{length } B^\circ C^\circ}$$

In other words,

$$\frac{\sqrt{8}}{c} = \frac{3}{10}$$

so that

$$3c = 10\sqrt{8}$$

$$c = \left(\frac{10}{3}\right)\sqrt{8}$$

Similarly, by Theorem III,

$$\frac{\text{length } AB}{\text{length } A^\circ B^\circ} = \frac{\text{length } BC}{\text{length } B^\circ C^\circ}$$

so that

$$\frac{1}{b} = \frac{3}{10}$$

$$3b = 10$$

$$b = \frac{10}{3}$$

Therefore the sides of triangle $A^\circ B^\circ C^\circ$ are of lengths 10, $\frac{10}{3}$, and $\frac{10}{3}\sqrt{8}$.

Table of
Powers, Roots,
and Reciprocals

N	N^2	N^3	$\sqrt{N}$	$\sqrt[3]{N}$	$1/N$	N	N^2	N^3	$\sqrt{N}$	$\sqrt[3]{N}$	$1/N$
1	1	1	1.000	1.000	1.0000	51	2601	132651	7.141	3.708	.0196
2	4	8	1.414	1.260	.5000	52	2704	140608	7.211	3.733	.0192
3	9	27	1.732	1.442	.3333	53	2809	148877	7.280	3.756	.0189
4	16	64	2.000	1.587	.2500	54	2916	157464	7.348	3.780	.0185
5	25	125	2.236	1.710	.2000	55	3025	166375	7.416	3.803	.0182
6	36	216	2.449	1.817	.1667	56	3136	175616	7.483	3.826	.0179
7	49	343	2.646	1.913	.1429	57	3249	185193	7.550	3.848	.0175
8	64	512	2.828	2.000	.1250	58	3364	195112	7.616	3.871	.0172
9	81	729	3.000	2.080	.1111	59	3481	205379	7.681	3.893	.0169
10	100	1000	3.162	2.154	.1000	60	3600	216000	7.746	3.915	.0167
11	121	1331	3.317	2.224	.0909	61	3721	226981	7.810	3.936	.0164
12	144	1728	3.464	2.289	.0833	62	3844	238328	7.874	3.958	.0161
13	169	2197	3.606	2.351	.0769	63	3969	250047	7.937	3.979	.0159
14	196	2744	3.742	2.410	.0714	64	4096	262144	8.000	4.000	.0156
15	225	3375	3.873	2.466	.0667	65	4225	274625	8.062	4.021	.0154
16	256	4096	4.000	2.520	.0625	66	4356	287496	8.124	4.041	.0152
17	289	4913	4.123	2.571	.0588	67	4489	300763	8.185	4.062	.0149
18	324	5832	4.243	2.621	.0556	68	4624	314432	8.246	4.082	.0147
19	361	6859	4.359	2.668	.0526	69	4761	328509	8.307	4.102	.0145
20	400	8000	4.472	2.714	.0500	70	4900	343000	8.367	4.121	.0143
21	441	9261	4.583	2.759	.0476	71	5041	357911	8.426	4.141	.0141
22	484	10648	4.690	2.802	.0455	72	5184	373248	8.485	4.160	.0139
23	529	12167	4.796	2.844	.0435	73	5329	389017	8.544	4.179	.0137
24	576	13824	4.899	2.884	.0417	74	5476	405224	8.602	4.198	.0135
25	625	15625	5.000	2.924	.0400	75.	5625	421875	8.660	4.217	.0133
26	676	17576	5.099	2.962	.0385	76	5776	438976	8.718	4.236	.0132
27	729	19683	5.196	3.000	.0370	77	5929	456533	8.775	4.254	.0130
28	784	21952	5.292	3.037	.0357	78	6084	474552	8.832	4.273	.0128
29	841	24389	5.385	3.072	.0345	79	6241	493039	8.888	4.291	.0127
30	900	27000	5.477	3.107	.0333	80	6400	512000	8.944	4.309	.0125
31	961	29791	5.568	3.141	.0323	81	6561	531441	9.000	4.327	.0123
32	1024	32768	5.657	3.175	.0313	82	6724	551368	9.055	4.344	.0122
33	1089	35937	5.745	3.208	.0303	83	6889	571787	9.110	4.362	.0120
34	1156	39304	5.831	3.240	.0294	84	7056	592704	9.165	4.380	.0119
35	1225	42875	5.916	3.271	.0286	85	7225	614125	9.220	4.397	.0118
36	1296	46656	6.000	3.302	.0278	86	7396	636056	9.274	4.414	.0116
37	1369	50653	6.083	3.332	.0270	87	7569	658503	9.327	4.431	.0115
38	1444	54872	6.164	3.362	.0263	88	7744	681472	9.381	4.448	.0114
39	1521	59319	6.245	3.391	.0256	89	7921	704969	9.434	4.465	.0112
40	1600	64000	6.325	3.420	.0250	90	8100	729000	9.487	4.481	.0111
41	1681	68921	6.403	3.448	.0244	91	8281	753571	9.539	4.498	.0110
42	1764	74088	6.481	3.476	.0238	92	8464	778688	9.592	4.514	.0109
43	1849	79507	6.557	3.503	.0233	93	8649	804357	9.644	4.531	.0108
44	1936	85184	6.633	3.530	.0227	94	8836	830584	9.695	4.547	.0106
45	2025	91125	6.708	3.557	.0222	95	9025	857375	9.747	4.563	.0105
46	2116	97336	6.782	3.583	.0217	96	9216	884736	9.798	4.579	.0104
47	2209	103823	6.856	3.609	.0213	97	9409	912673	9.849	4.595	.0103
48	2304	110592	6.928	3.634	.0208	98	9604	941192	9.899	4.610	.0102
49	2401	117649	7.000	3.659	.0204	99	9801	970299	9.950	4.626	.0101
50	2500	125000	7.071	3.684	.0200	100	10000	1000000	10.000	4.642	.0100

Table of Common Logarithms

x	0	1	2	3	4	5	6	7	8	9
1.0	.0000	.0043	.0086	.0128	.0170	.0212	.0253	.0294	.0334	.0374
1.1	.0414	.0453	.0492	.0531	.0569	.0607	.0645	.0682	.0719	.0755
1.2	.0792	.0828	.0864	.0899	.0934	.0969	.1004	.1038	.1072	.1106
1.3	.1139	.1173	.1206	.1239	.1271	.1303	.1335	.1367	.1399	.1430
1.4	.1461	.1492	.1523	.1553	.1584	.1614	.1644	.1673	.1703	.1732
1.5	.1761	.1790	.1818	.1847	.1875	.1903	.1931	.1959	.1987	.2014
1.6	.2041	.2068	.2095	.2122	.2148	.2175	.2201	.2227	.2253	.2279
1.7	.2304	.2330	.2355	.2380	.2405	.2430	.2455	.2480	.2504	.2529
1.8	.2553	.2577	.2601	.2625	.2648	.2672	.2695	.2718	.2742	.2765
1.9	.2788	.2810	.2833	.2856	.2878	.2900	.2923	.2945	.2967	.2989
2.0	.3010	.3032	.3054	.3075	.3096	.3118	.3139	.3160	.3181	.3201
2.1	.3222	.3243	.3263	.3284	.3304	.3324	.3345	.3365	.3385	.3404
2.2	.3424	.3444	.3464	.3483	.3502	.3522	.3541	.3560	.3579	.3598
2.3	.3617	.3636	.3655	.3674	.3692	.3711	.3729	.3747	.3766	.3784
2.4	.3802	.3820	.3838	.3856	.3874	.3892	.3909	.3927	.3945	.3962
2.5	.3979	.3997	.4014	.4031	.4048	.4065	.4082	.4099	.4116	.4133
2.6	.4150	.4166	.4183	.4200	.4216	.4232	.4249	.4265	.4281	.4298
2.7	.4314	.4330	.4346	.4362	.4378	.4393	.4409	.4425	.4440	.4456
2.8	.4472	.4487	.4502	.4518	.4533	.4548	.4564	.4579	.4594	.4609
2.9	.4624	.4639	.4654	.4669	.4683	.4698	.4713	.4728	.4742	.4757
3.0	.4771	.4786	.4800	.4814	.4829	.4843	.4857	.4871	.4886	.4900
3.1	.4914	.4928	.4942	.4955	.4969	.4983	.4997	.5011	.5024	.5038
3.2	.5051	.5065	.5079	.5092	.5105	.5119	.5132	.5145	.5159	.5172
3.3	.5185	.5198	.5211	.5224	.5237	.5250	.5263	.5276	.5289	.5302
3.4	.5315	.5328	.5340	.5353	.5366	.5378	.5391	.5403	.5416	.5428
3.5	.5441	.5453	.5465	.5478	.5490	.5502	.5514	.5527	.5539	.5551
3.6	.5563	.5575	.5587	.5599	.5611	.5623	.5635	.5647	.5658	.5670
3.7	.5682	.5694	.5705	.5717	.5729	.5740	.5752	.5763	.5775	.5786
3.8	.5798	.5809	.5821	.5832	.5843	.5855	.5866	.5877	.5888	.5899
3.9	.5911	.5922	.5933	.5944	.5955	.5966	.5977	.5988	.5999	.6010
4.0	.6021	.6031	.6042	.6053	.6064	.6075	.6085	.6096	.6107	.6117
4.1	.6128	.6138	.6149	.6159	.6170	.6180	.6191	.6201	.6212	.6222
4.2	.6232	.6243	.6253	.6263	.6274	.6284	.6294	.6304	.6314	.6325
4.3	.6335	.6345	.6355	.6365	.6375	.6385	.6395	.6405	.6415	.6425
4.4	.6435	.6444	.6454	.6464	.6474	.6484	.6493	.6503	.6513	.6522
4.5	.6532	.6542	.6551	.6561	.6571	.6580	.6590	.6599	.6609	.6618
4.6	.6628	.6637	.6646	.6656	.6665	.6675	.6684	.6693	.6702	.6712
4.7	.6721	.6730	.6739	.6749	.6758	.6767	.6776	.6785	.6794	.6803
4.8	.6812	.6821	.6830	.6839	.6848	.6857	.6866	.6875	.6884	.6893
4.9	.6902	.6911	.6920	.6928	.6937	.6946	.6955	.6964	.6972	.6981
5.0	.6990	.6998	.7007	.7016	.7024	.7033	.7042	.7050	.7059	.7067
5.1	.7076	.7084	.7093	.7101	.7110	.7118	.7126	.7135	.7143	.7152
5.2	.7160	.7168	.7177	.7185	.7193	.7202	.7210	.7218	.7226	.7235
5.3	.7243	.7251	.7259	.7267	.7275	.7284	.7292	.7300	.7308	.7316
5.4	.7324	.7332	.7340	.7348	.7356	.7364	.7372	.7380	.7388	.7396
x	0	1	2	3	4	5	6	7	8	9

x	0	1	2	3	4	5	6	7	8	9
5.5	.7404	.7412	.7419	.7427	.7435	.7443	.7451	.7459	.7466	.7474
5.6	.7482	.7490	.7497	.7505	.7513	.7520	.7528	.7536	.7543	.7551
5.7	.7559	.7566	.7574	.7582	.7589	.7597	.7604	.7612	.7619	.7627
5.8	.7634	.7642	.7649	.7657	.7664	.7672	.7679	.7686	.7694	.7701
5.9	.7709	.7716	.7723	.7731	.7738	.7745	.7752	.7760	.7767	.7774
6.0	.7782	.7789	.7796	.7803	.7810	.7818	.7825	.7832	.7839	.7846
6.1	.7853	.7860	.7868	.7875	.7882	.7889	.7896	.7903	.7910	.7917
6.2	.7924	.7931	.7938	.7945	.7952	.7959	.7966	.7973	.7980	.7987
6.3	.7993	.8000	.8007	.8014	.8021	.8028	.8035	.8041	.8048	.8055
6.4	.8062	.8069	.8075	.8082	.8089	.8096	.8102	.8109	.8116	.8122
6.5	.8129	.8136	.8142	.8149	.8156	.8162	.8169	.8176	.8182	.8189
6.6	.8195	.8202	.8209	.8215	.8222	.8228	.8235	.8241	.8248	.8254
6.7	.8261	.8267	.8274	.8280	.8287	.8293	.8299	.8306	.8312	.8319
6.8	.8325	.8331	.8338	.8344	.8351	.8357	.8363	.8370	.8376	.8382
6.9	.8388	.8395	.8401	.8407	.8414	.8420	.8426	.8432	.8439	.8445
7.0	.8451	.8457	.8463	.8470	.8476	.8482	.8488	.8494	.8500	.8506
7.1	.8513	.8519	.8525	.8531	.8537	.8543	.8549	.8555	.8561	.8567
7.2	.8573	.8579	.8585	.8591	.8597	.8603	.8609	.8615	.8621	.8627
7.3	.8633	.8639	.8645	.8651	.8657	.8663	.8669	.8675	.8681	.8686
7.4	.8692	.8698	.8704	.8710	.8716	.8722	.8727	.8733	.8739	.8745
7.5	.8751	.8756	.8762	.8768	.8774	.8779	.8785	.8791	.8797	.8802
7.6	.8808	.8814	.8820	.8825	.8831	.8837	.8842	.8848	.8854	.8859
7.7	.8865	.8871	.8876	.8882	.8887	.8893	.8899	.8904	.8910	.8915
7.8	.8921	.8927	.8932	.8938	.8943	.8949	.8954	.8960	.8965	.8971
7.9	.8976	.8982	.8987	.8993	.8998	.9004	.9009	.9015	.9020	.9025
8.0	.9031	.9036	.9042	.9047	.9053	.9058	.9063	.9069	.9074	.9079
8.1	.9085	.9090	.9096	.9101	.9106	.9112	.9117	.9122	.9128	.9133
8.2	.9138	.9143	.9149	.9154	.9159	.9165	.9170	.9175	.9180	.9186
8.3	.9191	.9196	.9201	.9206	.9212	.9217	.9222	.9227	.9232	.9238
8.4	.9243	.9248	.9253	.9258	.9263	.9269	.9274	.9279	.9284	.9289
8.5	.9294	.9299	.9304	.9309	.9315	.9320	.9325	.9330	.9335	.9340
8.6	.9345	.9350	.9355	.9360	.9365	.9370	.9375	.9380	.9385	.9390
8.7	.9395	.9400	.9405	.9410	.9415	.9420	.9425	.9430	.9435	.9440
8.8	.9445	.9450	.9455	.9460	.9465	.9469	.9474	.9479	.9484	.9489
8.9	.9494	.9499	.9504	.9509	.9513	.9518	.9523	.9528	.9533	.9538
9.0	.9542	.9547	.9552	.9557	.9562	.9566	.9571	.9576	.9581	.9586
9.1	.9590	.9595	.9600	.9605	.9609	.9614	.9619	.9624	.9628	.9633
9.2	.9638	.9643	.9647	.9652	.9657	.9661	.9666	.9671	.9675	.9680
9.3	.9685	.9689	.9694	.9699	.9703	.9708	.9713	.9717	.9722	.9727
9.4	.9731	.9736	.9741	.9745	.9750	.9754	.9759	.9763	.9768	.9773
9.5	.9777	.9782	.9786	.9791	.9795	.9800	.9805	.9809	.9814	.9818
9.6	.9823	.9827	.9832	.9836	.9841	.9845	.9850	.9854	.9859	.9863
9.7	.9868	.9872	.9877	.9881	.9886	.9890	.9894	.9899	.9903	.9908
9.8	.9912	.9917	.9921	.9926	.9930	.9934	.9939	.9943	.9948	.9952
9.9	.9956	.9961	.9965	.9969	.9974	.9978	.9983	.9987	.9991	.9996
x	0	1	2	3	4	5	6	7	8	9

Answers to Selected Exercises

CHAPTER 1: BASIC ALGEBRA

SECTION 1   PAGES 10–13

A.2. (a) $7 > 5$ (c) $x \geq 0$ (e) $-3 < z < -2$ (g) $c < 4 \leq d$
A.3. (a) 0 (c) π (e) 2 (g) -3.66 (i) $-14\pi + 2\pi^2$ **A.4.** (a) 7
(c) 26 (e) 70 (g) -50 (i) -19 **A.5.** (a) 0 (c) -1 (e) 3
B.2. (a) many correct answers, including $\frac{19}{63}, \frac{20}{63}, \frac{21}{63}, \ldots, \frac{34}{63}$ **B.4.** (a) $\geq$ (c) $\leq$
(e) $\leq$ **B.5.** (c) $b + c = a$ (e) a lies to the right of b (g) $a < b$

PAGES 14–15

A.1. (a) $.777 \cdots$ (c) $1.6428571428571 \cdots$ (e) $.052631578947368421052 \cdots$
C.1. (a) $\frac{37}{99}$ (c) $\frac{758679}{9900} = \frac{252893}{3300}$ (e) $\frac{5}{37}$

SECTION 2   PAGES 22–24

A.1. (a) 36 (c) 73 (e) 3 (g) $-\frac{125}{64}$ (i) $\frac{1}{3}$ **A.2.** (a) -112 (c) $\frac{81}{16}$
(e) $\frac{129}{8}$ **A.3.** (a) x^8 (c) $24x^7$ (e) $13z^2y^2$ (g) $384w^6$ (i) $216u^6v^6$
A.4. (a) x^7 (c) ce^9 (e) $b^2c^2d^6$ **A.5.** (a) $3^s/3^r$ (c) $1/a^3$
(e) $a + (1/a)$ (g) $6^s s^s / r^t$ (i) $a^{6t} b^{4t}$ **A.6.** (a) 11 (c) 0 (e) 6
(g) $\frac{1}{13}$ **A.7.** (a) c^3 (c) $\sqrt[5]{14abcd}$ (e) $14 + 3\sqrt{3}$ **A.8.** (a) $2ab$
(c) $3x^2y^4$ (e) ab^2 (g) $4xy$ (i) $2x^2y^4$ (k) y/x **B.1.** (a) $(7.9327)10^4$
(c) $2 \cdot 10^{-3}$ (e) $(5.963)10^{12}$ (g) $2 \cdot 10^{-12}$ **B.2.** (a) 48 (c) $.42$ (e) 42
B.3. (a) 2^6 (c) 2^{12} (e) 2^5 **B.4.** (a) Since $(\sqrt{7} - \sqrt{2})^2 = (\sqrt{7})^2 - 2\sqrt{7}\sqrt{2} + (\sqrt{2})^2 = 7 - 2\sqrt{14} + 2 = 9 - 2\sqrt{14}$, we conclude that $\sqrt{9 - 2\sqrt{14}} = \sqrt{7} - \sqrt{2}$.   (c) Since $(\sqrt{5} - \sqrt{2})^3 = (\sqrt{5} - \sqrt{2})^2(\sqrt{5} - \sqrt{2}) = (5 - 2\sqrt{5}\sqrt{2} + 2) \cdot (\sqrt{5} - \sqrt{2}) = 5\sqrt{5} - 10\sqrt{2} + 2\sqrt{5} - 5\sqrt{2} + 4\sqrt{5} - 2\sqrt{2} = -17\sqrt{2} + 11\sqrt{5}$, we have $\sqrt[3]{-17\sqrt{2} + 11\sqrt{5}} = \sqrt{5} - \sqrt{2}$.   **B.5.** many possible answers, including: (a) $3^2 + 4^2 \neq (3 + 4)^2$ (c) $3^2 \cdot 2^3 \neq (3 \cdot 2)^{2+3}$ (e) $5^{-2} \neq -5^2$ (g) $\sqrt[3]{8} + \sqrt[3]{27} = 2 + 3 = 5$, but $5 \neq \sqrt[3]{8 + 27}$ (i) $\sqrt{8 \cdot 2} \neq 4\sqrt{2}$

SECTION 3   PAGES 25–26

B.1. (a) Q, A (c) Z, Q, A (e) A (g) A

SECTION 4 PAGES 31–32

A.1. (a) -7 (c) 169 (e) -1 (g) $\pi - \sqrt{2}$ **A.2.** (a) $<$ (c) $>$
(e) $<$ (g) $=$ **A.4.** (a) 14.5 (c) 100 (e) $\pi + 3$ **B.3.** (d) b is closer to
0 than c is to 3 (f) $|x - c| = 5$ **B.4.** (a) c cannot be within 2 units of 1 *and* within 3
units of 12 at the same time **B.5.** (a) all real numbers x (c) $x \leq 0$
B.6. (a) $x = 1$ or -1 (c) $x = 1$ or 3 (e) $x = -\pi - 4$ or $-\pi + 4$ **B.7.** $|x - 1| =$
2 or 4; $|x| = 1$ or 5 **B.8.** $|x - 2| = 1$ or 7 **B.9.** (a) $-7 < x < 7$
(c) $-4 < x < -2$ (e) $x \geq 5$ or $x \leq -5$

SECTION 5 PAGES 39–41

A.1. (a) $8x$ (c) $-2a^2b$ (e) $-x^3 + 4x^2 + 2x - 3$ (g) $5u^3 + u - 4$
(i) $4z - 12z^2w + 6z^3w^2 - zw^3 + 8$ (k) $-3x^3 + 15x + 8$ (m) $-5xy - x$
A.2. (a) $2x^3 + 4x$ (c) $x^3y^2 - 6x^3y^3$ (e) $2x^3 - 6x^2y + 4xy^2$
(g) $-36x^8 + 21x^7$ (i) $-12a^2y^2 + 15ay^2$ **A.3.** (a) $x^2 - x - 2$ (c) $2x^2 +$
$2x - 12$ (e) $y^2 + 7y + 12$ (g) $-6x^2 + x + 35$ (i) $3y^3 - 9y^2 + 4y - 12$
A.4. (a) $y^2 - 64$ (c) $9x^2 - y^2$ (e) $x^2 + 12x + 36$ (g) $4x^2 + 12xy + 9y^2$
(i) $4s^4 - 81y^2$ (k) $16x^6 - 25y^4$ **A.5.** (a) $2c^3 - 7c^2 + 7c - 2$ (c) $2x^3 +$
$3x^2y - xy^2 + 2y^3$ (e) $5x^3 - 12x^2y + 19xy^2 - 6y^3$ (g) $-9y^3 + 15y^2 + 6y$
(i) $3y^3 + 2y^2 - 12y - 8$ **A.6.** (a) yes; leading coeff. 1; const. term 1; degree 3
(c) yes; leading coeff. 1; const. term -1; degree 3 (e) yes; leading coeff. 1; const. term -3;
degree 2 (g) no **A.7.** (a) quotient $3x^3 - 3x^2 + 5x - 11$; remainder 12
(c) quotient $x^2 + 2x - 6$; remainder $-7x + 7$ (e) quotient $5x^2 + 5x + 5$, remainder
zero **A.8.** (a) no (c) yes **B.1.** (a) 3 (c) -6 (e) 6
(g) 1 (i) 5 **B.2.** (a) $x - 25$ (c) $9 + 6\sqrt{y} + y$ (e) $\sqrt{3}x^2 + 4x + \sqrt{3}$
B.3. (a) $3ax^2 + (3b + 2a)x + 2b$ (c) $abx^2 + (a^2 + b^2)x + ab$ (e) $x^3 - (a +$
$b + c)x^2 + (ab + ac + bc)x - abc$ **B.5.** (a) 3^{4+r+t} (c) $x^{m+n} + 2x^n - 3x^m - 6$
(e) $2x^{4n} - 5x^{3n} + 8x^{2n} - 18x^n - 5$ **B.6.** (a) example: if $y = 4$, then $3(4 + 2) \neq$
$(3 \cdot 4) + 2$; correct statement: $3(y + 2) = 3y + 6$ (c) example: if $x = 2$,
$y = 3$, then $(2 + 3)^2 \neq 2 + 3^2$; correct statement: $(x + y)^2 = x^2 + 2xy + y^2$ (e) example: if $x = 2$, $y = 3$, then $(7 \cdot 2)(7 \cdot 3) \neq 7 \cdot 2 \cdot 3$; correct statement: $(7x)(7y) = 49xy$
(g) example: if $y = 2$, then $2 + 2 + 2 \neq 2^3$; correct statement: $y + y + y = 3y$
(i) example: if $x = 4$, then $(4 - 3)(4 - 2) \neq 4^2 - 5 \cdot 4 - 6$; correct statement:
$(x - 3)(x - 2) = x^2 - 5x + 6$ **C.1.** (a) If x is the chosen number, then adding one and
squaring the result gives $(x + 1)^2$. Subtracting one from the original number x and squaring
the result gives $(x - 1)^2$. Subtracting the second of these squares from the first yields:
$(x + 1)^2 - (x - 1)^2 = (x^2 + 2x + 1) - (x^2 - 2x + 1) = 4x$. Dividing by the original
number x now gives $\dfrac{4x}{x} = 4$. So the answer is always 4, no matter what number x is chosen.

PAGES 46–47

A.1. (a)
$$\begin{array}{r|rrrrr} 2 & 3 & -8 & 0 & 9 & 5 \\ & & 6 & -4 & -8 & 2 \\ \hline & 3 & -2 & -4 & 1 & \underline{|7} \end{array}$$
(c)
$$\begin{array}{r|rrrrr} -3 & 2 & 5 & 0 & -2 & -8 \\ & & -6 & 3 & -9 & 33 \\ \hline & 2 & -1 & 3 & -11 & \underline{|25} \end{array}$$

quotient $3x^3 - 2x^2 - 4x + 1$;   quotient $2x^3 - x^2 + 3x - 11$;
remainder 7   remainder 25

(e) $\underline{7|}$ 5 0 -3 -4 6   **(g)** $\underline{2|}$ 1 -6 4 2 -7

    35 245 1,694 11,830   2 -8 -8 -12

   $\overline{5\ \ 35\ \ 242\ \ 1,690\ \ |11,836}$ $\overline{1\ \ -4\ \ -4\ \ -6\ \ |-19}$

quotient $5x^3 + 35x^2 + 242x + 1690$; quotient $x^3 - 4x^2 - 4x - 6$;

remainder 11,836   remainder -19

B.1. **(a)** quotient $3x^3 + \frac{3}{4}x^2 - \frac{29}{16}x - \frac{29}{64}$; remainder $\frac{483}{256}$ **(c)** quotient $2x^3 - 6x^2 + 2x + 2$; remainder 1   **(e)** quotient $x^3 + 5x^2 - 6x + 1$; remainder 1   **B.2.** **(a)** $g(x) = (x + 4)(3x^2 - 3x + 1)$ **(c)** $g(x) = (x - \frac{1}{2})(2x^4 - 6x^3 + 12x^2 - 10)$ **B.3.** **(a)** quotient $x^2 - 2.15x + 4$; remainder 2.25

SECTION 6 PAGES 52–53

A.1. **(a)** $(x + 2)(x - 2)$ **(c)** $(3y + 5)(3y - 5)$ **(e)** $(9x + 2)^2$ **(g)** $(\sqrt{5} + x) \cdot (\sqrt{5} - x)$ **(i)** $(7 + 2z)^2$ **(k)** $(x^2 + y^2)(x + y)(x - y)$ **A.2.** **(a)** $(x + 3)(x - 2)$
(c) $(z + 3)(z + 1)$ **(e)** $(y + 9)(y - 4)$ **(g)** $(x - 3)^2$ **(i)** $(x + 5)(x + 2)$
(k) $(x + 9)(x + 2)$ **A.3.** **(a)** $(3x + 1)(x + 1)$ **(c)** $(2z + 3)(z + 4)$ **(e)** $9x(x - 8)$
(g) $(5x + 1)(2x - 2)$ **(i)** $(4u - 3)(2u + 3)$ **(k)** $(2x + 5y)^2$ **A.4.** **(a)** $(x - 5) \cdot (x^2 + 5x + 25)$ **(c)** $(x + 2)^3$ **(e)** $(2 + x)(4 - 2x + x^2)$ **(g)** $(-x + 5)^3$
(i) $(x + 1)(x^2 - x + 1)$ **(k)** $(2x - y)(4x^2 + 2xy + y^2)$ **A.5.** **(a)** $(x^3 + 2^3) \cdot (x^3 - 2^3) = (x + 2)(x^2 - 2x + 4)(x - 2)(x^2 + 2x + 4)$ **(c)** $(y^2 + 5)(y^2 + 2)$
(e) $(9 + y^2)(3 + y)(3 - y)$ **(g)** $(z + 1)(z^2 - z + 1)(z - 1)(z^2 + z + 1)$
(i) $(x^2 + 3y)(x^2 - y)$ **A.6.** **(a)** $(x + z)(x - y)$ **(c)** $(a + 2b)(a^2 - b)$
(e) $(x^2 - 8)(x + 4) = (x + \sqrt{8})(x - \sqrt{8})(x + 4)$ **A.7.** **(a)** $x^2 + 4x + 4 = (x + 2)^2$
(c) $z^2 + 3z + \frac{9}{4} = (z + \frac{3}{2})^2$ **(e)** $x^2 + 12x + 36 = (x + 6)^2$ **(g)** $2(x^2 + 2x + 1) = 2(x + 1)^2$ **(i)** $2(z^2 + 7z + \frac{49}{4}) = 2(z + \frac{7}{2})^2$ **B.1.** **(a)** $(2x - y)(x + 3y) + 3(2x - y) = (2x - y)(x + 3y + 3)$ **(c)** $(x - 3y)(x^2 + 3xy + 9y^2 + 1)$ **B.2.** **(a)** $(x + \frac{1}{8})(x - \frac{1}{8})$
(c) $(y + \frac{1}{6})(y - \frac{5}{6})$ **(e)** $(z + \frac{7}{4})(z + \frac{5}{4})$

SECTION 7 PAGES 58–60

A.1. **(a)** $\frac{9}{7}$ **(c)** $\frac{195}{8}$ **(e)** $\dfrac{x - 2}{x + 1}$ **(g)** $\dfrac{a + b}{a^2 + ab + b^2}$ **(i)** $1/x$

A.2. **(a)** $\frac{29}{35}$ **(c)** $\frac{121}{42}$ **(e)** $\dfrac{ce + 3cd}{de}$ **(g)** $\dfrac{b^2 - c^2}{bc}$ **A.3.** **(a)** $\dfrac{-1}{x(x + 1)}$

(c) $\dfrac{x + 3}{(x + 4)^2}$ **(e)** $\dfrac{2x - 4}{x(3x - 4)}$ **(g)** $\dfrac{x^2 - xy + y^2 + x + y}{x^3 + y^3}$

(i) $\dfrac{-6x^5 - 38x^4 - 84x^3 - 71x^2 - 14x + 1}{4x(x + 1)^3(x + 2)^3}$ **A.4.** **(a)** 2   **(c)** $2/3c$ **(e)** $3y/x^2$

A.5. **(a)** $\dfrac{12x}{x - 3}$ **(c)** $\dfrac{5y^2}{3(y + 5)}$ **(e)** $\dfrac{u + 1}{u}$ **(g)** $\dfrac{(u + v)(4u - 3v)}{(2u - v)(2u - 3v)}$ **A.6.** **(a)** $\frac{35}{24}$

(c) u^3/vw^2 **(e)** $\dfrac{x + 3}{2x}$ **(g)** $\dfrac{x^2y^2}{(x + y)(x + 2y)}$ **(i)** $\dfrac{cd(c + d)}{c - d}$ **A.7.** **(a)** $2\sqrt{5}/5$

(c) $\sqrt{70}/10$ **(e)** $\sqrt{x}/x$ **(g)** $\dfrac{r + 2\sqrt{rs} + s}{r - s}$ **(i)** $\dfrac{(u^2 - v^2)(\sqrt{u + v} + \sqrt{u - v})}{2v}$

B.1. **(a)** example: if $a = 1$, $b = 2$, then $\frac{1}{1} + \frac{1}{2} \neq \dfrac{1}{1 + 2}$; correct statement: $\dfrac{1}{a} + \dfrac{1}{b} = \dfrac{b + a}{ab}$ **(c)** example: if $a = 4$, $b = 9$, then $\left(\dfrac{1}{\sqrt{4} + \sqrt{9}}\right)^2 \neq \dfrac{1}{4 + 9}$; correct statement: $\left(\dfrac{1}{\sqrt{a}+\sqrt{b}}\right)^2 = \dfrac{1}{a+2\sqrt{ab}+b}$ **(e)** example: if $u=1$, $v=2$, then $\frac{1}{2}+$

$\frac{2}{1} \neq 1$; correct statement: $\dfrac{u}{v}+\dfrac{v}{u} = \dfrac{u^2+v^2}{vu}$ **(g)** example: if $x=4$, $y=9$, then

$(\sqrt{4}+\sqrt{9}) \cdot \dfrac{1}{\sqrt{4}+\sqrt{9}} \neq 4+9$; correct statement: $(\sqrt{x}+\sqrt{y}) \cdot \dfrac{1}{\sqrt{x}+\sqrt{y}} = 1$

CHAPTER 2: EQUATIONS AND INEQUALITIES

SECTION 1 PAGES 67–70

A.1. (a) $x=8$ (c) $z=-\frac{5}{6}$ (e) $y=-32$ (g) $x=-3$ (i) $x=\frac{42}{61}$
A.2. (a) $x=26$ (c) $x=\frac{5}{6}$ (e) $t=-\frac{5}{12}$ (g) $x=1$ (i) $x=-1$
A.3. (a) $x=1.23$ (c) $x=7.77$ **A.4.** (a) $b=\dfrac{2A}{h}-c$; $h \neq 0$ (c) $h=\dfrac{4V}{\pi d^2}$;

$d \neq 0$ (e) $v=1-\dfrac{b}{S}$; $v \neq 1$, $S \neq 0$ (g) $\dfrac{3b^2-12ab-a}{5a-b-2}$; $5a-b-2 \neq 0$

(i) $z = \dfrac{14}{(a+c)(a-b)}-b$; $a+c \neq 0$, $a-b \neq 0$ **B.1.** (a) $x=-\frac{5}{2}$
(c) $x=-\frac{3}{2}$ (e) $x=4$ **B.2.** (a) $c=1$ **B.3.** 91   **B.5.** 27   **B.7.** 30
B.9. $\frac{12}{13}$ hours   **B.11.** 8 ounces   **B.13.** 112.5 ounces   **B.15.** \$17.88
B.17 14%   **B.19.** 5   **B.21.** 24   **B.23.** 64, 66, 68, 70   **B.25.** 4:40 P.M.
B.27 12 mph; 30 miles

PAGES 77–80

A.1. (a) $k=4$ (c) $k=\frac{1}{2}$ **A.2.** (a) $k=16$ (c) $k=.012$ **A.3.** (a) $a=\dfrac{k}{b}$

(c) $p=\dfrac{k}{T}$ (e) $z=kxyw$ **A.4.** (a) $w=\dfrac{k}{d^2}$ (c) $d=k\sqrt{h}$ (e) $p=\dfrac{kw}{r^2}$

B.1. (a) $r=4$ (c) $t=1$ **B.2.** (a) $b=\frac{9}{4}=2.25$ (c) $x=\frac{10}{3}$
B.3. (a) $t=krs$ and $k=4$ (c) $B=\dfrac{k}{uv}$ and $k=12$ (e) $w=kxy^2$ and $k=2$

B.4. (a) $v=kT^3$ and $k=\frac{1}{4}$ (c) $p=\dfrac{kz^2}{r}$ and $k=4$ (e) $T=\dfrac{kpv^3}{u^2}$ and $k=16$

B.5. $u=50$ **B.7.** (a) $r=3$ **B.9.** $c=\frac{200}{3}$ **B.11.** (a) 14 pounds per square inch   **B.13.** .064 ohm   **B.15.** 3750 kg   **C.1.** (a) v is doubled   (b) v is multiplied by $\frac{1}{16}$

SECTION 2 PAGES 86–88

A.1. (a) $x=4$ or -3 (c) $x=-7$ or -2 (e) $y=-3$ or $\frac{1}{2}$ (g) $x=-5$ or $-\frac{1}{5}$ **A.2.** (a) $x=8$ or -8 (c) $z=\sqrt{56}$ or $-\sqrt{56}$ (e) $y=-2+\sqrt{5}$ or $-2-\sqrt{5}$ (g) $y=3$ **A.3.** (a) $x=5$ or -3 (c) $x=8$ or -4 (e) $t=\frac{1}{3}$ or -1 **A.4.** (a) $x=-5$ or -3 (c) $t=\dfrac{-2\pm\sqrt{2}}{2}$ (e) $u=\dfrac{-4\pm\sqrt{6}}{5}$

(g) $x=\dfrac{3\pm\sqrt{89}}{8}$ **A.5.** (a) 2   (c) 2   (e) 1   **A.6.** (a) $t=5$ or $-\frac{4}{3}$

(c) $x=\dfrac{-1\pm\sqrt{2}}{2}$ (e) $y=\dfrac{2\pm\sqrt{5}}{5}$ **A.7.** (a) $x \approx 1.824$ or   .47

(c) $x = 13.79$ **B.1.** **(a)** $x = -5$ or 1 or -3 or -1 **(c)** $x = \dfrac{-3 \pm \sqrt{21}}{2}$

B.2. **(a)** $k = 10$ or -10 **(c)** $k = 16$ **(e)** $k = 25$ **B.4.** **(a)** $(x-1)(x+2) = 0$,
or   equivalently, $x^2 + x - 2 = 0$ **(c)** $25x^2 - 30x + 9 = 0$
(e) $x^2 - \pi x - 2\pi^2 = 0$ **B.5.** **(a)** $c = \pm\sqrt{E/m}$; $m \neq 0$, $E/m \geq 0$
(c) $r = \dfrac{-\pi h \pm \sqrt{\pi^2 h^2 + 4A\pi}}{2\pi}$; $\pi h^2 + 4A \geq 0$ **(e)** $x = \dfrac{-y \pm \sqrt{49y^2 + 108}}{6}$

(g) $x = 3$ or $\dfrac{-2}{k}$; $k \neq 0$ **B.6.** **(a)** Since r and s are the solutions of $ax^2 + bx +$

$c = 0$, the quadratic formula shows that they must be the numbers $\dfrac{-b \pm \sqrt{b^2 - 4ac}}{2a}$. So

$r + s = \dfrac{-b + \sqrt{b^2 - 4ac}}{2a} + \dfrac{-b - \sqrt{b^2 - 4ac}}{2a} = \dfrac{-2b}{2a} = \dfrac{-b}{a}$.   **(c)** $x^2 - 2x - 1 =$

$(x - (1 + \sqrt{2}))(x - (1 - \sqrt{2}))$ **B.7.** $-17, -16$ or $16, 17$ **B.9.** 4 inches   **B.11.** 36
B.13. 3 feet   **B.15.** 12 hours   **B.17.** approximately 9.34 and 7.62 meters

SECTION 3   PAGES 93–94

A.1. **(a)** $x = \sqrt{5}$ or $-\sqrt{5}$ or $\sqrt{2}$ or $-\sqrt{2}$ **(c)** $z = \sqrt{2/3}$ or $-\sqrt{2/3}$
(e) $y = \sqrt{3 + \sqrt{2}}$ or $-\sqrt{3 + \sqrt{2}}$ or $\sqrt{3 - \sqrt{2}}$ or $-\sqrt{3 - \sqrt{2}}$ **(g)** $x = \sqrt{1 + \sqrt{2}}$ or
$-\sqrt{1 + \sqrt{2}}$ [*Note:* $1 - \sqrt{2}$ is negative, so it has no real square root]   **A.2.** **(a)** $x = 0$
or 4   **(c)** $x = -100$ or -7 or 2 or 7 **A.3.** **(a)** no   **(c)** yes   **(e)** no
A.4. **(a)** $x = 1$ or -1 or -3 **(c)** $x = 1$ or -1 or -5 **(e)** $x = -4$ or 1 or $\frac{1}{2}$
A.5. **(a)** $x = -3$ or   2   **(c)** $x = -2$ **(e)** no   rational   solutions
B.1. **(a)** $x = 1$ **(c)** $x = 0$ or 5 **(e)** $x = 0$ or $-1/2$ or $1/3$ **(g)** $x = 4$
(i) $x = 2$ or -1 **B.2.** **(a)** $x = 2$ or $(3 + \sqrt{5})/2$ or $(3 - \sqrt{5})/2$ **(c)** $x = -3$ or $-1/4$ or
$1/2$ **(e)** $x = 0$ or -7 or 1 **B.4.** **(a)** c is a solution of $x^n - c^n = 0$, so $x - c$ is a factor
of $x^n - c^n$ by the Factor Theorem.   **B.5.** **(a)** $k = 1$ **(c)** $k = 1$ **B.6.** **(a)** $x = 1$ or
2 or $-1/2$ **(c)** $x = 1$ or $1/2$ or $1/3$ **(e)** $x = -1$ or 2 **(g)** $y = 2/3$

PAGE 96

A.1. **(a)** between 2 and 3   **(c)** between -3 and -2 **(e)** between -5 and -4;
between -1 and 0; between 0 and 1; between 2 and 3

SECTION 4   PAGES 99–100

A.1. **(a)** 3, -3 **(c)** $-\frac{23}{11}$ **(e)** 9   **(g)** $\frac{17}{3}$ **B.1.** **(a)** $3 + \sqrt{8}$, $3 - \sqrt{8}$
(c) 2, -1 **(e)** -1, -4 **B.2.** **(a)** 6   **(c)** 3, 7   **(e)** no solutions since

the   left   side   is   *always*   positive   **(g)** $\frac{1}{3}$, -1 **B.3.** **(a)** $b = \sqrt{\dfrac{a^2}{A^2 - 1}}$

(c) $u = \sqrt{\dfrac{x^2}{1 - K^2}}$ **B.4.** **(a)** 8, $-27/8$ **(c)** 16   **(e)** 1, 81   **(g)** 1
B.5. **(a)** $\frac{1}{3}$, $-\frac{1}{2}$ **(c)** 1

SECTION 5   PAGES 104–106

A.1. **(a)** $(-\infty, -\frac{8}{5}]$ **(c)** $(1, \infty)$ **(e)** $(-\infty, \frac{4}{7})$ **B.1.** **(a)** $[-\frac{7}{17}, \infty)$
(c) $(-\infty, \frac{9}{5})$ **B.2.** **(a)** $(-\infty, 3)$ **(c)** $[1, \infty)$ **B.3.** **(a)** $[4, \infty)$
(c) $(-20, \infty)$ **B.4.** **(a)** $(2, 4)$ **(c)** $[-2, -\frac{3}{4}]$ **(e)** $[-1, \frac{1}{8})$
B.5. **(a)** $[-4, 8]$ **(c)** no solutions   **B.6.** **(a)** $[-\frac{4}{3}, 0]$ **(c)** $(\frac{7}{6}, \frac{11}{6})$

(e) $(-\frac{5}{2}, -\frac{1}{2})$ **B.7.** **(a)** $x < -2$ or $x > -1$ **(c)** $x \leq -\frac{11}{20}$ or $x \geq -\frac{1}{4}$ **(e)** $x < \frac{3}{7}$ or $x > \frac{5}{7}$ **B.8.** **(a)** $x < -\frac{53}{40}$ or $x > -\frac{43}{40}$ **(c)** $x < -\frac{7}{4}$ or $x > \frac{13}{4}$ **(e)** $[-\frac{4}{3}, \frac{8}{3}]$
B.9. **(a)** approximately $[.602, \infty)$ **(c)** approximately $(-\infty, -1.053)$ **B.10.** **(a)** all real numbers are solutions since $|2x + 1| \geq 0$ always

SECTION 6   PAGES 112–114

A.1. **(a)** $x < -2$ or $x > 1$ **(c)** $-1 \leq x \leq 0$ or $x \geq 1$ **(e)** $x < -\sqrt{7}$ or $x > \sqrt{7}$
(g) $x \leq -1$ or $0 \leq x \leq 5$ **B.1.** **(a)** $x > 1$ **(c)** $-\frac{3}{2} < x < -1$ **(e)** $x \leq -\frac{9}{2}$ or $x > -3$ **B.2.** **(a)** $-3 \leq x \leq 1$ or $x \geq 2$ **(c)** $x \leq -3$ or $-2 \leq x < 0$ or $x > 1$
(e) $x < -5$ or $x = -3$ or $1 < x < 2$ **B.3.** **(a)** $-3 < x < 1$ or $x \geq 5$
(c) $0 < x < 1$ **B.4.** **(a)** $-3 < x < -2$ **(c)** $x = 0$ or $1 < x < 2$ or $x > 3$
B.5. **(a)** $1 - \sqrt{2} \leq x \leq 1 + \sqrt{2}$ **(c)** $x \leq (1 - \sqrt{3})/2$ or $x \geq (1 + \sqrt{3})/2$
B.6. **(a)** $x \leq -\frac{7}{2}$ or $x \geq -\frac{5}{4}$ **(c)** $x < -5$ or $-5 < x < -\frac{4}{3}$ or $x > 6$
(e) $-\frac{1}{7} < x < 3$ **B.7.** **(a)** $-\sqrt{3} < x < -1$ or $1 < x < \sqrt{3}$ **(c)** $-3 < x < 3$
(e) $x < -\sqrt{6}$ or $x > \sqrt{6}$ **B.8.** **(a)** $x \leq -2$ or $-1 \leq x \leq 0$ or $x \geq 1$ **(c)** $0 < x < \frac{2}{3}$ or $2 < x < \frac{8}{3}$ **(e)** $x < -2$ or $1 < x < 4$ or $x > 7$ **B.9.** **(a)** $x \leq -5$ or $-4 \leq x \leq -\frac{1}{3}$ or $x \geq \frac{2}{3}$ **(c)** $-3 < x < (-5 - \sqrt{17})/4$ or $(-5 + \sqrt{17})/4 < x < \frac{1}{2}$ **B.10.** **(a)** $x^2 < x$ if $0 < x < 1$; $x^2 > x$ if $x < 0$ or $x > 1$ **B.11.**   51 and 399 (profit is 0 for 50 and 400 widgets)   **B.13.**   If h is the height, then h must satisfy: $-10 + 10\sqrt{13} < h < -10 + 10\sqrt{17}$ (approximately $26.06 < h < 31.23$). The base $b = h + 20$, so $46.06 < b < 51.23$ approximately.

CHAPTER 3:   BASIC ANALYTIC GEOMETRY

SECTION 1   PAGES 123–126

A.1. A $(-3, 3)$; C $(-2.3, 0)$; E $(0, 2)$; G $(2, 0)$; I $(3, -1)$ **A.3.** **(a)** $(-1.5, 4)$
(c) $(2.5, 6)$ **(e)** $(\frac{13}{4}, -\frac{1}{6})$ **A.4.** **(a)** yes, since $3(1) - (-2) - 5 = 0$ **(c)** yes, since $3(2) + 6 = 12$ **(e)** no, since $(3 - 2)^2 + (4 + 5)^2 \neq 4$ **A.5.** **(a)** $x = \frac{5}{7}$ and $y = -5$ **(c)** $x = \pm 1$ and $y = \pm 3$ **(e)** $x = -1$, $x = 15$, and $y = \pm\sqrt{15}$
A.6. **(a)** 13   **(c)** 5   **(e)** $\sqrt{2}|a - b|$ **B.4.** **(a)** the other vertices of possible squares are: $(6, 1)$, $(6, 5)$ and $(-2, 1)$, $(-2, 5)$ and $(4, 3)$, $(0, 3)$ **B.6.** **(a)** vertical straight line through $(3, 0)$ **(c)** straight line passing through $(0, 0)$ and bisecting the first and third quadrants   **(e)** all points in the first and third quadrants (coordinate axes *not* included)
B.7.

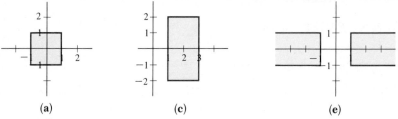

(a)   (c)   (e)

B.9. $10 + 5\sqrt{2}$ **B.10.** **(a)** $(0, 0)$, $(6, 0)$ **(c)** $(3, -5 + \sqrt{11})$, $(3, -5 - \sqrt{11})$
C.1. **(a)** $(0, -5)$ goes to $(0, 0)$; $(2, 2)$ goes to $(2, 7)$ **(c)** $(a, b + 5)$ **(e)** $(-4a, b - 5)$

SECTION 2   PAGES 135–137

A.1. **(a)** $\frac{5}{2}$ **(c)** 4   **(e)** $-\frac{8}{7}$ **(g)** $(\sqrt{5} + \sqrt{2})/7$ **(i)** $(1 - \pi)/(1 + \pi)$
A.4. **(a)** parallel   **(c)** perpendicular   **(e)** parallel   **B.3.** approx. 60.208 feet
B.5. **(b)** no   **B.6.** **(a)** yes   **B.8.** **(a)** 22   **(c)** −5   **(e)** 24

SECTION 3   PAGES 143–146

A.1. (a) $y - 5 = 1(x - 3)$, or equivalently, $y = x + 2$ (c) $y = -x + 8$ (e) $y = x/2 + \frac{5}{2}$ **A.2.** (a) $y = -x - 5$ (c) $y = -7x/3 + \frac{34}{9}$ (e) $y = x/8.7$, or equivalently, $y = 10x/87$ (g) $y - \sqrt{2} = \dfrac{\sqrt{6} - \sqrt{2}}{-\sqrt{2} - \sqrt{8}}(x - \sqrt{8})$ **A.3.** (a) $y = x + 2$ (c) $y = -4x + 2$ (e) $y = x/2 + 3$ **A.4.** m = slope, b = y-intercept: (a) $m = 2$, $b = 5$ (c) $m = -4$, $b = -\frac{7}{2}$ (e) $m = -\frac{3}{7}$, $b = -\frac{11}{7}$ **B.1.** (a) $y = 3x + 7$ (c) $y = 3x/2$ (e) $y = x - 5$ (g) $y = -x + 2$ (i) $y = 2$ (k) $y = x/3$ **B.2.** (a) parallel   (c) perpendicular   (e) perpendicular   **B.3.** (a) $k = -\frac{11}{3}$

B.8.

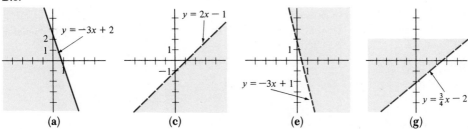

(a)   (c)   (e)   (g)

B.9.

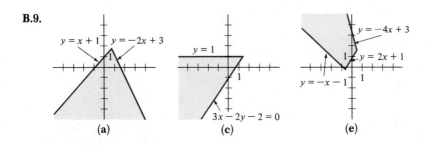

(a)   (c)   (e)

C.2. (a)   The distance from P to Q is 9400 feet.   (b) B is 88 feet from the road.

SECTION 4   PAGES 155–158

A.1. (a) $(x + 3)^2 + (y - 4)^2 = 4$ (c) $x^2 + y^2 = 2$ (e) $(x - 4)^2 + (y - 7)^2 = \frac{1}{4}$ (g) $(x - 3)^2 + (y - \frac{8}{3})^2 = 3$

A.2.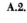

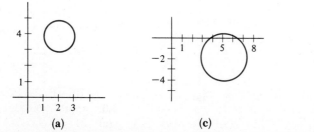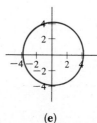

(a)   (c)   (e)

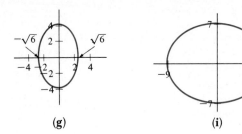

(g)   (i)

A.3. (a) $\dfrac{x^2}{49} + \dfrac{y^2}{4} = 1$ (c) $\dfrac{x^2}{81} + \dfrac{y^2}{100} = 1$

A.4. (a) 8π (c) $2\pi\sqrt{3}$ (e) $7\pi/\sqrt{3}$

A.5. (a) $\dfrac{x^2}{4} - \dfrac{y^2}{9} = 1$

B.1. (a) $(x-2)^2 + (y-2)^2 = 8$ (c) $(x-1)^2 + (y-2)^2 = 8$ (e) $(x-4)^2 + (y-3)^2 = 81$ (g) $(x+5)^2 + (y-4)^2 = 16$ **B.2.** (a) inside   (c) outside   (e) outside

B.3.

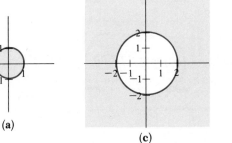

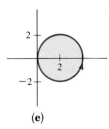

(a)   (c)   (e)

B.4.

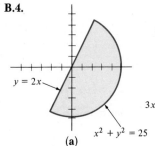

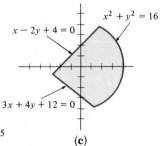

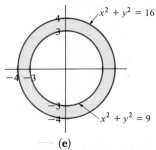

(a)   (c)   (e)

B.4.   **B.6.**

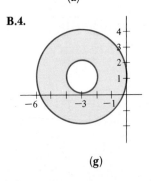

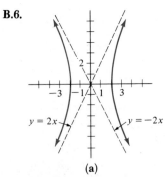

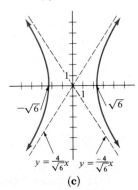

(g)   (a)   (c)

B.6.

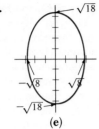

(e)

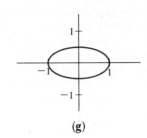

(g)

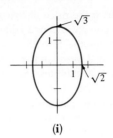

(i)

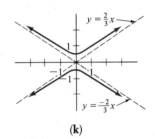

(k)

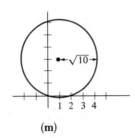

(m)

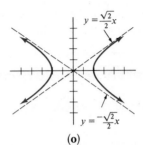

(o)

B.7. (a) $\Rightarrow$ means "implies." $a > b > 0 \Rightarrow \sqrt{a^2 - b^2} > 0$ and $a > 0 \Rightarrow e = \dfrac{\sqrt{a^2 - b^2}}{a} > 0.$

Furthermore, $a > 0$ and $b > 0 \Rightarrow b/a > 0 \Rightarrow b^2/a^2 > 0 \Rightarrow 1 + \dfrac{b^2}{a^2} > 1 \Rightarrow 1 > 1 -$

$\dfrac{b^2}{a^2} \Rightarrow 1 > \dfrac{a^2 - b^2}{a^2} = e^2 \Rightarrow 1 > e.$ **C.2.** $\sqrt{300} \approx 17.32$ feet

PAGES 162–163

A.1. (a) center $(-4, 3)$, radius $2\sqrt{10}$ (c) center $(-3, 2)$, radius $2\sqrt{7}$ (e) center $(-12.5, -5)$, radius $\sqrt{169.25}$ (g) center $(-1/4, 1/4)$, radius $\sqrt{13/8}$ **B.1.** (a) $x^2 + y^2 - 3y/2 - 1 = 0$ (c) $x^2 + y^2 - 2x - 4y - 5 = 0$

B.2.

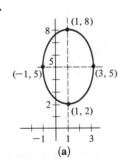

(a)

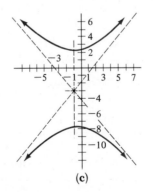

(c)

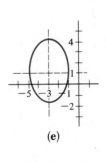

(e)

SECTION 5 PAGES 166–171

C.1. (a) 7 (c) 6 (e) 8 **C.2.** (a) 16.6 million (c) 1972 and 1985
(e) 1982, decreased; 1995, increased **C.3.** (a) Computronics (c) From March 10 to

March 20 the price of Synergistics *rose* approximately 23 dollars; the price of Computronics never rose more than 20 dollars in any *thirty*-day period.   **C.4.**   **(a)**   35   **(c)** $\frac{4500}{25} = 180$ dollars for the first 25   **(e)**   The first 20 cost the most.   **C.5.**   **(a)**   Approx. 13 miles   **(c)**   Car B went approximately 12 miles in the first 15 minutes and approximately 21 miles in the first 30 minutes. So car B went approximately $21 - 12 = 9$ miles between 15 and 30 minutes after start.   **(e)**   Car A traveled 40 miles in 60 minutes, so its average speed was $\frac{40}{60} = \frac{2}{3}$ miles per minute.   **(g)**   The steeper the graph is over an interval, the greater the average speed over that interval [why?].   **C.6.**   **(a)**   (iii) no change   **(c)**   The water level *rose* the fastest from noon to 3 P.M. (a ten-foot rise in 3 hours). It rose more slowly from 7:30 P.M. to midnight (a ten-foot rise in 4.5 hours).   **(e)**   The average *rate* of change in water level from 3 to 8 P.M. was $\frac{26}{5} = 5.2$ feet per hour. From approximately 5 to 6 P.M. the level fell approximately 5 feet, so the rate during that one hour was also 5 feet per hour.

CHAPTER 4: FUNCTIONS

SECTION 1   PAGES 178–180

A.1.   **(b)** $[-\frac{4}{3}] = -2, [-16\frac{1}{2}] = -17, [6.75] = 6, [2/3] = 0$ **B.2.**   **(a)**   tax on \$500 is 0; tax on \$6783 is \$119.15; tax on \$12,500 is \$405   **B.4.**   **(a)**   The domain is all *nonnegative* numbers. Let c and d be *different* numbers in the domain. The rule assigns $16c^2$ to c and $16d^2$ to d (see page 173). If we had $16c^2 = 16d^2$, then we would have $c^2 = d^2$, so that $c = \pm\sqrt{d^2} = \pm d$. Since c and d are both nonnegative, they cannot have opposite signs. So we would have $c = d$. This is impossible since c and d are different numbers. Thus it cannot happen that $16c^2 = 16d^2$ when $c \neq d$. Therefore the function is one-to-one. **B.6.**   **(a)**   domain $[-3, 3]$, range $[-4, 4]$ **(c)**   domain $[-2.5, 2]$, range $[-3, 2.5]$

SECTION 2   PAGES 188–192

A.1.   **(a)** $\sqrt{3} + 1$ **(c)** $\sqrt{11/2} - \frac{3}{2}$ **(e)** $\sqrt{\sqrt{2} + 3} - \sqrt{2} + 1$ **(g)**   4
A.2.   **(a)** $\frac{34}{3}$ **(c)** $\frac{59}{12}$ **(e)** $(a + k)^2 + 1/(a + k) + 2$ **(g)** $(2 - x)^2 + 1/(2 - x) + 2$
A.3.   **(a)**   8   **(c)** -1 **(e)** $s^2 + 2s$ **(g)** $t^2 - 1$ **(i)** $1/t^2 - 1$ **A.4.**   **(a)**   4
(c) $270 + \sqrt{14}$ **(e)**   11   **(g)** $|2 + x| + \sqrt{-x - 2} + x^2$ **(i)** $28 + \sqrt{3} - |2 - x| - \sqrt{x - 2} - x^2$

A.5.

	$f(2)$	$f(\frac{16}{3})$	$f(2) - f(\frac{16}{3})$	$f(r)$	$f(r) - f(x)$	$\dfrac{f(r) - f(x)}{r - x}$
(a)	2	$\frac{16}{3}$	$-\frac{10}{3}$	r	$r - x$	1
(c)	12	12	0	12	0	0
(e)	13	23	-10	$2r + 7$	$3(r - x)$	3
(g)	-2	$-\frac{208}{9}$	$\frac{190}{9}$	$r - r^2$	$r - r^2 - x + x^2$	$1 - r - x$
(i)	$\frac{1}{2}$	$\frac{3}{16}$	$\frac{5}{16}$	$1/r$	$1/r - 1/x$	$1/rx$

A.6.   **(a)** $f(-3) \approx .7$; $f(-\frac{3}{2}) \approx 2.1$; $f(0) \approx -2.8$; $f(1) \approx 0$; $f(\frac{5}{2}) \approx 1.8$; $f(4) \approx 1.6$
A.7.   **(a)** $f(-3) + f(-\frac{3}{2}) \approx .7 + 2.1 = 2.8$; $f(0) - f(2) \approx -2.8 - 3 = -5.8$ **(c)** $f(\frac{5}{2}) - f(3) = 3 - (-1) = 4$; $f(4) + 3f(-2) \approx .5 + 3(-1.8) = -4.9$ **A.8.**   **(b)** $T(3.6) = .18$; $T(0.6) = .03$ **B.1.**   **(b)**   (i) is true; (iii) is false   **B.2.**   **(a)**   (i), (ii), (iv) are true; (iii) is false for all $x \neq 0$ **(c)**   all are true   **B.3.**   **(a)**   all real numbers   **(c)**   all real numbers **(e)**   all real numbers   **(g)** $[0, \infty)$ **(i)**   all real numbers   **(k)**   all nonzero real num-

bers   **B.6.** **(a)** all real numbers   **(c)** all real numbers   **(e)** all real numbers
(g) $(-\infty, 1]$ **(i)** all real numbers *except* -2 and 3 **(k)** $[6, 12]$ **B.7.** **(a)** $x +$
Δx **(c)** 12   **(e)** $1/(x + \Delta x)$ **(g)** $x + \Delta x + 5$ **(i)** $x^2 + 2x\,\Delta x + (\Delta x)^2 + 3x +$
$3\,\Delta x - 7$ **B.8.** **(a)** 1   **(c)** 0   **(e)** $-1/(x(x + \Delta x))$ **(g)** 1   **(i)** $2x + \Delta x + 3$

B.9. **(a)**

	$\Delta x = 2$	$\Delta x = 1$	$\Delta x = .5$	$\Delta x = .1$	$\Delta x = .01$
(a)	1	1	1	1	1
(c)	0	0	0	0	0
(e)	$\dfrac{-1}{x^2 + 2x}$	$\dfrac{-1}{x^2 + x}$	$\dfrac{-1}{x^2 + .5x}$	$\dfrac{-1}{x^2 + .1x}$	$\dfrac{-1}{x^2 + .01x}$
(g)	1	1	1	1	1
(i)	$2x + 5$	$2x + 4$	$2x + 3.5$	$2x + 3.1$	$2x + 3.01$

(b) **(a)** 1   **(c)** 0   **(e)** $-1/x^2$ **(g)** 1   **(i)** $2x + 3$ **C.1.** **(a)** $d(0) = 0$;
$d(2) = 64$ **(c)** $d(2) = 64$; $d(4) = 256$ **(e)** 128 feet   **(g)** $d(t_2) - d(t_1)$
C.2. **(a)** **(i)** 42; **(v)** many possibilities, inluding 4 P.M.; **(vii)** lower

PAGES 195–196

A.1. $D(t) = \begin{cases} 55t \text{ if } t \le 2 \\ 100 + 45(t - 2) \text{ if } t > 2 \end{cases}$ **A.4.** $P(t) = .7t - 1800$, where $P =$ profit and
$t =$ number of pounds sold   **B.1.** **(a)** $c(x) = 5.75x + (45,000/x)$ **B.2.** **(a)** $N(p) =$
$17,500 - 100p$, where p is the price per hamburger in *cents* (not dollars) and N is the number
of hamburgers sold   **(c)** $D(p) = (17,500 - 100p)p - 40(17,500 - 100p) - 110,000$,
where p is the price in cents and D is the daily profit in cents.   **B.4.** $V(t) = t(16 - 2t) \cdot$
$(10 - 2t)$; maximum volume when $t = 2$

SECTION 3 PAGES 206–207

A.1.   **A.2.** see   **A.3.**   **A.5.**
                                 page 265

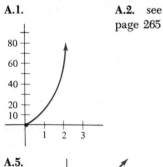   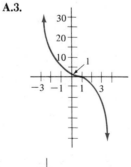   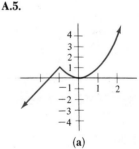

(a)

A.5.   **B.1.**

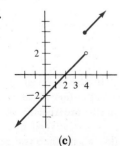   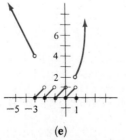   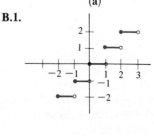

(c)   (e)

B.2.

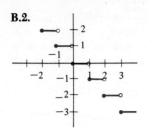 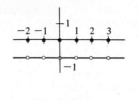

(a)   (c)

B.4. see page 282   **B.5.**

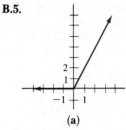

(a)

B.7.

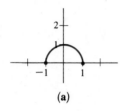 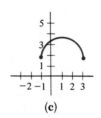

(a)   (c)

B.8.

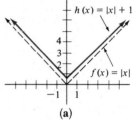

(a)

B.8.

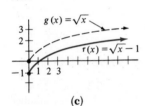 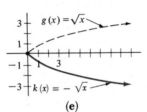 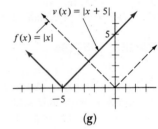

(c)   (e)   (g)

B.11.

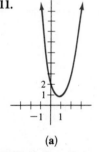 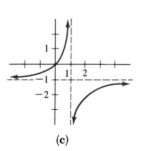 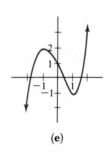

(a)   (c)   (e)

SECTION 4 PAGES 211–214

B.1. (a) 4   (c) 3.5   (e) 4.5   (g) 4   (i) 1, 5   (k) $[-3, 3]$
B.3. (a) $[-8, 9]$ (c) $-6.9, -3, 0, 3, 7$ (e) 1, 3, 5 and others   (g) $-3, 7$
(i) 1   **B.4.** (a) domain $f = [-6, 7]$ (c) $-1.4, -.2$ (e) $x = 3$ (g) $[-2, -1]$
and $[3, 7]$ **B.5.** (a) approx. $5000 - 17,000 = -12,000$ dollars (negative profit means a
loss of \$12,000)   (c) $12,000$ (f) profit on $5,000$ widgets is approx. 5000–
$22,000 = -17,000$ dollars [a loss]; the smallest number manufactured without a loss is approx. 14,500   **B.6.** (a) tem$(10) = 47°$ (c) 10:54 A.M. and 8:24 P.M. ($= 20.4$ hours)
(e) tem$(10) = 47°$, so $(10, 47)$ is on the graph; tem$(16) = 63.5°$, so $(16, 63.5)$ is on the graph.
The point $(10, 47)$ lies 16.5 units lower than $(16, 63.5)$.   (g) tem$(6 \cdot 2) =$ tem$(12) = 57$, but
tem$(2) = 38$, so that $6 \cdot$ tem$(2) = 6(38) = 228$.   (i) 10:54 A.M. ($= 10.9$ hours) and 8:24 P.M.
($= 20.4$ hours)

SECTION 5   PAGES 220–224

A.1.   (a), (c), (d), (f), (h) are symmetric with respect to the y-axis   **A.2.**   (a)   (i) yes, (ii) no, (iii) yes, (iv) no   **(c)**   (i)–(iv) no   **(e)**   (i) yes, (iv) no   **A.3.**   (a)   increasing on $[-2.5, 0]$ and $[1.5, 3]$, decreasing on $[-6, -2.5]$ and $[0, 1.5]$ **B.2.**   (a)   some possible answers are: (i) 4, (iii) 2; (v) all five   **(b)**   (i) 3, 5, and other pairs; (iii) 4, 2, and other pairs; (v) 1, 5, and other   pairs   **B.5.**   (a) $f(x + c) = f(x + 2c) = f(x + 3c) = f(x + 4c) = f(x + 5c) = k$ **(c)** $f(x + nc) = k$ **B.6.**   (a)   8   **(c)**   6   **B.8.**   (a)   If $0 < c < d \le 10$, then $c^2 < d^2$. Hence $c^2 + 3 < d^2 + 3$. But this says $f(c) < f(d)$. Thus if $0 < c < d \le 10$, then $f(c) < f(d)$. Therefore f is increasing on $(0, 10]$.   **(c)**   If $0 < c < d \le 10$, then $c^2 < d^2$. But $c^2 < d^2$ and $c < d$ imply that $c^2 + c < d^2 + d$. Hence $c^2 + c + 5 < d^2 + d + 5$. But this means $h(c) < h(d)$. Therefore h is increasing on $(0, 10]$.   **B.9.**   (a) $(c, -d)$ **(c)**   symmetric with respect to the x-axis

PAGES 226–227

A.1.   (a)   and   (c)   **A.2.**   (a), (b), (d), and (g)   **A.3.**   (a)   even   **(c)**   even **(e)**   neither

SECTION 6   PAGES 239–241

A.1.

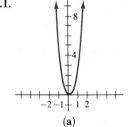

(a)

(c)

(e)

A.2.

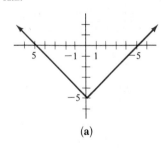

(a)

(c)

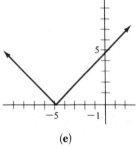

(e)

A.2.

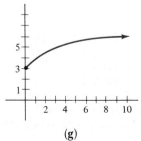

(g)

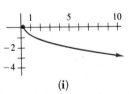

(i)

A.3.

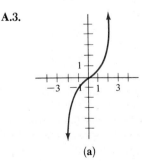

(a)

A.3.

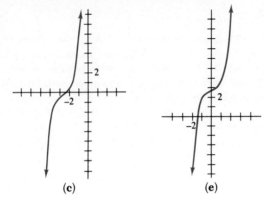

(c)   (e)

A.5.

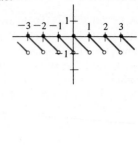

A.6.

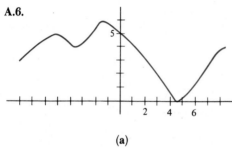

(a)   (c)

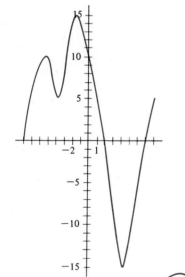

(e)

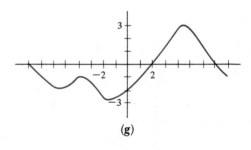

(g)

(i)

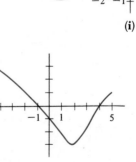

(k)

B.1.

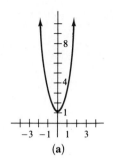

(a)

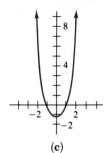

(c)

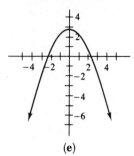

(e)

B.2.

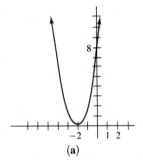

(a)

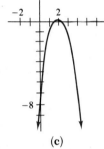

(c)

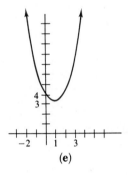

(e)

B.2.

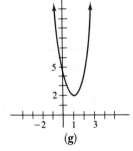

(g)

B.3.

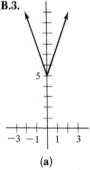

(a)

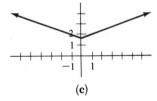

(c)

B.3.

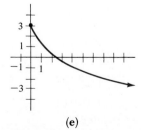

(e)

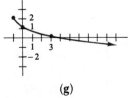

(g)

B.4.

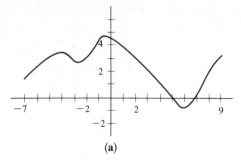

(a)

B.3.

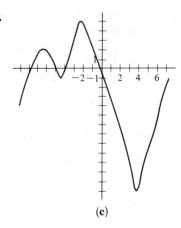

(c)

C.1.

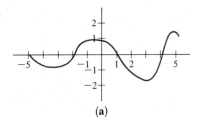

(a)

C.1.

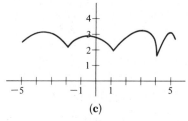

(c)

C.2.

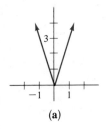

(a)

(c)

(e)

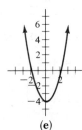

PAGES 246–247

A.1. (a) $(5, 2)$, upward   (c) $(1, 2)$ downward   (e) $(-\frac{3}{2}, \frac{3}{2})$, downward

A.2. (a) $(\frac{2}{3}, \frac{19}{3})$, downward   (c) $(\frac{1}{2}, \frac{1}{4})$, downward   (e) $(-\frac{1}{2}, \frac{3}{4})$, upward

(g) $(\frac{1}{2}, -\frac{1}{2})$, downward   **A.3.** $7, 500$

B.1.

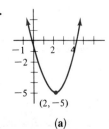

$(2, -5)$

(a)

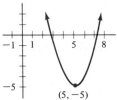

$(5, -5)$

(b)

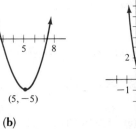

$(1, -1)$

(c)

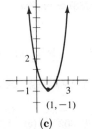

B.2. 0   **B.3.** 16   **C.1.** $t = \frac{5}{2}$, $h = 196$ **C.3.** $t = \frac{125}{8}$, $h = (125)^2/4 = 3906.25$
C.5. $A = \text{area} = hb/2$. Since $h + b = 30$, we have $A = hb/2 = (30 - b)b/2 = 15b - b^2/2$. Maximum area corresponds to the highest point (b, A) on the graph of the function $A = 15b - b^2/2$. This occurs when $b = 15$; hence $h = 30 - 15 = 15$.   **C.7.** If the base has side x and the height is y, then surface area $S = 2x^2 + 4xy$. Since $8x + 4y = 8$, we have $y = 2 - 2x$ and hence $S = 2x^2 + 4x(2 - 2x) = -6x^2 + 8x$. Maximum area occurs when $x = \frac{2}{3}$. Hence $y = 2 - 2(\frac{2}{3}) = \frac{2}{3}$.   **C.9.** \$3.50

SECTION 7 PAGES 253–257

A.1. (a) 0   (c) 30   (e) 42   **A.2.** (a) 49, 1, −8   (c) −25, 1, 4   (e) 5, 1, 0
A.3. (a) $x^2 + 6x + 8$ (c) $x + 6$ **A.4.** (a) $(g \circ f)(x) = |2x^2 + 2x - 2| + 2$;
$(f \circ g)(x) = 2(x - 1)^2 + 10|x - 1| + 11$ (c) $(g \circ f)(x) = (-3x + 2)^3$; $(f \circ g)(x) = -3x^3 + 2$ (e) $(g \circ f)(x) = (\sqrt[3]{x})^2 - 1$; $(f \circ g)(x) = \sqrt[3]{x^2 - 1}$ **A.7.** (a) $(f + g)(x) = 2x^2 + 2x + |x - 1| + 1$; $(f - g)(x) = 2x^2 + 2x - |x - 1| - 3$; $(g - f)(x) = |x - 1| - 2x^2 - 2x + 3$ (c) $(f + g)(x) = x^3 - 3x + 2$; $(f - g)(x) = -x^3 - 3x + 2$; $(g - f)(x) = x^3 + 3x - 2$ (e) $(f + g)(x) = \sqrt[3]{x} + x^2 - 1$; $(f - g)(x) = \sqrt[3]{x} - x^2 + 1$; $(g - f)(x) = x^2 - \sqrt[3]{x} - 1$ **A.8.** (a) $(f + g)(x + h) = 2(x + h)^2 + 2(x + h) + |x + h - 1| + 1$; $(fg)(x + h) = |x + h - 1|(2(x + h)^2 + 2(x + h) - 1) + 4(x + h)^2 + 4(x + h) - 2$
(c) $(f + g)(x + h) = (x + h)^3 - 3(x + h) + 2$; $(fg)(x + h) = -3(x + h)^4 + 2(x + h)^3$
(e) $(f + g)(x + h) = \sqrt[3]{x + h} + (x + h)^2 - 1$; $(fg)(x + h) = \sqrt[3]{x + h}(x + h)^2 - \sqrt[3]{x + h}$
A.9. (a) $(fg)(x) = |x - 1|(2x^2 + 2x - 1) + 4x^2 + 4x - 2$; $\left(\dfrac{f}{g}\right)(x) = \dfrac{2x^2 + 2x - 1}{|x - 1| + 2}$;
$\left(\dfrac{g}{f}\right)(x) = \dfrac{|x - 1| + 2}{2x^2 + 2x - 1}$ (c) $(fg)(x) = -3x^4 + 2x^3$; $\left(\dfrac{f}{g}\right)(x) = \dfrac{-3x + 2}{x^3}$; $\left(\dfrac{g}{f}\right)(x) = \dfrac{x^3}{-3x + 2}$ (e) $(fg)(x) = (\sqrt[3]{x})x^2 - \sqrt[3]{x}$; $\left(\dfrac{f}{g}\right)(x) = \dfrac{\sqrt[3]{x}}{x^2 - 1}$; $\left(\dfrac{g}{f}\right)(x) = \dfrac{x^2 - 1}{\sqrt[3]{x}}$
B.1. (a) $f(-4) = -3$, $g(-4) = -1$; $f(0) = 1$, $g(0) = 1.3$; $f(2) = 1$, $g(2) = 1.3$; $f(4) = -2$, $g(4) = 0$
B.2. (a)

x	1	2	3	4	5
$(g \circ f)(x)$	4	2	5	4	4

(c)

x	1	2	3	4	5
$(f \circ f)(x)$	1	3	3	5	1

B.3. The given function is $B \circ A$, where A and B are the functions listed here. In some cases other correct answers are possible.   (a) $A(x) = x^2 + 2$, $B(x) = \sqrt[3]{x}$ (c) $A(x) = 7x^3 - 10x + 17$, $B(x) = x^7$ (e) $A(x) = x^2 - \sqrt{x} + 2$, $B(x) = |x|$ (g) $A(t) = t + 2$, $B(t) = t\sqrt{t^2 - 5}$ (i) $A(x) = 3x^2 + 5x - 7$, $B(x) = 1/x$ **B.5.** (a) $(f \circ g)(x) = (\sqrt{x})^3$, domain $[0, \infty)$; $(g \circ f)(x) = \sqrt{x^3}$, domain $[0, \infty)$ (c) $(f \circ g)(x) = \sqrt{5x + 10}$, domain $[-2, \infty)$; $(g \circ f)(x) = 5\sqrt{x + 10}$, domain $[-10, \infty)$ (e) $(f \circ g)(x) = \dfrac{1}{x^2 + 1}$, domain all real numbers; $(g \circ f)(x) = \dfrac{1}{x^2} + 1$, domain all nonzero real numbers   **B.7.** (a) $f(x^2) = 2x^6 + 5x^2 - 1$ **C.1.** (a) $A(81) = 50,000$; $T(11.5) = 85°$; 65,000 at 4 P.M.; $T(8.5) = 72$; $A(T(12)) = A(88) \approx 62,500$ (c) approximately 9:30–11:30 A.M.

CHAPTER 5: POLYNOMIAL AND RATIONAL FUNCTIONS

SECTION 1 PAGES 261–263

A.1. (a) 7,   −3   (c) 2,   −2   **A.2.** (a) 2   (c) 6   (e) −30
A.3. (a) 170, 802   (c) 5, 935, 832   (e) $\frac{55}{16} = 3.4375$ **A.4.** (a) 0 has multiplicity

54, $-\frac{4}{5}$ has multiplicity 1   **(c)**   0 has multiplicity 15, π has multiplicity 14 and $\pi + 1$ has multiplicity 13   **B.1.**   many correct answers, including: **(a)** $(x - 1)(x - 7)(x + 4)$ **(c)** $(x - 1)(x - 2)^3(x - \pi)^2$ **C.1.**   **(a)**   small; large   **(c)**   (i) $x = \frac{1}{8}$ inch [for example, a baby shrew]; (ii) $x = \frac{5}{2}$ inches [for example, a field mouse]; (iii) $x = 60$ inches [for example, a human   **(e)**   It could eat its own weight once every 600 days. For comparison, an average size human who ate his or her own weight once every 600 days would eat approximately one and a half pounds of food per week. If this food were one pound of bread and a half pound of cheese, it would provide about 2800 calories per week, that is, 400 calories per day. But the minimum subsistance level for such a human is approximately 1500 calories per day.

SECTION 2   PAGES 274–276

A.3.

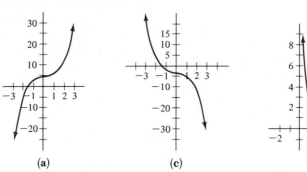

B.1.

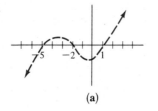

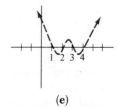

B.3.   **(a)**   increasing
         (c)   increasing

B.5.

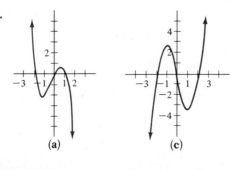

B.7.

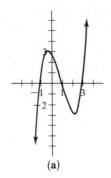

(a)

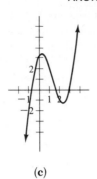

(c)

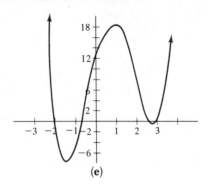

(e)

PAGE 278

A.1. (a)

x	10	50	100	250
$f(x) = x^3$	1000	125,000	1,000,000	15,625,000
$g(x) = 10x^2$	1000	25,000	100,000	625,000

(c)

x	3000	5000	10,000
$k(x) = 50x^3$	1,350,000,000,000	6,250,000,000,000	50,000,000,000,000
$t(x) = x^4/100$	810,000,000,000	6,250,000,000,000	100,000,000,000,000

B.1. yes, at $(100,100000)$

SECTION 3   PAGES 295–297

A.1. (a) all real numbers except -2 (c) all real numbers except -1 (e) all real numbers except $0, 1, -1$

A.3.

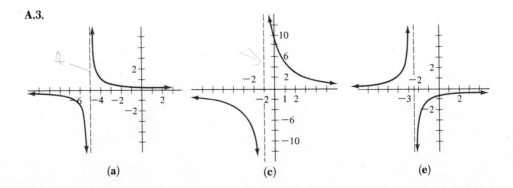

(a)   (c)   (e)

A.3.

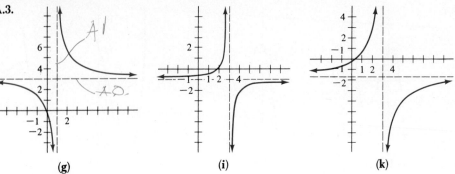

(g)   (i)   (k)

A.4. **(a)** 3, 2   **(c)** 5, 2   **(e)** 3   **B.1.** One such function is $f(x) = \dfrac{4x - 4}{x - 4}$. More

generally, for any nonzero number a, the graph of $f(x) = \dfrac{ax - a}{\dfrac{a}{4}x - a}$ passes through the given

points.

B.3.

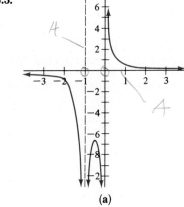

(a)

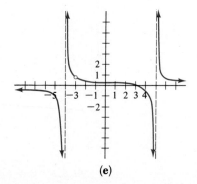

(c)

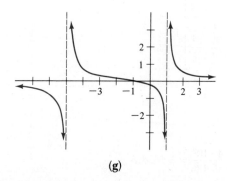

(e)   (g)

B.4.

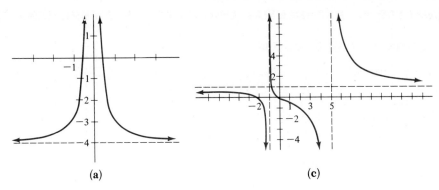

(a)   (c)

B.5.

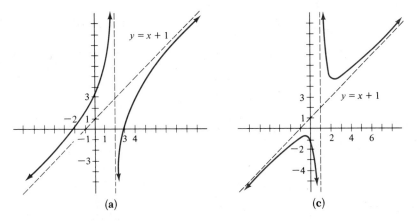

(a)   (c)

B.5.

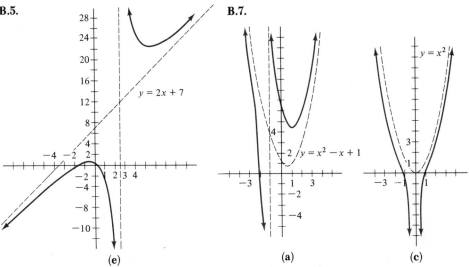

(e)   (a)   (c)

B.7.

C.1. (a) $\dfrac{4 \cdot 10^2}{(6.4)^2} = 9.765625$ (c) no roots

CHAPTER 6: EXPONENTIAL AND LOGARITHMIC FUNCTIONS

SECTION 1 PAGES 303–304

A.1. (a) $100,000$ (c) $7^3/2^3 = \frac{343}{8}$ (e) $100,000$ **A.2.** (a) $2^{4/3}$ (c) $2^{8/3}$
(e) $2^{1/2}$ **A.3.** (a) $(a^2 + b^2)^{1/3}$ (c) $a^{3/16}$ (e) $4t^{27/10} = 4t^{2.7}$
B.1. (a) $x^{7/6} - x^{11/6}$ (c) $x - y$ (e) $x + y - (x + y)^{3/2}$ **B.2.** (a) $(x^{1/3} + 3) \cdot$
$(x^{1/3} - 2)$ (c) $(x^{1/2} + 3)(x^{1/2} + 1)$ (e) $(x^{2/5} + 9)(x^{1/5} + 3)(x^{1/5} - 3)$ **B.3.** (a) $\frac{1}{2}$
(c) 1 (e) $1/49ab$ (g) a^x (i) $b^{x/4}$ **B.4.** (a) $\dfrac{1}{x^{1/5}y^{2/5}}$ (c) 1

(e) $c^{5/3} + \dfrac{1}{c^{5/3}} - 2$ **B.7.** (a) $x = 7$ or -9 (c) $x = 2$ or 6

SECTION 2 PAGES 310–312

A.1. many possible answers, including $x = 1.07$ and $x = 60$ **A.2.** (a) 512 (c) 2
(e) $\sqrt[4]{3}$

A.3.

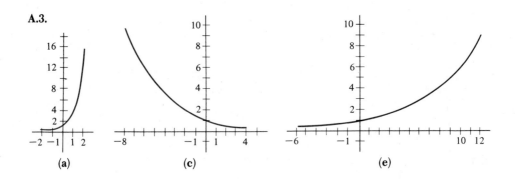

(a)   (c)   (e)

A.4. (a) $\dfrac{10^x(10^{\Delta x} - 1)}{\Delta x}$ (c) $3^{-x}\left(\dfrac{3^{-\Delta x} - 1}{\Delta x}\right)$ (e) $2^x\left(\dfrac{2^{\Delta x} - 1}{\Delta x}\right) + 2^{-x}\left(\dfrac{2^{-\Delta x} - 1}{\Delta x}\right)$
A.5. (a) e^{3x+1} (c) $5^{2x} - 5^{-2x}$

B.1.

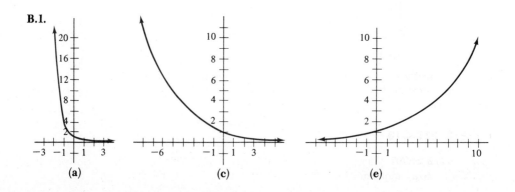

(a)   (c)   (e)

B.2.

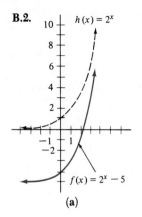

(a)

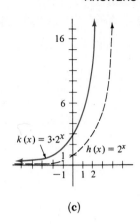

(c)

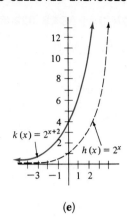

(e)

B.3.

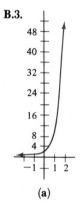

(a)

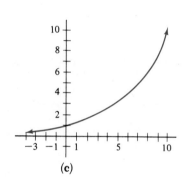

(c)

B.3.

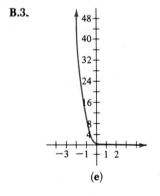

(e)

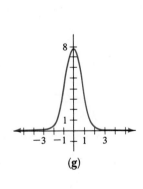

(g)

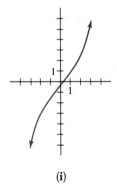

(i)

B.6. (a) neither   (c) even   (e) even   **B.8.** 13 hours   **B.10.** (a) 100 kg
(b) approximately 139.3 kg, 163.2 kg and 186.5 kg   **C.2.** (c) slower   (e) $t(x)$ grows
more slowly   **C.4.** (a) $P(x) = 2^x/100$

PAGES 317–318

A.1. $\sqrt{2}/2 \approx .707$ grams   **A.3.** (a) $814.45   (c) $824.35   **B.2.** approximately
6.992%   **B.4.** approximately .444 billion years, that is, 444,000,000 years

SECTION 3 PAGES 329–332

A.1. (a) 4   (c) 6   (e) $-\frac{2}{3}$ (g) 7   **A.2.** (a) 4   (c) $-\frac{3}{2}$ (e) -6
(g) -8 **A.3.** (a) $\log_{10}(.01) = -2$ (c) $\log_{10}\sqrt[3]{10} = \frac{1}{3}$
(e) $\log_{10} 27.3 \approx 1.4367$ (g) $\log_{10} r = 7k$ (i) $\log_{10} y = x^2 + 2$
A.4. (a) $\log_5 625 = 4$ (c) $\log_2(\frac{1}{8}) = -3$ (e) $\log_b 3379 = 14$ (g) $\log_e .0183 \approx$
-4 (i) $\log_a c = -b$ **A.5.** (a) $10^4 = 10,000$ (c) $10^{2.86} \approx 750$
(e) $10^{-.097} \approx .8$ (g) $10^b = a$ (i) $10^{z+w} = x^2 + 2y$ **A.6.** (a) $2^{1/2} = \sqrt{2}$
(c) $8^{-2/3} = \frac{1}{4}$ (e) $e^{1.099} \approx 3$ **A.7.** (a) $\sqrt{43}$ (c) 4.7   (e) $\sqrt{x^2 + y^2}$
(g) 14   (i) 931   **A.8.** (a) -4 (c) 6   (e) -1 (g) 5/4   (i) -4
A.9. (a) 4   (c) 3/4   (e) 3/2   **A.10.** (a) .43   (c) .26   (e) .10
(g) .53   (i) .7   **A.11.** (a) $\log_e(x^2 y^3)$ (c) $\log_e(x - 3)$ (e) $\log_e(x^{-7})$
B.1. (a) $-.039$ (c) $-.595$ (e) 1.32   (g) .878   (i) 1.88
B.2. (a) true   (c) true   (e) false   (g) false   **B.4.** (a) 5   (c) 2
(e) 1   (g) $\sqrt{1.01}$ **B.5.** (a) $\pm\sqrt{10,001}$ (c) 3   (e) $\sqrt{11}/3$ **B.6.** (a) 1
and 100   (c) $\frac{1}{10}$ and 1000   (e) 5^5 and $\frac{1}{5}$ **B.8.** (a) 4.0969   (c) 7.301
(e) 5.699

PAGES 339–340

A.1. each characteristic is underlined: (a) $\underline{0}.0043$ (c) $\underline{1}.6590$ (e) $\underline{3}.8965$
(g) $0.9614 - 4$ (i) $\underline{7}.7582$ **A.2.** (a) .3702   (c) 2.6701   (e) $0.9276 - 4$
(g) $0.8826 - 1$ (i) 6.7262   **A.3.** (a) 2.22   (c) 89.7   (e) .0662
A.4. (a) 7.544   (c) 197,500   (e) .00005485   **A.5.** (a) $x \approx 438$
(c) $x \approx 29.75$ (e) $z \approx .02329$ **A.6.** (a) 3.149   (c) 1.285   (e) 24,230,000
(g) 9.68   **B.1.** (a) 2728   (c) .007762   (e) 15.11

SECTION 4 PAGES 345–346

A.1. (a) $b = 10$ (c) $b = 2$ **A.2.** (a) $(-1, \infty)$ (c) $(-\infty, 0)$ (e) $(0, \infty)$
(g) all x such that $x < -1$ or $x > 1$ (i) $(2, \infty)$

A.3.

B.2. (a) all x
except $x = 0$
(c) all positive x
(e) all x greater
than 1

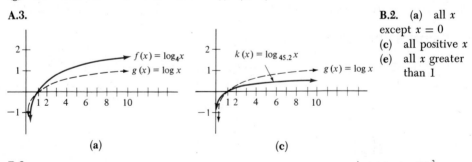

(a)   (c)

B.3.

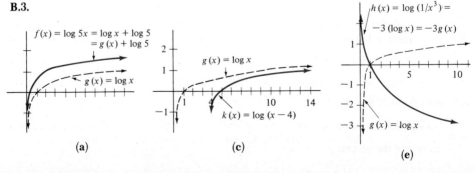

(a)   (c)   (e)

B.4.

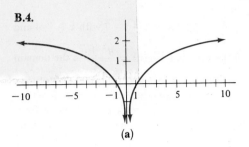

(a)

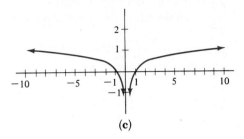

(c)

B.4.

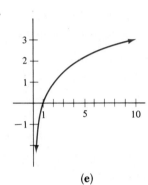

(e)

B.5.

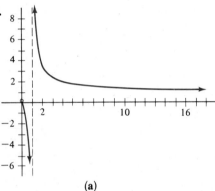

(a)

B.7. $A = -9,\ B = 10$ **C.1.** (a) x must be doubled   (c) The bill increases \$1.28 from $L = 8$ to $L = 9$ and increases \$2, 621.44 from $L = 19$ to $L = 20$.

PAGES 348–349

A.1. (a) 2   (c) approx. 2.54   **B.1.** (a) 71.2, 66.8, 64.0, 62.0   (b) 16 months
B.2. (a) 77   (c) 13 weeks, 34 weeks, 90 weeks   **B.3.** approximately 199.53 and 7.94

SECTION 5 PAGES 356–358

A.1. (a) $(f \circ g)(x) = f(g(x)) = f(x - 1) = (x - 1) + 1 = x$ and $(g \circ f)(x) = g(f(x)) = g(x + 1)$
$= (x + 1) - 1 = x$ (c) $(f \circ g)(x) = f\left(\dfrac{1 - x}{x}\right) = \dfrac{1}{\left(\dfrac{1 - x}{x}\right) + 1} = \dfrac{1}{\dfrac{(1 - x) + x}{x}} = x$

and $(g \circ f)(x) = g\left(\dfrac{1}{x + 1}\right) = \dfrac{1 - \dfrac{1}{x + 1}}{\dfrac{1}{x + 1}} = \dfrac{\dfrac{(x + 1) - 1}{x + 1}}{\dfrac{1}{x + 1}} = x$ (e) $(f \circ g)(x) = f(\sqrt[5]{x}) =$

$(\sqrt[5]{x})^5 = x$ and $(g \circ f)(x) = g(x^5) = \sqrt[5]{x^5} = x$ (g) $(f \circ g)(x) = f(\log_e x) = e^{\log_e x} = x$ and
$(g \circ f)(x) = g(e^x) = \log_e e^x = x$ **B.1.** (a) The rule of f is "multiply by 5, then add 1," so
the rule of the inverse g is "subtract 1, then divide by 5." Hence $g(x) = \dfrac{x - 1}{5}$.   (c) Rule
of g is "take the cube root," so $g(x) = \sqrt[3]{x}$.   (e) Rule of g is "add 1, then divide by 2, then
take the cube root, and finally subtract 4," so $g(x) = \sqrt[3]{\dfrac{x + 1}{2}} - 4$.   **B.2.** (a) $y = -x$, so
$x = -y$ and the rule of the inverse g is $g(y) = -y$ (c) $y = (x^5 + 1)^3$, so $x = \sqrt[5]{\sqrt[3]{y} - 1}$
and the rule of the inverse g is $g(y) = \sqrt[5]{\sqrt[3]{y} - 1}$ (e) $y = \dfrac{1}{2x + 1}$, so $x = \dfrac{1}{2}\left(\dfrac{1}{y} - 1\right) =$

$\dfrac{1-y}{2y}$ and the rule of the inverse g is $g(y) = \dfrac{1-y}{2y}$ (g) $y = \sqrt{4x-7}$ with $x \geq 7/4$ and

$y \geq 0$, so $x = \dfrac{y^2+7}{4}$ with $y \geq 0$ and the rule of the inverse g is $g(y) = \dfrac{y^2+7}{4}$; the domain

of g is all $y \geq 0$ **B.3.** There are several correct answers for each part, including these:
(a) one restricted function is $f(x) = |x|$ with $x \geq 0$ (so that $f(x) = x$); inverse function:
$g(y) = y$ with $y \geq 0$ (c) one restricted function is $f(x) = -x^2$ with $x \leq 0$; inverse function $g(y) = -\sqrt{-y}$ with $y \leq 0$. Another restricted function is $f(x) = -x^2$ with $x \geq 0$; inverse function $h(y) = \sqrt{-y}$ with $y \leq 0$ (e) one restricted function is $f(x) = \dfrac{x^2+6}{2}$ with

$x \geq 0$; inverse function $g(y) = \sqrt{2y-6}$ with $y \geq 3$ (g) one restricted function is

$f(x) = \dfrac{1}{x^2+1}$ with $x \leq 0$; inverse function $g(y) = -\sqrt{\dfrac{1}{y}-1} = -\sqrt{\dfrac{1-y}{y}}$ with $0 < y \leq 1$

B.4.

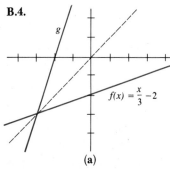

(a)

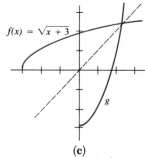

(c)

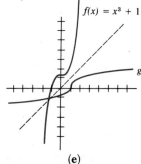

(e)

B.5.

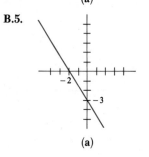

(a)

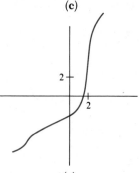

(c)

C.1. Let $y = f(x) = mx + b$. Since $m \neq 0$, we can solve for x and obtain $x = \dfrac{y-b}{m}$. Hence

the rule of the inverse function g is $g(y) = \dfrac{y-b}{m}$, and we have: $(f \circ g)(y) = f(g(y)) =$

$f\left(\dfrac{y-b}{m}\right) = m\left(\dfrac{y-b}{m}\right) + b = y$ and $(g \circ f)(x) = g(f(x)) = g(mx+b) =$

$\dfrac{(mx+b)-b}{m} = x$.   **C.2.** (a) Adding 2, dividing by 7, and taking reciprocals are inverti-

ble.   (c) In part (a) taking absolute values is not invertible; in parts (c), (e), (g) squaring is
not invertible.

PAGE 361

B.1. (a) Neither because the graph lies below the x axis when $x < 3$ and above it when
$x > 3$ (see Figure 5–28 on page 281)   **C.2.** (a) Yes, it has slope $\frac{1}{2}$.   (c) The inverse has
negative slope.

SECTION 6   PAGES 366–368

A.1. (a) $x = 4$ (c) $x = 1$ (e) $x = -\frac{1}{9}$ (g) $x = \frac{1}{2}$ or $x = -3$ (i) $x = -2$ or
$x = -\frac{1}{2}$ **A.3.** (a) $x = \log 5/\log 3 \approx 1.465$ (c) $x = \log 2 \approx .301$ (e) $x =$
$(\log 20 - \log 4)/\log 7 = \log 5/\log 7 \approx .827$ **A.4.** (a) $x = \log 3/(\log 3 - \log 2) = \log 3/$
$\log 1.5 \approx 2.7095$ (c) $x = \dfrac{\log 3 - 5 \log 5}{\log 5 + 2 \log 3} \approx -1.825$ (e) $x = \dfrac{\log 2 - \log 3}{3 \log 2 + \log 3} \approx -.1276$

A.5. (a) $x = 0$ or $x = 1$ (c) $x = 0$ (e) $x = \log 2/\log 4 = \log 2/(2 \log 2) =$
$1/2$ or $x = \log 3/\log 4 \approx .792$ (g) $x = 0$ or $x = (2 \log 5)/\log 2 \approx 4.644$ **B.1.** (a)
$x = \log_5(3 + 2\sqrt{2})$ or $x = \log_5(3 - 2\sqrt{2})$ (c) $x = \log_5(t + \sqrt{t^2 - 1})$ or $x = \log_5(t - \sqrt{t^2 - 1})$ **B.2.** (a) $x = \ln(2 + \sqrt{3})$ or $x = \ln(2 - \sqrt{3})$ (c) $x = \frac{1}{2} \ln\left(\dfrac{t+1}{t-1}\right)$

B.3. (a) $\log 2/\log 1.07 \approx 10.245$ years   (c) $\dfrac{\log 2}{365\left[\log\left(1 + \dfrac{.07}{365}\right)\right]} \approx 9.9$ years

B.5. (a) $\log 3/\log 1.05 \approx 22.5$ years   **B.7.** $5,000/(1.0125)^{36} \approx \$3,197.05$

B.9. $\dfrac{(5730)(\log .64)}{-(\log 2)} \approx 3,689.3$ years old   **B.11.** $\dfrac{(3.6)(\log .15)}{-(\log 2)} \approx 9.853$ days

B.13. $\dfrac{(5730)(\log .49)}{-(\log 2)} \approx 5897$ years old

CHAPTER 7 THE COMPLEX NUMBERS

SECTION 1   PAGES 375–379

A.1. (a) $8 + 2i$ (c) $-2 - 10i$ (e) $-\frac{1}{2} - 2i$ (g) $\left(\dfrac{\sqrt{2} - \sqrt{3}}{2}\right) + 2i$

A.2. (a) $1 + 13i$ (c) $-10 + 11i$ (e) $-21 - 20i$ (g) 4 **A.3.** (a) $-i$
(c) i (e) i **A.4.** (a) $\bar{z} = 1 - i$, $\bar{w} = -2i$, $\overline{zw} = -2 - 2i$ (c) $\bar{z} = 4 + 5i$;
$\bar{w} = 2 + 3i$, $\overline{zw} = -7 + 22i$

A.5.

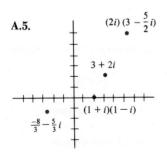

$(2i)(3 - \frac{5}{2}i)$

$3 + 2i$

$(1 + i)(1 - i)$

$\frac{-8}{3} - \frac{5}{3}i$

B.1. (a) $\frac{5}{29} + \frac{2}{29}i$ (c) $\frac{-1}{3}i$ (e) $\frac{12}{41} - \frac{15}{41}i$
(g) $-2 - \frac{7}{2}i$ **B.2.** (a) $\frac{-5}{41} - \frac{4}{41}i$ (c) $\frac{10}{17} - \frac{11}{17}i$ (e) $\frac{31}{130} + \frac{27}{130}i$ **B.3.** (a) $\frac{7}{10} +$
$\frac{11}{10}i$ (c) $\frac{-113}{170} + \frac{41}{170}i$ (e) $\frac{1}{25} - \frac{57}{25}i$ **B.4.** many correct answers, including $z = 1$,
$w = i$; in this case $|z + w| = |1 + i| = \sqrt{2}$, but $|z| + |w| = 1 + 1 = 2$ **B.5.** (a) 13
(c) $\sqrt{3}$ (e) 12 (g) $2\sqrt{10}$ (i) $1/\sqrt{17}$ **B.6.** -1 **B.7.** (a) $x = 2$,
$y = -2$ (c) $x = -\frac{3}{4}$, $y = \frac{3}{2}$

B.8.

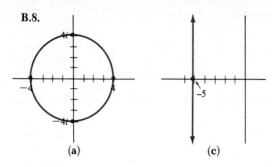

(a)   (c)

C.1. (a) $\dfrac{z + \bar{z}}{2} = \dfrac{(q + bi) + (a - bi)}{2} = \dfrac{2a}{2} = a = \text{Re}(z).$ **C.2.** $\dfrac{1}{z} = \left(\dfrac{a}{a^2 + b^2}\right) -$

$\left(\dfrac{b}{a^2 + b^2}\right)i$ **C.3.** (a) $\bar{z} = a - bi;$ $z + \bar{z} = (a + bi) + (a - bi) = 2a$, which is a real

number since a is one. (c) $\bar{w} = c - di;$ $\bar{z} + \bar{w} = (a - bi) + (c - di) = (a + c) -$
$(b + d)i = (\overline{z + w})$ **C.4.** (a) $\bar{z} = a - bi;$ $\qquad |\bar{z}| = \sqrt{a^2 + (-b)^2} = \sqrt{a^2 + b^2} = |z|$
(c) $zw = (ac - bd) + (bc + ad)i;$ $\qquad |zw| = \sqrt{(ac - bd)^2 + (bc + ad)^2} =$
$\sqrt{a^2c^2 - 2abcd + b^2d^2 + b^2c^2 + 2abcd + a^2d^2}$ $\quad = \quad \sqrt{a^2c^2 + b^2d^2 + b^2c^2 + a^2d^2} =$

$\sqrt{a^2(c^2 + d^2) + b^2(c^2 + d^2)} = \sqrt{(a^2 + b^2)(c^2 + d^2)}$ $\qquad$ (e) $\dfrac{z}{w} = \dfrac{a + bi}{c + di} \cdot \dfrac{c - di}{c - di} =$

$\left(\dfrac{ac + bd}{c^2 + d^2}\right) + \left(\dfrac{bc - ad}{c^2 + d^2}\right);$ $\quad \left|\dfrac{z}{w}\right| \quad = \quad \sqrt{\left(\dfrac{ac + bd}{c^2 + d^2}\right)^2 + \left(\dfrac{bc - ad}{c^2 + d^2}\right)^2} \quad =$

$\sqrt{\dfrac{(ac + bd)^2 + (bc - ad)^2}{(c^2 + d^2)^2}} \quad = \quad \sqrt{\dfrac{a^2c^2 + b^2d^2 + b^2c^2 + a^2d^2}{(c^2 + d^2)^2}} \quad =$

$\sqrt{\dfrac{(a^2 + b^2)(c^2 + d^2)}{(c^2 + d^2)^2}} = \sqrt{\dfrac{a^2 + b^2}{c^2 + d^2}}$ **C.6.** (a) b/a (c) $y - b = (d/c)(x - a)$

SECTION 2   PAGES 385–387

A.1. (a) $6i$ (c) $\sqrt{14}\,i$ (e) $-4i$ **A.2.** (a) $11i$ (c) $(\sqrt{15} - 3\sqrt{2})i$
(e) $-4\sqrt{3}$ (g) $\frac{2}{3}$ **A.3.** (a) $-41 - i$ (c) $(2 + 5\sqrt{2}) + (\sqrt{5} - 2\sqrt{10})i$
(e) $(15 + \sqrt{2}) + (5\sqrt{2} - 3)i$ (g) $\frac{1}{3} - \frac{\sqrt{2}}{3}i$ **B.1.** (a) $x = 1 + 2i$ or $1 - 2i$
(c) $x = \frac{1}{5} + \frac{2}{5}i$ or $\frac{1}{5} - \frac{2}{5}i$ (e) $x = 2$ or $-\frac{3}{2}$ **B.2.** (a) $x = 3$ or $\frac{-3}{2} + \frac{3\sqrt{3}}{2}i$
or $\frac{-3}{2} - \frac{3\sqrt{3}}{2}i$ (c) $x = -2$ or $1 + \sqrt{3}i$ or $1 - \sqrt{3}i$ (e) $x = 1$ or i or -1 or $-i$ **B.3.**
many correct answers, including: (a) $x^2 - 4x + 5$ (c) $x^3 - 6x^2 + 13x - 10$
(e) $x^3 + x^2 + x + 1$ **B.4.** (a) $i, -i, 3, -2$ (c) $2 - i, 2 + i, i, -i$ **B.5.** many
correct answers, including: (a) $x^2 - 2x + 5$ (c) $x^6 - 5x^5 + 8x^4 - 6x^3$
B.6. (a) $x = \frac{3}{5} + \frac{1}{5}i$ (c) $x = \frac{3}{7} + \frac{2}{7}i$ (e) $x = \frac{-11}{2} + \frac{3}{2}i$ (g) $x = -i$
B.7. (a) $x = \dfrac{-1}{2}i + \dfrac{\sqrt{7 + 12i}}{2}$ or $\dfrac{-1}{2}i - \dfrac{\sqrt{7 + 12i}}{2}$ (c) $x = \dfrac{1 + \sqrt{3}}{2} + 2i$ or

$\dfrac{1 - \sqrt{3}}{2} + 2i$ (e) $x = (\frac{-3}{4} - \frac{3}{4}i) + (1 - i)\sqrt{7 - 8i}$ or $(\frac{-3}{4} - \frac{3}{4}i) - (1 - i)\sqrt{7 - 8i}$

B.8. many correct answers, including: (a) $x^2 - (1 - i)x + (2 + i)$ (c) $x^2 - 2x + (1 + 2i)$

CHAPTER 8: TOPICS IN ALGEBRA

SECTION 1   PAGES 398–402

A.1. (b) and (c)   **A.2.** neither of them   **B.1.** (a) $x = \frac{11}{5}$, $y = -\frac{7}{5}$ (c) $x = \frac{6}{5}$, $y = \frac{13}{5}$ (e) $x = -\frac{7}{8}$, $y = \frac{5}{16}$ **B.2.** (a) $x = \frac{66}{5}$, $y = \frac{18}{5}$ (c) $x = -6$, $y = 54$
B.3. (a) $x = 4$, $y = 1$, $z = 2$ (c) $x = -\frac{17}{3}$, $y = \frac{68}{3}$, $z = \frac{22}{3}$ (e) $x = \frac{3}{2}$, $y = \frac{3}{2}$, $z = -\frac{3}{2}$ **B.4.** (a) $z = t$, $y = -1 + \frac{1}{3}t$, $x = 2 - \frac{4}{3}t$, where t is any real number   (c) $z = 0$, $y = t$, $x = 1 - 2t$, where t is any real number   **B.5.** (a) $x = 1$, $y = 2$ (c) no solutions   (e) no solutions   **B.6.** (a) dependent   (c) inconsistent   (e) inconsistent   **B.7.** (a) $x = 5$, $y = 6$, $z = 0$, $w = -1$ (c) no   solutions
B.8. (a) $x = \frac{7}{11}$, $y = -7$ (c) $x = \frac{1}{2}$, $y = \frac{1}{3}$, $z = -\frac{1}{4}$ (e) $x = -\frac{3}{4}$, $y = \frac{10}{3}$, $z = \frac{5}{2}$
B.9. (c) $w = 0$, $z = s$, $y = 2 - 3s$, $x = -1 + 2s$, where s is any real number
(e) $v = r$, $w = -r$, $z = s$, $y = t$, $x = -2t - 3s - 4r$, where r, s, t are any real numbers
B.10. (a) $x \approx .1845341968$, $y \approx -.6239742478$ **B.11.** $a = -\frac{7}{20}$, $b = -\frac{19}{20}$, $c = \frac{23}{10}$
B.12. (a) $f(x) = (\frac{-7}{6})x^2 + \frac{37}{6}x - 7$ (c) $f(x) = \frac{3}{2}x^2 - \frac{1}{2}x$ **B.13.** (a) $x = 3$, $y = 9$ or $x = -1$, $y = 1$
B.14. (a) $x = 1$, $y = -3$ or   (c) $x = 4$, $y = 3$ or   (e) $x = -3$, $y = 4$ or
   $x = -3$, $y = 5$ $x = -4$, $y = 3$ or $x = 1$, $y = 0$
                $x = \sqrt{21}$, $y = -2$ or
                $x = -\sqrt{21}$, $y = -2$

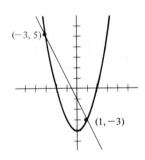
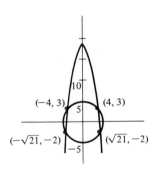
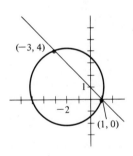

B.15. 13 and 19   **B.17.** no   **B.19.** 10 quarters, 28 dimes, 14 nickels   **B.21.** $x = 550$ mph, $y = 50$ mph   **B.23.** 12 liters of the 18%; 18 liters of the 8%   **B.25.** 4 hours for R, 12 hours for S, 6 hours for T

SECTION 2   PAGES 411–414

A.1. (a) -29 (c) $\frac{17}{2}$ (e) 13 (g) -13 (i) -26 **B.1.** (a) $x = 2, y = 3$, $z = -1$ (c) $x = -2$, $y = -1$, $z = 4$ (e) $w = t$, $z = -4t$, $y = 3t$, $x = 8t$, where t is any real number   (g) $x = -1$, $y = 1$, $z = -3$, $w = -2$ **B.2.** (a) $\begin{pmatrix} 10 & -3 \\ 3 & 7 \end{pmatrix}$
(c) $\begin{pmatrix} 2 & \frac{1}{2} \\ \frac{13}{2} & \frac{9}{2} \end{pmatrix}$ (e) $\begin{pmatrix} 3 & 5 \\ 7 & 9 \end{pmatrix}$ **B.3.** (a) $\begin{pmatrix} 14 & 9 \\ 8 & 7 \end{pmatrix}$ (c) $\begin{pmatrix} 7 & 9 \\ 3 & 5 \end{pmatrix}$ (e) $\begin{pmatrix} 1 & 2 \\ -6 & 10 \end{pmatrix}$
B.5. (a) $AB = \begin{pmatrix} 1 & 2 \\ 3 & 4 \end{pmatrix}\begin{pmatrix} -1 & 4 \\ 5 & 2 \end{pmatrix} = \begin{pmatrix} 9 & 8 \\ 17 & 20 \end{pmatrix}$, but $BA = \begin{pmatrix} -1 & 4 \\ 5 & 2 \end{pmatrix}\begin{pmatrix} 1 & 2 \\ 3 & 4 \end{pmatrix} = \begin{pmatrix} 11 & 14 \\ 11 & 18 \end{pmatrix}$

(c) If $A = \begin{pmatrix} 0 & 2 \\ 0 & 0 \end{pmatrix}$, then $A^2 = \begin{pmatrix} 0 & 2 \\ 0 & 0 \end{pmatrix}\begin{pmatrix} 0 & 2 \\ 0 & 0 \end{pmatrix} = \begin{pmatrix} 0 & 0 \\ 0 & 0 \end{pmatrix}$. (e) $A + B = \begin{pmatrix} 3 & 1 \\ 0 & 9 \end{pmatrix}$, so

$(A + B)^2 = \begin{pmatrix} 3 & 1 \\ 0 & 9 \end{pmatrix}\begin{pmatrix} 3 & 1 \\ 0 & 9 \end{pmatrix} = \begin{pmatrix} 9 & 12 \\ 0 & 81 \end{pmatrix}$; but $A^2 + 2AB + B^2 = A^2 + AB + AB + B^2 =$

$\begin{pmatrix} 2 & -1 \\ 3 & 5 \end{pmatrix}\begin{pmatrix} 2 & -1 \\ 3 & 5 \end{pmatrix} + \begin{pmatrix} 2 & -1 \\ 3 & 5 \end{pmatrix}\begin{pmatrix} 1 & 2 \\ -3 & 4 \end{pmatrix} + \begin{pmatrix} 2 & -1 \\ 3 & 5 \end{pmatrix}\begin{pmatrix} 1 & 2 \\ -3 & 4 \end{pmatrix} +$

$\begin{pmatrix} 1 & 2 \\ -3 & 4 \end{pmatrix}\begin{pmatrix} 1 & 2 \\ -3 & 4 \end{pmatrix} = \begin{pmatrix} 1 & -7 \\ 21 & 22 \end{pmatrix} + \begin{pmatrix} 5 & 0 \\ -12 & 26 \end{pmatrix} + \begin{pmatrix} 5 & 0 \\ -12 & 26 \end{pmatrix} + \begin{pmatrix} -5 & 10 \\ -15 & 10 \end{pmatrix} = \begin{pmatrix} 6 & 3 \\ -18 & 84 \end{pmatrix}$

B.7. (a) $ad - bc - dx + cy + hx - ay$ **B.10.** (a) $x = -\frac{9}{31}$, $y = \frac{7}{31}$
(c) $x = \frac{39}{41}, y = \frac{22}{41}$ (e) $x = 4, y = 2$ **B.11.** (a) and (d)

SECTION 3 PAGES 420–422

A.1. (a) 720 (c) 220 **A.2.** (a) 0 (c) 64 (e) 3,921,225
A.3. (a) $x^5 + 5x^4y + 10x^3y^2 + 10x^2y^3 + 5xy^4 + y^5$ (c) $a^5 - 5a^4b + 10a^3b^2 -$
$10a^2b^3 + 5ab^4 - b^5$ (e) $32x^5 + 80x^4y^2 + 80x^3y^4 + 40x^2y^6 + 10xy^8 + y^{10}$
B.2. (a) $x^3 + 6x^2\sqrt{x} + 15x^2 + 20x\sqrt{x} + 15x + 6\sqrt{x} + 1$ (c) $1 - 10c + 45c^2 -$
$120c^3 + 210c^4 - 252c^5 + 210c^6 - 120c^7 + 45c^8 - 10c^9 + c^{10}$ **B.3.** (a) 56
(c) $-8i$ **B.4.** (a) $10x^3y^2$ (c) $35c^3d^4$ (e) $\frac{35}{8}u^{-5}$ **B.5.** (a) 4032
(c) 160 **B.6.** $\frac{-63}{8}$ **B.8.** (b) *Hint:* $0^n = (1 - 1)^n$ **B.9.** (a) $\cos^4\theta +$
$4i\cos^3\theta\sin\theta - 6\cos^2\theta\sin^2\theta - 4i\cos\theta\sin^3\theta + \sin^4\theta$ (b) $\cos 4\theta + i\sin 4\theta$ (c) $\cos 4\theta =$
$\cos^4\theta + \sin^4\theta - 6\cos^2\theta\sin^2\theta$; $\sin 4\theta = 4\cos\theta\sin\theta(\cos^2\theta - \sin^2\theta)$ **B.10.** (a) $f(x + h) -$
$f(x) = \binom{5}{1}x^4h + \binom{5}{2}x^3h^2 + \binom{5}{3}x^2h^3 + \binom{5}{4}xh^4 + \binom{5}{5}h^5$ (c) $\binom{5}{1}x^4 = 5x^4$ since all the terms involving h are very, very close to 0 when h is small enough (e) If h is very close to 0, then
$\dfrac{f(x + h) - f(x)}{h}$ is approximately equal to $\binom{12}{1}x^{11} = 12x^{11}$ (f) If h is very close to 0, then

$\dfrac{f(x + h) - f(x)}{h}$ is approximately equal to $\binom{n}{1}x^{n-1} = nx^{n-1}$

SECTION 4 PAGES 431–433

A.1. (a) 24 (c) 40,320 (e) 132 **A.2.** (a) 91 (c) 3,764,376
B.1. (a) $n(n - 1) = n^2 - n$ (c) n (e) $(n^2 - n)/2$ **B.2.** (a) $n = 11$
(c) $n = 9$ (e) $n = 7$ **B.3.** 40,320 **B.5.** 24 **B.6.** (a) 120 **B.7.** 3024
B.9. (a) 1,860,480 **B.11.** 7,290,000 **B.13.** 192 **B.15.** 1,048,576
B.17. (a) 12 (c) 50,400 **B.19.** 1260 **B.21.** 56 **B.23.** 56
B.24. (a) 2,598,960 **B.25.** 56 **B.27.** $\binom{11}{4}\binom{7}{3} = 11,550$
B.29. (a) $\binom{5}{3}\binom{7}{2} = 210$ **B.30.** (a) $13\binom{4}{2} = 78$ (c) $\binom{4}{2}\binom{48}{3} + \binom{4}{3}\binom{48}{2} + \binom{4}{4}\binom{48}{1} = 108,336$
C.1. (a) 2 (c) 24 **C.3.** 479,001,600 **C.5.** 76,204,800

SECTION 5 PAGES 441–443

B.1. (a) *Step 1:* for $n = 1$ the statement is $1 = 2^1 - 1$, which is true. *Step 2:* Assume the statement is true for $n = k$: that is,

$$1 + 2 + 2^2 + 2^3 + \cdots + 2^{k-1} = 2^k - 1$$

Add 2^k to both sides, and rearrange terms:

$$1 + 2 + 2^2 + 2^3 + \cdots + 2^{k-1} + 2^k = 2^k - 1 + 2^k$$

$$1 + 2 + 2^2 + 2^3 + \cdots + 2^{k-1} + 2^{(k+1)-1} = 2^k + 2^k - 1 = 2(2^k) - 1$$

$$1 + 2 + 2^2 + 2^3 + \cdots + 2^{k-1} + 2^{(k+1)-1} = 2^{k+1} - 1$$

But this last line says that the statement is true for $n = k + 1$. Therefore by the Principle of Mathematical Induction the statement is true for every positive integer n.

Note: Hereafter, in these answers, Step 1 will be omitted if it is trivial (as in B.1. (a)) and only the essential parts of Step 2 will be given.

B.1. **(c)** Assume that the statement is true for $n = k$:

$$1 + 3 + 5 + \cdots + (2k - 1) = k^2$$

Add $2(k + 1) - 1$ to both sides:

$$1 + 3 + 5 + \cdots + (2k - 1) + (2(k + 1) - 1) = k^2 + 2(k + 1) - 1 = k^2 + 2k + 1 = (k + 1)^2$$

The first and last parts of this equation say that the statement is true for $n = k + 1$.

B.1. **(e)** Assume that the statement is true for $n = k$:

$$1^2 + 2^2 + 3^2 + \cdots + k^2 = \frac{k(k + 1)(2k + 1)}{6}$$

Add $(k + 1)^2$ to both sides:

$$1^2 + 2^2 + 3^2 + \cdots + k^2 + (k + 1)^2$$

$$= \frac{k(k + 1)(2k + 1)}{6} + (k + 1)^2$$

$$= \frac{k(k + 1)(2k + 1) + 6(k + 1)^2}{6} = \frac{(k + 1)[k(2k + 1) + 6(k + 1)]}{6}$$

$$= \frac{(k + 1)[2k^2 + 7k + 6]}{6} = \frac{(k + 1)(k + 2)(2k + 3)}{6}$$

$$= \frac{(k + 1)[(k + 1) + 1][2(k + 1) + 1]}{6}$$

The first and last parts of this equation say that the statement is true for $n = k + 1$.

B.2. **(a)** Assume the statement is true for $n = k$:

$$\frac{1}{2} + \frac{1}{4} + \frac{1}{8} + \cdots + \frac{1}{2^k} = 1 - \frac{1}{2^k}$$

Add $\dfrac{1}{2^{k+1}}$ to both sides:

$$\frac{1}{2} + \frac{1}{4} + \frac{1}{8} + \cdots + \frac{1}{2^k} + \frac{1}{2^{k+1}} = 1 - \frac{1}{2^k} + \frac{1}{2^{k+1}} = 1 + \frac{-2 + 1}{2^{k+1}} = 1 - \frac{1}{2^{k+1}}$$

The first and last parts of this equation say the statement is true for $n = k + 1$.

B.3. Assume the statement is true for $n = k$:

$$\left(1 + \frac{1}{1}\right)\left(1 + \frac{1}{2}\right)\left(1 + \frac{1}{3}\right) \cdots \left(1 + \frac{1}{k}\right) = k + 1$$

Multiply both sides by $1 + \dfrac{1}{k + 1}$:

$$\left(1 + \frac{1}{1}\right)\left(1 + \frac{1}{2}\right)\left(1 + \frac{1}{3}\right) \cdots \left(1 + \frac{1}{k}\right)\left(1 + \frac{1}{k + 1}\right)$$

$$= (k + 1)\left(1 + \frac{1}{k + 1}\right) = (k + 1) + 1$$

Therefore the statement is true for $n = k + 1$.

B.4. **(a)** Assume the statement is true for $n = k$: $k + 2 > k$. Adding 1 to both sides, we have: $k + 2 + 1 > k + 1$, or equivalently, $(k + 1) + 2 > (k + 1)$. Therefore the statement is true for $n = k + 1$. **(c)** Assume the statement is true for $n = k$: $3^k > 3k$. Multiplying both sides by 3 yields: $3 \cdot 3^k > 3 \cdot 3k$, or equivalently, $3^{k+1} > 3 \cdot 3k$. Now since $k \geq 1$, we know that $3k \geq 3$ and hence that $2 \cdot 3k \geq 3$. Therefore $2 \cdot 3k + 3k \geq 3 + 3k$, or equivalently, $3 \cdot 3k \geq 3k + 3$. Combining this last inequality with the fact that $3^{k+1} > 3 \cdot 3k$, we see that $3^{k+1} > 3k + 3$, or equivalently, $3^{k+1} > 3(k + 1)$. Therefore the statement is true for $n = k + 1$. **(e)** Assume the statement is true for $n = k$: $3k > k + 1$. Adding 3 to both sides yields: $3k + 3 > k + 1 + 3$, or equivalently, $3(k + 1) > (k + 1) + 3$. Since $(k + 1) + 3$ is certainly greater than $(k + 1) + 1$, we conclude that $3(k + 1) > (k + 1) + 1$. Therefore the statement is true for $n = k + 1$.

B.5. Assume that the statement is true for $n = k$:

$$c + (c + d) + (c + 2d) + \cdots + (c + (k - 1)d) = \frac{k(2c + (k - 1)d)}{2}$$

Adding $c + kd$ to both sides, we have

$$c + (c + d) + (c + 2d) + \cdots + (c + (k - 1)d) + (c + kd)$$

$$= \frac{k(2c + (k - 1)d)}{2} + c + kd$$

$$= \frac{k(2c + (k - 1)d) + 2(c + kd)}{2} = \frac{2ck + k(k - 1)d + 2c + 2kd}{2}$$

$$= \frac{2ck + 2c + kd(k - 1) + 2kd}{2} = \frac{(k + 1)2c + kd(k - 1 + 2)}{2}$$

$$= \frac{(k + 1)2c + kd(k + 1)}{2} = \frac{(k + 1)(2c + kd)}{2}$$

$$= \frac{(k + 1)(2c + ((k + 1) - 1)d)}{2}$$

Therefore the statement is true for $n = k + 1$.

B.7. **(a)** Assume the statement is true for $n = k$; then 3 is a factor of $2^{2k+1} + 1$; that is, $2^{2k+1} + 1 = 3M$ for some integer M. Thus $2^{2k+1} = 3M - 1$. Now

$$2^{2(k+1)+1} = 2^{2k+2+1} = 2^{2+2k+1} = 2^2 \cdot 2^{2k+1} = 4(3M - 1) = 12M - 4 = 3(4M) - 3 - 1$$

$$= 3(4M - 1) - 1$$

From the first and last terms of this equation we see that $2^{2(k+1)+1} + 1 = 3(4M - 1)$. Hence 3 is a factor of $2^{2(k+1)+1} + 1$. Therefore the statement is true for $n = k + 1$. **(c)** Assume the statement is true for $n = k$: 64 is a factor of $3^{2k+2} - 8k - 9$. Then $3^{2k+2} - 8k - 9 = 64N$ for some integer N so that $3^{2k+2} = 8k + 9 + 64N$. Now

$$3^{2(k+1)+2} = 3^{2k+2+2} = 3^{2+(2k+2)} = 3^2 \cdot 3^{2k+2} = 9(8k + 9 + 64N).$$

Consequently,

$$3^{2(k+1)+2} - 8(k + 1) - 9 = 3^{2(k+1)+2} - 8k - 8 - 9 = 3^{2(k+1)+2} - 8k - 17$$

$$= [9(8k + 9 + 64N)] - 8k - 17$$

$$= 72k + 81 + 9 \cdot 64N - 8k - 17 = 64k + 64 + 9 \cdot 64N$$

$$= 64(k + 1 + 9N)$$

From the first and last parts of this equation we see that 64 is a factor of $3^{2(k+1)+2} - 8(k + 1) - 9$. Therefore the statement is true for $n = k + 1$.   **B.9.** First observe that for every $n \geq 1$ we have $x_{n+1} = \sqrt{2 + x_n}$. Assume the statement is true for $n = k$, that is, assume $x_k < 2$. Then $(x_{k+1})^2 = (\sqrt{2 + x_k})^2 = 2 + x_k < 2 + 2 = 4$. Since $(x_{k+1})^2 < 4$ we must have $x_{k+1} < 2$. Therefore the statement is true for $n = k + 1$.   **B.10.**   (a)   false; counterexample: $n = 9$ (c)   true; proof: since $(1 + 1)^2 > 1^2 + 1$, the statement is true for $n = 1$.   Assume   the   statement   is   true   for $n = k$: $(k + 1)^2 > k^2 + 1$.   Then $[(k + 1) + 1]^2 = (k + 1)^2 + 2(k + 1) + 1 > k^2 + 1 + 2(k + 1) + 1 = k^2 + 2k + 2 + 2 > k^2 + 2k + 2 = k^2 + 2k + 1 + 1 = (k + 1)^2 + 1$. The first and last terms of this inequality say that the statement is true for $n = k + 1$.   Therefore by induction the statement is true for every positive integer n.   (e)   false; counterexample: $n = 3$
B.11.   (a)   The statement is true for $n = q$ by Property (i). Consequently, by Property (ii) (with q in place of k), the statement must also be true for $n = q + 1$. By Property (ii) again (with $q + 1$ in place of k), the statement must also be true for $n = (q + 1) + 1 = q + 2$. Repeated use of Property (ii) shows that the statement is true for $n = (q + 2) + 1 = q + 3$, for $n = (q + 3) + 1 = q + 4$, for $n = q + 5$, and so on.   (c)   Since $2 \cdot 5 - 4 > 5$, the statement is true for $n = 5$. Assume the statement is true for $n = k$ (with $k \geq 5$): $2k - 4 > k$. Adding 2 to both sides shows that $2k - 4 + 2 > k + 2$, or equivalently, $2(k + 1) - 4 > k + 2$. Since $k + 2 > k + 1$, we see that $2(k + 1) - 4 > k + 1$. So the statement is true for $n = k + 1$. Therefore by the Extended Principle of Mathematical Induction the statement is true for all $n \geq 5$.   (e)   Since $2^2 > 2$, the statement is true for $n = 2$. Assume that $k \geq 2$ and that the statement is true for $n = k$: $k^2 > k$. Then $(k + 1)^2 = k^2 + 2k + 1 > k^2 + 1 > k + 1$. The first and last terms of this inequality show that the statement is true for $n = k + 1$. Therefore by induction, the statement is true for all $n \geq 2$.   (g)   Since $3^4 = 81$ and $2^4 + 10 \cdot 4 = 16 + 40 = 56$, we see that $3^4 > 2^4 + 10 \cdot 4$. So the statement is true for $n = 4$. Assume that $k \geq 4$ and that the statement is true for $n = k$: $3^k > 2^k + 10k$. Multiplying both sides by 3 yields: $3 \cdot 3^k > 3(2^k + 10k)$, or equivalently, $3^{k+1} > 3 \cdot 2^k + 30k$. But $3 \cdot 2^k + 30k > 2 \cdot 2^k + 30k = 2^{k+1} + 30k$. Therefore $3^{k+1} > 2^{k+1} + 30k$. Now we shall show that $30k > 10(k + 1)$. Since $k \geq 4$, we have $20k \geq 20 \cdot 4$, so that $20k \geq 80 > 10$. Adding $10k$ to both sides of $20k > 10$ yields: $30k > 10k + 10$, or equivalently, $30k > 10(k + 1)$. Consequently, $3^{k+1} > 2^{k+1} + 30k > 2^{k+1} + 10(k + 1)$. The first and last terms of this inequality show that the statement is true for $n = k + 1$. Therefore the statement is true for all $n \geq 4$ by induction.   **C.2.**   After one time period the total amount $T(1)$ is the sum of the amount invested (namely, P dollars) and the interest earned on this amount in one time period (namely, rP); that is, $T(1) = P + rP = P(1 + r) = P(1 + r)^1$. So the statement $T(x) = P(1 + r)^x$ is true for $x = 1$. Assume that this statement is true for $x = k$. This means that the total amount after k time periods is $T(k) = P(1 + r)^k$. At the end of the next time period (the $(k + 1)$st) the new total $T(k + 1)$ will be the sum of the amount at the beginning of the period (namely, $T(k)$) and the interest earned by this amount in one time period (namely, $rT(k)$); that is,

$$T(k + 1) = T(k) + rT(k) = P(1 + r)^k + rP(1 + r)^k = (P + rP)(1 + r)^k = P(1 + r)(1 + r)^k$$
$$= P(1 + r)^{k+1}.$$

The first and last terms of this equation show that the statement is true for $x = k + 1$. Therefore by induction it is true for every positive integer x.

Index

Note: Page numbers followed by "fn" indicate footnotes.